Neck and Back Pain
The Scientific Evidence of
Causes, Diagnosis, and Treatment

Neck and Back Pain

The Scientific Evidence of Causes, Diagnosis, and Treatment

Editors

Alf L. Nachemson, M.D., PH.D.
Professor
Department of Orthopaedics
University of Göteborg, Sweden
Department of Orthopaedics
Georgetown University
Washington, D.C., USA

Egon Jonsson, PH.D.
Professor
The Swedish Council on Technology
Assessment in Health Care (SBU)
Stockholm, Sweden

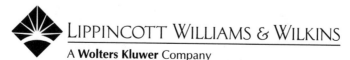

LIPPINCOTT WILLIAMS & WILKINS
A **Wolters Kluwer** Company

Philadelphia · Baltimore · New York · London
Buenos Aires · Hong Kong · Sydney · Tokyo

Acquisitions Editor: Robert A. Hurley
Developmental Editor: Kerry Barrett
Production Editor: Jeff Somers
Manufacturing Manager: Colin Warnock
Cover Designer: Mark Lerner
Compositor: The PRD Group
Printer: R. R. Donnelley, Crawfordsville

© **2000 by the Swedish Council on Technology Assessment**
in Health Care (SBU)
Published by Lippincott Williams & Wilkins
530 Walnut Street
Philadelphia, PA 19106 USA
LWW.com

Printed in the USA

Library of Congress Cataloging-in-Publication Data

Neck and back pain : the scientific evidence of causes, diagnosis, and treatment / editors, Alf L. Nachemson, Egon Jonsson.
    p. ; cm.
  Includes bibliographical references and index.
  ISBN 0-7817-2760-X (alk. paper)
    1. Backache. 2. Neck pain. 3. Exercise therapy. I. Nachemson, Alf L. II. Jonsson, Egon.
    [DNLM: 1. Neck Pain—diagnosis. 2. Back Pain—diagnosis. 3. Back Pain—therapy. 4. Neck Pain—therapy. WE 708 N3645 2000]
  RD771.B217 N43 2000
  617.5′64—dc21
                                  00-023914

---

10 9 8 7 6 5 4 3 2 1

To Ann and Louise

Contents

Contributing Authors

Carl-Axel Carlsson, M.D., Ph.D. *Professor, Department of Neurosurgery, University Hospital, Lund, Skrattmåsgången 22, 42669 V Frölunda, Sweden*

Lars Englund, M.D. *Department of Public Health and Caring Sciences, Family Medicine Section, Uppsala University, Uppsala Science Park, 75185 Uppsala, Sweden*

Silvia Evers, M.Sc. *Department of Health Organisation, Policy and Economics, University of Maastricht, P.O. Box 616, 6200 MD Maastricht, The Netherlands*

J. N. Alastair Gibson, M.D., F.R.C.S. *Consultant Orthopaedic Surgeon, Clinical Research Unit, Princess Margaret Rose Orthopaedic Hospital, Edinburgh EH10 7ED, United Kingdom*

Mariëlle Goossens, Ph.D. *Economist, Institute for Rehabilitation Research, Zandbergsweg 111, 6432 CC, Hoensbroek, The Netherlands*

Inga Grant, M.Sc. *Research Fellow, Clinical Research Unit, Princess Margaret Rose Orthopaedic Hospital, Edinburgh EH10 7ED, United Kingdom*

Karin Harms-Ringdahl, Dr. Med. Sci. *RPT, Professor, Departments of Physical Therapy and Rehabilitation Medicine, Karolinska Institute Huddinge and Karolinska Hospitals, 17176 Stockholm, Sweden*

Jan Hoving, P.T., M.T., M.Sc. *Institute for Research in Extramural Medicine, Vrije Universiteit, van der Boechorstraat 7, 1081 BT Amsterdam, The Netherlands*

Egon Jonsson, Ph.D. *Professor and Director, Swedish Council on Technology Assessment in Health Care (SBU), Box 5650, 11486 Stockholm, Sweden*

Steven J. Linton, Ph.D. *Program for Behavioral Medicine, Department of Occupational and Environmental Medicine, Örebro Medical Center, 70181 Örebro, Sweden*

Alf Nachemson, M.D., Ph.D. *Professor, Department of Orthopaedics, Sahlgrenska University Hospital, 41345 Göteborg, Sweden; Research Professor, Department of Orthopaedics, Georgetown University, Washington, D.C.*

Anders I. Norlund, M.L., B.Sc., Ph.D. *Swedish Council on Technology Assessment in Health Care, Tyrgatan 7, Box 5650, S-11486 Stockholm, Sweden*

Margareta Söderström, M.D., Ph.D. *Associate Professor, Department of Family Medicine, Göteborg University, Vasa sjukhus, 41133 Göteborg, Sweden*

Maurits W. van Tulder, Ph.D. *Senior Researcher, Institute for Research in Extramural Medicine, Vrije Universiteit, van der Boechorstraat 7, 1081 BT Amsterdam, The Netherlands*

Eva Vingård, M.D., Ph.D.   *Section of Personal Injury Prevention, Karolinska Institutet, Box 12718, 11294 Stockholm, Sweden*

Gordon Waddell, D.Sc., M.D., F.R.C.S.   *Orthopaedic Surgeon, The Glasgow Nuffield Hospital, Glasgow G12 OPJ, Scotland*

Hazel Waddell, M.A.   *Department of Social Work and Social Policy, University of Glasgow, Glasgow G12 OPJ, Scotland*

Preface

For nearly half a century I have tried to uncover the mysteries of common back pain. Now, at the dawn of a new millennium, a somewhat clearer picture of the most common pain problem of the human frame is emerging. This is why this book was written with friends and colleagues from several different areas of health care.

Only through a collaborative effort will we be able to solve the back pain enigma. Contributions from specialists in sociology, psychology, epidemiology, economics, and social policy have helped to paint the larger picture. Contributions by the more traditional health specialists such as primary care physicians, orthopaedic- and neurosurgeons, and physical therapists have helped with the basic underlying patient problem: understanding spinal pain and its treatment.

In time, it is possible that input from genetics and microbiology will be able to modulate peripheral as well as central nociception and also aging of the intervertebral discs. Until then, however, it is our hope that this evidence-based book will help all of us to better handle the back pain problem, to encourage and treat our patients with better result, to change our social framework for improved general and spinal health, and to guide future research endeavors into areas where they are most needed.

The direction from today's available studies is fairly clear: examine, encourage, exercise, pay attention to psychosocial deterrents to function, involve the workplace in rehabilitation of those with work disability. Moderate insurance benefits to sustainable levels and remove, if possible, the adversarial situations arising from issues of work-related injury.

We are also in the beginning of The Bone & Joint Decade 2000–2010 for Prevention and Treatment of Musculoskeletal Disorders, endorsed by professional societies, governments, and the World Health Organization, with the aim of restoring quality of life to people with bone and joint disease and injury throughout the world.

Just as we accept that no one past the age of 35 wins a gold medal in an Olympic athletic event, some mechanically taxing workplaces may be difficult for a patient with an aging spine. Policies should be made to accommodate this fact, to find work suitable also for those with back pain—work actually can be remedial. Politicians, union leaders, and patients must all understand this life-saving message. Early disability pension endangers your life. "The new welfare state should help and encourage people of working age to work where they are capable of doing so" (Blair).

On a personal note, I thank all my teachers and collaborators who have helped me understand sociology, epidemiology, psychology, biology, and biomechanics, enabling me and my colleagues to improve treatment for our patients. Lastly, let me express my appreciation of my family, who for years have suffered from "indirect" back pain.

Alf Nachemson

Preface

I am by no means a specialist on back pain—I am not even a medical doctor. Nevertheless, for more than ten years I have been working in close relationship with Alf Nachemson on precisely the subject of back pain. Why?

It is a reflection of "The new medicine—something different" as Lewis Thomas once wrote. There is a need to broaden the basis for clinical decision-making to include synthesis of findings from research, not only in medicine but also in behavioral sciences and in the economics of health care. Also, the research on ethical and social implications of the diffision and use of medical technologies needs to be considered. Therefore, dealing with the scientific facts published in the tens of thousands of manuscripts of the literature requires multidisciplinary skills. This effort, in short, is a reflection of the current shift from opinion-based towards evidence-based medicine.

The present synthesis of the scientific literature on back pain was made by a multidisciplinary, critical mass of scholars. It has been a privilege to belong to this group. On a personal level I have been struck by many of our findings. The most surprising, I believe, is the fact that so little research of high scientific validity has been done on such a huge and common problem. One way of illustrating this is the fact that the total financial cost of back pain is about three times higher than the total cost of all forms of cancer diseases. Another is the fact that of all randomized trials in medicine, only 0.2 percent concern back pain.

All of us in this group did this job on the initiative of The Swedish Council on Technology Assessment in Health Care (SBU) which is constantly running about twenty projects on the evidence-base for different medical practices. There are many more such multidisciplinary groups around the world. Although SBU is permeated by a critical view on scientific evidence, the group on back pain contributed much to the development of improved working procedures in the future projects of the agency. The main target groups for SBU, and indeed for this book, are the general public, the patients, health policy makers, and the professionals. I sincerely hope that this book somehow improves the situation for people with back pain.

I thank the scientifically knowledgeable and socially talented group of people who made this book possible. Especially, I thank my friend Alf Nachemson.

Egon Jonsson

Acknowledgment

Without the assistance of numerous individuals involved with literature search, manuscript preparation, and typing, this book could not have been completed. In particular we thank our hardworking and diligent secretaries, both in Göteborg and in Stockholm, and the Editors at Lippincott Williams & Wilkins.

Neck and Back Pain: The Scientific Evidence of Causes, Diagnosis, and Treatment, edited by Alf Nachemson and Egon Jonsson. Published by Lippincott Williams & Wilkins, Philadelphia 2000.

1

Introduction

Alf Nachemson

Department of Orthopaedics, Sahlgrenska University Hospital, Göteborg, Sweden

GENERAL PRINCIPLES

In 1991, the Swedish Council on Technology Assessment in Health Care (SBU) published a monograph on the causes, diagnoses, and treatment of back pain (55) that summarized current knowledge at that time. It was mostly a single author's review of knowledge about back pain up to 1990.

Since then, the methodology for evaluation of scientific studies in medicine has undergone a revolution. We have seen the birth of the Cochrane Collaboration (22,29) and the emergence of several new journals on evidence-based diagnosis and treatment of the most common clinical ailments afflicting humankind.

Because back pain, including neck and lower back pain, continues to be extremely common, with a high prevalence and wide socioeconomic consequences all over the industrialized world, it was deemed necessary to reevaluate the problem in depth, by using more stringent criteria for inclusion of scientific articles in the evaluation of admissible evidence for treatment efficacy, as well as for causality and diagnosis. In addition, improved literature search methods are at hand.

In the 1990s, numerous guidelines were published in various countries around the world (1,9,16,34,35,48,58,59,65,66,71,75,77,79,80,85), many professional organizations produced consensus guidelines (17,20,50,53,77), and the Cochrane Collaboration of Systematic Reviews, which started in 1992, has now more than 3,000 collaborators worldwide (29). In 1995, the Cochrane Collaboration Back Review Group for Spinal Disorders was started with the help of Institute for Work and Health and the SBU (12,84).

Because of continued public interest in the problem, its commonality, and continued diversity in treatment methods, some of which had no proven efficacy, a reevaluation was deemed necessary even though, for the majority of patients, the true origin of pain remains unknown.

Advances in molecular biology, new knowledge of the human genome with possible influences on our understanding of both pain and aging, have just barely reached spinal structures. Another decade of such research in these areas will most likely provide better solutions to the problem; reports from the first few experimental studies are now available (8,47,86).

Now, however, there is enough evidence from good scientific studies to state clearly that a whole new treatment paradigm has emerged, resulting from randomized controlled studies (RCTs), metaanalytic reviews, and guidelines, all published since 1991.

As stated by Frank et al., "New evidence gives new hope—if we can just get all the players onside" (39).

With the continued increasing influx of valid scientific literature and the emerging complexity of the problem of back pain, this book is the result of several years of work by collaborators representing many different medical specialties, as well as physical therapists, psychologists, and economists. The overwhelming burden of scrutinizing the enormous literature on back pain in search of hard evidence also necessitates some division of tasks. Even though each chapter in this book has separate authors, the group as a whole has worked together to obtain a balance of content and general conclusions, again based on up-to-date methodology in reviewing the literature.

It is our hope that this effort will further better understanding and treatment for the large majority of patients who suffer from pain syndromes in the neck and the lower back. A discussion of pain in the middle thoracic part of the spine is left out because of its rarity.

That a need exists for a scientific evaluation of treatment for neck and low back pain should be obvious from Table 1.1, and, with few exceptions, most practitioners who treat these patients agree that some evidence of efficacy and effectiveness is necessary. It is also true, however, as described in Chapter 10, that strong personal beliefs of the practitioner and of the patient can influence the results of treatment. In addition, we have different perceptions, cultures, and social influences in various countries, and these variations explain, for example, the different outcomes of acupuncture treatment for low back pain in China versus those in Great Britain (33).

Practitioners, in particular those treating patients with pain syndromes, thus should have not only the (sometimes weak or equivocal) evidence at hand, but also some knowledge of the personal beliefs and societal influences on their patients. This ap-

TABLE 1.1. *Examples of different methods for treatment of back pain*

Acupuncture	Laser therapy
Anthroposophic medicine	Magnet therapy
Back school	Manipulation
Balneotherapy	Massage
Bed rest	Medication
Behavioral therapy	Meditation
Body awareness therapy	Mobilization
Biofeedback	Moxibustion
Cardiovascular fitness training	Multimodal rehabilitation
Connective tissue massage	Nerve blocks
Corsets	Ointments
Crutches	Relaxation techniques
Cupping	Spa treatment
Diet	Stretching
Disc injections	Surgery, various types
Electrotherapy	Taping
Epidural anesthesia	Therapeutic conversation
Exercises	Thermotherapy
Facet blocks and denervation	Traction
Healing	Transcutaneous electrical nerve stimula-
Herbal medicine	tion, high and low frequency
Holistic therapy	Trigger point injections
Homeopathy	Ultrasound
Hydrotherapy	Vibrator
Injections of saline, water, local anesthetics	X-ray therapy
Ionic modulation	Zone therapy
Iontophoresis	

proach also emphasizes the need for empathy toward patients and their problems. This important part of any patient consultation and treatment is further elaborated in Chapter 18.

By *back pain,* we in this book mean painful conditions in the neck and lower back that may or may not radiate to the limbs. These symptoms are so common that they can be regarded as a natural part of life, and with few exceptions, they strike everyone, everywhere in the world sometime during life. In the medical sense, back pain is rarely a symptom of serious disease. For most patients, our knowledge of the true cause of spinal pain is insufficient. Causal therapy is therefore virtually nonexistent, but as with fever, another common condition, we have means to abate the symptoms.

As long as we have had interpretable communications from our ancestors, back pain has been described (3). It was not until the early 1930s, however, that the symptom was thought to emanate from spinal structures, through the description of disc herniation (51). Unfortunately, these authors labeled it an injury, "ruptured disc," but the event, although sometimes dramatic, cannot be distinguished pathoanatomically from the normal aging process. In addition, we now know that disc herniation can be found in more than 50% of persons 30 to 50 years old (11,13) without symptoms, including symptoms in the past and for the next several years (14,15). Before the mid-1930s, back pain was mostly labeled "rheumatic," whereas in medieval times, it was regarded as punishment by evil spirits.

In the early part of the twentieth century and lingering well into the 1980s, the leading principle of back pain treatment was rest; in some cases, several days of bed rest was advocated (3,55,88). As in many other specialties of medicine, this principle has been proven erroneous, even counterproductive (88). This has been demonstrated not only for "aging" processes causing symptoms but also for true injuries, such as muscle and tendon ruptures and fractures.

As elucidated in several chapters in this book, physicians and other professionals who treat patients with back pain all have their own models of pathogenesis, and they all try to correct, based on these models, what they presume is wrong (26). Without true knowledge of the cause of a patient's pain, success rates vary, not surprisingly, and they are disappointing most of the time when they are subjected to strict studies, as demonstrated in Chapters 11 to 17.

With our present knowledge, it could be stated that part of the enormous scope of the problem is *iatrogenic,* that is, created by these various professional views, and that includes all of us treating back pain sufferers. Allan and Waddell (3) even accused physicians of being responsible for low back disability in their patients, on the grounds that bed rest was the mainstay of treatment, contrary to the results of several current randomized trials (88).

The proponents of rest based their views on Thomas' dictum from the late 1800s that rest was the treatment when something was injured, ruptured, or broken (3). This view, embraced first by orthopedic surgeons and then by other specialists treating back pain, also influenced benevolent politicians who wanted to help patients who were ordered not to work by their physicians. This approach led to the development of the high disability rates resulting from back pain that are now seen in most industrialized societies (55,56).

The concentration solely on the presumed structural features of the symptoms of spinal pain created a model that totally missed the important psychosocial part of the personal experience of pain. Pain was always interpreted as a sign of disease or injury, and although this interpretation is probably true for most patients with acute back pain, it becomes less true for patients with chronic back pain (17,18). Our understanding of the complex mechanisms of pain is also increasing (see Chapters 3 and 7).

As mentioned in Chapter 2, it is clear that we need a shift of paradigm from a pure pathoanatomic model to a more biopsychosocial model of disease and pain in particular. Functional disability, particularly work disability, and pain are not directly related (37). Loss of working ability depends in varying degrees on patients' and societies' attitudes and beliefs. Thus, in many studies, psychologic factors have been demonstrated to be more important than physical changes in the spine in patients with disability resulting from back pain (see Chapter 3).

With the commonality of spinal symptoms, pain, and diminution of ability to work, it has been nearly impossible to pinpoint specific mechanical or other factors that elicit a patient's symptoms. Neck and back pain is common in all professions and is equally frequent following various recreational and vocational activities. Many studies show no specific event causing back pain (42,55). When we look at disability resulting from spinal pain, a different picture emerges, again influenced by societal views and levels of insurance, but also to some extent influenced by the workplace, where both physical and psychologic stressors are important (see Chapters 3 to 6).

In Sweden as in the rest of the industrialized world, spinal pain has been a prevalent cause of lost work time. The incidence in Sweden peaked toward the end of the 1980s when, in a population of 8.5 million persons, 30 million sick days were paid, and the number of persons permanently disabled by back pain was 52,000 (55). Fortunately for patients and society alike, this picture was changed (Chapters 20 and 21), partly resulting from political interactions and partly because of increased medical knowledge spread by guidelines such as the 1991 SBU report and others mentioned earlier.

The variety of treatment methods offered patients with back pain (Table 1.1) should raise some eyebrows. It has become increasingly important to evaluate methods that show efficacy either for "curing" or for diminishing back pain (26). In the last 10 years, the medical profession has woken up to its shortcomings with regard to the effects of many types of treatment for many different diseases including back pain, partly the result of the quest for evidence-based practice (25,27,28).

In Sweden, the most common treatment modalities for patients with subacute back pain (employees disabled for 4 weeks), according to one study (43), are as follows, in descending order: physical therapy; physical modalities (heat or cold, ultrasound, massage); manipulation and mobilization; back school; transcutaneous electrical nerve stimulation; multimodal rehabilitation programs; and surgery.

The demand for evidence-based medicine has escalated from many parts of society in the last 10 years. *Evidence-based medicine* is an approach to practicing medicine in which the clinician is aware of the evidence in support of his or her clinical practice and the strength of that evidence (67,82). Evidence-based health care promotes the collection, interpretation, and integration of valid, important, and applicable patient-reported, clinician-observed, and research-derived evidence. The best available evidence, moderated by patients' circumstances and preferences, is applied to improve the quality of clinical judgments and to facilitate cost-effective health care (67). In Sweden, the SBU has been largely responsible for the promotion of this type of medicine, for information on the results of these analyses, and for the distribution of this information to the medical profession and to society at large (4,41,69,70).

The science of evidence synthesis is fairly new and is still developing. The methods used in most of the SBU reports on various diagnostic and treatment modalities for

TABLE 1.2. *Methods used in the Swedish Council on Technology Assessment in Health Care*

Type of study	High quality	Medium quality	Low quality
Metaanalysis of several randomized controlled trials	Thorough reanalysis of original data from all studies	< >	Based on two or three studies and only reported results
Prospective and randomized study	Large, well-controlled, multicenter study with adequate description of protocols, materials, and methods and treatment techniques	< >	Randomized studies with few patients with lack of statistical power; poor description of patients; large "drop out"; poor description of techniques; poor nonvalidated outcome measures
Prospective study without randomization	Well-defined questions; large patient material (>60); adequate statistical methods; adequate follow-up numbers and time	< >	Few patients; ill-defined questions; short personal follow-up
Retrospective study	Large consecutive patient material well described and analyzed with adequate statistical methods; long follow-up time; preferably unbiased observer	< >	Few patients not followed sufficient time
Review article	Proper good studies, clearly focused questions with thorough search for relevant studies described as well as inclusion criteria	< >	Review of expert opinions
Other studies			

certain common ailments have been published (70) (Table 1.2), but nevertheless they merit a short description.

Because spinal pain has such wide social and personal implications, this book is broad in its content, as can be seen by the various headings of the different chapters, more so than the usual medical textbooks on back pain. The reason for this should be obvious. To achieve the most helpful approach to the individual patient, as well as to society at large, it is of the utmost importance that everyone involved in this biopsychosocial problem take responsibility based on current knowledge. By this, we mean that patients, politicians, employers, employees, and all medical personnel, as well as the media, must be aware and must act in accordance with the currently available scientific evidence.

REVIEW OF THE LITERATURE

This book on neck and back pain—its causes, diagnosis, treatment, and social and economic implications—presents scientific background information derived from relevant studies in various fields in which different types of studies have been evaluated using modern epidemiologic principles. Our patients will not be well served by strongly held opinions that are unsupported by scientific evidence.

We have used some previous guidelines and published reviews of treatment efficacy available from the Cochrane Library (21). When necessary, because of time gaps between the aforementioned publications and the writing of this book, relevant articles that we retrieved from EMBASE, MEDLINE, and other sources have been evaluated by at least two persons (usually those responsible for the apposite chapters), and results have been added to the previously performed evidence syntheses.

This work has been ongoing for 4 years. The whole group has met altogether eight times for 2 days each, and individual meetings among authors of the various chapter groups have been more numerous. At the onset of this collaborative effort, a special tutorial on how to evaluate the literature was attended by all the members.

The number of published studies on various aspects of back pain has increased exponentially during the past 10 years; a MEDLINE search from 1995 to 1997 provides 2,000 new references on back pain alone. For the busy clinician, it is impossible to distill all this "evidence" and to identify reliable data. Unfortunately, the traditional belief in authoritative reviews to guide our practice has been found unreliable because these reviews often exhibit important biases (2,6,10,38,53,58,61,62,67,68,82). This situation has resulted over the last 10 years in an increased awareness that we need a more systematic approach based on valid methodologic criteria to judge the content of the articles (10,19,83,89). To synthesize the evidence, preparing and maintaining this systematic review are considerable tasks that require time, effort, and financial support (54,67). Usually, such support emanates from government agencies such as SBU, from large pharmaceutical companies, or from private insurers. An international initiative was established to coordinate ongoing reviews. The *Cochrane Collaboration* was established in England in 1992 to promote systematic collection, review, and synthesis of the literature (29). It is named after British epidemiologist Archie Cochrane (22), who challenged the medical community to: "organize a critical summary by specialty, to be updated periodically, of all relevant randomized controlled trials." Various subspeciality interest groups have convened, one of them being the *Back Review Group,* from which much of the evidence synthesis brought forward in the treatment chapters has been adapted (12,84).

The first literature synthesis on back problems that was widely quoted was the 1987 "Scientific Approach to the Assessment and Management of Activity-Related Spinal Disorders: A Monograph for Clinicians. Report of the Quebec Task Force on Spinal Disorders" (58), in which an epidemiology and biostatistics professor, Walter Spitzer, of McGill University in Montreal, Quebec, Canada, convened a board of 20 collaborators to evaluate the literature up to 1985 with the objective of basing its recommendation on the scientific evidence available. The review of relevant publications focused on two aspects in the studies: type and quality. Several data banks were consulted, and more than 7,000 articles in various languages were identified and, after scrutinizing of abstracts, were reduced to around 700 articles of possible relevance.

A quality evaluation by all the members, specifically trained for the topic, reduced this number to around 450 remaining publications, which were classified in four groups: RCTs, cohort and case-control studies, descriptive studies without control groups, and literature reviews. Less than 1% of the 7,000 studies retrieved up to the end of 1985 consisted of RCTs. Fortunately, by the end of 1997, this number had increased considerably, to approximately 500, even though the quality was sometimes disappointing (see Chapters 11 to 17).

As mentioned earlier, the 1990s brought forward more stringent criteria for evidence synthesis (23), and biostatistical and epidemiologic research continues (32,44,52,76,78).

TABLE 1.3. *Recommendations of the United States Agency for Health Care Policy and Research: Panel ratings of available evidence supporting guidelines statements*

A. Strong research-based evidence (multiple relevant and high-quality scientific studies)
B. Moderate resarch-based evidence (one relevant, high-quality scientific study or multiple adequate scientific studies)
C. Limited research-based evidence (at least one adequate scientific study in patients with low back pain)
D. Panel interpretation of information that did not meet inclusion criteria as research-based evidence

Moreover, numerous articles and books have been published, guiding the individual reader to a better understanding of these more stringent criteria for review articles and for the increasing number of RCTs and case-control trials (5,62,67,72). We have, when at all possible, tried to adhere to these modern principles by which some methodologic criteria should be fulfilled in each trial brought forward: methods of treatment allocation, withdrawal and dropout rate, patient-blinded method if possible, nonbiased outcome assessor, and intention-to-treat analysis, for example (44,52,84).

The Agency for Health Care Policy and Research in the United States was the first body to implement a thorough literature search and to use evidence synthesis with metaanalysis for the problem of spinal disorders and pain (9). These guidelines, as well as many ensuing recommendations, have been criticized for being too strict (46,73,81), and in the United States, they even initiated political action and the writing of an antithetical book (40). None of these actions, however, brought forward any new scientific evidence, but merely emphasized the time-honored clinical freedom, which will be partly eliminated in the coming years, based on evidence of poor effectiveness.

Thus, more stringent criteria than in the Quebec report were used in the more recent scientific guideline, and the statistical method of metaanalysis was adopted when several RCTs were available. When RCTs were not available, then the appropriateness method initially developed by the Rand Corporation was used (74). The ensuing recommendations were classified as in Table 1.3. Most ensuing guidelines that have tried to be evidence-based (in contrast to consensus recommendations) have used this type of grading, also adopted with slight modifications by the SBU and used in this book (Table 1.4).

Metaanalysis is the process of combining study results that can be used to draw conclusions about therapeutic effectiveness or to plan new studies (44,49,63,78). The final product of such an analysis has both quantitative and qualitative elements because it takes into account the numeric results and the sample sizes of the individual studies as well as the more subjective issues such as quality, extent of bias, and strength of the study design. Metaanalysis is a systematic reviewing strategy for addressing research questions that is especially useful when results from several studies disagree with regard to magnitude or direction of the effect, when sample sizes are individually too

TABLE 1.4. *Grading of evidence used in this book*

A. Support from metaanalysis or systematic review of good quality of two or more studies
B. Support from one or more randomized controlled trials or good observational studies
C. Insufficient or inconclusive evidence (no or poor randomized controlled trials or observational studies)
D. No acceptable scientific support from available studies

small to detect an effect, or when a large trial is too costly and time consuming to perform.

It has become obvious from various observational studies on prognosis and from RCTs on treatment efficacy that a need exists for temporal definition of spinal pain problems of unknown origin (10,24,30,37,64). In accordance with most reviews (1,9,87,88), we have agreed to the following definitions:

Acute neck or back pain: 0 to 3 weeks' duration of pain and/or disability.
Subacute neck or back pain: 4 to 12 weeks' duration of pain and/or disability.
Chronic neck or back pain: more than 12 weeks' duration of pain and/or disability.
Recurrent problems: patients seeking help after at least 1 month of not seeking care or being on sick leave after at least 1 month of working.

Earlier reports on the natural history of back pain showed a relatively rapid recovery for most patients (80% within 1 month) (55,56,58). Such studies, however, were mostly based on insurance surveillance data mirroring a return to function. Studies of primary care patients both in Great Britain and the United States demonstrated a slower recovery, with approximately one-fourth of patients still having some problems after 1 year (24,30,87). Recurrences of pain were also common although not always disabling.

In addition, in each chapter a brief description is given on the literature that was scrutinized, search methodologies and date when the search was terminated, and the specific databases that were searched. Some of the chapters in this book are narrative in construction because no or few scientific studies can be performed or alternatively have not been found. In these chapters, however, after the literature search, the best available studies are described, as agreed on by the chapter authors (45).

Within different types of studies, the scientific quality can also vary and can influence the weight of the evidence. This can be tabulated, as was done by the SBU (70) (Table 1.3). The main questions to answer for the validity of an RCT (44,52,61) are as follows:

1. Was the assignment of patients to treatment really randomized and was the randomization concealed?
2. Were all the patients entered into the trial accounted for at its conclusion?
3. Were they analyzed in the group to which they were randomized?

There are also some other points to address:

1. Were the patients and clinicians kept "blind" to the treatment group to which they were being allocated? This is sometimes impossible, such as in trials of surgical versus conservative treatment, but the outcome assessor potentially could and should be blinded.
2. Compared with the experimental treatment group, were the groups treated equally, that is, given the same amount of attention? This is particular important when evaluating treatment of nonspecific pain conditions.
3. Were the groups similar at the start of the trial?

Evidence-based medicine is certainly not restricted to RCTs and metaanalysis. It involves tracking down the best external evidence with which to answer the clinical questions. You can obtain these data from systematic reviews or from primary case-control, cohort, or even clinical follow-up studies, provided some basic principles are followed.

For example, in the area of diagnostic tests when we need to find the accuracy of such tests without a gold standard, we need to find proper cross-sectional studies of patients clinically suspected of having a relevant disorder, and these studies cannot be randomized trials. For a question about prognosis, we need proper follow-up studies of patients assembled at a uniform early point in the clinical course of the disease. In addition, some indirect evidence can come from basic science, which is now slowly enhancing our understanding of pain and of the aging of connective tissues.

All questions about therapy do not require randomized trials. This concept was summarized by Eddy and Jackson: "Treatment can be considered efficacious if outcomes are obvious, dramatic, immediate and cannot be explained by any other factors." (31) Unfortunately, when it comes to the proper diagnosis or treatment of spinal disorders in which pain is the only "objective finding," no such efficacious methods exist.

Judging the relevance of nonrandomized studies, we have also adopted strict rules for inclusion. There must be a clear description of the patients and interventions with valid intake and outcome measures, as well as an adequate sample size and a nonbiased personal follow-up after an adequate length of time after treatment. In general, this requires a minimum of 3 to 6 months for a nonoperative procedure, whereas for an intervention such as surgery, a period of 2 years is the minimum required. Some authors actually even advocate longer follow-up periods (7,36).

The collaborators of this book have agreed to follow a grading system similar to most other guidelines and also recommended by SBU. Our statements based on evidence can, of course, also have a negative meaning (i.e. evidence of no effect).

Several grading schemes exist, none proven "better" than the next (61,84). In addition, the methods of evaluating an RCT, questions of blinding the reviewer to the author and journal of publication, are being subjected to scientific studies (52).

Evidence synthesis is a developing specialty, and the results brought forward in this book should not be looked on as written in stone, but rather as recommendations based on currently available admissible studies of neck and low back pain. Our recommendations should also be modulated by patients' preferences and societal circumstances as part of the most important empathic approach by the practitioner (60).

Based on the strength of the evidence, our conclusions can either be positive or negative. In the chapters on sociology, epidemiology, and various risk factors for neck and low back pain, different grading systems for the evidence have been used, mainly because of a lack of RCTs. These systems are described in the respective chapters.

The outcome of an acceptable RCT shows the possible efficacy of a treatment method. Effectiveness of this particular method, which is an important next step for patients, practitioners, and politicians, means that the treatment method in question also is acceptable, applicable, and generalizable to a larger group of patients in a society; that is, it has a demonstrable, beneficial effect in general practice.

Admittedly few studies of effectiveness exist in medicine, and the field of back pain is no exception. Without well-controlled RCTs, however, everyone—patients, practitioners, and politicians—is left with clinical experience that is proven to be wrong too frequently (68,82).

REFERENCES

1. Accident Rehabilitation and Compensation Insurance Corporation and the National Health Committee. New Zealand acute low back pain guide. Wellington, New Zealand: ACC and the National Health Committee, 1997.
2. Advisory Group on Health Technology Assessment for the Director of Research and Development.

Assessing the effects of health technologies: principles-practice-proposals. London: Research and Development Division, Department of Health, 1992.

3. Allan DB, Waddell G. An historical perspective on low back pain and disability. *Acta Orthop Scand Suppl* 1989;60:1–23.

4. Alvegard T, Blomgren H, Einhorn J, et al. *Radiotherapy in Sweden.* SBU structured abstracts. Stockholm: SBU (Swedish Council on Technology Assessment in Health Care), 1995–1996.

5. Ashcroft RE, Chadwick DW, Clark SRI, et al. Implications of sociocultural contexts for the ethics of clinical trials. *Health Technol Assess* 1997;1:1–65.

6. Assendelft WJJ, Koes BW, Knipschild PG, et al. The relationship between methodological quality and conclusions in reviews of spinal manipulation. *JAMA* 1995;274:1942–1948.

7. Atlas SJ, Deyo RA, Keller RB, et al. The Maine Lumbar Spine Study. III: 1-year outcomes of surgical and nonsurgical management of lumbar spinal stenosis. *Spine* 1996;21:1787–1794.

8. Baranauskas G, Nistri R. Sensitization of pain pathways in the spinal cord: cellular mechanisms. *Prog Neurobiol* 1998;54:349–365.

9. Bigos S, Bowyer O, Braen, et al. Acute low-back problems in adults. Clinical practice guideline no. 14. AHCPR Publication no 95-0642. Rockville, MD: Agency for Health Care Policy and Research, Public Health Service, United States Department of Health and Human Services, 1994.

10. Bloch R. Methodology in clinical back pain trials. *Spine* 1987;12:430–432.

11. Boden SD. The use of radiographic imaging studies in the evaluation of patients who have degenerative disorders of the lumbar spine. *J Bone Joint Surg Am* 1996;78:114–124.

12. Bombardier C, Esmail R, Nachemson AL, et al. The Cochrane Collaboration Back Review Group for Spinal Disorders. *Spine* 1997;22:837–840.

13. Boos N, Rieder R, Schade V, et al. The diagnostic accuracy of magnetic resonance imaging, work perception, and psychosocial factors in identifying symptomatic disc herniations. *Spine* 1995;20:2613–2625.

14. Boos N, Semmer N, Elfering A, et al. Natural history of individuals with asymptomatic disc abnormalities in MRI. *Spine* 2000; in print.

15. Borenstein D, O'Mara J, Boden S, et al. A 7 year follow-up study of the value of lumbar spine MR to predict the development of low back pain in aymptomatic individuals. Presented at: International Society for the Study of the Lumbar Spine, 26th Annual Meeting, Hawaii, 1999.

16. Borkan J, Reis S, Ribak J, et al. *Guidelines for the treatment of low back pain in primary care.* Tel Aviv: Israeli Low Back Pain Guidelines Group, 1995.

17. Burton AK, Waddell G. Clinical guidelines in the management of low back pain. *Baillieres Clin Rheumatol* 1998;12:17–35.

18. Burton KA. Spine update. Back injury and work loss: biomechanical and psychosocial influences. *Spine* 1997;22:2575–2580.

19. Chalmers IG, Collins RE, Dickersin K. Controlled trials and meta-analyses can help resolve disagreements among orthopaedic surgeons [Editorial]. *J Bone Joint Surg Br* 1992;74:641–643.

20. *Clinical practice guidelines of the Finnish Medical Association Duodecim.* Malmivaara A, ed. Helsinki: Finnish Medical Association, 1998.

21. Cochrane library http://www.cochranelibrary.net (Health Communication Network).

22. Cochrane A. *Effectiveness and efficacy: random reflections on health services.* London: Nuffield Provincial Hospitals Trust, 1972:1–98.

23. Cochrane handbook. How to conduct a cochrane systematic review. In: Mulrow CD, Oxman A, eds. *The Cochrane Collaboration Handbook.* San Antonio: The Cochrane Collaboration, 1997:1–277.

24. Croft P, Macfarlane GJ, Papageorgiou AC, et al. Outcome of low back pain in general practice: a prospective study. *BMJ* 1998;316:1356–1359.

25. Croft P, Papageorgiou A, McNally R. Low back pain. In: Stevens A, Raferty J, eds. *Health care needs assessment.* Oxford: Radcliffe Medical Press, 1997:129–182.

26. Deyo RA. Practice variations, treatment fads, rising disability: do we need a new clinical research paradigm? *Spine* 1993;18:2153–2162.

27. Deyo RA. Promises and limitations of the patient outcome research teams: the low-back pain example. *Proc Assoc Am Physicians* 1995;107:3.

28. Deyo RA. Low-back pain: low-back pain is at epidemic levels. Although its causes are still poorly understood, treatment choices have improved, with the body's own healing power often the most reliable remedy. *Sci Am* 1998;Aug:29–33.

29. Dickersin K, Manheimer E. The Cochrane Collaboration: evaluation of health care and services using systematic reviews of the results of randomized controlled trials. *Clin Obstet Gynecol* 1998;41:2:315–331.

30. Dionne CE, Koepsell TD, Von Korff M, et al. Predicting longterm functional limitations among back pain patients in primary care settings. *J Clin Epidemiol* 1997;50:31–43.

31. Eddy DM, Jackson WY. Medicine, money and mathematics. *Am Coll Surg Bull* 1992;77:36–49.

32. Emerson JD, Burdick E, Hoaglin DC, et al. An empirical study of the possible relation of treatment differences to quality scores in controlled randomized clinical trials. *Control Clin Trials* 1990;11:339–352.

33. Ernst E, White AR. Acupuncture for back pain: a meta-analysis of randomized controlled trials. *Arch Intern Med* 1998;158:2235–2241.

34. Evans G, Richards S. *Low back pain: an evaluation of therapeutic interventions.* Bristol, England: Health Care Evaluation Unit, University of Bristol, Dept of Social Medicine, 1996.
35. Faas A, Chavannes AW, Koes AW, et al. NHG practice guideline: low back pain [Translated]. *Huisars Wet* 1996;39:18–31.
36. Fishbain DA, Cutler RB, Rosomoff HL, et al. Impact of chronic pain patients' job perception variables on actual return to work. *Clin J Pain* 1997;13:197–206.
37. Fordyce WE, ed. *Back pain in the workplace: management of disability in nonspecific conditions.* Seattle: IASP Press, 1995.
38. Fowkes FGR, Fulton PM. Critical appraisal of published research: introductory guidelines. *BMJ* 1991;302:1136–1140.
39. Frank J, Sinclair S, Hogg-Johnson S, et al. Preventing disability from work-related low-back pain: new evidence gives new hope–if we can just get all the players onside. *Can Med Assoc J* 1998;158:1625–1631.
40. Gonzales EG, Materson RS. *The nonsurgical management of acute low back pain: cutting through the AHCPR guidelines.* New York: Demos Vermande, 1997.
41. Goodman C. *Literature searching and evidence interpretation for assessing health care practices: SBU, the Swedish Council on Technology Assessment in Health Care.* Stockholm: Norstedts Tryckeri, 1993.
42. Hall H, McIntosh G, Wilson L, et al. Spontaneous onset of back pain. *Clin J Pain* 1998;14:129–133.
43. Hansson E, Hansson T, Bergendorff S, et al. *Rygg och nacke 3.* Stockholm: International Social Security Association Report, 1999.
44. Jadad AR, McQuay HJ. Meta-analyses to evaluate analgesic interventions: a systematic qualitative review of their methodology. *J Clin Epidemiol* 1996;49:235–243.
45. Johansson C, Johnell O, Jonsson R, et al. *Bone density measurement.* SBU structured abstracts. Stockholm: SBU, 1996.
46. Johnson L. Outcomes analysis in spinal research: how clinical research differs from outcomes analysis. *Orthop Clin North Am* 1994;25:205–213.
47. Jones G, White C, Sambrook P, et al. Allelic variation in the vitamin D receptor, lifestyle factors and lumbar spinal degenerative disease. *Ann Rheum Dis* 1998;57:94–99.
48. Kendall NAS, Linton SJ, Main CJ. *Guide to assessing psychosocial yellow flags in acute low back pain: risk factors for long-term disability and work loss.* Wellington, New Zealand: Accident Rehabilitation and Compensation Insurance Corporation of New Zealand and the National Health Committee, 1997.
49. L'Abbé KA, Detsky AS, O'Rourke K. *Meta-analysis in clinical research.* Chicago: The American Academy of Orthopaedic Surgeons, Department of Research, Outcomes and Effectiveness in Musculoskeletal Research, 1993.
50. Manniche C, Ankjaer-Jensen A, Fog A, et al. *Ondt i ryggen: en kortlaegning av problemets forekomst og oplaeg til dets håndtering i et MTV-perspektiv.* Copenhagen: Sundshedsstyrelsen, 1997.
51. Mixter WJ, Barr JS. Rupture of the intervertebral disc with involvement of the spinal canal. *N Engl J Med* 1934;211:210–215.
52. Moher D, Jadad AR, Tugwell P. Assessing the quality of randomized controlled trials. *Int J Technol Assess Health Care* 1996;12:195–208.
53. Mörk Hansen T, Bendix T, Bünger CD, et al. Laendesmerter: klaringsrapport fra dansk selskap for intern medisin. *Uqeskr Laeqer* 1996;158 [Suppl 4]:1–18.
54. Muir Gray JA. *Evidence-based healthcare: how to make health policy and management decisions.* New York: Churchill Livingstone, 1997.
55. Nachemson A. *Ont i ryggen orsaker diagnostik och behandling.* Stockholm: SBU (Swedish Council on Technology Assessment in Health Care), 1991.
56. Nachemson A. Newest knowledge of low back pain: a critical look. *Clin Orthop* 1992;279:7–20.
57. Nachemson A, LaRocca H. Editorial. *Spine* 1987;12:427–429.
58. Nachemson A, Spitzer WO, Leblanc FE, et al. Scientific approach to the assessment and management of activity-related spinal disorders: a monograph for clinicians. Report of the Quebec Task Force on Spinal Disorders. *Spine* 1987;12 [Suppl]:S1–S59.
59. NHS executive. *Clinical guidelines: using clinical guidelines to improve patient care within the NHS.* London: NHS Executive, 1997.
60. Owens DK. Spine update: patient preferences and the development of practice guidelines. *Spine* 1998;23:1073–1079.
61. Oxman AD. Checklists for review articles. *BMJ* 1994;309:648–651.
62. Oxman AD, Cook DJ, Guyatt GH. The medical literature: users' guides to the medical literature. VI. How to use an overview. *JAMA* 1994;272:1367–1371.
63. Roach HI, Shearer JR, Archer C. Invited article: the choice of an experimental model. *J Bone Joint Surg Br* 1989;71:549–53.
64. Roos H, Roos E, Ryd L. On the art of measuring. *Acta Orthop Scand* 1997;68:1–5.
65. Rosen M, Breen A, Hamann W, et al. Report of a clinical standards advisory group committee on back pain. London: Her Majesty's Stationery Office, 1994.
66. Royal College of General Practitioners. *The development and implementation of clinical guidelines. report of the clinical guidelines working group.* London: Royal College of General Practitioners, 1995.

67. Sackett DL, Richardson WS, Rosenberg W, et al. *Evidence-based medicine: how to practice and teach EBM.* New York: Churchill Livingstone, 1997.
68. Sackett DL. Clinical epidemiology rounds: how to read clinical journals. I. Why to read them and how to start reading them critically. *Can Med Assoc J* 1981;124:555–558.
69. SBU (Swedish Council on Technology Assessment in Health Care). *Kritisk analys inom medicinen: rapport från en konferens augusti 1991.* Stockholm: SBU, 1992.
70. SBU (Swedish Council on Technology Assessment in Health Care). Grading of scientific quality. *Vetenskap Praxis* 1996;3:5.
71. Schott A-M, Nizard R, Mainsonneuve H, et al. Methods used to develop clinical guidelines in France: the example of common lumbosciatic syndrome. *Rev Rhum Engl Ed* 1996;63:830–836.
72. Schulz KF. Unbiased research and the human spirit: the challenges of randomized controlled trials [Editorial]. *Can Med Assoc J* 1995;153:783–786.
73. Shapiro S. Is meta-analysis a valid approach to the evaluation of small effects in observational studies? [Commentary] *J Clin Epidemiol* 1997;50:223–229.
74. Shekelle PG, Schriger DL. Evaluating the use of the appropriateness method in the agency for health care policy and research clinical practice guideline development process. *Health Serv Res* 1996;31:4453–468.
75. Smeele IJM, Van den Hoogen JMM, Mens JMA, et al. NHG practice guideline: lumbosacral radicular syndrome. Translated version from *Huisarts Wet* 1996;39:78–89.
76. Smith GD, Egger M. Commentary incommunicable knowledge? Interpreting and applying the results of clinical trials and metaanalyses. *J Clin Epidemiol* 1998;51:289–295.
77. Spitzer WO, Skovron ML, Salmi LR, et al. Scientific monograph of the Quebec Task Force on Whiplash-Associated Disorders: redefining "whiplash" and its management. *Spine* 1995;20 [Suppl]:8S–73S.
78. Spitzer WO. Meta-meta-analysis: unanswered questions about aggregating data [Editorial]. *J Clin Epidemiol* 1991;44:2:103–107.
79. Statens helsetilsyn 7–95, IK-2508. *Vondt i ryggen. Hva er det? Hva gjör vi?* Oslo, Norway: Statens helsetilsyn, 1995.
80. Steven ID (chairperson). *Guidelines for the management of back-injured employees.* Australia: Work-Cover Corporation, 1993.
81. Stirrat GM, Farrow SC, Farndon J, et al. The challenge of evaluating surgical procedures. *Ann R Coll Surg Engl* 1992;74:80–84.
82. Trial and error. *Economist* 1998;Oct 31:93.
83. Tugwell PX. Clinical epidemiology rounds: how to read clinical journals. III. To learn the clinical course and prognosis of disease. *Can Med Assoc J* 1981;124:869–872.
84. van Tulder MW, Assendelft JJ, Koes BW, et al. Method guidelines for systematic reviews in the cochrane collaboration back review group for spinal disorders. *Spine* 1997;22:2323–2330.
85. Victorian Workcover Authority. *Guidelines for the management of employees with compensable low back pain.* Melbourne, Australia: Victorian Workcover Authority, 1996.
86. Videman T, Leppävuori J, Kaprio J, et al. Intragenic polymorphisms of the vitamin d receptor gene associated with intervertebral disc degeneration. *Spine* 1998;23:2477–2485.
87. von Korff M, Saunders K. The course of back pain in primary care. *Spine* 1996:21:2833–2837.
88. Waddell G, Feder G, Lewis M. Systematic reviews of bed rest and advice to stay active for acute low back pain. *Br J Gen Pract* 1997;47:647–652.
89. Waddell G, Feder G, McIntosh A, et al. *Low back pain evidence review.* London: Royal College of General Practitioners, 1996.

Neck and Back Pain: The Scientific Evidence
of Causes, Diagnosis, and Treatment, edited
by Alf Nachemson and Egon Jonsson.
Published by Lippincott Williams & Wilkins,
Philadelphia 2000.

2

A Review of Social Influences on Neck and Back Pain and Disability

Gordon Waddell* and Hazel Waddell†

*Department of Orthopaedics, The Glasgow Nuffield Hospital, Glasgow, Scotland;
†Department of Social Work and Social Policy, University of Glasgow,
Glasgow, Scotland

Aristotle, in the fourth century BC, recognized that "man is by nature a social animal" and laid out the principles of social influence and persuasion. Halliday (73) pointed out that this concept is as true of illness as of any other human behavior, that illness is very much a social phenomenon and depends on its social context: the foundation of social medicine. It is now widely recognized that spinal pain and disability can only be understood and managed according to a biopsychosocial model (174,175). Low back disability depends to some extent on the degree of objective physical impairment, but all analyses show that it depends to a much greater extent on psychosocial factors. Psychosocial factors play a particularly important role in the development of chronic pain and disability (see Chapter 3). Physical and psychologic issues may be most important for pain, but it may be hypothesized that social issues may be even more important for disability and work loss. Back pain and neck pain always occur in a particular social setting, which may influence pain, disability, and work loss. Social interactions are potentially two-way: Low back pain and disability may affect other people and society; conversely, the way in which other people react and the provisions society makes may affect the individual's illness behavior.

Allan and Waddell (1) reviewed the history of low back pain and disability over the last 3,500 years. They suggested that low back pain has not changed throughout recorded human history, but what has changed is how low back pain is understood and managed. Over the past century, and particularly in the past 20 years, there has been a marked increase in chronic disability, sick certification, and invalidity benefits attributed to nonspecific low back pain in all Western countries. This has occurred in the absence of any evidence of change in the physical pathology or prevalence of back pain or in the neurophysiology or psychology of these patients. It may be hypothesized that this change is cultural, and it may be best understood as a social epidemic.

THE SICK ROLE

A *social role* is a set of expectations about what a person should do or how he or she should behave. These expectations are the individual's, other people's, and society's.

The onset of illness always triggers a social process that, in turn, shapes the person's response to the ailment. The sick role is not a medical condition or a diagnosis, but rather a status accorded to the individual by other members of society that may be variably associated with a medical condition. The individual must accept and assume the sick role. Often, particularly for work loss or financial support, there must also be medical certification to legitimize the role.

Parsons (133) analyzed illness as a social phenomenon and tried to define the social rights and duties of the person in the sick role. He started from the assumption that sickness is something unfortunate that occurs without the individual's control and involves some degree of helplessness.

Rights:

The sick person is exempt from responsibility for incapacity.

The sick person is relieved from normal social duties and responsibilities.

The sick person is entitled to special attention and support. On the other hand, anyone who claims these rights when not "really" sick is judged to be malingering.

Duties:

The sick person accepts that to be sick is undesirable, and the obligation is to try to get well.

The sick person is obliged to seek professional help and to cooperate in the process of getting well. Therefore, health professionals and society disapprove of those who do not try to get well.

The concept of the sick role takes illness beyond mere disease and sees illness as part of the much broader relationship between the individual and society. Health professionals should not regard themselves as being above or outside this system. If anything, health professionals interpret and enforce the sick role conditions more rigidly than do other members of society.

Parsons (133) based these ideas on acute physical illness, and this analysis must be modified for chronic pain and disability, which cannot be understood purely in terms of physical disease and treatment. The concept of chronic illness modifies expectations of health care and "getting well," nor does physical analysis fit well with chronic disability in which the person's beliefs and behavior may be part of the problem. Waddell et al. (176) offered a modified analysis of the sick role for chronic pain and disability by redefining the following rights and duties:

Rights:

The sick person is not responsible for the original physical problem.

The sick person may modify normal social obligations to a degree proportionate to the illness.

Duties:

The sick person recognizes that to be ill is undesirable and is obliged to reduce illness behavior and disability as much as possible.

The sick person must share responsibility for his or her own health and disability.

This approach also recognizes that the sick role is not static but dynamic, and it may change with time and at different stages of the illness. It allows scope for adapting and coping. What is a normal sick role in acute illness, as in Parsons' original model, may even become maladaptive in chronic illness. It means some shift in responsibility from health professionals to the individual. It raises questions about the relative rights and duties of the sick role and about society's attitudes and obligations to the chronically sick person.

Many of these questions are now in flux. New understanding of low back pain and disability and its management undermines the old Parsonian sick role of a simple social perspective on physical disease (95), but it does not diminish the importance of these issues. In addition, the sick role applies equally to a nonspecific symptom such as back pain and a clear-cut disease such as cancer, even if to a varying degree. Serious physical diseases such as cancer may inexorably cause illness and death, but in the process, different victims may have different lives and sick roles and even vary greatly in the manner of their dying.

METHODS

Aims and Definitions

The aim of this chapter is to review the literature about social influences on neck and back pain and disability. Because of the nature of this literature, some of the studies are about pain in general (although in most of these studies a large proportion of the patients have low back pain), but as far as possible, the present review focuses on information available on neck and back pain.

For the purpose of this review, *social influences* are defined as external influences resulting from relationships or interactions with other people, either individually, as a group, or collectively with society.

Literature Search

The first stage of the literature retrieval started with a MEDLINE search from 1980 to 1996. The search strategy combined back pain, neck pain, and whiplash injuries with costs, cost analysis, health insurance, workers' compensation, claims, and legal issues and identified 287 titles. Many additional references came from Dr. Alf Nachemson's and Dr. Gordon Waddell's extensive personal bibliographies and from other members of this book's economics group. Dr. George Mendelson also supplied an international bibliography of more than 700 references and abstracts on medicolegal aspects of pain and the effect of compensation, for which we are extremely grateful.

Initially, two members of the economics group (G. Waddell and M. Goossens) each independently reviewed the abstracts and selected those that met the search criteria. In general, if *either* reviewer thought a reference was of possible relevance, it was included, unless it was already known to the other and was excluded after discussion.

The second stage of the literature retrieval was a series of further searches of MEDLINE, EMBASE, and PSYCLIT from 1985 to December 1997 for specific social topics. *Back pain, neck pain,* and *musculoskeletal disorders* were combined with all *socioeconomic factors (exploded), job satisfaction, pensions* and *retirement, family,* and *spouse.* MEDLINE identified 400 references, EMBASE identified 97, and PSYCLIST identified 61, although there were many duplicates, and fewer than 15% of these references were new and relevant additions to the review. In view of the high reliability of the initial search and the limited decisions required about content, further selection of articles from these searches and citation tracking was carried out by one author (G. Waddell) and then was checked by the other author and by other members of the economic group for inclusions and completeness.

However, more than 50% of this material is not included in computerized databases but is in nonindexed sources or the "gray" literature. Even what is in computerized databases is poorly indexed and is difficult to retrieve. More than half the final references came from citation tracking of the reference lists of all the articles retrieved. Certain issues were by necessity allocated to other chapters and were excluded from the present review, although social, psychologic, and work-related factors are obviously closely interrelated:

- Physical demands of work and physical risk factors for back pain (see Chapter 6).
- Individual psychologic factors such as general attitudes and beliefs, distress, coping strategies, and illness behavior (see Chapter 5).
- Job satisfaction and psychosocial aspects of work (see Chapter 5).
- Social security and socioeconomic data in different countries and international comparisons (see Chapter 19).

Altogether, approximately 6,000 possible titles, abstracts, or full papers were considered, to identify 167 relevant papers that provide actual social data, reviews, or theoretic analysis and are included in the present review. Most of the remaining publications were not included because they only provided "clinical experience," anecdotal information, or opinion.

Social influences may potentially have different effects on pain, disability, and work loss, which must each be considered separately, though some reviews have failed to do so. Gender issues must also be considered, because social roles and influences may be different in men and women. Gender may be more important to these social influences than it is for the physical or psychologic dimensions. Unfortunately, however, this review found relatively little evidence on gender issues.

Methodologic Quality of the Studies

The 171 articles from the first stage of the literature search were each reviewed independently by two members of the economic group (G. Waddell, M. Goossens, or A. Nachemson and either E. Jonsson or L-Å Marké) to judge if they contained socioeconomic data relevant to neck or low back pain. The fundamental criteria was whether they actually presented data, rather than just clinical experience or opinion. Because of the generally poor methodologic quality of most of the literature in this field, it was decided not to set any arbitrary quality for inclusion or we would have excluded most of the material. There was 95% agreement on which articles to include, and all disagreements were resolved by discussion between the reviewers without requiring adjudication. Several theoretic and review articles that did not include original data were also used for background material.

Goossens and Nachemson independently tried to assess the quality of the selected articles using the methodologic checklist described in the cost-effectiveness analysis (see Chapter 19). This worked reasonably well for cost-effectiveness, but it proved impractical for most of the other social material. Such methodologic checklists were originally designed for randomized controlled trials of treatment and had already been modified to deal with cost-effectiveness. They are simply not applicable to most of this social material. Moreover, this material is varied in nature and content, and generally, it is of a low scientific standard that meets few standard quality measures. In practice, attempts to apply the checklist gave results of "not applicable" or "not met" and did not produce any meaningful scores.

It is important to emphasize the low scientific standard of most of the material throughout most of this social review, with the main exception of psychosocial aspects of work. Most of the studies in many areas are descriptive or cross-sectional, and few longitudinal and even fewer experimental studies have been reported.

RESULTS

Culture

Culture is "that complex whole which includes knowledge, belief, art, morals, law, custom and any other capabilities and habits acquired by the individual as a member of society, and that affects their entire lifestyle," to paraphrase Fabrega and Tyma (53). More specific to this context, it is the broad, shared pattern of values, attitudes, and behaviors that may interact with low back pain and disability. These may vary in different societies, in different subcultures of a society, or in a society over time.

Zborowski (188) is frequently quoted as the author of a classic study of the effect of culture in the United States in patients with chronic spinal pain who were receiving workers' compensation. Experimental pain *threshold* is more or less the same irrespective of nationality, sex, age, or social background, which affects pain *expression* and *tolerance.* Zborowski's clinical observation of patients of Jewish, Italian, Irish, and "old American" background showed that different cultural backgrounds were associated with different beliefs about pain, coping strategies, expressions of pain, and response to health care. He also suggested that culture may be more strongly related to attitudes and beliefs about pain, whereas individual background and peer pressure may be more strongly related to pain behavior.

There was considerable interest on the effect of culture on pain from the 1940s to the 1960s, as reviewed by Wolff and Langley (181) and Fabrega and Tyma (53). Elton and Stanley (50) gave a more modern and succinct summary. There appear to be marked differences in pain experience and behavior in different cultural and ethnic groups and consistencies within each group. These findings suggest that pain may be a less well-defined experience than commonly believed, so individuals may depend on normative standards that are in part the product of social learning. The present search found few more recent studies (since Elton and Stanley [50] in 1982) about the effect of culture on back pain and none on neck pain.

Honeyman and Jacobs (81) gave a dramatic example of the effect of culture on back pain in Australian aboriginals. On close questioning, nearly one-third of the men and one-half of the women admitted to long-term back pain, but they kept their pain "private" and did not show much public expression of pain, communicate it to others, or seek health care. That society appeared to have strong cultural pressures about tolerating and not displaying pain.

Svensson (160) in Göteborg, Sweden, made one of the earliest studies of socioeconomic factors and low back pain that showed an association between reported low back pain, foreign citizenship, and increased sickness-related absence from work. Ekberg et al. (48,49) in Sweden found that immigrant status was significantly associated with neck and shoulder symptoms (odds ratio [OR], 4.9), sick leave (10% of variance), and poor response to rehabilitation. Eden et al. (47), also in Sweden, found that immigrant status, low socioeconomic status, lower educational level, and heavy manual work were associated with increased early retirement for all reasons. Wood et al. (184) also found that a workers' compensation program in western Australia showed a 71.1%

return to work in workers with English as their native language, but the rate was only 41.1% in immigrant workers whose preferred language was not English. However, Hewson et al. (76) studied patients with back pain who were receiving workers' compensation in Australia and found little evidence for the commonly accepted stereotype of immigrant workers. Most of the accident vulnerability of these workers and their response to treatment could be accounted for by the nature of their employment, referral patterns, and ability to communicate. Elton and Stanley (50) also studied 70 male patients with chronic pain who were undergoing a cognitive-behavioral treatment program in the United States and found that those patients of "Anglo-Saxon" background had a neutral or positive attitude to such treatment, whereas those of "European" background generally had a more guarded or negative reaction; 92% of Anglo-Saxon patients but only 14% of European patients obtained greater than 50% pain relief. Keel et al. (90,91) discussed the situation of foreign workers in Switzerland and suggested that an accumulation of negative factors contributed to chronic pain and disability and could seriously hinder rehabilitation. However, these investigators concluded that these negative factors were related to the position of these patients as foreign workers rather than to their cultural background.

The randomized controlled trial of early rehabilitation by Lindstrom et al. (104) in Göteborg only found statistically significant results in patients born in Sweden, whereas foreign workers showed no such benefit (Table 2.1). However, many cultural, educational, language, and employment factors may be associated with immigrant status, and that trial did not provide any information on possible causes of this effect. Lofvander et al. (107) in Sweden carried out a randomized controlled trial of rehabilitation in young immigrants with chronic benign pain and showed that a rehabilitation program tailored to meet their specific needs could produce a significant improvement in the number of patients on sick leave.

Volinn (171) reviewed epidemiologic surveys of back pain in different countries, and Deyo (42) commented on the methodologic problems of such international comparisons. In most high-income areas such as Europe and the United States, the annual prevalence of reported back pain is about 20% to 40%. In low-income countries, urban populations have a comparable level of 23% to 35%, but rural populations report a prevalence of only 7% to 18%, despite the much harder and more physically demanding lives of rural workers. However, even in low-income and middle-income countries, selected groups of workers in "enclosed workshops" report a prevalence of back pain of 38% to 68%. Understanding such studies across different languages and cultures is problematic, and it is difficult to know whether the questions were exactly the same or how people in different cultures chose to answer. These surveys may provide more

TABLE 2.1. *Effect of immigrant status on response to an early active intervention program in Göteborg*

	Born in Sweden		Not born in Sweden	
	Intervention	Control	Intervention	Control
Sickness days	208 +/− 195	367 +/− 282	341 +/− 278	339 +/− 273
	$p = .0001$		NS	
Early retirement	9%	32%	31%	26%

NS, not significant.
From Lindstrom I, Areskong B, Nunes JF. *Rygghälsan rapport 2.* Göteborg: Göteborgs sjukvård, 1996, with permission; Nachemson A, personal communication.

TABLE 2.2. *Percentage of adolescents reporting back pain in different countries*

Country	Age 11		Age 13		Age 15	
	Boys	Girls	Boys	Girls	Boys	Girls
Finland	1	2	1	1	2	3
Poland	2	3	2	4	2	5
Austria	3	3	5	8	8	8
Scotland	4	5	6	8	9	10
Spain	4	8	5	9	7	12
Wales	5	8	6	9	8	13
Norway	3	3	5	10	10	13
Hungary	4	5	4	8	6	14
Canada	8	8	12	14	12	16
Belgium	7	7	8	13	9	22

Data from King A, Coles B. The health of Canada's youth: views and behaviours of 11-, 13- and 15-year olds from 11 countries. Ottawa: Health and Welfare Canada, 1992.

information about how different groups *report* their pain than about the physical condition of their backs or the neurophysiology of their pain. Nevertheless, urbanization and rapid industrialization seem to be associated with increased reports of back pain.

King and Coles (93) found a marked variation of self-reported pain in adolescents in different European countries and in Canada that ranged from 3% for girls aged 15 years in Finland to 22% in Belgium (Table 2.2).

Skovron et al. (157) studied sociocultural factors in Belgium, which is divided into two culturally different—French-speaking and Flemish-speaking—areas, although members of both cultures share a common health care and social security system. On multivariate analysis, these investigators found that cultural background was weakly associated with history (adjusted OR, 1.30; 95% confidence interval [CI], 1.14 to 1.47) and first occurrence (OR, 1.81; 95% CI, 1.37 to 2.38) of back pain but not daily back pain (OR, 1.05 NS), with the French-speaking population having the higher risk. These investigators suggested that sociocultural factors may influence the reporting of back pain but not the risk of chronicity after low back pain develops. In a parallel study, they found no cultural variation in migraine and suggested that cultural influences may be greater on nonspecific symptoms than on more specific physical conditions (Szpalski, personal communication). Further analysis of that back pain study by Szpalski et al. (161) found that various social factors were associated with health beliefs and consulting behavior, but there was no significant difference between French-speaking and Flemish-speaking people.

Burton et al. (25) studied Flemish-speaking nurses in Belgium and the Netherlands and found significant but relatively slight differences in psychosocial variables. These investigators found no difference in the point prevalence of low back pain or in associated absence from work, but the Dutch nurses were more positive about pain, work, and activity, and they showed less depressive symptoms. Szpalski (personal communication) related that finding to unsettled industrial conditions in Belgian health care at that time.

The frequently quoted study by Carron et al. (30) compared patients at multidisciplinary pain clinics in the United States and New Zealand and suggested that although the frequency and intensity of pain were similar, patients in the United States reported a greater emotional and behavioral impact of their pain. However, these were both highly selected groups of patients with different local referral patterns, a feature that makes it impossible to draw any conclusions.

In summary, neck pain and back pain are common to all societies, but different cultural groups do not seem to perceive or to respond to this pain in the same way. All the available evidence suggests that social and cultural attitudes and beliefs, pressures, and learning may be more important. Attitudes and beliefs about back pain, expectations, and the meanings attached to pain seem to vary in different societies and over time. Culture may be associated with how people express pain and emotions and pain behavior and with whether and how they communicate their pain to others, including health professionals. Culture may be associated with how people seek and respond to treatment. However, there is a risk to this kind of ethnic stereotyping. Cultural patterns are not fixed but fluid. Zborowski (188) found that as his different groups became Americanized, they changed their attitudes and behavioral patterns to conform to their new society. Stereotyping also ignores the great individual variation in learning and experience about pain and illness within each cultural group.

Little evidence exists on the role of culture in neck pain, although in principle it seems likely to be comparable to its role in low back pain. Other evidence suggests that culture has major effects on gender roles, but this review did not find any evidence specific to neck or back pain. Unfortunately, despite the probable importance of cultural influences on back pain, there is little evidence on which cultural issues are most important, on how they operate, or on how they can be modified.

Family and Social Support

The *family* is the primary unit of society and the one in which the earliest and most powerful social learning occurs. The family unit and the "significant other" provide the most immediate and powerful social feedback and reinforcement. Investigators have suggested that the family should be viewed as the primary unit of health care. Of all illness episodes, 70% to 90% are handled outside the formal health care system, and how a person interprets and deals with his or her symptoms is largely based on formal and informal consultation with family members.

Cobb (36) reviewed the role of social support as a moderator of life *stress*, which could help to maintain health in the face of life's crises and change. In 1929 and 1950, Cannon (28) and Selye (155), respectively, developed the theory that stress could disturb the stable homeostasis on which health depends and so could *cause* diseases of adaptation. Hinkle (77) reviewed more recent evidence. Maes et al. (111) and Lundberg (110) extended the concept to more modern ideas of how environmental stress may influence the onset, course, and outcome of any disease, within a biopsychosocial model of illness. Stress depends on actual or perceived disparity between environmental demands and the individual's ability to cope; its impact depends on the balance among the level of stress, the individual's ability to cope, and social support. This forms a major part of the theoretic basis for how work and family demands and support may modify the impact of neck and back pain. This concept is considered further under psychosocial aspects of work (see Chapter 5), but here let us consider the evidence on the influence of the family.

The literature on the family's role in the development and maintenance of chronic pain is extensive. Narrative reviews of this literature have been published

(21,59,134,169), although little of it is specific to neck or back pain, and research on the role of the family in acute pain has been minimal.

Studies on family structure, such as size, birth order, and early loss of a family member, do not give consistent results of any magnitude. Many studies report that patients with chronic pain tend to come from families with a higher incidence of pain and illness, and some studies also report concordance of pain sites with other family members. This finding has led to theories that early learning in the family and modeling may modify adult pain experiences and behavior.

Bradley et al. (21) suggested that families may exert their influence in three ways. First, family members may act as models for health and illness behaviors, particularly for children. Second, family members may reinforce pain behavior. Third, physical and sexual abuse may increase the risk for developing pain problems, although the mechanism is unclear. (Abuse is reviewed in Chapter 5.) In the first mechanism, it is hypothesized that "dysfunctional family systems" may promote, permit, and maintain chronic pain and disability. In the second mechanism, operant conditioning theory suggests that the family may also act as a powerful behavioral reinforcer. Fordyce (63) first applied behavioral principles to pain and suggested that there is always powerful positive or negative social reinforcement of pain behavior that determines whether or not that behavior will continue. Attention, sympathy, and social support encourage the individual to express the pain and feelings about it and to continue the pain behavior. Ignoring pain expressions and behavior, rejecting emotions, withholding social support, and expecting the person to fulfill social duties all discourage the communication of pain. The present search found few more recent studies about the relationship of family factors with neck or back pain since the aforementioned reviews in 1986 and 1987 (59,135,169).

Balague et al. (6) looked at how school children report pain. They found little evidence that family background actually affects the occurrence of back pain, but family background does seem to influence children's attitudes, reporting of symptoms, and behavior. As children grow up, social peer groups may become equally or even more influential.

Hasvold and Johnsen (75) surveyed nearly 2,000 adults in Norway to explore gender differences in neck and shoulder symptoms and family-learned illness behavior. They found that females in the family and brothers and sisters were the main family members who imprinted the way in which children deciphered these symptoms later in life. That pattern was later influenced relatively little by the spouse.

Feuerstein et al. (55) made a multivariate analysis of the relationship among general stress, family and work environment, psychologic distress, and pain experience in 33 patients with chronic low back pain and 35 matched, healthy controls. The patients had more family problems. Family and work characteristics were more closely associated with the affective and evaluative dimensions of pain. Increased family conflict was associated with increased pain and distress, whereas increased family independence was associated with increased pain but less distress. These findings suggest that stress and operant mechanisms act in the family, whereas operant and distraction mechanisms play a greater role in work influences.

Naidoo and Pillay (128) studied 15 patients with chronic low back pain and 15 matched, healthy controls. The patients had lower scores on family cohesion, independence, and organization and higher scores on family conflict, and these family support scores showed weak positive or negative correlations with severity of pain.

Trief et al. (168) examined the relationship between social support and depression in 48 patients with chronic low back pain. Patients who perceived that they had more social support and better quality of family environment were significantly less depressed ($p < .01$). On regression analysis, social support accounted for about 10% of the variance of the Beck depression score.

Baldwin et al. (7) analyzed first return to work and subsequent work loss in 8,690 patients in Ontario who had received Workers' Compensation Board payments. Marital status had opposite effects on the duration of first work absence for men and women. All else being equal, married men had shorter absences and married women had longer absences than unmarried men and women. However, marital status had no significant association, in men or in women, with failure ever to return to work, repeat absences, or the chance of eventually giving up work.

Muramatsu et al. (126) carried out a longitudinal 3-year study of social support, with complex mathematical modeling, in Japanese people aged 60 years and older. These investigators found that instrumental support was associated with a lower risk of new-onset back pain, but emotional support was associated with an increased risk of new-onset pain and reduced the chance of recovery.

Tarsh and Royston (164) reported exploratory, follow-up interviews of 35 highly selected patients with chronic pain (50% with back pain) who were involved in litigation and who had "compensation neurosis." These investigators suggested that the family could play a major role in the process and identified four patterns, although they often overlapped: family overprotectiveness, providing the family with a role, family "total belief," and role change and entrenchment.

In summary, Turk et al. (169) considered that much of this family research is weak methodologically, that many of the results are inconclusive, and that assessment remains true. Most of the available evidence is about chronic pain in general; although some of these studies are on patients with low back pain, many include a high proportion of patients with low back pain, and the results all appear similar. There is no evidence specifically about neck pain, although in principle we have no reason to believe that it is any different. There is little evidence on acute pain or on routine primary care patients. It is possible that genetic factors could have some influence on the physical condition of the back and the prevalence of back pain, although evidence is minimal. Men and women have different gender roles in the family, but there is limited evidence on how this affects neck or back pain.

Despite all these limitations, the available evidence suggests that family influences may be associated with treatment outcome and the development and maintenance of chronic pain and disability. Different aspects of family support and reinforcement may theoretically have positive or negative effects, either promoting wellness behavior and staying at work or promoting illness behavior. This review suggests that, for most routine patients with back pain, good family and social support may be associated with better recovery and less disability (Table 2.3), but for a few patients with chronic pain, physical or sexual abuse or spouse reinforcement (Table 2.4) may be associated with more chronic pain and disability. For most routine patients, any influence may be relatively weak, but for a few patients with chronic pain, it may be stronger. Unfortunately, despite the potential importance of family issues, there is little evidence on exactly which family influences are most important, how they operate, or how they can be modified.

Considerable evidence shows unanimously that the spouse's reaction can modify the behavior of patients with chronic pain. Most of these studies are of highly selected groups of patients or of experimental situations, and there is very little information

TABLE 2.3. Studies on the influence of social support on neck and back pain and disability

Study	Country	Subjects	Design	Dependent variable	Measure of social support	Allowance for confounders	Results
Reisbord and Greenland, 1985 (137)	US	2,782 enrollees HMO	Cross-sectional	LBP	Married versus separated/divorced/widowed	Age, gender, education	18.1% versus 28.8%
Biering-Sorensen and Thomsen, 1986 (12)	Denmark	920 gen population	Longitudinal	Recurrent or persistence of LBP	Living alone	General health social habits work and leisure	Men + in multivariate analysis Women NS
Bergenudd and Nilsson, 1988 (11)	Sweden	575 55 year old gen population	Cross-sectional	Point prevalence LBP	"Social network"	*	NS
Bigos et al., 1991 (13)	US	3,020 aircraft workers	Longitudinal	Report low back injury	Family APGAR	Demographic, medical, work distress	NS
Cats-Baril and Frymoyer, 1991 (32)	US	14,407 gen population	Cross-sectional	Disability	Divorced or widowed	Age, socioeconomic	LBP NS Disability 1.22
Volinn et al., 1991 (172)	US	Industrial insurance claims	Cross-sectional	Work loss >90 days	Widowed or divorced with no children	Demographic and socioeconomic	Men 2.11 (1.30–3.44) Women 2.54 (1.55–4.16)
Lancourt and Kettelhut, 1992 (98)	US	134 WCB patients	Longitudinal	Return to work	Family stability	Clinical employment	NS
Lehmann et al., 1993 (102)	US	55 orthopaedic patients off work 4 weeks	Longitudinal	Chronic disabling LBP	Marital status	Demographic, work, clinical	$P < .01$
Cheadle et al., 1994 (33)	US	28,473 workers' comp claims (all causes)	Cross-sectional	Duration of total temporary disability Work absence for LBP	Divorced or widowed	Demographic, clinical, social, work	0.90 (0.85–0.94) 0.87 (0.76–1.0)
Linton and Buer, 1995 (105)	Sweden	63 female employees	Case-control		Duke social support	Psychologic	NS
Isacsson et al., 1995 (84)	Sweden	621 retired men age 68–69	Cross-sectional	Daily neck or back pain	Social anchorage, instrumental support	Previous work physical and psychosocial	OR 2.0 (1.2–3.4) OR 1.7 (1.0–2.7)
Klapow et al., 1995 (94)	US	965 male orthopedic patients (veterans) (>6/12 LBP)	Cross-sectional	Chronic pain syndrome	Satisfaction with social support networks	Pain, disability distress, and psychosocial	Positive
Foppa and Noack, 1996 (62)	Switzerland	850 employed	Cross-sectional	Back pain	Poor social network	Personal, health, work, psychosocial	NS
Baldwin et al., 1996 (7)	Canada	8,690 injured workers (WCB)	Cross-sectional plus retrospective sickness records	First return to work Subsequent work loss	Married	Multiple	Men: return to work sooner Women return to work later
Muramatsu et al., 1997 (126)	Japan	2,200, aged 60+	Longitudinal	Back pain	Instrumental and emotional support	Health, social and behavioral	NS Positive Negative

APGAR, American Pediatric Gross Assessment Record; HMO, health maintenance organization; LBP, low back pain; NS, not significant; OR, odds ratio; WCB, Workers' Compensation Board.

23

TABLE 2.4. *Studies on the influence of the spouse on pain behavior*

Study	Country	Subjects	n	Study design	Results
Block et al., 1980 (18)	US	Chronic pain management program patients >8 months	20	Patients report of pain levels while observed by spouse versus observed by neutal observer	Patients with solicitous spouses report higher pain level when observed by spouse than with neutral observer. Patients with nonsolicious spouses report lower pain level when observed by spouse than with neutral observer.
Flor et al., 1987 (58)	US	Chronic pain management program patients	32	Multiple regression of patient and spouse questionnaires	Spouse reinforcement was associated with duration and impact of pain on spouse's life and positive spouse attitudes but not spouse's assessment of pain level or marital satisfaction. Spouse solicitousness accounted for about 30% of variance of pain level. Spouse "punishment" accounted for about 30% of variance of activity level.
Romano et al., 1989 (141)	US	Chronic low back pain patients >6 months	83	Patient and spouse questionnaires	A stronger relationship was noted for female than for male spouses. In male patients, poorer spouse marital satisfaction is associated with patient depression. In male patients, spouse depression is associated with more depression and poorer marital satisfaction in patients.
Kerns et al., 1990 (92)	US	Chronic pain patients referred to rehabilitation program	106	Regression analysis of patient and spouse questionnaires	A solicitous response by spouse accounted for 6% of pain severity. Interaction between solicitous responses and spouse marital satisfaction also had significant effect.
Saarijärvi et al., 1990 (146,147)	Finland	Primary care patients with chronic low back pain	63	Patient and spouse questionnaires	In female patients, marital dissatisfaction was associated with higher levels of pain and disability (20% of variance) and distress (>50% of variance). In male patients, marital dissatisfaction and distress were much less closely related.
Lousberg et al., 1992 (109)	Netherlands	Chronic low back pain patients	42	Patients did treadmill test with and without spouse present	Patients with solicitous spouses report more pain and walk a shorter time in the presence of the spouse than patients with nonsolicitous spouses. However, there were considerable methodologic problems in measure solicitousness.

24

Study	Country	Sample	N	Method	Results
Romano et al., 1992 (142) Romano et al., 1995 (143)	US	Chronic pain management program patients Control couples	50* 33	Patients and spouses (and control couples) videotaped while doing common household tasks	Spouses' solicitous responses to nonverbal pain behaviors predicted 30% of variance of pain behaviors patients with higher pain levels. Spouses' solicitous responses to nonverbal pain behaviors predicted 20% of variance of disability in more depressed patients. Significantly less patient pain behavior occurred after spouses' aggressive behaviors ($p < .05$).
Schwartz et al., 1994 (151)	US	Male chronic back pain patients	34	20-minute exercise cycling with spouse support, immediately after maritally focused stress interview or neutral talking control; pain report and blood pressure	Marital stress led to earlier termination of physically demanding tasks.
Flor et al., 1995 (61)	Germany	Chronic low back pain patients; matched controls	17 15	Cold pressure test with and without spouse present, and with different verbal interactions; reported pain and lumbar muscle electromyogram.	Spouse solicitousness associated with heightened pain perception but no effect on lumbar muscle activity.
Fernandez and McDowell, 1995 (54)	US	Selected chronic pain management program patients	12	Spouse recorded pain behaviors and healthy behaviors and patients recorded contingent reinforcers over 2 weeks	Hyperbolic relationship. Recorded contingent reinforcements accounted for 86% of the variance of recorded pain behaviors and 76% of the variance of recorded healthy behaviors.
Schwartz et al., 1996 (152)	US	Male chronic back pain patients	61	Patient and spouse questionnaires	Patients respond to marital conflict with increased pain behavior, which, in turn, is associated with more negative affect and more punitive behaviors by the spouse. Spouse punitive behaviors are associated with higher self-reported levels of pain and functional and psychosocial impairment on the Sickness Impact Profile.

on the importance or magnitude of these effects in "normal" patients with neck and back pain in everyday life. A separate literature, not reviewed here, discusses how chronic pain conversely affects the spouse and the family (17,60,134,153,169).

Social Class

The use of social class is a crude attempt to measure social influences on back pain and disability. Most surveys on back pain in the United Kingdom use a simple classification of social class based mainly on occupation.

     I. Professional groups such as doctors, lawyers, and scientists.
    II. "Intermediate" groups such as teachers, nurses, and self-employed shop-keepers.
   III. Skilled occupations:
IIINM. Skilled, nonmanual groups such as clerical workers.
 IIIM. Skilled manual groups such as tradesmen.
   IV. Partly skilled groups such as process workers in industry or transport workers.
    V. Unskilled groups such as laborers and cleaners.

This classification is really twofold. It is partly occupational, with a major division between manual and nonmanual work, and that may be why it usually shows stronger results in men than in women. It is also partly socioeconomic and serves as a proxy for all facets of social disadvantage, such as education, housing, and income, in both men and women. Many studies focusing on social class use more sophisticated classification systems, but they still generally reflect the broad division between manual and nonmanual occupations (3).

The oldest statistics on health inequalities in the world are the United Kingdom Registrar General's occupational mortality tables from the end of the nineteenth century, whereas the earliest figures on morbidity are from the Department of Health in Scotland in the early 1930s. There is now wide recognition that low income and social disadvantage are associated with inequalities in health (3,15,88), and these factors affect not only mortality but all aspects of health status and morbidity (3,16,88). The present search identified various studies on the association of back pain and social class.

Gyntelberg (71) in Denmark made one of the first observations of a relationship between social status and low back pain. Walsh et al. (177) provided the most detailed data on the relation between back pain and social class in the United Kingdom (Table 2.5). In men, the prevalence of back pain, disability, and work loss all increased

TABLE 2.5. *Relation between back pain and social class*

Prevalence	Social class	Men		Women	
		I–II	IV–V	I–II	IV–V
Back pain	1 year	23%	42%	No trend	
	Lifetime	51%	65%	No trend	
Low back disability	1 year	2.9%	8.1%	1.9%	6.2%
	Lifetime	No trend		No trend	
Work loss due to back pain	1 year	5.6%	13.9%	No trend	
	Lifetime	22.3%	38.5%	No trend	

Data from Walsh K, Cruddas M, Coggon D. Low back pain in eight areas of Britain. *J Epidemiol Community Health* 1992;46:227–230.

TABLE 2.6. *Relation between social class and giving up work*

Social class	Percentage who said they gave up work because of back pain
I–II	2%
III	4%
IV–V	11%

Data from *The Which Report on back pain.* London: Consumer's Association, 1985.

between social classes I to II and IV to V. Women, however, had little variation with social class, and only the 1-year prevalence of disability showed a pattern similar to that in men. In complete and unexplained contrast, however, there was no trend in lifetime disability with social class in either men or women.

Croft and Rigby (39) tried to disentangle the socioeconomic relationships. In men, the only link seemed to be with unskilled manual labor. Women in the lowest income category (OR, 1.6; 95% CI, 1.2 to 2.1) and those with less formal education (OR, 1.5; 95% CI, 1.0 to 2.1) also had more back pain, and in them, it seemed to be related to social disadvantage. It was not possible to say what aspects of social environment, lifestyle, or attitudes and behavior were most relevant. Papageorgiou et al. (132) found that lower social status (social classes IV and V) and perceived inadequacy of income were strong predictors of seeking health care for back pain.

Mason (117) found little relation between the prevalence of back pain or disability and social class. However, there was a marked increase in work loss between the nonmanual social classes I to IIINM and the manual classes IIIM to V. A higher proportion of both men and women in the manual classes blamed their back pain on work. They were also more likely to lie down with back pain. In employed people with back pain, about 4% in the nonmanual classes and 8.7% in the manual classes reported that they did not work at least 1 day in the last 4 weeks because of back pain. The Consumer's Association (37) also found corresponding figures of 14% and 23% for the number who reported that they had lost time from work with back pain in the last year. There was a marked social gradient in those whose stated reason for giving up work was back pain (Table 2.6).

Skovron et al. (157) used a similar classification of five social classes in Belgium and found no difference in the lifetime prevalence of low back pain. However, social class was associated with the prevalence of daily back pain, which ranged from 31% in the highest social class to 48% in the lowest class (OR, 0.43; 95% CI, 0.27 to 0.70, $p < .001$) and remained significant on multivariate analysis. Further analysis of the same study by Szpalski et al. (161) found that social class had a significant association with health care use. Visiting a health professional for back pain ranged from 62.4% of the highest social class to 70.6% in the lowest social class. Lower social class was also associated with taking more medication and an increased likelihood of having radiographs and back surgery.

Similar data have been published on the relationship of low income and social deprivation with back pain in United States. A large health insurance survey (137) found that the self-reported prevalence of back pain increased from 13% in professional and managerial workers to 21% in laborers ($p < .0001$), although in multivariate analysis controlling for other demographic measures, only gender, education, and marital status remained significant. Once again, however, social class was more strongly related to what happens to people after they have back pain. Cats-Baril and Frymoyer (32) analyzed National Health and Nutrition Examination Survey I data from the general United States population. They found that stopping work for health reasons (not solely back pain) was significantly related to low family income, lower education level, an unpleasant working environment, and increasing age over 45 years. Volinn et al. (173) found that three socioeconomic factors–unemployment rate, percentage receiving food stamps, and per capita income–accounted for about one-third of the variance in the regional benefit claim rate for back pain. In a second study, Volinn et al. (172) showed that three socioeconomic factors were associated with increased risk of chronicity: age, wages, and lack of family support in the form of being either widowed or divorced with no children. The Nam-Powers Socioeconomic Index was also significant for men: N-PSI higher than 50, only 5.4% of men lost work for 90 days or more; N-PSI less than 17, 10.1% of men lost work for 90 days or more (OR, 1.97, calculated from published data).

Badley and Ibanez (5) looked at socioeconomic risk factors for musculoskeletal disorders in Canada and found that, apart from gender, they were much the same for back disability, other musculoskeletal disabilities, and nonmusculoskeletal disabilities. Lower income was associated with more disability, although the relationship was slightly weaker for back disability (adjusted OR, 2.28; 95% CI, 1.93 to 2.70) than for arthritis (OR, 2.69) or nonmusculoskeletal disability (OR, 2.70).

In Sweden, formal classification of social class has not been used in public statistics since the 1960s, although the underlying issues of educational level, work type, income, poverty, and social deprivation remain (3,88). In the Norrtalje MUSIC study, Hogstedt et al. (79) found that certain lower socioeconomic groups had an OR of up to 1.9 of seeking health care for new-incident low back pain, a ratio that varied among men, full-time working women, and part-time working women. However, none of the ORs reached statistical significance, and on multivariate analysis the relationship with social class disappeared. Because of the limited nature of the social class data, these results were considered to be inconclusive. Viikari-Juntura et al. (170) made a lifelong follow up of 154 patients in Finland and found that socioeconomic status of the family in adolescence bore no relation to neck and shoulder pain or low back pain in adult life.

In summary, there is conflicting evidence for a relationship between the prevalence of back pain and lower social class, and any association is probably weak. There is strong and consistent evidence that back pain is associated with more work loss in people of lower social class. The relationship with social class is more consistent in men but less clear in women. The main problem is in determining the significance of these findings. Social class is a crude index, which deals with a host of social, educational, occupational, economic, lifestyle and psychosocial influences, and corresponding social attitudes and behavior, any and all of which may bear a relation to work loss associated with back pain. It is probably partly a matter of manual work, particularly in men. It is probably also a matter of social disadvantage in both men and women, although it is not clear exactly which aspects of that disadvantage are important or how they affect back pain. Virtually no data on social class and neck pain have been reported.

Education

Many international studies show a similar association between lower education level and a higher prevalence of back pain, although a few studies disagree. Several studies show, without exception, an association between lower education and more work loss attributed to back pain. Many of these studies emphasize the interrelation among lower social class, lower level of education, and heavy manual work, but few try to unravel it.

In a careful analysis, Makela (112) concluded that education was simply an indirect measure of heavy work, work stress, and work injury. In an equally careful study, Deyo and Tsui-Wu (43) found that education did have an independent association. Viikari-Juntura et al. (170) made one of the few longitudinal studies and found no link between intelligence or socioeconomic status in adolescence and low back symptoms in adult life. Dione et al. (44) made a much shorter 2-year study of education and back-related disability in adults. As had most previous studies, these investigators found that people with less than 13 years of schooling had more disability. More important was what happened over the next 2 years. Disability tended to improve, particularly in those with more education, but it did not improve as much in those with less education. These authors also considered possible mechanisms to explain the relationship and suggested that occupational and psychologic factors are more important than health care access or use. Straaton et al. (159) also found that higher education level was significantly associated with better rehabilitation outcome.

Job Satisfaction and Psychosocial Aspects of Work

There is extensive evidence reviewed in Chapter 3 that job satisfaction and certain psychosocial aspects of work are associated with increased self-reports of neck and low back pain. From the perspective of the present chapter, the possibility should be considered whether these psychosocial aspects of work may act to at least some extent as social *influences* on the reporting of pain, pain behavior, and disability, rather than necessarily as "risk factors" in a causal sense.

Employer-Management Strategies and Industrial Relations

Cooper and Marshall (38) and Arnold et al. (2) pointed out that work stress not only produces symptoms in the individual worker, but also produces organizational symptoms such as high absenteeism, high labor turnover, poor industrial relations, poor quality control, and poor work safety.

Beale and Nethercott (8) showed that the threat of redundancy was associated with workers reporting more illness, seeking more health care, and having significantly longer periods of absence, particularly for men and for workers who had previously consulted their family doctor infrequently. Clemmer and Mohr (35) examined rates of reported work-related low back strains, low back impact injuries, and non-low back injuries in a petroleum drilling company from 1979 to 1985. Lost time for low back strains increased at times of threatened layoffs, but the incidence of low back impact injuries remained constant. These investigators suggested that the most likely explanation lies in worker response to possible layoffs and uncertain future employment.

Hunt and Habeck (82) reviewed different managerial approaches to reducing back injury claims and disability. These researchers concluded that ergonomic approaches and wellness orientation were not effective. Disability case monitoring could actually be counterproductive, probably because it is adversarial. They found that safety training and active safety leadership and proactive return to work programs appeared to be most effective, probably because they all improve relationships between the worker and the employer or supervisor. Various authors have stressed the importance of good relations between the worker and the employer, supervisor, and fellow workers. There should be mutual respect and trust. There should be regular communication, reinforcing the worker's importance and value. There should be cooperation and support. In principle, it is widely believed that good industrial relations will increase the chances of successful rehabilitation and return to work.

A survey of low back disability in the United Kingdom Royal Air Force by Mitchell (125) suggested that good employee-employer relations and the ready availability of modified work can minimize the amount of sickness absence. Baldwin et al. (7) analyzed work loss after occupational injury in 8,690 patients receiving Workers' Compensation Board payments in Ontario, Canada. All else being equal, the availability of light work and reduced hours was associated with an increased chance of going back to work in the first place, but it bore no relation to the chances of further absences or eventually giving up work. The availability of modified equipment had no significant association with any of these outcomes. Loisel et al. (108) in Quebec, Canada, tested this more scientifically in a randomized controlled trial of patients who had lost work for more than 4 weeks because of back pain. They showed that a combination of clinical and occupational interventions produced the best chances of return to work. However, the specific effect of the occupational intervention accounted for the most important part of this result, with a rate ratio for return to work of 1.91 (95% CI, 1.18 to 3.10, $p <$ .01). The occupational intervention consisted of sickness surveillance followed by an occupational medicine and ergonomic assessment, which included a worksite evaluation involving both union and management representatives. All parties agreed on ergonomic improvements to the worksite directed toward stable return to work.

Robertson and Keeve (139) analyzed injury claim rates in the United States in three plants in different states during 1973 to 1980 and found that these rates were not explained by worker attributes or work exposure. Changes in claim rates were largely explained by increases in workers' compensation greater than inflation. In addition, however, Occupational Safety and Health Administration inspections were followed by substantially reduced numbers of objectively verifiable injuries in the next year and significant reduction in days lost because of injury. The relationship with inspections remained significant even after allowing for changes in the compensation rates. (This study refers to all injuries and not only to back injuries.)

Catchlove and Cohen (31) found that 60% of patients with chronic pain whose treatment program included specific directives about return to work did actually return, compared with 25% of those who received similar treatment but no specific directives. Wood (182) got the supervisor to phone workers who were home from work with acute back pain and say: "How are you? We are thinking about you. You are a vital part of the team. Your work is important and your job is waiting for you." That simple act of communication reduced the number who stayed away from work on a long-term basis from 7.1% to 1.7%. In summary, there is limited but suggestive evidence that good and bad industrial relations can be associated with altered rates of reporting low back injuries and the amount of sickness absence.

Unemployment

In current Western society, work, in the form of gainful employment, occupies a major place in most people's lives. The primary purpose may be to provide financial status and security, but it also defines the individual and his or her role in society. Work provides the following:

- Income.
- Activity.
- Occupation and structure of time.
- Creativity and mastery.
- Social interaction.
- Sense of identity.
- Sense of purpose.

All workers have these to varying degrees, although the relative importance of each element varies with the individual and the job.

If work is such an important part of the modern social fabric, it is not surprising that loss of work and unemployment are catastrophic. Unemployment causes the loss of all the social and emotional advantages of work. It undermines the individual's whole social position and status and is one of the greatest personal failures in a material society. Welfare status involves loss of social value, loss of respect, and isolation. It is not surprising that unemployment causes pessimism, depression, and fatalism. Unemployment, poverty, and social deprivation lead to poor physical and mental health, with increased suicide and mortality rates, as reviewed systematically by Janlert (88). A huge, prospective, 10-year study in Denmark showed that the mortality rate among the unemployed was two to three times higher at all age groups, mainly through violent deaths (accidents and suicide) and alcohol-related deaths, although also from cardiovascular disease (85). Lack of work causes loss of physical fitness and increased weight, psychologic distress and depression, and loss of work-related attitudes and habits, all of which are associated with low back disability. Janlert (88) pointed out that this is not entirely a question of unemployment's causing ill health: Ill health also increases the chance of unemployment. However, Martikainen (115) in Finland found that even allowing for health status at the start of unemployment and considering only the "healthy unemployed," the relative risk for mortality was still 2. So there is an element of health selection among those who become unemployed, but unemployment then causes poorer health. That study was conducted at a time of relatively low unemployment, but unemployment in Finland then rose rapidly from 3.2% in 1990 to 12.4% in 1992. Martikainen and Valkonen (116) found that the mortality ratios for men and women unemployed for the first time in 1990 were 2.11 (95% CI, 1.76 to 2.53) and 1.61 (1.09 to 2.36), respectively, but for those unemployed for the first time in 1992, the corresponding ratios fell to 1.35 (1.16 to 1.56) and 1.30 (0.97 to 1.75). These investigators suggested that the association between unemployment and poor health weakened as the general unemployment rate increased, when there was less selection involved in becoming unemployed, and unemployment became more socially "normal."

Selander et al. (154) in Sweden analyzed Social Insurance data on 915 people who were listed as sick for 90 days or more in Stockholm, Sweden, during 1992. Of these people, 20% were already unemployed when they first reported sick. The odds of going on to a temporary disability pension were about three times greater for the unemployed, with a particularly high risk for younger people aged 16 to 39 years (crude OR, 6.88, calculated from published data). The greatest difference in the unemployed was the frequency of psychiatric diagnoses–50% in unemployed men and 37% among unemployed women. This study gave limited information on a small subsample of people with back pain that did not permit any more detailed analysis, but it did not show any significant difference in the number of unemployed sick who were certificated for back pain.

Table 2.7 gives data from the United Kingdom on back pain in persons who are unemployed compared with the employed. It shows little difference in the prevalence of back pain in those who are unemployed. The unemployed do seek slightly more health care for back pain, but the most dramatic increase is in sick certification. Department of Social Security statistics from the United Kingdom show that nearly half the benefits paid for back pain go to people who were not employed when they started these benefits. These statistics should be interpreted with caution, however, because some of these claimants may have lost their jobs due to back pain before starting invalidity benefit, and it is not possible to separate cause and effect.

RFV statistical data from 1993 confirmed that local unemployment in Sweden had a high negative correlation for the outcome of long-term sickness absence in men: A weak labor market led to longer absences. One explanation may be that attempts at rehabilitation are considered less meaningful in times of high unemployment. For women, higher rates of unemployment led to increased risk of early retirement. The explanation of these different results for men and for women may be their differential employment; more men are employed in the private sector, and more women work in the public sector. The different effects from unemployment may be interpreted as one of societal economic development for men, that is, the state of the market, but as one of structural problems for women, that is, the tendency for women to stay unemployed for longer periods because market changes only slowly affect the public sector.

There are several North American studies of unemployment and back pain. Volinn et al. (173) carried out a small area analysis in Washington State that showed that disabling back pain was related to unemployment rate, the percentage of persons receiving food stamps, and income. Cheadle et al. (33) also found that unemployment was a significant factor in multivariate analysis of the duration of work loss in 28,472 workers' compensation claims in the same state. Hurwitz and Morgenstern (83) analyzed the 1989 United States National Health Interview Survey and found that the unemployed had an OR of 1.33 (1.16 to 1.53) for a disabling back condition, but in that cross-sectional analysis, it was not possible to distinguish cause and effect.

Enterline (51) showed that the general sickness absence rate over time is inversely

TABLE 2.7. *Relation between back pain and lack of employment*

	Employed	Not employed
Prevelance of back pain		
Point prevalence	11%	9%
1 year prevalence	37%	42%
Lifetime prevalence	65%	62%
Medical care for back pain in the past year	13%	20%
Sickness certification for the last 4 weeks because of low back pain	1%	20%

Data from Mason V. The prevalence of back pain in Great Britain. Office of Population Censuses and Surveys, Social Survey Division (now Office of National Statistics). London: Her Majesty's Stationery Office, 1994:1–24.

proportional to the unemployment rate. In that early study in 1966, he found that, on an average day, about 7% of workers in the United States were not at work, either unemployed or sick. As unemployment rates rose, so sickness rates fell, and vice versa. Brooker et al. (23) made a similar, more recent analysis of macroeconomic forces ("the business cycle") and back claim rates in Ontario from 1975 to 1993. Both back pain claims and other acute musculoskeletal claims increased during boom times and fell during periods of recession, inversely with unemployment rates. The relationship was slightly clearer when one used a combination of the current unemployment rate and the unemployment rate for the previous 3 months. It was similar in different industry sectors. From the end of the World War II, Sweden aimed to have a labor market policy that activated the unemployed. However, during the 1990s, the unemployment rate in Sweden has risen to levels that had not been seen since the 1920s, and sickness absence rates have also changed. RFV statistical analysis in 1993 found that each 1% increase of unemployment was associated with a 4% decrease of days of sickness absenteeism, or -0.9 days, whereas a more recent RFV statistical analysis, covering the period from 1987 to 1993, found that this relationship was significant for levels of unemployment between 1% and 5%, that is, the levels that used to be normal in Sweden before the 1990s.

Thomason (166) found that an interaction between increased benefit levels and the unemployment rate was related to the transition from temporary to permanent disability status in the workers' compensation system. Cheadle et al. (33) reviewed five studies including their own that showed higher duration of sickness absence in areas with high unemployment rates, although all those studies were about sickness absence for all causes, and the effect was modest (0.88; 95% CI, 0.82 to 0.95).

Sanderson et al. (149) studied a selected group of patients at an orthopedic surgeon's back clinic. These investigators found that disability (assessed using the Oswestry disability questionnaire) was related to both employment status and litigation, but unemployment was the more important factor. Of the unemployed, 79% had an Oswestry score greater than 40, compared with 40% of those who were still employed. However, it was not possible to distinguish cause and effect.

Stopping work because of back pain is ultimately a decision made by the worker, with or without the advice or agreement of a health professional or employer. Enterline (51) suggested that when a worker falls ill, he or she is more likely to stay away from work if there is:

• Little risk of losing his or her job (because of low unemployment and labor shortage).
• Little or no economic loss (because of continued pay or good wage replacement rates).
• Little or no disapproval from fellow workers and supervisors, a factor closely linked to little or no disruption of the work.

The decision to stay home from work depends on the relative attractiveness and price of the alternatives. Higher unemployment rates produce greater competition for available work and higher selection criteria by employers. More jobs are also now shorter term with greater turnover of labor, a feature that increases the frequency with which workers must seek and gain jobs. Any degree of mental or physical incapacity, whether from age or illness, or a poor sickness record, may make it harder to obtain or hold work than in better economic times when work is more readily available. A mild degree of incapacity may then cause adoption of the sick role in a person who would otherwise have been able to continue to work without symptoms being a health problem. Brooker et al. (23) discussed alternative hypotheses about how the economic climate may influence the composition of the workforce, the work environment, work stress, and the risk of injury.

Over the past decade or two, there has also been a change in attitudes to disability, which has become much more socially acceptable. This change has been supported by policy attempts to improve the social facilities and status of disabled people. For the disabled, this has clearly been helpful. It means, however, that entry to disability status has also become more socially acceptable. Sickness and disability may now appear to be more socially acceptable than unemployment. Over the same period, pain per se has also become acceptable as a basis for chronic disability and benefits (64). Enterline (51), of the United States, commented that in the 1950s and 1960s, "the right not to go to work when feeling ill appears to be part of a social movement that has swept across Europe."

Sickness benefits are generally financially better than unemployment benefits and may have less social stigma, and there are suggestions that many doctors collude to help their patients by giving certification of illness for social rather than medical reasons (138). Chew and May (34) looked at the dilemma the family doctor faces in such a situation. These investigators suggested that back pain may be a social resource for some patients, a concept that has major implications for how patient and doctor approach the consultation.

- Chronic low back pain permits withdrawal from normal social obligations.
- These patients recognize that the doctor is not able to help, but they view the doctor as a resource through which their social and economic inactivity can be legitimized.
- These patients do recognize the relation between psychosocial factors and pain.
- Chronic low back pain involves both the patient and the doctor in negotiating conflicting roles.

In summary, three longitudinal studies in times of relatively low unemployment (5% to 6%) showed an inverse relationship between unemployment and sickness absence. Numerous cross-sectional studies showed that in times or areas of high unemployment, increased unemployment rates are associated with increased sickness certification and disability benefits. This finding suggests that unemployment may have different effects in different situations. When unemployment rates are high and job security is low, there may be more pressure on workers to stay at work when they feel unwell, and that may reduce absenteeism from back pain. However, once someone is under threat of layoff or loss of his or her job, there may be social and financial advantages to sickness and disability benefits, which may increase sickness certification for back pain among those who are not employed.

There is no evidence available about the association of unemployment with neck pain. Some evidence suggested gender differences in patterns of unemployment, but this review did not provide evidence on whether or how this is related to neck or back pain.

Early Retirement

Chapter 19 shows that the greatest social security problem over the past one to two decades is the increasing trend to early retirement, often on medical grounds. Incapacity for work, sickness certification, and sickness benefits related to low back pain are a particular problem in people older than about 50 years, in whom these factors are associated with early retirement. The present review covers the background literature on early retirement. Although low back pain is one of the most common health reasons given for early retirement, this is part of a more general problem and is not unique to back pain.

Since the 1970s, economists have carefully examined retirement patterns and trends and have sought to identify and measure the factors that influence the timing of retirement, although much of that research is technical and inaccessible to nonspecialist readers. Leonesio (103) provided a nontechnical review of this economic evidence. The present search identified some studies on low back pain and early retirement.

Astrand and Isacsson (4) studied 391 male employees in a Swedish pulp and paper company in 1961 and then followed them for 22 years. Sick leave in their sample was low. There were 30 cases of early retirement with a diagnosis of back disorder on the retirement certificate. Perhaps surprisingly, report of back pain at baseline did not predict early retirement for back pain, although back abnormalities on physical examination were a weak predictor. Rothenbacher et al. (144) also carried out a longitudinal study of prognostic factors for early retirement among employees in the construction industry in Germany. Reported back pain or sciatica led to a relative risk of 1.6 (1.3 to 2.1) of early retirement. An abnormal clinical finding in the spine led to a relative risk of 1.8 (1.4 to 2.2), and a recorded medical diagnosis of a back condition led to a relative risk of 1.5 (1.2 to 1.8).

There are several other Swedish studies. Eden et al. (47) studied 453 early-retirement pensioners and compared them with matched controls. Low socioeconomic status, lower educational level, heavy manual work, and immigrant status were associated with increased early retirement. Eden et al. (46) found that early retirement was followed by a deterioration in self-reported health status in men of all ages and in women aged 25 to 54 years, although it improved in women aged 55 to 64 years. However, these studies did not provide separate data on back or neck pain. Berg et al. (10) found no significant difference in the prevalence of neck or back symptoms in male manual or office workers before and after retirement. Ostberg and Samuelsson (131) found that women aged 62 to 64 years had improved subjective health and fewer musculoskeletal symptoms after retirement, and the prevalence of back complaints fell from 47% to 31%.

Harkapaa (74) in Finland followed 476 patients with chronic low back pain for 4.5 years and found that, in that group, back pain accounted for 51% of the early retirements. Older age and psychologic measures were the best predictors of early retirement, irrespective of the initial level of low back disability or treatment. Mansson and Israelsson (113) undertook health screening of 123 men aged 48 to 50 years and reviewed them again 4 to 8 years later after they had received early disability pensions, most commonly for musculoskeletal disorders (41%), mental illness (17%), and cardiovascular disease (16%). The most striking difference from the control group was the number of pensioners with raised γ-glutamyltransferase levels, a finding suggesting high alcohol intake. The persons with the highest levels were associated with increased reports of back pain, both before and even more so after retirement.

Baldwin et al. (7) analyzed first return to work and subsequent work loss in 8,690 patients receiving workers' compensation benefits in Canada who were injured in 1974 to 1986 and who were examined by a physician in 1989 to 1990 for permanent partial disability assessment. All else being equal, back injuries were associated with longer first work absences than other injuries in men but not in women, and they were associated with a higher chance of failing ever to return to work, more repeat absences, and a higher chance of eventually giving up work in both men and women. All else being equal, increasing age was associated with a longer duration of first absence, a higher chance of failing ever to return to work, and a higher chance of multiple absences and eventually giving up work in both men and women.

Leonesio (103) provided a comprehensive review of retirement in the United States. Data from 1995 showed an even pattern of retirement between the ages of 55 and 70 years, although for men this accelerated as they entered their early 60s, with slight peaks of retirement at about age 62 and 65 years. Labor force participation fell from 81% at age 55 years to 20% at age 70 years for men and from 62% to 11% for women. Since World War II, there has been a trend to retire earlier, although by 1995 the most popular retirement age in the United States was still 62 years. The major change has been in the number of people who continue working well after age 65 years: Labor force participation by all men age 65 years or older fell from 49% in 1948 to 22% in 1974 to about 10% in 1995. Perhaps surprisingly from a European perspective, however, about 7% of men and 3% of women in the United States are still working at age 75 years. Moreover, many male heads of household who spent most of their adult life working for a single employer only partially retire in their later working years, and one-fourth of those who completely retire subsequently take other employment. Overall, about one-third of adults in the United States work part-time at some stage of their later working life, for an average of about 20 hours per week over an average of 5 years.

The largest United States database available at present is the Social Security Administration's Retirement History Study, a study of approximately 11,000 Americans who were 58 to 63 years old in 1969 and who were followed for 10 years until 1979, by which time most of them had retired. In future, there should be further data from the Health and Retirement Study of approximately 5,000 couples and 2,400 unmarried persons who were 51 to 61 years old when they were interviewed in 1992 and who are now being followed until at least the year 2004 (89).

There are obvious economic constraints on when retirement becomes an option; however, decisions about work, retirement, and leisure are not solely economic, but also are all part of how people decide to use their time. The basic work-leisure choice and the secondary decision about how much to work depend on the balance between the financial and other rewards of work, alternative sources of income available, financial needs, and the other attractions but also financial needs for leisure activities. Economists produce statistical models and empiric analyses to support this type of decision-making framework (70,103). Job opportunities, social pressures, and health also influence the decision, and it must be viewed in a dynamic model as part of a whole lifecycle. However, retirement and particularly early retirement are often a voluntary decision, and there may be wide variation in how individuals respond to these various influences.

Leosenio (103) reviewed some empiric studies that suggest that, in the United States, the availability of a Social Security pension is a major factor in the timing of retirement, although the actual level of payments has a relatively modest effect. For example, a 10% increase in retirement benefit may lower the average retirement age by about 1 month. The best estimate is that Social Security accounts for the current popularity of retirement at 62 and 65 years of age in the United States and overall has probably reduced the average age of retirement for men by several months. An earlier analysis in the United Kingdom (187) reached similar conclusions: People do respond to economic incentives, but age, gender, and poor health are much stronger influences.

However, most of these analyses fail to allow for private pensions, which are a key source of retirement income for a significant portion of the population, and the structure of the pension plan may be much more important. Kotlikoff and Wise (96) studied one Fortune 500 company in the United States and suggested that the provisions of the firm's pension plan were the major factor in the timing of early retirement, much greater than any Social Security considerations, although Social Security conditions may also contribute to the peak in retirements at age 65 years. The influence of financial incentives varies with a person's health status: Poor health may lead to higher financial benefits; persons in poor health are more likely to respond to financial incentives; persons in poor health are more sensitive to negative job characteristics. Moreover, these economic studies seem to accept that health is a completely independent variable and assume cause and effect. They fail to allow for the interactions among psychosocial aspects of work, financial incentives, and health complaints. Nevertheless, overall, age and health often appear to overshadow financial incentives in the decision to retire.

Gustman et al. (70) reviewed economic research on company pensions in the United States that suggests that many issues are important (Table 2.8), although these investigators concluded that the evidence was insufficient to determine the relative weight to attach to these variables.

The percentage of women working in the United States rose from 28% in 1940 to 57% in 1991, and women now make up 45% of the United States labor force. However, most of the research on retirement is about men, and there are relatively few studies on the retirement decisions of older women. Weaver (179) reviewed 13 studies, although he urged that the results should be interpreted with caution because of the limited data, many of which are dated, and methodologic weaknesses. Generally, however, these studies show that married women's decisions about retirement seem to be related more to the financial rewards of work, but not to the levels of financial benefits after retirement. This finding may be partly explained by a lack of linkage between earnings and benefits for many married women, a feature that may act as a deterrent to retirement. Husbands and wives may often reach joint retirement decisions, and a married woman is less likely to continue working once her husband retires, just as a married man is less likely to continue working once his wife retires. The family, the presence of dependent children or parents, and the husband's health appear to play little part in the decision. This finding is perhaps surprising, but it may be the result of conflicting effects: increased need for the woman in the home versus increased

TABLE 2.8. *Behavioral motivations for employer-provided pensions*

Worker motivations	Tax-preferred retirement savings, often inflation proofed
	Convenience and economies of scale
	Insurance against incapacity and other contingencies
	Union preference
Employer motivations	Human resource tool:
	Regulate retirement
	Reduce worker turnover other than retirement
	Productivity incentive
Outcomes of supply-demand interactions	Pension plan structure and conditions
	Patterns of retirement
	Worker selection, motivation, turnover
	Wage bargaining

Adapted from Gustman AL, Mitchell OS, Steinmeier TL. The role of pensions in the labor market: a survey of the literature. *Ind Labor Rel Rev* 1994;47:417–438, with permission.

financial need for her to work and increased attractions of getting out of the home. Virtually, no data are available on the relation of women's health to retirement decisions. Moreover, few data exist on unmarried women, although their retirement decisions may be more similar to those of men. The current United States Health and Retirement Study of couples should in due course provide much better data on all these issues, as should the United States National Longitudinal Survey of Mature Women, which has now been running for about 30 years, with many of the subjects now about retirement age.

Poole (136) assessed the process and outcome of retirement resulting from ill health in six large organizations in the United Kingdom. Rates of retirement resulting from ill health varied from 20 to 250 per 10,000 contributing members per annum. In different organizations, the rate of early retirement rose progressively after age 40 or 45 years, but in two organizations that provided gender-specific data, women showed a more even spread, with another slight peak in their late 20s and early 30s. Musculoskeletal and minor psychiatric illnesses were the most common medical reason given for early retirement. In four organizations, the modal age and length of service at retirement coincided with enhancement in benefits.

Hobbs (78) studied sickness absence and medical retirement in the police service in England and Wales, with similar findings. He found a high level of sickness absence of about 5.5% of days lost in both police officers and civilian support staff and an extremely high level of retirement on medical grounds, most commonly because of musculoskeletal conditions and stress-related disorders. In 1996 to 1997, between 16% and 77% of all police retirements in different police forces were on medical grounds, a finding reflecting the wide variation in management and culture in different forces. After government concern, medical retirement had fallen from a national average of 59% in 1991, but it was still 43% in 1996 to 1997. This was partly because there is no formalized alternative to assist departure from the police, and Hobbs (78) identified a particular problem of retirement on medical grounds that preempted disciplinary proceedings. Retirement on medical grounds was also closely related to pension entitlement. Bourne (20) made a parallel study of the London Metropolitan Police Service, with similar findings, and discussed approaches to the management of long-term sickness absence.

Poole (136) pointed out that the granting of retirement benefits on grounds of ill health is often not determined solely by illness. Different organizations make more or less use of early retirement on health grounds as a method of terminating employment or alternative methods of redundancy whether compulsory, voluntary, or forced, disciplinary proceedings, or early retirement on nonhealth grounds. He suggested that doctors may be subject to organizational pressures and conflicts of interest in reaching these decisions.

A Department of Social Security study in the United Kingdom (52) studied 1,545 new recipients of long-term sickness benefits. "Among recipients aged 50+, their health condition appeared to be only one of several considerations in determining their attitudes towards returning to work. Attitudes to work appear to change quite dramatically around aged 50. It would appear that personal considerations and labor market conditions play a prominent role in shaping the attitudes of recipients aged 50+."

Once again, the changes seem to be more social than biologic (40). Older people may have more difficulty coping with back pain, with heavy physical work, and especially with the combination of these factors. However, any biologic change in the back with age seems to be only part of the story. Early retirement because of back pain occurs not only in workers with heavy jobs. Over the last two decades, in which there has been a marked increase in long-term incapacity and early retirement attributed to back pain, no evidence indicates any change in back pain, and the number of people in heavy manual jobs has fallen.

In summary, many of these studies suggest that back pain is only one element in early retirement on health grounds, and it is often associated with comorbidities, psychologic problems, and social factors. With present data, it is not possible to determine the relative importance of these various elements linking employment status, low back disability, and early retirement. It is probably always multifactorial, and the relative importance of different elements varies in each individual. Back pain and disability may contribute to incapacity for work and job loss. The physical, mental, and social ill effects of loss of employment may interact with and may aggravate low back pain and disability. There may be social and financial advantages to sickness certification, sickness benefits, and retirement on medical grounds. Conversely, the common symptom of back pain may be used to cover other reasons for sickness absence or early retirement. On the evidence available at present, the balance of probabilities is that the physical state of the back is the least important.

No data are available on early retirement associated with neck pain. This review and social security data in Chapter 21 show major gender differences in early retirement.

Workers' Compensation

Before going any further, it is important to stress that true *malingering,* or the complete fabrication of symptoms that do not exist, is extremely rare. Most workers have entirely "genuine" physical pain, although reasonable people may reasonably disagree about the degree of recovery, the level of disability, and the appropriate duration of time lost from work.

Few issues around back pain have given rise to more controversy than the question of compensation and secondary gain. *Secondary gain* is a vague term that suggests the person is somehow rewarded economically, physically, or emotionally as a result of an injury or illness (56,57).

All illness involves some secondary gains. Illness may provide an excuse for avoiding all kinds of activities and may lead to increased social support. For some people, it may provide an emotional crutch to deal with life's problems. Some people simply do not have the emotional and social resources to deal with life, particularly in times of adversity. Some people are passive and dependent, and health professionals offer a ready source of support. There is another group of people who have always coped remarkably well, but when illness does strike, they never manage to return to their previous hyperactive state. They then have difficulty adjusting and "never seem to get over it." That does not mean that any of these people consciously contrives the situation. They are not malingering. They have genuine symptoms. It is just that they are not able to cope with them well and may continue to varying degrees in the sick role.

Too often, however, discussions about secondary gain focus on money and imply malingering. Any benefit such as disability payments or a concerned family member then casts suspicion on the legitimacy of the patient's symptoms. If treatment fails, secondary gain makes a good excuse. This is all a circular argument, which may say more about the bias of the observer than the motivation of the patient. No one raises questions of secondary gain about the patient with a cerebrovascular accident.

These discussions also usually neglect that secondary gains are balanced by secondary losses (56). Money is only one part of the secondary gains and losses of stopping work and going sick, and it is probably not the most important. Loss of all the other social benefits of working, loss of financial and social status, and the major change from a working role to a sick role are probably all more important. For most patients, these losses greatly outweigh any emotional gains. Even if the argument is confined to money, the value of compensation should not be overestimated. Danson (41) showed that the mean wage replacement rate for temporary total disability under United States workers' compensation ranged from 63.9% in 1960 to 67.9% in 1985. Nagi and Hadley (127) showed that 82% of disabled people in the United States were worse off financially than when they were working, 17% had little change, and only 1.5% were better off financially. That has not changed. Few patients in the United Kingdom who are home sick with low back pain are better off financially than when they were working. Half receive less than 50% of their previous net earnings, and only one in eight receives more than 80% of previous net earnings (52). In a personal series, only 5% of our patients with back pain were financially better off while sick than when working, and these few were generally part-time or poorly paid workers whose wages were so low that they gave little financial incentive to work at all. Looking at their whole social situation, most people who are home from work with back pain are much worse off in many ways. Workers' compensation and other social security benefits are an inadequate replacement.

Against that background, however, financial gain is a major motivating force in a material society. All humans respond to financial incentives and disincentives. Indeed, all health professionals make much greater secondary gains from back pain than any patient ever did.

Several studies show that injuries that occur at work lead to significantly longer work loss than comparable nonwork injuries. Sander and Meyers (148) studied railroad workers who lost time from work and who returned to work with restrictions after a back injury. They found that the average time lost from work after a work injury was 14.2 months compared with 4.9 months for a comparable nonwork injury. The results were comparable for those who had a lumbosacral sprain or strain and for those who had back surgery, even if different in magnitude. Leavitt (99) studied patients from orthopedic office practices and compared 1,373 patients who had a back injury sustained at work with 417 who had a nonwork injury. Of those injured at work, 23.7% lost more than 12 months of work compared with 13.2% of those with a nonwork injury. However, work-related injury involves many factors other than the receipt of workers' compensation.

Most of the evidence about compensation is based on studies of workers' compensation in the United States and to a lesser extent in Canada and Australia. Workers' compensation is a no-fault system that covers about 90% of all workers in the United States.

There is little change in the incidence of serious workplace injuries, but since the 1960s and 1970s, there has been a rapid rise in the number of claims for work-related injuries leading to loss of time from work (185). Between 1971 and 1991, the number of workers who lost time from work for all work-related injuries and illnesses increased from 3.3 to 4 per 100 workers per annum, whereas the amount of time lost increased from 48 to 90 days per 100 workers per annum (72). National Council for Compensation Insurance data showed an 80% increase in the number of claims during the 1980s and a marked shift toward soft tissue injuries such as sprains, strains, and low back claims, although the *proportion* of low back injuries only increased slightly from 29.2% to 31.8% (129). Butler et al. (26) analyzed that shift and suggested that most of it was due to the "moral hazard" of altered claims behavior.

Miller (124) was one of the first to calculate, in 1976, that benefits of more than about 50% to 55% of wages were associated with an increase in the days of disability claimed by insured persons, and his report to the United States House of Representatives Committee on Ways and Means is still frequently quoted. There have been many such studies, reviewed and analyzed by Loeser et al. (106). The evidence is not fully consistent, and not all studies show any effect. However, their best available literature synthesis suggested that a 10% increase in workers' compensation benefits is associated with a 1 to 11% increase in the number of claims and a 2 to 11% increase in the average duration of claims. That is an average increase of 2 to 5 days lost from work because of back pain. These findings are similar for "verifiable" injuries such as fractures, as well as more subjective, soft tissue injuries.

Kreuger (97) analyzed United States Population Survey data on workers' compensation. He found that a 10% increase in benefits was associated with about a 7% increase in claim rate. The waiting period to qualify for claims (at that time 7 days or less in all states) had a substantial negative relation to the claim rate. Time-series analysis showed that the growth in claims during the 1970s corresponded reasonably well to the growth in real benefits over that period.

Ruser (145) analyzed a longitudinal data set from 2,798 manufacturing establishments. He found that increased workers' compensation benefits were associated with increased frequency of most nonfatal injuries but no change in the frequency of fatal injuries. Higher benefits were also more likely to be associated with days lost from work after an injury.

Baldwin et al. (7) analyzed first return to work and subsequent work loss in 8,690 Workers' Compensation Board patients in Ontario, Canada. All else being equal, a higher wage replacement rate was associated with longer first absence in women but not in men. However, the chances of a successful return to work, subsequent absences, and eventual giving up of work were all unrelated to the wage replacement rate in both men and women.

Meyer et al. (122) in the United States reported a natural experiment when two states increased the maximum weekly benefit under workers' compensation by approximately 50%. Effectively, benefits were only increased for high-earning workers, but there was no change in benefits for low-earning workers. For all injuries, duration of work loss increased for those eligible for the higher benefits but remained unchanged for those whose benefits did not change. For back pain, one of the states showed a highly significant change, but the other showed no change.

Hadler et al. (72) made a detailed comparison of 505 patients receiving workers' compensation benefits and 861 patients who were not receiving workers' compensation who sought health care for an acute episode of low back pain. The patients receiving compensation described their jobs as more physically demanding and were more likely to have lost time from work in the month before seeking health care. The patients receiving compensation had slower subjective recovery, but there was no significant difference in recovery of function or return to work. This delay was independent of the severity of their back pain, perception of job demand, or type of health care.

Several studies have looked at the nature rather than the amount of compensation payments. The study by Carron et al. (30) comparing patients at multidisciplinary pain clinics in United States and New Zealand also commented on the different compensation systems in these two countries. However, as discussed previously, the highly selected nature of the patients and the different local referral patterns make it impossible to draw any valid conclusions.

Jamison et al. (86,87) in Tennessee looked at patients with chronic low back pain who were attending a pain control center and compared patients receiving time-limited workers' compensation with those receiving unlimited disability payments. Time-limited payments were generally received during the initial period that a patient was receiving medical treatment after an accident. Once maximum medical outcome was achieved, there was settlement, and no further benefits were given. Unlimited compensation consisted of regular financial disability benefits for an indefinite period until the worker felt able to return to work. This study showed that patients with unlimited compensation took more analgesics, showed more pain behavior and physician-rated symptom dramatization, and were less likely to return to work. However, these were two completely different groups of patients, and those receiving unlimited benefits were older and had been away from work for 18 months longer. The two groups of patients were not comparable, and it is not possible to draw any conclusions about the effect of the two types of payment.

Greenough and Fraser (68) looked at lump sum settlements under the South Australian workers' compensation scheme. This study had major strengths and major weaknesses. The strengths were careful control for clinical factors and injury severity, as well as 96% follow-up at 4 years. However, the weaknesses were that this was a selected group of patients referred to a single surgeon's practice, the authors did not allow for any of the other work-related factors that could influence return to work (see later), and they did not perform any kind of multivariate analysis. On univariate analysis, these investigators found that in men, only 49% of patients receiving compensation returned to work compared with 89% of patients not receiving compensation. For women, the corresponding figures were 54% and 93%. More important to the present discussion, these researchers looked at the effect of lump sum payments, wherein liability for any one incident could be commuted either at the initiation of the worker or indirectly by the insurance company. They found that a much lower proportion of patients receiving workers' compensation who received lump sum payments returned to work (men, 35%; women, 46%) than those who received continued, regular payments (men, 85%; women, 80%). However, they again did not make any allowance for other work or injury-related factors that could influence return to work. The authors also pointed out themselves that this was a different group of patients, with an increased incidence of previous claims, dispute concerning their injury, and disputed claims that had been stopped unilaterally by the insurance company. These factors all imply differences in the nature of the claim, the disability, and the worker. Any conclusions from this particular Australian workers' compensation situation cannot be extrapolated more generally.

Wood et al. (183) made one of the most detailed mathematic analyses of the method of settlement of 8,232 workers' compensation claims in Western Australia and found that lump sum settlement was associated with substantially higher costs. In particular, lump sum settlement of a common law action was associated with a fourfold increase in costs. Various forms of lump sum settlement of the workers' compensation claim were also associated with increased costs, although not to the same degree. However, eligibility for lump sum settlement depended on the type of injury, recurrent history, and the nature of the claim. Once again, it is not possible to separate the effect of the method of payment from these associated factors or to extrapolate from this the particular Australian workers' compensation situation. (This study covers all injuries and not only neck and back injuries.)

Thomason (166) analyzed the transition from temporary to permanent disability under the workers' compensation system in New York State. He suggested that claimants exercise some discretion in the pursuit of a permanent disability claim. He found that the higher the financial benefits of permanent disability status and the lower the uncertainty of achieving it, the more likely claimants were to pursue and achieve permanent disability status.

Worrall et al. (186) also made a highly mathematic analysis of the transition from temporary to permanent disability under the workers' compensation system in Massachusetts and Illinois. These investigators also found that the structure of benefits and increase in financial benefits could be associated with a sizable increase in permanent disability claims.

Clinical studies of workers' compensation in the literature show a striking dichotomy. At one extreme, some pain clinic studies and experts say that there is no clinical difference between patients receiving compensation and those not receiving compensation. At the other extreme, some medicolegal experts, who are mainly orthopedic surgeons, imply that many of the claimants they see are little short of frank malingerers. The difference seems to be a combination of case selection and observer bias, in both directions.

Rohling et al. (140) made the most careful review of this literature, although they cautioned that most studies were in pain clinic settings, and the results may not apply to more routine compensation patients. They found 32 studies that gave usable data on 3,802 compensated and 3,849 noncompensated patients. Patients receiving compensation consistently reported more pain, although the difference was small, about 6%. The review by Rohling et al. (140) and another review by Walsh and Dumitru (178) concluded that compensation does seem to be associated with delayed clinical recovery: The outcomes of conservative treatment, back surgery, and chronic pain rehabilitation programs are consistently poorer in patients receiving compensation, but there is conflicting evidence on the magnitude of this difference, with estimates ranging from 0% to 30%. Many studies show little difference in the physical findings and levels of distress in patients receiving compensation. Some studies suggest that compensated patients are more depressed. To put this in context, 75% to 90% of compensated patients do respond well to health care and do recover and return to work rapidly.

This situation is not unique to back or neck pain. Binder and Rohling (14) showed a similar effect in patients with mild head injury. Their metaanalysis of 17 studies of 2,353 patients showed that patients with financial incentives reported more symptoms and disability, with a moderate effect size of 0.47.

Economists often play down the role of health care and psychosocial factors in their studies, just as health care providers often overlook economic and administrative issues. Yet disability, health care, and compensation are closely linked. No hard data are available on the influence of health care and its providers on the submission and duration of claims, although clinical decisions certainly have a major impact on health care costs and on compensation duration and costs. However, this relationship works both ways. Gardner and Butler (66) extended their analysis of "moral hazard" to show the impact of workers' compensation on health care. Simmonds and Kumar (156) carried out an experimental study of 69 physical therapists who each viewed three videotaped assessments of patients with low back pain. Knowledge of the patients' workers' compensation status did not influence the therapists' assessment of the physical findings but did influence their judgment of prognosis, which could bias their approach to the patient and management. Taylor et al. (165) suggest that compensation may even influence patients' and professionals' decisions about back surgery. Before passing judgment on how compensation incentives influence workers, consideration should also be given to how these incentives influence employers, health professionals, and lawyers.

It is also too easy to assume that this is all a direct effect of compensation, but that does not allow for other differences in these patients. Leavitt (100) pointed out that compensated patients usually have heavier physical jobs and are generally younger, are male, have less education, are of a lower social class, and are more often immigrants. These patients comprise a different occupational, economic, and social group. Their selection and referral patterns are also different. These differences may have a more direct and much greater impact on their clinical progress and return to work than compensation itself. There is conflicting evidence on this from multivariate analyses. Dworkin et al. (45) found that employment status was most strongly related to the outcome of pain management, and compensation or litigation did not add anything. Sanderson et al. (149) found that both unemployment and compensation were related to disability, but employment status was most important. Leavitt (100) showed the importance of job demands, but found that work-related injury and compensation were associated with more prolonged disability, even after allowing for job demands. Nagi and Hadley (127) hypothesized that in patients with more severe physical injuries, social factors are less important, but in those with less severe injuries, higher education, higher income, greater loss of income, and greater number of dependents seemed to be associated with higher motivation to return to work.

Burns et al. (24) provided empirical evidence to support this concept. Patients receiving workers' compensation who had no previous back surgery and low levels of pain responded as well to a multidisciplinary pain program as noncompensated patients. The subgroup of patients receiving workers' compensation who had undergone previous surgery and who had high pain levels had poor results. These investigators suggested that moderating and mediating factors are more important than compensation itself.

Overall, the level of compensation is probably a small factor in the decision to stop work and is only one factor in maintaining the sick role (Table 2.9). As already noted, there have been great changes in attitudes to work and disability and compensation over recent decades. Rapid change has occurred in conditions of employment, with much more unemployment, job insecurity, and job turnover. The average job tenure

TABLE 2.9. *Socioeconomic issues in workers' compensation*

Work demands
Work environment
Availability of modified work
Income
Job security
Advancement and career potential
Pension
Natural job attrition
Job availability
Compensation

TABLE 2.10. *Relation of compensation to low back pain and disability*

Relation of compensation level to claims
  There is no evidence that compensation changes the actual injury rate.
  10% increase in compensation level is associated with a 1%–11% increase in claims rate.
  10% increase in compensation level is associated with a 2%–11% increase in duration of disability.
  This affects "verifiable" injuries such as fractures as much as more subjective, soft tissue injuries.
Relation of compensation to surgical outcome
  Compensated patients are less likely to have a good result of back surgery.
  These findings have been criticized because
    These men often have heavier physical jobs.
    They may receive overaggressive surgical intervention.
  Despite that, more than 75% of compensated patients do return to their previous work after primary
    surgery for a well-defined disc prolapse.
Relation of compensation to rehabilitation outcome
  Compensated patients respond less well to pain management and rehabilitation.
  These findings have been criticized because
    There are methodologic flaws in many of these studies. They are often small samples of highly se-
      lected patients with poor diagnostic criteria. Follow-up is poor. There is failure to allow for other
      factors such as job demands.
    Differences are small.
  Despite that, many compensated patients do benefit.

in the United States is now less than 3 years. This shift has inevitably changed attitudes to work, employers, and unemployment. These changed attitudes are all probably much more important than the actual level of compensation.

In summary, most of this evidence is on workers' compensation in United States and, to a lesser extent, in Canada and Australia, and it may not apply equally to other sickness benefit systems. There is no evidence that compensation increases the amount of back pain or changes the condition of anyone's back. There is little doubt that compensation does affect what people do when they have back pain, but it does not cause the pain or create the situation in these patients. It is only one, and probably one of the less powerful, social influences on whether they find themselves in this situation and what they do to get out of it. The best available literature suggests that a 10% increase in workers' compensation benefits is associated with a 1% to 11% increase in the number of claims and a 2% to 11% increase in the average duration of claims (Table 2.10). There is insufficient evidence to draw any conclusions about the type of benefit payments and, in particular, about regular payments or lump sum settlements. Compensated patients consistently report more pain, although the difference is small, about 6%. Many studies show little difference in the physical findings and levels of distress in patients receiving compensation. The outcomes of conservative treatment, back surgery, and chronic pain rehabilitation programs are consistently poorer in compensated patients, but there is conflicting evidence on the magnitude of this effect, with estimates ranging from 0% to 30%. All this evidence deals with statistical associations in groups of patients, a method that is quite different from attributing motives or judging the individual patient. To put this in context, 75% to 95% of patients receiving compensation do respond well to health care and do recover and return to work rapidly, whereas secondary losses usually greatly outweigh secondary gains.

It is also too easy to assume that this is all a direct effect of compensation, but that does not allow for other differences in these patients. Patients receiving workers' compensation usually have heavier physical jobs and are generally younger, male, less well educated, of lower social class, and are more likely to be immigrants. They form a different occupational, economic, and social group, and their selection and referral patterns are different. These differences may have a more direct and much greater relation to their clinical progress and return to work than compensation itself.

There is an astonishing lack of data on the effect of workers' compensation on neck injuries. Few data are available on gender issues, and most of the foregoing studies are largely of male workers. Some published reviews are suggested as a starting point for more detailed reading of differing views about compensation (9,19,22,26,56,57, 114,120,121,180).

Litigation: Adversarial Medicolegal Proceedings

Litigation is defined as the act of carrying out a lawsuit, and the key element in all European and North American systems is the adversarial nature of the legal proceedings and the associated medicolegal evidence. This usually takes the form of personal injury litigation, which in all European and North American countries may proceed independently of incapacity for work, health care, workers' compensation, and social security issues.

Anecdotal clinical and legal experience shows general agreement that some claimants magnify or exaggerate their symptoms and disability to varying degree during medical assessment carried out specifically for legal proceedings. So the judicial process insists on cross-checking the claimant's self-report of symptoms and disability against some other form of evidence such as the nature and severity of the initial injury, health care sought and received, objective clinical evidence of impairment, or independent functional capacity evaluation. This evidence is also weighed in the balance of judicial assessment of the claimant's credibility.

Many articles on workers' compensation, for example, that by Greenough and Fraser (68), extend the discussion to the deleterious effects of litigation and adversarial legal proceedings. However, there is actually little direct evidence on the impact of such legal proceedings.

Several workers' compensation studies have commented on the negative effect of a lawyer's involvement in the claim, but they generally have not presented any data, and none of them have allowed for the fact that there must have been differences in the accident, the claim, the worker, or the disability that led to a lawyer's involvement. Several studies of workers' compensation included patients involved in litigation (27,30,68,101). However, these were a minority of patients in all of these studies, no data were presented separately for these patients, and it is unjustifiable to extrapolate any conclusions about workers' compensation to litigation. The present search identified 14 studies that provided data specifically about litigation, 4 on neck pain, 5 on low back pain, and 5 on various types of injuries or pain but usually including a large proportion of spinal pain.

Schutt and Dohan (150) followed-up 67 patients for 6 to 26 months after accidental neck injury and found no difference in the proportion with symptoms whether litigation was continuing, litigation was settled, or litigation was not pursued. Hohl (80) reexamined 146 patients after soft tissue injury to the neck resulting from traffic injuries and found no difference in the proportion who were free of symptoms at 5 years. More of those patients whose litigation was settled within 6 months became symptom free than those whose litigation lasted longer, but that finding may simply reflect earlier settlement of legal proceedings in the patients with less severe conditions who recovered faster. Norris and Watt (130) found that litigation was associated with more persistent symptoms after whiplash injury to the neck, but they also found that patients with clinically more severe cases were more likely to sue. Gore and Sepic (67) found that continuing or completed litigation had no effect on the outcome of cervical fusion.

Peck et al. (135) compared pain reports of two groups of patients receiving workers' compensation for work-related injuries (although these were not all back injuries): 105 who also had personal litigation proceedings related to their accidents and 103 who did not. The personal, work, and injury characteristics of the two groups were similar. These investigators found no difference in the severity of pain, pain behavior, or health care consumption. Mendelson (119) compared 47 patients with chronic low back pain who were involved in personal injury litigation and 33 control subjects who were not and found no difference in the level of reported pain and similar levels of psychologic disturbance. Guest and Drummond (69) found no difference in severity of pain but did find higher levels of anxiety and depressive symptoms in patients with chronic low back pain who were still receiving compensation compared with those who had settled their claims. Unfortunately, none of this group of studies looked at clinical outcome or return to work.

Sanderson et al. (149) found that patients at a surgical back clinic who were involved in litigation reported higher levels of disability, with an average Oswestry score of 32.4 compared with 26.6 for patients not involved in litigation. However, the difference was not significant, and as previously noted, this was a highly selected group of patients in whom it was not possible to distinguish cause and effect.

Tait et al. (162) analyzed the interaction of employment status and litigation in patients with chronic pain who were attending a multidisciplinary pain center. These investigators compared 99 patients who were working, 15 who were working and in litigation, 53 who were receiving workers' compensation, and 34 who were receiving workers' compensation and were in litigation. Patients in litigation reported more pain and more disability. There were significant interactions with psychologic distress: Working patients who were in litigation reported more distress than nonlitigants, whereas patients receiving workers' compensation who were in litigation reported less distress than nonlitigants. These investigators suggested that litigation may function as a coping response for patients who are distressed by the adversarial nature of the workers' compensation system.

Solomon and Tunks (158) studied patients at a chronic pain clinic, the majority of whom had spinal pain. Eighty patients were involved in litigation, either industrial litigation (workers' compensation claims, appeals, and tribunals) or civil litigation for a personal injury claim, and were compared with 47 nonlitigating control subjects. On multivariate analysis, litigation was the primary predictor of depressive symptoms but had no significant relation to the amount of medication taken, the amount of time spent lying down, or return to work. However, Mayou et al. (118) studied posttraumatic stress disorder and other psychologic outcomes in patients 5 years after motor vehicle accident injury (31% of whom had whiplash) and found no significant association with compensation proceedings.

Trief and Stein (167) studied 81 patients with chronic low back pain who underwent a 6-week behavioral treatment program. Patients who had pending litigation for compensation showed significantly less improvement in psychologic distress and behavioral measures, although they did still show worthwhile improvement.

Talo et al. (163) studied 60 patients with chronic pain at a residential multidisciplinary treatment center in Finland and compared those with workers' compensation litigation or other accident litigation with patients with active or completed litigation. These investigators found no differences in physical or psychologic disorders. There was a trend for fewer patients receiving workers' compensation to return to work, but this did not reach statistical significance in the relatively small groups. Active or completed litigation made no difference to the findings.

Gallagher et al. (65) found that neither workers' compensation status nor litigation was associated with return to work in 92 unemployed patients at a low back pain clinic or in 77 applicants for Social Security disability benefits.

There is a myth, promoted by and commonly attributed to an early article by Miller in 1961 (123) and still shared by many medical practitioners and lawyers, that once litigation is settled, many claimants are "cured by a verdict," their symptoms and disability improve, and they return to work. Mendelson (120) reviewed a large number of international follow-up studies that showed that this concept is not true. However adversarial legal proceedings may aggravate or perpetuate symptoms or disability, by the time settlement occurs, often after several years, the clinical and social pattern is set and generally does not change dramatically.

In summary, the present review found limited and conflicting evidence on litigation. Most studies are on selected clinical series, often from highly selected referral situations, and it is difficult to generalize the results. It is possible that litigation may influence reports of symptoms and disability and the clinical presentation in the medicolegal context, but it does not appear to be associated with any significant increase in the severity of pain or distress in the clinical situation. There is insufficient evidence to assess whether or to what extent litigation may be associated with any difference in clinical outcomes, disability, or return to work.

Social Security Benefits

The completely separate and enormous literature on social security is reviewed in Chapter 21.

CONCLUSION

Neck pain and back pain are real and have a physical cause in the neck or back. All this evidence indicates that social issues may *influence* these symptoms and what people do about them, but that does not imply that the symptoms are not real or that they are imaginary or faked.

There is extensive, although scientifically often poor-quality, evidence that social factors may influence the reporting of back and neck pain, pain behavior, disability, sickness absence, and early retirement. There is suggestive evidence that some of these interactions may be potentially powerful and at least in some situations may be more important than any physical abnormality in the neck or back. On the evidence available at present, and remembering the limitations and weaknesses of much of that evidence, it may be hypothesized that the key social influences lie in the area of individual, group, and society in general's attitudes and beliefs about work, about back pain and its relationship to work, about sickness absence, about welfare benefits, and about retirement. These findings are not unique to neck or back pain, but they form part of much wider social issues.

However, this review must end with a strong note of caution. These social influences are complex and interacting, difficult to define, and harder to measure, and they may or may not be open to modification. Many may be powerful but may only apply to a few people. Most of the evidence on social influences is of low scientific quality, is cross-sectional, and demonstrates only associations, rather than necessarily causal relationships. It mainly relates to low back pain and disability: There is much less evidence on neck pain, although in principle the findings are likely to be similar. Gender is associated with different social roles and influences, but data on gender differences in these social influences are limited. This is a subjective, narrative review. Readers are strongly advised to consider the evidence for themselves and to form their own judgments on whether they regard the interpretation and conclusions as reasonable.

Despite these caveats, it is possible that understanding these social influences may be the key to controlling the current epidemic of chronic disability, sickness certification, and social security benefits associated with neck and back pain. There is a need for much more high-quality research into which social factors are most important, including the mechanisms by which they work, the interactions between them, the magnitude of their effect, and the ways in which they may be modified. Any proposal to change social policy must recognize the limitations of the scientific evidence and our understanding and must be made with caution and restraint.

ACKNOWLEDGMENTS

Certain sections of this review are adapted and developed with permission from Waddell G: *The back pain revolution.* Edinburgh: Churchill Livingstone, 1998, which provides a more comprehensive review of the biopsychosocial model of low back pain and disability.

REFERENCES

1. Allan DB, Waddell G. An historical perspective on low back pain and disability. *Orthop Scand* 1989; 60 [Suppl 234]:10–23.
2. Arnold J, Robertson IT, Cooper CL. *Work psychology,* 3rd ed. London: Pitman, 1998.
3. Arve-Pares B, ed. *Inequality in health: a Swedish perspective.* Stockholm: Socialvetenskapliga forskningsradet, 1998.
4. Astrand N-E, Isacsson S-O. Back pain, back abnormalities and competing medical, psychological, and social factors as predictors of sick leave, early retiral, unemployment, labor turnover and mortality: a 22 year follow up of male employees in a Swedish pulp and paper company. *Br J Ind Med* 1988; 45:387–395.
5. Badley EM, Ibanez D. Socioeconomic risk factors and musculoskeletal disability. *J Rheumatol* 1994;21:515–522.
6. Balague F, Skovron M-L, Nordin M, et al. Low back pain in school children. A study of familial and psychological factors. *Spine* 1995;20:1265–1270.
7. Baldwin ML, Johnson WG, Butler RJ. The error of using returns-to-work to measure the outcomes of health care. *Am J Ind Med* 1996;29:632–641.
8. Beale N, Nethercott S. Certificated sickness absence in industrial employees threatened with redundancy. *BMJ* 1988;296:1508–1510.
9. Bellamy R. Compensation neurosis. *Clin Orthop* 1997;336:94–106.
10. Berg M, Sanden A, Torell G, et al. Persistence of musculoskeletal symptoms: a longitudinal study. *Ergonomics* 1988;31:1281–1285.
11. Bergenudd H, Nilsson B. Back pain in middle age. An occupational workload and psychologic factors: an epidemiologic survey. *Spine* 1988;13:58–60.
12. Biering-Sorensen F, Thomsen C. Medical, social and occupational history as risk indicators for low-back trouble in a general population. *Spine* 1986;11:720–723.
13. Bigos SJ, Battie MC, Spengler DM, et al. A prospective study of work perceptions and psychosocial factors affecting the report of back injury. *Spine* 1991;16:1–6.
14. Binder LM, Rohling ML. Money matters: a meta-analytic review of the effects of financial incentives on recovery after closed head injury. *Am J Psychiatry* 1996;153:7–10.

15. Black D. Inequalities in health: report of a working group chaired by Sir Douglas Black. London: Department of Social Security, Her Majesty's Stationery Office, 1980.

16. Blaxter M. Health and social class: evidence on inequality in health from a national survey. *Lancet* 1987;2:30–33.

17. Block AR, Boyer SL. The spouse's adjustment to chronic pain: cognitive and emotional factors. *Soc Sci Med* 1984;19:1313–1317.

18. Block AR, Kremer EF, Gaylor M. Behavioral treatment of chronic pain: the spouse as a discriminative cue for pain behavior. *Pain* 1980;9:243–252.

19. Boden LI. Work disability in an economic context. In: Moon SD, Sauter SL, eds. *Beyond biomechanics: psychosocial aspects of musculoskeletal disorders in office work.* London: Taylor and Francis, 1996:287–293.

20. Bourne J. The management of sickness absence in the Metropolitan Police Service. London: Her Majesty's Stationery Office, 1997.

21. Bradley LA, McDonald-Haile J, Jaworski TM. Assessment of psychological status using interviews and self-report instruments. In: Turk DC, Melzack R, eds. *Handbook of pain assessment.* New York: Guilford Press, 1992:193–213.

22. Brena SF, Chapman SL. Pain and litigation. In: Wall PD, Melzack R, eds. *Textbook of pain.* Edinburgh: Churchill Livingstone, 1984:832–838.

23. Brooker A-S, Frank JW, Tarasuk VS. Back pain claims rates and the business cycle. *Soc Sci Med* 1997;45:429–439.

24. Burns JW, Sherman ML, Devine J, et al. Association between workers' compensation and outcome following multidisciplinary treatment for chronic pain: roles of mediators and moderators. *Clin J Pain* 1995;11:94–102.

25. Burton AK, Symmonds TL, Zinzen E, et al. Is ergonomic intervention alone sufficient to limit musculo-skeletal problems in nurses? *Occup Med* 1997;47:25–32.

26. Butler R, Durbin D, Helvacian N. Increasing claims for soft tissue injuries in workers compensation: cost shifting and moral hazard. *J Risk Uncertainty* 1996;13:73–87.

27. Cairns D, Mooney V, Crane P. Spinal pain rehabilitation: inpatient and outpatient treatment results and development of predictors for outcome. *Spine* 1984;9:91–95.

28. Cannon WB. *Bodily changes in pain, hunger, fear and rage: an account of recent researches in the function of emotional excitement.* New York: Appleton 1929.

29. Carr-Hill R. The inequalities in health debate: a critical review of the issues. *J Soc Policy* 1987; 16:509–542.

30. Carron H, DeGood DE, Tait R. A comparison of low back pain patients in the United States and New Zealand: psychosocial and economic factors affecting severity of disability. *Pain* 1985;21:77–89.

31. Catchlove R, Cohen K. Effects of a directive return to work approach in the treatment of workman's compensation patients with chronic pain. *Pain* 1982;14:181–191.

32. Cats-Baril WL, Frymoyer JW. Demographic factors associated with the prevalence of disability in the general population. *Spine* 1991;16:671–674.

33. Cheadle A, Franklin G, Wolfhagen C, et al. Factors influencing the duration of work-related disability: a population-based study in Washington State Workers Compensation. *Am J Public Health* 1994; 84:190–196.

34. Chew CA, May C. The expert patient and the benefits of back pain. Paper presented at the Back Pain Management Meeting, Chester, England, 1997.

35. Clemmer DI, Mohr DL. Low back injuries in a heavy industry. II: labor market forces. *Spine* 1991; 16:831–834.

36. Cobb S. Social support as a modulator of life stress. *Psychosom Med* 1976;38:300–314.

37. Consumer's Association. *The Which Report on back pain.* London: Consumer's Association, 1985.

38. Cooper CL, Marshall J. Occupational sources of stress: a review of the literature relating to coronary heart disease and mental health. *J Occup Psychol* 1976;49:11–28.

39. Croft PR, Rigby AS. Socioeconomic influences on back problems in the community in Britain. *J Epidemiol Community Health* 1994;48:166–170.

40. CSAG. Clinical Standards Advisory Group Report on back pain. London: Her Majesty's Stationery Office, 1994.

41. Danson PM. The determination of workers compensation benefit levels. In: Durbin D, Borba PS, eds. *Workers compensation insurance: claims costs, prices and regulation.* Boston: Kluwer Academic, 1993;1–24.

42. Deyo RA. Point of view on Volinn E: The epidemiology of low back pain in the rest of the world: a review of surveys in low and middle income countries. *Spine* 1997;22:1754.

43. Deyo RA, Tsui-Wu Y-J. Functional disability due to back pain. *Arthritis Rheum* 1987;30:1247–1253.

44. Dione C, Koepsell TD, Von Korff M, et al. Formal education and back-related disability: in search of an explanation. *Spine* 1995;20:2721–2730.

45. Dworkin RH, Handlin DS, Richlin DM, et al. Unraveling the effects of compensation, litigation and employment on treatment response in chronic pain. *Pain* 1985;23:49–59.

46. Eden L, Ejlertsson G, Leden I. Health and health care utilisation among early retirement pensioners with musculoskeletal disorders. *Scand J Prim Health Care* 1995;13:211–216.
47. Eden L, Ejlertsson G, Lamberger B, et al. Immigration and socio-economy as predictors of early retirement pensions. *Scand J Soc Med* 1994;22:187–193.
48. Ekberg K, Wildhagen I. Long-term sickness absence due to musculoskeletal disorders: the necessary intervention of work conditions. *Scand J Rehabil Med* 1996;28:39–47.
49. Ekberg K, Bjorkqvist B, Malm P, et al. Case-control study of risk factors for disease in the neck and shoulder area. *Occup Environ Med* 1994;51:262–266.
50. Elton D, Stanley G. Cultural expectations and psychological factors in prolonged disability. *Adv Behav Med* 1982;2:33–42.
51. Enterline PE. Social causes of sick absence. *Arch Environ Health* 1966;12:467–473.
52. Erens B, Ghate D. Invalidity benefit: a longitudinal study of new recipients. Department of Social Security research report number 20. London: Her Majesty's Stationery Office, 1993:1–127.
53. Fabrega H, Tyma S. Language and cultural influences in the description of pain. *Br J Med Psychol* 1976;49:349–371.
54. Fernandez E, McDowell JJ. Response-reinforcement relationship in chronic pain syndrome: applicability of Hernstein's law. *Behav Res Ther* 1995;3:855–863.
55. Feuerstein M, Sult S, Houle M. Environmental stressors and chronic low back pain: life events, family and work environment. *Pain* 1985;22:295–307.
56. Fishbain DA. Secondary gain concept: definition problems and its abuse in medical practice. *Am Pain Soc J* 1994;3:264–273.
57. Fishbain DA, Rosomoff HL, Cutler RB, et al. Secondary gain concept: a review of the scientific evidence. *Clin J Pain* 1995;11:6–21.
58. Flor H, Kerns RD, Turk DC. The role of spouse reinforcement, perceived pain, and activity levels of chronic pain patients. *J Psychosom Res* 1987;31:251–259.
59. Flor H, Turk DC, Rudy TE. Pain and families. II: assessment and treatment. *Pain* 1987;30:29–45.
60. Flor H, Turk DC, Scholz B. Impact of chronic pain on the spouse: marital, emotional and physical consequences. *J Psychosom Res* 1987;31:63–71.
61. Flor H, Breitinstein C, Birbaumer N, et al. A psychophysiological analysis of spouse solicitousness towards pain behaviors, spouse interaction and pain perception. *Behav Ther* 1995;26:255–272.
62. Foppa I, Noack RH. The relation of self-reported back pain to psychosocial, behavioral, and health-related factors in a working population in Switzerland. *Soc Sci Med* 1996;43:1119–1126.
63. Fordyce WE. *Behavioral methods for chronic pain and illness.* St. Louis: CV Mosby, 1976.
64. Fordyce W, ed. *Back pain in the workplace: report of an IASP task force.* Seattle: IASP Press, 1995.
65. Gallagher RM, Williams RA, Skelly J, et al. Workers' compensation and return-to-work in low back pain. *Pain* 1995;61:299–307.
66. Gardner HH, Butler RJ. A human capital perspective for cumulative trauma disorders. In: Moon SD, Sauter SL, eds. *Beyond biomechanics: psychosocial aspects of musculoskeletal disorders in office work.* London: Taylor and Francis, 1996:233–249.
67. Gore DR, Sepic SB. Anterior cervical fusion for degenerated or protruded discs: a review of 146 patients. *Spine* 1984;9:667–667.
68. Greenough CG, Fraser RD. The effects of compensation on recovery from low back injury. *Spine* 1989;14:947–955.
69. Guest GH, Drummond PD. Effect of compensation on emotional state and disability in chronic back pain. *Pain* 1992;48:125–130.
70. Gustman AL, Mitchell OS, Steinmeier TL. The role of pensions in the labor market: a survey of the literature. *Ind Labor Rel Rev* 1994;47:417–438.
71. Gyntelberg F. One year incidence of low back pain among male residents of Copenhagen aged 40–59. *Dan Med Bull* 1974;21:30–36.
72. Hadler NM, Carey TS, Garrett J. The influence of indemnification by workers' compensation insurance on recovery from acute backache: North Carolina Back Pain Project. *Spine* 1995;20:2710–2715.
73. Halliday JL. Psychological factors in rheumatism: a preliminary study. *BMJ* 1937;1:213–217.
74. Harkapaa K. Psychosocial factors as predictors for early retirement in patients with chronic low back pain. *J Psychosom Res* 1992;36:553–559.
75. Hasvold T, Johnsen RIN. Headache and neck or shoulder pain: family learnt illnesses behaviour? The Bardu Muscoloskeletal Study, 1989–1990. *Fam Pract* 1996;13:242–246.
76. Hewson D, Halcrow J, Brown CS. Compensable back pain and migrants. *Med J Aust* 1987;147:280–284.
77. Hinkle LE. Stress and disease: the concept after 50 years. *Soc Sci Med* 1987;25:561–566.
78. Hobbs P. *Lost time: the management of sickness absence and medical retirement in the police service.* HMIC Thematic Inspection Report. London: Her Majesty's Inspectorate of Constabulary, 1997.
79. Hogstedt C, Lundberg I, Vingard E, et al. Some observations on the influence of the physical work environment on the inequity in health. Personal communication from E Vingard, 1998.
80. Hohl M. Soft tissue injury of the neck in automobile accidents: factors influencing prognosis. *J Bone Joint Surg Am* 1974;56:1675–1682.

81. Honeyman PT, Jacobs EA. Effects of culture on back pain in Australian aboriginals. *Spine* 1996; 21:841–843.
82. Hunt HA, Habeck RV. The Michigan Disability Prevention Study. Lansing, MI: Michigan Department of Labor, 1993.
83. Hurwitz EL, Morgenstern H. Correlates of back problems and back-related disability in the United States. *J Clin Epidemiol* 1997;50:669–681.
84. Isacsson A, Hanson BS, Ranstam J, et al. Social network, social support and the prevalence of neck and low back pain after retirement: a population study of men born in 1914 in Malmo, Sweden. *Scand J Soc Med* 1995;23:17–22.
85. Iversen L, Sabroe S. Psychological well-being among unemployed and employed people after a company cl;osedown: a longitudinal study. *J Soc Issues* 1988;44:141–152.
86. Jamison RN, Matt DA, Parris WC. Effects of time-limited vs unlimited compensation on pain behavior and treatment outcome in low back pain patients. *J Psychosom Res* 1988;32:277–283.
87. Jamison RN, Matt DA, Parris WC. Treatment outcome in low back pain patients: do compensation benefits make a difference? *Orthop Rev* 1988;17:1210–1215.
88. Janlert U. Unemployment as a disease and diseases of the unemployed. *Scand J Work Environ Health* 1997;23 [Suppl 3]:79–83.
89. Juster FT, Suzman R. An overview of the health and retirement study. *J Hum Res* 1995;30 [Suppl]:S7–S56.
90. Keel P. Prevalence and persistence of back pain in foreign workers: class or culture-induced? *Ther Umsch* 1992;49:616–622.
91. Keel P, Calanchini C. Chronic backache in migrant workers from Mediterranean countries in comparison to central European patients: demographic and psychosocial aspects. *Schweiz Med Wochenschr* 1989;119:22–31.
92. Kerns RD, Haythornthwaite J, Southwick S, et al. The role of marital interaction in chronic pain and depressive symptom severity. *J Psychosom Res* 1990;34:401–408.
93. King A, Coles B. The health of Canada's youth: views and behaviours of 11-, 13- and 15-year olds from 11 countries. Ottawa: Health and Welfare Canada, 1992.
94. Klapow JC, Slater MA, Patterson TL, et al. Psychosocial factors discriminate multidimensional clinical groups of chronic low back pain patients. *Pain* 1995;62:349–355.
95. Kleinman A. *The illness narratives: suffering, healing and the human condition.* New York: Basic Books, 1988.
96. Kotlikoff LJ, Wise DA. Employee retirement and a firm's pension plan. In: Wise DA, ed. *The economics of ageing.* Chicago: University of Chicago Press, 1989.
97. Kreuger A. Incentive effects of workers compensation insurance. *J Public Economics* 1990;41:73–99.
98. Lancourt J, Kettelhut M. Predicting return to work for lower back pain patients receiving worker's compensation. *Spine* 1992;17:629–640.
99. Leavitt F. The role of psychological disturbance in extending disability time among compensated back injured workers. *J Psychosom Res* 1990;34:447–453.
100. Leavitt F. The physical exertion factor in compensable work injuries: a hidden flaw in previous research. *Spine* 1992;17:307–310.
101. Leavitt F, Garron DC, McNeill TW, et al. Organic status, psychological disturbance and pain report characteristics in low back pain patients on compensation. *Spine* 1982;7:398–402.
102. Lehmann TR, Spratt KF, Lehmann KK. Predicting long term disability in low back injured workers presenting to a spine consultant. *Spine* 1993;18:1103–1112.
103. Leonesio MV. The economics of retirement: a non-technical guide. *Soc Secur Bull* 1996;59:29–50.
104. Lindstrom I, Areskong B, Nunes JF. Rygghälsan. Rapport Z. Göteborgs sjukvård, (Publ). Göteborg, Sweden, 1996.
105. Linton SJ, Buer N. Working despite pain: factors associated with work attendance versus dysfunction. *Int J Behav Med* 1995;2:252–262.
106. Loeser JD, Henderlite SE, Conrad DA. Incentive effects of workers compensation benefits: a literature synthesis. *Med Care Res Rev* 1995;52:34–59.
107. Lofvander M, Engstrom A, Theander H, Furhoff AK. Rehabilitation of young immigrants in primary care. A comparison between two treatment models. *Scand J Prim Health Care* 1997;15:123–128.
108. Loisel P, Abanhaim L, Durand P, et al. A population based randomized clinical trial on back pain management. *Spine* 1997;22:2911–2918.
109. Lousberg R, Schmidt AJ, Groenman NH. The relationship between spouse solicitousness and pain behavior: searching for more experimental evidence. *Pain* 1992;51:75–79.
110. Lundberg U. Methods and applications of stress research. *Technol Health Care* 1995;3:3–9.
111. Maes S, Vingerhoets A, Van Heck G. The study of stress and disease: some developments and requirements. *Soc Sci Med* 1987;25:561–566.
112. Makela M. Common musculoskeletal syndromes: prevalence, risk indicators and disability in Finland. Helsinki: Publications of the Social Insurance Institution, 1993;ML123:1–162.
113. Mansson NO, Israelsson B. Middle-aged men before and after disability pension: health screening profile with special emphasis on alcohol consumption. *Scand J Soc Med* 1987;15:185–189.

114. Marcus EH. Compensation payment: blessing or curse? *Med Trial Tech Q* 1983;29:319–323.
115. Martikainen PT. Unemployment and mortality among Finnish men 1981–5. *BMJ* 1990;301:407–411.
116. Martikainen PT, Valkonen T. Excess mortality of unemployed men and women during a period of rapidly increasing unemployment. *Lancet* 1996;348:909–912.
117. Mason V. The prevalence of back pain in Great Britain. Office of Population Censuses and Surveys, Social Survey Division (now Office of National Statistics). London: Her Majesty's Stationery Office, 1994:1–24.
118. Mayou R, Tyndel S, Bryant B. Long-term outcomes of motor vehicle accident injury. *Psychosom Med* 1997;59:578–584.
119. Mendelson G. Compensation, pain complaints and psychological disturbance. *Pain* 1984;20:169–177.
120. Mendelson G. *Psychiatric aspects of personal injury claims.* Springfield, IL: Charles C Thomas, 1988.
121. Mendelson G. Compensation and chronic pain [Editorial]. *Pain* 1992;48:121–123.
122. Meyer B, Viscusi W, Durbin D. Workers compensation and injury duration: evidence from a natural experiment. *Am Econ Rev* 1995;85:322–340.
123. Miller H. Accident neurosis. *BMJ* 1961;1:919–925, 992–998.
124. Miller JH. Preliminary report on disability insurance to the Committee on Ways and Means of the US House of Representatives. Washington, DC: United States Government Printing Office, 1976.
125. Mitchell JN. Low back pain and the prospects for employment. *J Soc Occup Med* 1985;35:91–94.
126. Muramatsu N, Liang J, Sugisawa H. Transitions in chronic low back pain in Japanese older adults: a sociomedical perspective. *J Gerontol B Psychol Sci Soc Sci* 1997;52:S222–S234.
127. Nagi SZ, Hadley LW. Disability behavior: income chang and motivation to work. *Ind Labor Rel Rev* 1972;25:223–233.
128. Naidoo P, Pillay YG. Correlations among general stress, family environment, psychological distress, and pain experience. *Percept Motor Skills* 1994;78 [Spec Issue]:1291–1296.
129. NCCI Workers compensation back claim study. Florida: National Council on Compensation Insurance, 1992:1–25.
130. Norris SH, Watt I. The prognosis of neck injuries resulting from rear-end vehicle collisions. *J Bone Joint Surg Br* 1983;65:608–611.
131. Ostberg H, Samuelsson S-M. Occupational retirement in women due to age: health aspects. *Scand J Soc Med* 1994;22:90–96.
132. Papageorgiou AC, Macfarlane GJ, Thomas E, et al. Psychosocial factors in the workplace: do they predict new episodes of low back pain? *Spine* 1997;22:1137–1142.
133. Parsons T. *The social system.* New York: Free Press, 1951.
134. Payne B, Norfleet MA. Chronic pain and the family: a review. *Pain* 1986;26:1–22.
135. Peck CJ, Fordyce WE, Black RG. The effect of pendency of claims for compensation upon behavior indicative of pain. *Wash Law Rev* 1978;53:251–278.
136. Poole CJM. Retirement on grounds of ill health: cross sectional survey in six organisations in United Kingdom. *BMJ* 1997;314:929–932.
137. Reisbord LS, Greenland S. Factors associated with self-reported back pain prevalence: a population based study. *J Chronic Dis* 1985;38:691–702.
138. Ritchie J, Ward K, Duldig W. A qualitative study of the role of GPs in the award of invalidity benefit. Department of Social Security research report no. 18. London: Her Majesty's Stationery Office, 1993:1–72.
139. Robertson LS, Keeve JP. Worker injuries: the effect of workers' compensation and OSHA inspections. *Health Politics Policy Law* 1983;8:581–597.
140. Rohling ML, Binder LM, Langhinrichsen-Rohling J. Money matters: a meta-analytic review of the association between financial compensation and the experience and treatment of chronic pain. *Health Psychol* 1995;14:537–547.
141. Romano JM, Turner JA, Clancy SL. Sex differnces in the relationship of pain patient dysfunction to spouse adjustment. *Pain* 1989;39:289–295.
142. Romano JM, Turner JA, Friedman LS, et al. Sequential analysis of chronic pain behaviors and spouse responses. *J Consult Clin Psychol* 1992;60:777–782.
143. Romano JM, Turner JA, Jensen MP, et al. Chronic pain patient-spouse behavioral interactions predict patient disability. *Pain* 1995;63:353–360.
144. Rothenbacher D, Brenner H, Arndt V, et al. Disorders of the back and spine in construction workers: prevalence and prognostic value for disability. *Spine* 1997;22:1481–1486.
145. Ruser J. Workers compensation and the distribution of occupational injuries. *J Hum Res* 1993; 28:593–617.
146. Saarijarvi S, Rytokoski U, Karppi SL. Marital satisfaction and distress in chronic low-back pain patients and their spouses. *Clin J Pain* 1990;6:148–152.
147. Saarijarvi S, Hyyppa MT, Lehtinen V, et al. Chronic low back pain patient and spouse. *J Psychosom Res* 1990;34:117–122.
148. Sander RA, Meyers JE. The relationship of disability to compensation status in railroad workers. *Spine* 1986;11:141–143.

149. Sanderson PL, Todd BD, Holt GR, et al. Compensation, work status, and disability in low back pain patients. *Spine* 1995;20:554–556.
150. Schutt CH, Dohan FC. Neck injury to women in auto accidents: a metropolitan plague. *JAMA* 1968;206:2689–2692.
151. Schwartz L, Slater MA, Birchler GR. Interpersonal stress and pain behaviors in patients with chronic pain. *J Consult Clin Psychol* 1994;62:861–864.
152. Schwartz L, Slater MA, Birchler GR. The role of pain behaviors in the modulation of marital conflict in chronic pain couples. *Pain* 1996;65:227–233.
153. Schwartz L, Slater MA, Birchler GR, et al. Depression in spouses of chronic pain patients: the role of patient pain and anger, and marital satisfaction. *Pain* 1991;44:61–67.
154. Selander J, Marnetoft S-U, Bergroth A, et al. Unemployment among the long-term sick. *Eur J Phys Med Rehabil* 1996;6:150–153.
155. Selye H. *The physiology and pathology of exposure to stress.* Montreal: Acta, Inc, 1950.
156. Simmonds M, Kumar S. Does knowledge of a patient's workers' compensation status influence clinical judgments? *J Occup Rehabil* 1996;6:93–107.
157. Skovron ML, Szpalski M, Nordin M, et al. Sociocultural factors in back pain: a population based study in Belgian adults. *Spine* 1994;19:129–137.
158. Solomon P, Tunks E. The role of litigation in predicting disability outcomes in chronic pain patients. *Clin J Pain* 1991;7:300–304.
159. Straaton KV, Maisiak R, Wrigley JM, et al. Musculoskeletal disability, employment, and rehabilitation. *J Rheumatol* 1995;22:505–513.
160. Svensson H-O. Low back pain in forty to forty-seven year old men. II. Socio-economic factors and previous sickness absence. *Scand J Rehabil Med* 1982;14:55–60.
161. Szpalski M, Nordin M, Skovron ML, et al. Health care utilisation for low back pain in Belgium. *Spine* 1995;20:431–442.
162. Tait RC, Chibnall JT, Richardson WD. Litigation and employment status: effects on patients with chronic pain. *Pain* 1990;43:37–46.
163. Talo S, Hendler N, Brodie J. Effects of active and completed litigation on treatment results: workers' compensation patients compared with other litigation patients. *J Occup Med* 1989;31:265–269.
164. Tarsh MJ, Royston C. A follow-up study of accident neurosis. *Br J Psychiatry* 1985;146:18–25.
165. Taylor VM, Deyo RA, Ciol M, et al. Surgical treatment of patients with back problems covered by workers' compensation versus those with other sources of payment. *Spine* 1996;21:2255–2259.
166. Thomason T. The transition from temporary to permanent disability: the evidence from New York State. In: Durbin D, Borba PS, eds. *Workers compensation insurance: claims costs, prices and regulation.* Boston: Kluwer Academic, 1993:69–97.
167. Trief P, Stein N. Pending litigation and rehabilitation outcome of chronic low back pain. *Arch Phys Med Rehabil* 1985;66:95–99.
168. Trief P, Carnrike CLM, Drudge O. Chronic pain and depression: is social support relevant? *Psychol Rep* 1995;76:227–236.
169. Turk DC, Flor H, Rudy TE. Pain and families. I. Etiology, maintenance and psychosocial impact. *Pain* 1987;30:3–27.
170. Viikari-Juntura E, Vuori J, Silverstein BA, et al. A life-long prospective study on the role of psychosocial factors in neck-shoulder and low back pain. *Spine* 1991;16:1056–1061.
171. Volinn E. The epidemiology of low back pain in the rest of the world: a review of surveys in low and middle income countries. *Spine* 1997;22:1747–1754.
172. Volinn E, Koevering DV, Loeser JD. Back sprain in industry: the role of socioeconomic factors in chronicity. *Spine* 1991;16:542–548.
173. Volinn E, Lai D, McKinney S, et al. When back pain becomes disabling: a regional analysis. *Pain* 1988;33:33–39.
174. Waddell G. A new clinical model for the treatment of low back pain. *Spine* 1987;12:632.
175. Waddell G. *The back pain revolution.* Edinburgh: Churchill Livingstone, 1998.
176. Waddell G, Pilowsky I, Bond M. Clinical assessment and interpretation of abnormal illness behaviour in low back pain. *Pain* 1989;39:41–53.
177. Walsh K, Cruddas M, Coggon D. Low back pain in eight areas of Britain. *J Epidemiol Community Health* 1992;46:227–230.
178. Walsh NE, Dumitru D. The influence of compensation on recovery from low back pain. *Occup Med* 1988;3:109–121.
179. Weaver DA. The work and retirement decisions of older women: a literature review. *Soc Secur Bull* 1994;57:3–24.
180. Weighill VE, Buglass D. An updated review of compensation neurosis. *Pain Manage* 1989;2:100–105.
181. Wolff B, Langley S. Cultural factors and the response to pain: a review. *Am Anthropologist* 1968;70:494–501.
182. Wood DJ. Design and evaluation of a back injury prevention program within a geriatric hospital. *Spine* 1987;12:77–82.

183. Wood G, Morrison D, MacDonald S. Factors influencing the cost of workers' compensation claims: the effects of settlement method, injury characteristics, and demographics. *J Occup Rehabil* 1993;3:201–211.
184. Wood G, Morrison D, MacDonald S. Rehabilitation programs and return to work outcomes. *J Occup Health Safety Aust N Z* 1995;11:125–137.
185. Worrall JD. Compensation costs, injury rates and the labor market. In: Worral JD, ed. *Safety and the work force.* Ithaca, NY: ILR Press, Cornell University, 1983:1–17.
186. Worrall JD, Durbin D, Appel D, et al. The transition from temporary total to permanent partial disability: a longitudinal analysis. In: Durbin D, Borba PS, eds. *Workers compensation insurance: claims costs, prices and regulation.* Boston: Kluwer Academic, 1993:51–67.
187. Zabalza A, Pissarides C, Barton M. Social Security and the choice between full-time, part-time work and retirement. *J Public Economics* 1980;14:245–276.
188. Zborowski M. Cultural components in responses to pain. *J Soc Issues* 1952;8:16–30.

Neck and Back Pain: The Scientific Evidence of Causes, Diagnosis, and Treatment, edited by Alf Nachemson and Egon Jonsson. Published by Lippincott Williams & Wilkins, Philadelphia 2000.

3

Psychological Risk Factors for Neck and Back Pain

Steven J. Linton

Program for Behavioral Medicine, Department of Occupational and Environmental Medicine, Örebro Medical Center, Örebro, Sweden

Long-term pain from the spinal region is a common, debilitating problem associated with considerable suffering. Neck or back pain may result in functional problems, but it may also influence us psychologically, such as by triggering anxiety, fear, or a depressive mood. Likewise, psychologic factors may influence the way we perceive pain. For example, if we are anxious about seeing a dentist, this anxiety may lower our threshold for pain. As logical as this may seem, the inclusion of psychologic factors in consideration of neck and back pain is relatively new. However, modern views do underscore the multidimensional aspects of pain in which psychology is one of several factors that reciprocally interact. Consequently, the historical split between pain as purely psychologic and pain as purely physical now appears to be naive. As a result, inclusion of psychologic factors in an analysis of neck and back pain should expand our knowledge and should help to provide new ways of dealing with the problem that ultimately will benefit individual patients.

A multidimensional approach to the understanding of pain has gained acceptance, and it places psychologic factors firmly in the realm of pain research and practice. Although a great deal of research has been conducted, and many ideas have been put forth on the role of psychologic factors in neck and back pain, there is a need to review this work to ascertain our current knowledge. We may ask what the specific role of psychologic factors is in the origin and development of chronic neck and back pain. Indeed, psychologic variables have often been highlighted, particularly in chronic back pain. The question is how well these ideas are supported by the research facts. To enhance understanding of the material, a short introduction into the theory of psychologic processes in pain perception and behavior is presented.

AIM

The aim of this chapter is to review systematically the evidence concerning psychologic factors in neck and back pain. The following questions are posed: Is there evidence that psychologic variables are risk factors for neck and back pain? Have psychologic variables been shown to be involved in the etiology of these problems? Have psychologic variables been shown to be involved in the development of chronic problems?

PSYCHOLOGY OF PAIN

The role of psychologic factors in pain perception may be vividly underscored by imagining various painful events, such as bad scrapes or cuts. Each of these images may bring to mind unpleasant memories and negative emotions. Each may tend to be associated with specific adjectives. Yet these emotional reactions to pain are but one psychologic aspect. Taken together, psychologic factors are currently viewed as important determinants in pain perception and behavior. Indeed, our knowledge has expanded greatly since the days when pain associated with no apparent lesion was cast to the realms of psychology.

Today, psychologic processes are thought to play a central role in the complex process of attending to, interpreting, and reacting to noxious stimuli. The *gate-control theory of pain* is a landmark because it underscores the complexity of pain and expands pain from an entirely sensory phenomenon to a multidimensional one (55,68,71). The gate-control theory divides pain into sensory (physiologic), affective (motivational), and evaluative (cognitive) dimensions and thereby integrates physiologic and psychologic aspects. It laid the foundation for the biopsychosocial model (67,76). In fact, this model integrates peripheral stimuli with psychologic ones on the cortical level (e.g., depression or anxiety) in pain perception and emphasizes the idea that pain is an ongoing chain of events that are modifiable by ascending and, above all, descending activity in the central nervous system. Consequently, psychologic processes are not merely a reaction to pain, but they are an integral part of pain perception.

Research on neck and back pain problems then has attempted to explain specific aspects of the problem in relation to various psychologic factors. Although psychologic factors have often been considered as mere correlates of a pain problem, the relationship between psychologic factors and pain is extraordinarily complex. There is consequently reason to consider the possibility that psychologic variables are involved in the *process* of pain perception and behavior, and, therefore, in some cases and forms, may be causal. The difficult task of untangling the relationship between psychologic variables and pain has been a tedious one that remains incomplete. Even if a psychologic variable is not causally linked to a pain problem, it may be of help in controlling or alleviating the pain.

A Model

Various models of pain perception have evolved over the years, and each has stressed certain psychologic aspects. The interested reader will find an abundant literature on the subject (17,24,43,55,66). A basic model to aid in understanding the role of psychologic factors in pain perception is briefly presented here (14,65,70).

Pain may be said to consist of cognitive (sometimes labeled subjective), behavioral, and physiologic components that interact with, but do not necessarily correspond to, each other completely. As a result, there is reciprocal involvement such that these components mutually affect one another. For example, a trauma may significantly influence cognitive appraisal and the emotional reaction of hurt, which, in turn, may be expressed in behavior such as a verbal complaint and the taking of medication. Likewise, cognitions such as the belief that movement may cause further injury may influence both behavior (e.g., avoidance) and physiology (e.g., a stress reaction).

Psychologic variables may intervene at different places in the process of pain perception and behavior (44). Some factors may *predispose* a person, whereas others may act as a *trigger*, that is, may initiate the problem. Psychologic factors are often involved in maintaining or catalyzing the problem. Learning, for example, may result in lifestyle changes that appear adaptive, but that maintain the problem in the long run. Moreover, some factors, such as depression, may be related to *treatment prognosis*. Finally, *buffer factors* such as social support and active coping strategies may help people to withstand problems. Certain factors, such as anxiety or depression, may well be involved in several of these stages, whereas other variables may be specific to one stage.

Time is an important concept. The length of suffering is crucial for understanding the psychologic processes because cognition and behavior are greatly influenced by experience, that is, learning.

Figure 3.1 presents a "cross-sectional" view of pain perception featuring cognitions and learning (44). This model stresses the role of appraisal and beliefs that complement the roles of coping and learning. As the model illustrates, the first step is to attend to the noxious stimulus. This, in part, is controlled by psychologic factors, such as whether a person's attention is focused inward or outward. In the second step, an appraisal of the stimulus is made. This attribution is influenced by a host of psychologic factors and previous experience and is complicated. The noxious stimulus is given meaning and is evaluated, such as for whether it is harmful or unusual. This process, in turn, influences coping strategies, that is, the way we "plan" to deal with the pain. These cognitive processes, according to the model, are important prerequisites to the

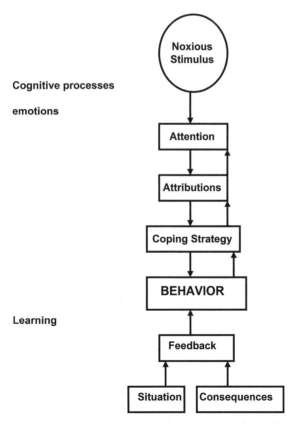

FIGURE 3.1. A model of pain perception depicting some important psychological factors including cognitions and behavior. (From Linton SJ. The role of psychological factors in back pain and its remediation. *Pain Rev* 1994; 1:231–243, with permission.)

next step, which is behavior. However, these cognitive processes are not always conscious "thought" and may occur automatically.

Learning factors operate and influence "pain" behaviors just as they do any other behavior (16,32–34,68,71). Consequently, behaviors designed to cope with a pain problem are influenced by the situation in which they occur, as well as by the consequences. Although the rules governing learning are specific and intricate, simply put, behaviors that successfully reduce or eliminate pain will tend to increase in frequency in similar situations. Similarly, behaviors that do not reduce the pain or that increase the pain will tend to decrease in frequency. An example of how learning may affect pain behaviors is the *avoidance paradigm*. In the first stage, respondent conditioning occurs, so stimuli such as a certain place, situation, or activity (e.g., lifting) elicit a response such as increased anxiety, fear, and muscle tension. In the second stage, this stimulus is experienced as a "threat" ("Please help me lift this piano"), and this sets the stage for an avoidance response. The behavioral response of avoiding the situation is reinforced by the consequences, that is, a reduction in anxiety, tension, and pain (42,74,77). This paradigm, moreover, is related to certain cognitions such as *catastrophizing,* in which the patient systematically exaggerates and makes negative interpretations. This paradigm has received considerable attention as a partial explanation of disability, and the term *fear-avoidance* has been coined.

REVIEW METHODOLOGY

Literature Search

To identify as many relevant articles as possible, three databases were searched. These were MEDLINE (1985 to September 1998), PsychInfo (1967 to September 1998) and ArbLine. The MEDLINE search strategy was to include articles about psychologic aspects and treatment of neck pain, back pain, or musculoskeletal pain. Because many of the psychologic factors are not believed to be disease specific, evidence regarding "mixed" populations were included when a substantial number of participants reported neck or back pain problems. Therefore, the following words were employed in the search: behavior or psychotherapy, adaptation, psychologic, probability, risk factors, predictors, prognosis, self-care, exercise therapy, back school, health education. The search was restricted to include randomized controlled trials, review articles, comparative studies, follow-up studies, prospective studies, evaluation studies, and clinical trials because all these may include risk factor analyses. This search resulted in 550 citations in MEDLINE. The PsychInfo strategy was similar and included back and neck pain and prevention, predictors, and risk factors, as well as treatment. This search produced 152 citations. A similar ArbLine search gave 14 citations.

Finally, articles and reviews were perused to identify additional relevant citations that may not be included in these database searches. In all, more than 900 articles were identified.

REVIEW PROCEDURE

This review is organized such that review articles in the literature are examined first, and then key articles, as well as articles published after the period covered in the reviews, are evaluated. Critical and systematic reviews were given precedence.

To ensure a relatively high level of quality, studies employing broad measures and a prospective design were given priority. Cross-sectional and case-control studies were secondary and were considered primarily if no prospective studies were available. Relevant studies using other designs provide important data, but they are subject to a host of bias factors. The criteria for inclusion ensure a minimum methodologic standard, although the level is more generous than some reviews that employ quality ratings.

A table of quality studies was subsequently constructed to provide an overview of the current data specific to neck and back pain. This table was used to summarize the best current information.

Finally, conclusions are based on the findings of the review articles in addition to the results of the tables. Each conclusion has been evaluated with regard to the level of evidence supporting it. A grading system has been employed in which level A evidence indicates support from a systematic review of good quality or two or more good-quality studies, whereas level B represents support from one or more randomized controlled trials or a good observational study. Level C means that data are insufficient or inconclusive, and level D means that no acceptable studies are available.

Limitations

Although every effort has been made to include all relevant articles and to appraise them in a fair and scientific way, there are several limitations to the present review. First, the search may not have identified all articles. Some journals are not, for example, included in the databases used in the search. Furthermore, because the area is not strictly defined, authors may not have used terms included in our search strategy. Consequently, some important articles may not have been identified.

A second problem involves the criteria for inclusion in the evaluation. Methodologic criteria have been suggested (64,72). However, although there is considerable agreement concerning the basic criteria, the exact weight of each aspect may be debated. Quality ratings were therefore not applied. Although this approach may lead to the inclusion of studies of questionable merit, the criteria employed do establish a basic and relatively high standard, but nevertheless avoid the problem of eliminating valuable studies because of low ratings.

Third, summarizing studies in tables inevitably results in the loss of information that may color interpretation. Thus, the investigation's aim and setting, for example, may become blurred even though these issues are important. Finally, studies summarized in tables tend to be evaluated simplistically, for example, as "positive" or "negative," although reality is considerably more complex. Conclusions may be drawn in a "box score" fashion that may not do justice to the differences between among. Taken together, these factors represent limitations that need to be considered when one reads the evaluation.

PSYCHOLOGIC RISK FACTORS

Psychologic factors may be related to the onset, development, and treatment outcome of neck and back pain problems. A large body of evidence examines the role of psychologic factors. However, the measures used and the study designs have varied greatly, thus making direct comparisons difficult (20,69,78). These problems may include selection bias, inappropriate comparison groups (design), inappropriate use of tests, intercorrelation of measures, and overinterpretation of correlational data. Moreover, some studies have included other categories of variables such as workplace factors, demographics, physical examinations, and lifestyle, whereas others have not.

Including these variables allows one to evaluate the *relative* effects of each factor, and therefore, the results may also be statistically adjusted to control for intercorrelations and the effects of other types of variables. Often, investigators have used a large number of psychosocial variables that may be suspected to be correlated. Thus, there are methodologic problems in collapsing these data to provide simple answers about whether a certain variable is "important." Further, the labeling of factors is usually arbitrary. Whether a factor is called "anxiety," "fear-avoidance," or "distress" depends on the authors' framework. A final point is the problem of using self-ratings for measuring both the independent and dependent variables. For example, some studies employ ratings of the perceived work environment as the independent variable and self-ratings of pain as the dependent variable. Because pain may also affect one's perception of work, using self-ratings as both the independent and the dependent variable introduces possible bias and may inflate risk estimates. Despite these difficulties, there is a need to evaluate critically the many studies conducted to date to ascertain the role of psychologic variables in neck and back pain.

REVIEW ARTICLES

Tremendous numbers of studies have implicated psychosocial variables as risk factors in the onset of acute neck or back pain, in the development of pain to a subacute or chronic state, or in treatment prognosis. Fortunately, several review articles are already available that summarize a large portion of these data and provide structure that, at least in part, takes into consideration the methodologic factors noted earlier.

Several review articles were identified and examined (2,3,13,17,18,19,20,28,30,35, 36,44,46,63,65,68,69,78). The reviews have different aims and methods, and there are considerable differences in approach that are reflected in the review method and conclusions drawn. For example, the reference lists of three reviews were compared (2,69,78). These references mirror both the articles considered in the review as well as the framework for the presentation. The Bigos review included 45 citations, but only 7 of these appeared in the Turk review, even though his reference list comprised no less than 130 references. Similarly, only 2 citations in the Weiser review, which included 97 publications, also appeared in the Bigos review. This finding points out important differences in how articles are retrieved as well as differences in aim and inclusion criteria. Two of the reviews listed earlier, for example, looked specifically at psychosocial factors, whereas Bigos et al. looked at all risk factors. Thus, it is important to examine several reviews carefully to obtain a picture of the effects of psychologic variables on neck and back pain. Let us examine the systematic reviews, as well as some key current studies.

Specific Reviews

Weiser and Cedraschi, 1992

Weiser and Cedraschi (78) reviewed the literature concerning psychosocial factors in chronic pain in which back pain has been the dominant focus. In particular, these investigators were interested in risk factors and conducted a systematic review, and a summary of their results is presented in Table 3.1 The search strategy is not described, but 16 predictive studies were identified.

These studies employed various populations including healthy (3), acute (4), recur-

TABLE 3.1. *A summary of significant psychosocial predictors of low back pain*

Study	Population		Prediction variables	Outcome
Barnes et al., 1988	Recurrent	−	Pain level	Return to work
		−	Depression	
		−	Premorbid pessimism	
		+	Cooperation scale	
		−	Hypochondriasis scale	
		+	Levels of compensation	
Bigos et al., 1991	Healthy	+	Hysteria	Report of back injury
		+	Psychopathy	
		+	Schizophrenia	
		+	Low back pain	
		−	Work perceptions	
Cats-Baril and Frymoyer, 1991	Acute	+	Job characteristics (including compensation)	Work status
Cauford et al., 1990	Acute	+	Life events	Onset of pain in patients "with a certain cause of pain," related to seeking treatment in patients with "specific diagnosis"
Deyo and Diehl, 1988	Acute	+	"Always feel sick"	Pain level Compensation seeking Number of visits to a physician
		−	"Always feel sick"	Physical + psychologic improvement
Hurri, 1989	Recurrent	+	Work satisfaction	Return to work Spontaneous recovery
Gallagher et al., 1989	Recurrent	−	Hysteria scale	Return to work
		+	Internal health locus of control	
Lacroix et al., 1990	Acute	−	Hysteria	Return to work
		−	Hypochondriasis scale	
		+	Patient's understanding of his back condition	
Leino, 1989	Healthy	+	Stress symptoms	Musculoskeletal complaints
		+	Musculoskeletal complaints	Stress symptoms
Leino and Lyyra, 1990	Healthy	+	Work stress	Musculoskeletal complaints in blue-collar workers
		−	Social support	
Polatin et al., 1989	Chronic	−	Pain intensity	Response to treatment
		−	Depression	
		−	Premorbid pessimism	
		+	Job characteristics	
Rosenstiel and Keefe, 1983	Chronic	+	Cognitive coping and suppression	Functional impairment
		−	Helplessness	Adjustment to pain
		+	Diverting attention or praying	Report of pain
Sandstrom and Esbjornsson, 1986	Recurrent	+	Beliefs about return to work	Return to work
Spinhoven and Linssen, 1991	Chronic	−	Perceived control as a coping strategy	Pain level
Turner et al., 1987	Chronic	+	Pain levels	Pain level
		+	Primary stress or coping responses	Functional capacity
Waddell et al., 1984	Chronic	+	Psychologic distress	Disability
		+	Inappropriate symptoms and signs	

+, significant positive relationship; −, significant negative relationship.
From Weiser S, Cedraschi C. Psychological issues of the prevention of chronic low back pain: a literature review. *Baillieres Clin Rheumatol* 1992;6:657–684, with permission.

TABLE 3.2. *A summary table from the Turk review*

Predicted		Failed to Predict
History of anxiety, depression, psychologic distress, psychologic care		
Frymoyer et al., 1980 Frymoyer et al., 1983 Frymoyer et al., 1985 Vallfors, 1985		Lanier and Stockton, 1988 Leavitt, 1990 Leino and Magni, 1993
Anxiety/fear avoidance		
Murphy and Cornish, 1984 Sandstrom & Esbjornsson, 1986 Philips et al., 1991 Dworkin et al., 1992	Waddell et al, 1993 Klenerman et al., 1995 Williams et al., 1995	Gatchel et al., 1995a Gatchel et al., 1995b
Current depression		
Frymoyer and Cats-Baril, 1987 Bigos et al., 1991 Dworkin et al., 1992 Leino and Magni, 1993 Magni et al., 1993	Von Korff et al., 1993 Magni et al., 1994 Weickgenant et al., 1994 Williams et al., 1995	Lehmann et al., 1993 Gatchel et al., 1995a Gatchel et al., 1995b
Lassitude, malaise, loneliness		
Derebery and Tulis, 1983 Sander and Meyers, 1986 Haddad, 1987 Deyo and Diehl, 1988	Greenough and Fraser, 1989 Bigos et al., 1991 Fordyce et al., 1992 Gatchel et al., 1995a,b	Lacroix et al., 1990
Personality disorders		
Gatchel et al., 1995 (at 6 months)		Gatchel et al., 1995a (at 12 months)
Alcohol and substance abuse		
Sandstrom et al., 1984 Vallfors, 1985 Frymoyer and Cats-Baril, 1987 Greenwood et al., 1990	Atkinson et al., 1991 Polatin et al., 1993 Williams et al., 1995	
Maladaptive coping		
Lancourt and Kettelhut, 1992 Hasenbring et al., 1994 Linton et al., 1994 Weickgenant et al., 1994	Burton et al., 1995 Klenerman et al., 1995 Linton and Buer, 1995	
Passive cognition		
Philips et al., 1991	Linton and Buer, 1995	
Back pain		
Bergquist-Ullman, 1977 Biering-Sorensen, 1983 Singer et al., 1987 Feuerstein and Thebarge, 1991 Radanov et al., 1991	Lancourt and Kettelhut, 1992 Potter and Jones, 1992 Tate, 1992 Weickgenant et al., 1994 Gatchel et al., 1995a	Murphy and Cornish, 1984 Hellsing et al., 1994
Perceived stress/stressful life events		
Frymoyer et al., 1980 Feuerstein et al., 1985 Vallfors, 1985 Greenwood et al., 1990	Feuerstein and Thebarge, 1991 Lancourt and Kettelhut, 1992 Klenerman et al., 1995	

TABLE 3.2. Continued

Predicted		Failed to Predict
Heightened somatic concern		
Klenerman et al., 1995		
Disease conviction		
Cats-Baril and Frymoyer, 1991 Dworkin et al., 1992	Hazard et al., 1996	Murphy and Cornish, 1984
Perceptions of poor health		
Biering-Sorenson, 1986 Deyo and Diehl, 1988	Linton et al., 1994 Linton and Buer, 1995	
Perceived severity of illness or disability		
Tait et al., 1988 Lacroix et al., 1990	Feuerstein and Thebarge, 1991 Hazard et al., 1996	Lehmann et al., 1993
Job dissatisfaction		
Westrin et al., 1972 Bergquist-Ullman and Larsson, 1977 Frymoyer and Cats-Baril, 1987 Bigos et al., 1991	Cats-Baril and Frymoyer, 1991 Skovron et al., 1994 Williams et al., 1995	Lehmann et al., 1993

From Turk DC. The role of demographic and psychosocial factors in transition from acute to chronic pain. In: Jensen TS, Turner JA, Wiesenfeld-Hallin Z, eds. *Proceedings of the 8th World Congress on Pain, Progress in Pain Research and Management,* vol 8. Seattle: IASP Press, 1997, with permission.

rent (4), and chronic (5) samples. As shown in Table 3.1, various factors have been found to be related to outcome, and outcome in itself has been measured in several ways. These investigators found that psychologic distress as measured by questionnaires and personality inventories (e.g., traits seen in the Minnesota Multiphasic Personality Inventory [MMPI]) are related to outcome. Patients with acute pain who are preoccupied with their symptoms and are depressed and anxious fare more poorly than others. Cognitive factors such as coping and illness beliefs were related to recovery in chronic sufferers, and some evidence was found for a relationship in the development of the problem. Job satisfaction and stress were also found to be related to outcome. The authors underscored the need for methodologic rigor and multicausal models to explain the development and maintenance of chronic problems. This review provides a good overview of the field, but some publications have since appeared, and the review does not specify inclusion criteria.

Turk, 1997

A specific review of the role of psychosocial factors in the transition from acute to chronic pain was reported by Turk (69). Most of these studies deal with low back pain, but the criteria for including studies were not reported. Table 3.2 summarizes the results of Turk's review.

Pain severity at the time of acute onset was found to be a significant predictor of later pain and disability in 10 of 12 studies concerning back pain. Because pain is subjective and is influenced certain factors other than disease, it was considered a psychosocial variable.

The terms *distress* and *affective distress* refer to psychobiologic and emotional reactions. A history of anxiety, depression, or psychologic treatment was weakly established as a risk factor (Table 3.2), but anxiety, fear, and depression at the time of acute pain were clearly related to the development of chronic problems in certain well-conducted studies. Psychologic distress of a less dramatic type, such as evidenced by loneliness, lassitude (fatigue, lack of interest), or malaise (bodily discomfort), was also shown to predict the development of chronic pain in 9 studies. Substance abuse was shown to be related to the transition from acute to chronic pain in 7 studies, and Turk found no study contradicting this relationship. Maladaptive coping strategies and passive cognitions were also related to chronicity in all the studies located. Perceived stress was found to be related to the development of long-term problems in 7 studies. Finally, various forms of concern about poor health were shown to be related to chronicity of pain in 12 of the 14 studies reviewed.

The only psychosocial workplace factor included in Turk's review was job dissatisfaction. He found that seven of eight studies reported a predictive relationship between job dissatisfaction and the development of chronicity.

Turk pointed out certain factors that may help to explain some of the discrepancies in findings. These include the sample composition and size, severity of the injury or disease, measures of predictors, time of outcome, outcome criteria, study design, and possible treatment received between initial assessment and outcome. He also emphasized the difficulties in simply aggregating studies that have addressed this field.

Despite the inherent difficulties in comparing studies, Turk asserted that some conclusions may be drawn. These include the following:

1. Psychosocial factors are better predictors of chronicity than are clinical or physical factors.
2. Studies of risk factors often account for limited amounts of variability, a finding underscoring the complexity of pain and the outcomes being predicted.
3. "Clearly, chronicity is determined by many factors that interact in a reciprocal way across time." A list of such variables includes pain severity, emotional distress, substance abuse, anxiety and depression, perceived stress, coping resources, social support, job satisfaction, and perceived health.

Bongers et al., 1993

A closer look at psychosocial factors at work was provided by Bongers and associates (3). Although psychosocial work factors are reviewed in Chapter 5, this review is included briefly to provide a broad picture including workplace factors. These authors searched OSH_ROM, CIS-DOC, PsychInfo, and MEDLINE for articles analyzing the relationship between musculoskeletal disorders and psychosocial factors at work (demands and control, social support, individual characteristics, stress, and physical and behavioral health indicators). Only studies related to factors at work and the development of problems were reviewed, and thus prognostic studies, as well as those of factors outside work, were excluded. Finally, some sort of comparison group was required. Cross-sectional studies were analyzed separately from longitudinal and prospective studies because the latter have a stronger design. In all, these investigators analyzed 44 cross-sectional and 15 longitudinal studies; some of these studies reported on more than one pain location and are therefore included in more than one area. Of these studies, 22 adjusted their results for physical load.

The review by Bongers et al. found that the results for back, neck, and musculoskeletal pain (not specified or mixed) were surprisingly similar. Thirty studies that included data on back pain were found in their review, and 9 of these studies were prospective. By comparison, 15 studies reporting on neck pain were found, and 5 of these employed prospective designs. Because the authors concluded that the results were similar regardless of pain site, an overview of the result is presented (by them) in Table 3.3, in which they also have taken consideration of the weight of the evidence. They found that the

TABLE 3.3. *Summary of the epidemiologic evidence for the relationship between psychosocial factors, personal characteristics, stress, and musculoskeletal disease*

	Cross-sectional studies (N)	Longitudinal studies (N)	BP	NP/SP	MP	Total
Psychosocial factors at work: demands and control	28	2	+/−	?	+	+
Monotonous work			+	+	+	+
Time pressure			+/−	+	+	+
High concentration			−	?	?	?
High responsibility			−	?	−	?
Poor work content			+	+	?	+/−
High workload			?	+/−	+	+
Lack of clarity			?	?	−	?
Few opportunities to take breaks			−	?	−	−
Low control, autonomy			?	?	+	+
Psychosocial factors at work: social support	15	2	+	+/−	+	+
Poor social support by colleagues			+	+/−	+	+
Poor social support by superiors			?	+/−	+	+/−
Demand and support variables combined			+	+	?	+
Individual characteristics	15	9	+/−	?	?	?
Neuroticism			+/−	?	?	?
Type A behavior			+	+	+	+
Extrovert personality			?	−	?	?
Depression			+/−	?	?	?
Coping styles			−	?	?	?
Attitude toward own health			+/−	?	+	+
Low social class			+/−	−	?	−
Low educational level			+/−	+/−	?	+/−
Stress symptoms	24	8	+	+	+	+
Worry, tension, anxiety, nervousness			+	+	+	+
Physical stress symptoms			+	?	?	?
Tiredness and exhaustion			+/−	?	?	+/−
High perceived work stress			+	+	+	+
Low job satisfaction			+/−	+/−	?	+/−
Physiologic parameters			?	?	?	?
Physical and behavioral health indicators	8	8	+	?	?	+
Poor physical health			+	?	?	+
Respiratory disease or cough			+	?	?	+
Stomach trouble			+	?	?	+
Cardiovascular disease			+/−	?	?	+/−
Headache			+/−	?	?	+/−
Use of medication			+	?	?	+
Use of medical services			+	?	?	+

+, positive evidence for an association; −, association absent, +/−, conflicting data; ?, too little information; BP, back pain; MP, symptoms of the musculoskeletal system, no location specified (neck or shoulder and back or all musculoskeletal sites); NP/SP, neck or shoulder pain.

From Bongers PM, de Winter CR, Kompier MA, et al. Psychosocial factors at work and musculoskeletal disease. *Scand J Work Environ Health* 1993;19:297–312.

studies support a relationship between pain and job demands, job control, monotonous work, perceived workload, and work under time pressure. Lack of social support and low control were also concluded to be risk factors.

Family Factors

One potentially important area not included in the foregoing reviews because prospective studies were not found is the *family*. Although there are no prospective studies, Bradley and associates (4) reviewed the evidence on the role of the family and pointed out that family members may be influential in three ways. First, family members may be models for illness and health behaviors, particularly for children. Second, family members may provide important reinforcement for sick behavior. Third, physical and/or sexual abuse may increase the risk for developing pain problems, although the exact mechanism is not clear. Abuse has been suggested to be a risk factor for a variety of pain problems (4). More recently, it has been linked to musculoskeletal pain problems, in particular back pain (10,50,80).

It has been extraordinarily difficult to establish a firm link between abuse and neck and back pain, given the sensitive nature of the variable and the large number of possible confounding variables such as substance abuse, social class, and education. Ethical, practical, and sensitivity problems have preempted prospective studies. Nevertheless, a population-based study shed some light on the relationship because this investigation compared those having no back or neck pain (n = 449) with those having mild pain (n = 229) and those having more pronounced pain (n = 271) (45). The rate of reported abuse was much lower for men than for women; however, the increased risk for having pronounced pain for men reporting sexual abuse was slightly increased, but the confidence interval fell below unity (odds ratio [OR], 1.56; confidence interval [CI], 73–3.38).

For women, conversely, the report of abuse was associated with a fourfold increase in the risk of reporting pronounced pain (OR, 4.2; CI, 2.39–7.36). Similar results were found for physical abuse. Thus, there is some evidence that sexual or physical abuse is related to the development of more pronounced or chronic problems.

SUMMARY AND EVALUATION OF KEY STUDIES

To complement the reviews already conducted, prospective, English-language articles published in international journals that have examined the relationship between psychosocial factors and neck or back pain were selected (Table 3.4). These studies represent a body of well-conducted investigations that shed light on the most recent developments in the field. Nevertheless, the variables included and the populations studied are unique for each study. The search for prospective studies located 36 investigations (Table 3.4).

Various "personality" factors such as traits on the MMPI were measured in eight studies (2,21–23,25,59,61,73). However, although four studies found a significant relationship, four did not. No support was found for a "pain-prone" personality. The significant findings seemed related to personality disorders, as noted by Gatchel et al. (21), in whose study axis I personality disorders involving depression and anxiety emerged. This is consistent with findings described later concerning an individual's psychologic functioning.

Stress, distress, or anxiety was reported on in 11 investigations (5,8,12,21,37,38,41, 49,53,54,58). All 11 studies found a significant relationship, although the study by Estlander et al. (12) found only a weak relationship.

Mood and depression were investigated in 16 reports in Table 3.4 (7,9,11,12,26,31,37, 41,49,51,52,53,54,59,60,75). Fourteen of these studies reported reliable relationships indicating that depressed mood increases the risk of pain problems.

Cognitive functioning, including fear-avoidance beliefs and coping strategies, were reported on in nine investigations (5,26,27,37,47,49,58,60,61). Eight of these studies have found a significant relationship.

Finally, pain behavior and function were studied as risk factors in seven studies (21, 26,29,38,49,56,79). Six of these studies reported a significant relationship suggesting that high levels of pain behavior and dysfunction serve as a risk factor for future back pain problems.

Example Studies

Three prospective studies may serve as detailed illustrations of current research employing prospective designs. Burton and associates (5) studied 252 consecutive patients with a new episode of low back pain and followed them 1 year. At consultation, patients received a standardized clinical examination, and an interview history was taken. A battery of questionnaires said to measure pain experience, disability, distress, pain beliefs, fear-avoidance, and coping strategies was also obtained. Patients were then treated in a standard manner. One year later, participants completed a questionnaire measuring pain and disability, and the outcome measure was disability (Roland and Morris disability score). Multiple regression analyses were used to deal with the large numbers of data, and possible intercorrelations and models were developed for all patients, those with acute, as well as those with subacute pain at initial presentation. The psychologic variables were by far the most potent predictors in each of these three models. The analysis for acute pain provided the best prediction because 69% of the variance was accounted for by five variables: the catastrophizing coping strategy, somatic distress, straight leg raising, the hoping and praying coping strategy, and leg pain. The authors concluded that the results ". . . show that the psychologic status of the patient at presentation has a much stronger influence on outcome than does conventional clinical information." Catastrophizing, for example, was found to be seven times more important than the best clinical or historical variables.

Klenerman and associates (37) studied 300 patients with acute low back pain and made assessments again at 2 and at 12 months. These investigators assessed a variety of medical and psychosocial entities. They found that patients who had not recovered by 2 months were likely to develop chronic pain. Multiple regression was used to isolate predictors, and psychologic factors were found to be highly related to outcome. In fact, clusters of measures they labeled "fear-avoidance" were the best predictors of pain and disability at 12 months. These variables alone correctly classified 66% of the sample, whereas using all variables increased the accuracy to 88%.

A 10-year follow-up study of employees shed light on the role of psychologic factors in back pain (40). Questionnaires and a clinical examination were administered at the Valmet engineering factories in Jyväskylä, Finland. A total of 411 subjects completed both pretest and 10-year follow-up evaluations. At pretest, the psychosocial variables, especially "mental overstrain" and physical workload, were all found to be related to pain, as well as clinical findings made by a physical therapist. Prospectively, the score on

TABLE 3.4. *Prospective-longitudinal studies of psychosocial risk factors from 1991 to present*

Study (ref.)	Population	Design	Predictors	Outcome	Comments
Bigos et al., 1991 (1)	3,020 (1,223 participated, Boeing workers, 22% female)	Prospective 3 yr	Enjoyment of work: −; MMPI(hys): +; Work relation: − (1 + 2 best predictors)	Reported injury	Study controlled for other factors
Burton et al., 1995 (5)	252 LBP, primary care; 48% female	Prospective 1 yr	Distress: +; Catastrophizing: +; Pain intensity: +; Praying/hoping: +; Dysfunction: +	Disability (Roland and Morris)	Strong design. 76% correctly classified; psychosocial factors better predictors than standard medical/history variables
Cats-Baril et al., 1991 (6)	252 patients, new episode LBP; % female not stated	Prognostic 3 and 6 mo	Work, i.e., satisfaction, status: −; Perceived injury as compensable: −	Working	Predictive model with psychosocial factors correctly predicts 89%
Cherkin et al., 1996 (7)	219 primary care patients LBP; % female ??	Prospective ?? mo	Educational level: −; Depression: +	Symptom satisfaction	
Croft et al., 1996 (8)	4,501 (same as above)	Prospective 12 mo	Distress: −	New episodes of pain	1.8 increase even when bias factors controlled
Dionne et al., 1997 (9)	569 primary care, LBP; % female ??	Prospective ??? mo	Somatization: +; Depression: +	Disability	?
Engel et al., 1996 (11)	1,059 primary care, LBP; 53% female	Prospective 12 mo	Depression: +; Pain: +	Costs	Pain status and disc disorders strong predictors, depression also predicted high costs
Estlander et al., 1998 (12)	452 forestry-industry workers with neck, shoulder or back pain	Prospective 24 mo	Distress: 0; Depression: 0; Self-efficacy: 0; Work prognosis: 0; Disability: +; Work characteristics: 0	Change in pain status	Distress, self-efficacy, depression, and work prognosis were significant in univariate analyses; all had pain at baseline
Fishbain et al., 1997 (15)	128 patients with back pain > 6 mo 57% female	Prospective 30 mo (work assessed retrospectively)	Gender: +; Intent to work: +; Job stress: +; Age: +; Education: +; Belief that work is dangerous: +	Work status	75% correctly classified at 30 mo
Gatchel et al., 1994 (23)	152 chronic LBP; 36% female	Prospective prognosis 12 mo	Psychopathology: 0	Return to work	If psychopathology is addressed, it does not affect outcome

Study	Population	Design	Predictors	Outcome	Comments
Gatchel, 1995 (21)	324 acute LBP; 36% female	Prospective 6 mo	Pain and disability score: + Axis I depression, anxiety, substance abuse disorders: 0 Axis II personality disorder: + MMPI Hys: +	Return to work	Pain and disability important predictors even when injury severity and work controlled for; 87% correctly classified
Gatchel et al., 1995 (22)	421 patients with acute back pain; 38% female	Prospective 3, 6, 9, 12 mo	Pain and disability: − Psychopathology: 0 MMPI: −	Job status	91% correctly classified robust psychologic factor psychopathology does not predispose MMPI not related to a new episode
Hansen et al., 1995 (25)	673 general population; 43% female	Prospective 10 and 20 yr	MMPI: 0	Back pain	
Hasenbring et al., 1994 (26)	111 acute disc prolapse; 38% female	Prognostic 6 mo	Depression: + Avoidance: + Nonverbal pain behavior: + Search of social support: +	Pain intensity, recurrence, early retirement	Psychosocial variables correctly classified 70%, whereas all variables classified = 86%; psychosocial variables most important
Hazard et al., 1996 (27)	166 LBP injury report; % female not stated	Prospective measure within 15 d, 3-mo outcome	Pain intensity: + Job demands: + Perceived future problem: + Relations at work: + Perceived chance of work at 6 months: + Blame: +	Working	11 questions were good predictors. 94% sensitivity, 84% specificity
Hellsing et al., 1994 (29)	121 acute neck/back pain; 48% female	Prospective 1 yr	Additional function: 0 Pain intensity: 0 Monotonous work: + Depression: +	Sick leave	
Junge et al., 1995 (31)	164 secondary care, LBP; % female ??	Prospective ??		Response to surgery	
Klenerman et al., 1995 (37)	300 acute LBP; 50% female	Prospective measures at 1 and 8 wk to predict 12 mo	Fear-avoidance beliefs: + Psychosocial variables (distress, experienced disability, depression, pain intensity): +	Pain and disability, sick leave	66% correctly classified with only fear-avoidance variables, 88% with all variables
Lehmann et al., 1993 (39)	55 acute LBP; 33% female	Prospective 6 mo	Pain: 0 Job satisfaction/work: 0 History: 0 Function: 0	Time to return to work	Small N provides limited power
Leino and Hänninen, 1995 (40)	902 workers; 32% female	Prospective 10 yr	Work content: − Work control: 0 Work relationships: − Mental strain: −/0	Symptoms or physical therapy examination	Psychosocial factors were predictive even when age, gender, class, and workload were controlled

TABLE 3.4. Continued

Study (ref.)	Population	Design	Predictors	Outcome	Comments
Leino and Magni, 1993 (41)	607 employees; 36% female	Prospective 3-, 5-yr periods	Depressive symptoms: + Distress: +	Musculoskeletal pain	Effects of depression were general as they predicted pain at various sites
Linton et al., 1999 (47)	449 pain-free general population; 49% female	Prospective 1 yr	Fear-avoidance: + Catastrophizing: +	New episode of spinal pain, activity hindered	Fear-avoidance produce an OR = 2.04 for pain, whereas catastrophizing was 1.5
Linton and Halldén, 1998 (49)	142 acute spinal pain; 65% female	Prospective 6 mo	Work: − Pain: + Fear-avoidance: + Activities of daily living: − Coping: 0 Job satisfaction: − Perceived future: − Stress/anxiety: + Mood: −	Pain, function, sick leave	The best predictors for sick leave were fear-avoidance, perceived future pain, perceived work function, stress, and earlier sick leave
Magni et al., 1993 (51)	2,341 general population (representative 25–74 yr olds); 57% female	Prospective 8 yr	Depression: +	Chronic pain	Depression increased the risk for MSP by two- to threefold
Magni et al., 1994 (52)	2,324; 57% female	Prospective 8 yr	Depression: +	Chronic pain	Depression related to pain (OR = 2.14) and pain related to depression (OR = 2.85)
Main et al., 1992 (53)	567 patients with LBP referred to orthopedic clinic (107 included in follow-up); 51% female	Prognosis 1–4 yr	Depression: + Distress (MSPQ): + DRAM: +	Disability	Scores on DRAM highly related to future disability
Mannion et al., 1996 (54)	403 volunteers, no pain; 92% female	Prospective 6, 12, 18 mo	Distress: + Depression: + Health locus of control: 0	Back pain, pain-absenteeism, consultation	Distress and depression were good predictors, but presence at beginning so not causal
Öhlund et al., 1996 (56)	103 patients LBP, subacute	Prospective prognosis	Pain drawing: +	Return to work	
Papageorgiou et al., 1997 (57)	4,501 general population; 55% females	Prospective 12 mo	Three questions: 1. Job satisfaction: − 2. Relations at work: 0 3. Sufficient money: −	New episode of back pain	Dissatisfied were twice as likely to experience a new episode

72

Study	Sample	Design	Variables	Pain status	Comments
Philips & Grant, 1991 (58)	117 acute back; 57% female	Measures at pre-3 and 6 mo	Pain intensity: + Pain quality: + Negative cognitions: + Anxiety: + Impact (SIP): +	Pain status	80% correctly classified
Pietri-Taleb et al., 1994 (59)	1,015 men; <7 d neck pain	3 yr	Hysteria: + Neuroticism: + Depression: +	Severe neck pain	Complex interaction between occupation and results; other parts of Maudsley and Mid-dlesex not significant
Potter & Jones, 1992 (60)	45 patients at 4 wk pain female; % not stated	Prospective followed 26 wk	Pain intensity: + Depression: +	Pain	
Radanov et al., 1994 (61)	117 whiplash	Longitudinal 3, 6, 12 mo	Passive coping: + Personality: 0 Cognitive failure: 0	Symptoms	Personality nor psychoneuro-logic variables did not predict outcome
Viikari-Juntura et al., 1991 (73)	154 general population; 47% female	Prospective measures taken in adolescence	Intelligence: 0 Alexithymia: 0 Social confidence: 0	Neck or back pain as adult (M = 37 yrs)	Personality etc. in childhood did not predict future problem
Von Korff et al., 1993 (75)	803 health maintenance organization enrollees	Prospective 3 yr	Depression: 0 Number of pain conditions: +	Back pain onset	Depression related to chest and headache pain, but not directly to back pain onset; number of pain sites was pre-dictive
Werneke et al., 1993 (79)	183 LBP patients off work; 33% female	Prognostic 3 mo	Behavioral signs test: −	Return to work	All 8 behavioral signs signifi-cantly higher for the "failed" group at discharge

+, positive relationship; −, negative relationship; 0, no relationship; DRAM, Distress and Risk Assessment Method; LBP, low back pain; MMPI, Minnesota Multiphasic Personality Inventory; MSPQ, Modified Somatic Perception Questionnaire; SIP, Sickness Impact Profile.

social relations at work produced the most consistent relationship with musculoskeletal morbidity. Poor satisfaction with social relationships at work was an antecedent to pain symptoms and findings. For blue collar workers, pain was also predicted by work content, work control, and "mental overstrain." Interestingly, physical load was not associated with morbidity. The findings were similar regardless of anatomic region, and this led the authors to suggest a general musculoskeletal reactivity to psychosocial factors. Psychosocial work factors were then found to be related to and predicted musculoskeletal problems including neck and back pain.

The data on risk factors have been applied such that attempts at identifying people "at risk" have been made. This is one "gold standard" test of whether the risk factors identified are actually important. (The other method is modification of risks that lead to improvements.) At least four attempts have been made to develop a screening procedure to identify people at risk for developing long-term problems. Main (53) developed a questionnaire based on measures of depression and distress (DRAM) and showed that it accurately identified patients seeking orthopedic care who were at risk of a poor outcome. Gatchel (21) employed a battery of instruments with patients seeking help for acute back pain in primary care and followed them 6 months to determine return-to-work status. They found that scores on a pain and disability measure, personality disorders, and scale 3 (Hys) of the MMPI were important factors that correctly classified 87% of the patients.

The Vermont Screening Questionnaire (27) consists of 11 systematically selected questions and is oriented toward predicting future compensation among people filing an injury report. A study of 163 people assessed within 15 days of having filed an injury report had 94% sensitivity and 84% specificity in identifying those with long-term disability. However, this study only predicted absenteeism in a group filing an injury claim, and the study suffered from a large dropout or refusal rate.

As a final example, a screening questionnaire has been developed based on a variety of psychosocial risk factors and includes 24 items covering background, function, fear-avoidance beliefs, pain experience, work, and reactions to pain (48,49). The questionnaire was tested on 137 consecutive primary care patients with acute or subacute neck and/or back pain problems. A median split of the total score demonstrated a sensitivity of 87% and a specificity of 75% for three classes of sickleave outcome, whereas chance would be 33%.

The studies on screening all show significantly higher levels of classification than chance. Although the levels are surprisingly high given the nature of the problem, they are still rough estimates, and several possible problems may be encountered when dealing with patients in clinical settings. Furthermore, the studies thus far have not tested the instruments on new, independent populations in whom we may expect the accuracy to decrease. Nevertheless, these data suggest that screening questionnaires employing psychosocial variables may be a valuable tool in the identification of patients at risk for developing long-term disability.

CONCLUSIONS ABOUT RISK FACTORS BASED ON THE EVIDENCE

The following conclusions are based primarily on the evaluation of the prospective studies in Table 3.4. However, the published reviews summarized earlier were also considered. The authors of the various reviews drew similar conclusions, although the degree varied. This finding indicates good consistency. The following conclusions have been derived, and the level of evidence indicated as described earlier and in Chapter 1:

1. There is strong evidence that psychosocial variables are strongly linked to the transition from acute to chronic pain disability: level A evidence.
2. There is strong evidence that psychologic factors can be associated to the reporting of the onset of back and neck pain: level A evidence.
3. There is strong evidence that psychosocial variables generally have more impact than biomedical or biomechanical factors on back pain disability: level A evidence.
4. There is no evidence to support the idea of a "pain-prone" personality, and the results are mixed with regard to personality and personality traits as risk factors: level C evidence.
5. There is strong evidence that attitudes, cognitions, and fear-avoidance beliefs are strongly related to the development of pain and disability: level A evidence.
   a. There is strong evidence that passive coping is strongly related to pain and disability: level A evidence.
   b. There is strong evidence that pain cognitions such as catastrophizing are strongly related to pain and disability: level A evidence.
   c. There is little evidence concerning acute pain: level C evidence.
6. There is strong evidence that depression, anxiety, distress, and related emotions are strongly related to pain and disability: level A evidence.
7. There is limited evidence that sexual and/or physical abuse may be related to chronic pain and disability: level C evidence.
8. There is evidence that poor self-perceived health is moderately related to chronic pain and disability: level A evidence.
9. There is evidence that psychosocial factors are moderate predictors for long-term pain and disability Level A/B evidence.

Implications

The results of this review suggest the need for major changes in the way in which we view and clinically deal with neck and back pain disability. The data clearly show that psychosocial factors are important not only in the development of long-term disability resulting from neck and back pain, but also in the earliest stages. Consequently, approaches to prevention, initial treatment, and rehabilitation may benefit from incorporating this knowledge into practice. The research indicates that psychosocial factors are not simply an "overlay," but rather they are an integral part of the pain disability process that includes emotional, cognitive, and behavioral aspects. Because psychosocial factors were found to have more impact on disability than biomedical variables, treatment and preventive approaches that only address biomedical factors may be questionable. Rather, psychosocial factors may need to become a normal part of a comprehensive assessment and treatment routine even in patients with early neck and back pain. Including psychosocial factors in medical practice may give insight into the patient's problem and may provide new avenues for treatment and management. Moreover, preventive efforts may benefit greatly from incorporating these factors into their programs.

RESEARCH NEEDS

- Research that delves into the mechanisms by which psychologic factors affect pain and disability, that is, how these factors work.

- Development and testing of theories that incorporate and integrate psychologic risk factors, that is, why they are important.
- Screening instruments to use the risk factors for early identification of patients at risk of developing chronic problems.
- Development of assessment techniques for clinical and research purposes.
- Research into the actual process of the development of long-term pain and disability, that is, longitudinal studies that provide insight into critical aspects of this development.

REFERENCES

1. Bigos SJ, Battié MC, Spengler DM, et al. A prospective study of work perceptions and psychosocial factors affecting the report of back injury. *Spine* 1991;16:1–6.
2. Bigos S, Holland J, Webster M, et al. A methodological literature analysis concerning prevention and risks of reporting back injury claims and complaints at work. Presented at the Orthopaedic Research Foundation, Chicago, 1996.
3. Bongers PM, de Winter CR, Kompier MA, et al. Psychosocial factors at work and musculoskeletal disease. *Scand J Work Environ Health* 1993;19:297–312.
4. Bradley LA, McDonald-Haile J, Jaworski TM. Assessment of psychological status using interviews and self-report instruments. In: Turk DC, Melzack R, eds. *Handbook of pain assessment.* New York: Guilford Press, 1992.
5. Burton AK, Tillotson KM, Main CJ, et al. Psychosocial predictors of outcome in acute and subchronic low back trouble. *Spine* 1995;20:722–728.
6. Cats-Baril WL, Frymoyer JW. Identifying patients at risk of becoming disabled because of low-back pain: the Vermont Rehabilitation Engineering Center predictive model. *Spine* 1991;16:605–607.
7. Cherkin DC, Deyo RA, Street JH, et al. Predicting poor outcome for back pain seen in primary care using patients' own criteria. *Spine* 1996;21:2900–2907.
8. Croft PR, Papageorgiou AC, Ferry S, et al. Psychologic distress and low back pain: evidence from a prospective study in the general population. *Spine* 1996;20:2731–2737.
9. Dionne CE, Koepsell TD, Von Korff M, et al. Predicting long-term functional limitations among back pain patients in primary care settings. *J Clin Epidemiol* 1997;50:31–43.
10. Drossman DA, Leserman J, Nachman G, et al. Sexual and physical abuse in women with functional or organic gastrointenstinal disorders. *Ann Intern Med* 1990;113:828–833.
11. Engel CC, von Korff M, Katon WJ. Back pain in primary care: predictors of high health-care costs. *Pain* 1996;65:197–204.
12. Estlander AM, Takala EP, Viikari-Juntura E. Do psychological factors predict changes in musculoskeletal pain: a prospective, two-year follow-up study of a working population. *J Occup Environ Med* 1998;40:445–453.
13. Evans G, Richards S. *Low back pain: an evaluation of therapeutic interventions.* Bristol, UK: Health Care Evaluation Unit, University of Bristol, 1996.
14. Feuerstein M, Beattie P. Biobehavioral factors affecting pain and disability in low back pain: mechanisms and assessment. *Phys Ther* 1995;75:267–280.
15. Fishbain DA, Cutler RB, Rosomoff HL, et al. Impact of chronic pain patients' job perception variables on actual return to work. *Spine* 1997;13:197–206.
16. Fordyce WE. *Behavioral methods for chronic pain and illness.* St. Louis: CV Mosby, 1976.
17. Fordyce WE. *Back pain in the workplace: management of disability in nonspecific conditions. A report of the Task Force on Pain in the Workplace of the IASP.* Seattle: IASP Press, 1995.
18. Frymoyer JW. Lumbar disk disease: epidemiology. *Instr Course Lect* 1992;41:217–223.
19. Frymoyer JW. Predicting disability from low back pain. *Clin Orthop* 1992:101–109.
20. Gamsa A. the role of psychological factors in chronic pain: a half centrury of study. *Pain.* 1994;57:5–15.
21. Gatchel RJ, Polatin PB, Kinney RK. Predicting outcome of chronic back pain using clinical predictors of psychopathology: a prospective analysis. *Health Psychol* 1995;14:415–420.
22. Gatchel RJ, Polatin PB, Mayer TG. The dominant role of psychosocial risk factors in the development of chronic low back pain disability. *Spine* 1995;20:2702–2709.
23. Gatchel RJ, Polatin PB, Mayer TG, et al. Psychopathology and the rehabilitation of patients with chronic low back pain disability. *Arch Phys Med Rehabil* 1994;75:666–670.
24. Gatchel RJ, Turk DC. *Psychological approaches to pain management: a practitioner's handbook.* New York: Guilford Press, 1996.
25. Hansen FR, Biering F Sr, Schroll M. Minnesota Multiphasic Personality Inventory profiles in persons with or without low back pain: a 20-year follow-up study. *Spine* 1995;20:2716–2720.
26. Hasenbring M, Marienfeld G, Kuhlendahl D, et al. Risk factors of chronicity in lumbar disc patients:

a prospective investigation of biologic, psychologic, and social predictors of therapy outcome. *Spine* 1994;19:2759–2765.

27. Hazard RG, Haugh LD, Reid S, et al. Early prediction of chronic disability after occupational low back injury. *Spine* 1996;21:945–951.

28. Heliövaara M. Risk factors for low back pain and sciatica. *Ann Med* 1989;21:257–264.

29. Hellsing AL, Linton SJ, Ka M. A prospective study of patients with acute back and neck pain in Sweden. *Phys Ther* 1994;74:116–124.

30. Himmelstein JS, Andersson GB. Low back pain: risk evaluation and preplacement screening. *Occup Med* 1988;3:255–269.

31. Junge A, Dvorak J, Ahern S. Predictors of bad and good outcomes of lumbar disc surgery: a prospective clinical study with recommendations for screening to avoid bad outcomes. *Spine* 1995;20:460–468.

32. Keefe FJ, Blumenthal JA. *Assessment strategies in behavioral medicine.* New York: Grune & Stratton, 1982.

33. Keefe FJ, Brown C, Scott DS, et al. Behavioral assessment of chronic pain. In: Keefe FJ, Blumenthal JA, eds. *Assessment strategies in behavioral medicine.* New York: Grune & Stratton, 1982.

34. Keefe FJ, Williams DA. Pain behavior assessment. In: Turk DC, Melzack R, eds. *Handbook of pain assessment.* New York: Guilford Press, 1992.

35. Kelsey JL, Golden AL. Occupational and workplace factors associated with low back pain. *Occup Med* 1988;3:7–16.

36. Kendall NAS, Linton SJ, Main CJ. *Guide to assessing psychosocial yellow flags in acute low back pain: risk factors for long-terms disability and work loss.* Wellington, NZ: Accident Rehabilitation & Compensation Insurance Corporation of New Zealand and the National Health Committee, 1997.

37. Klenerman L, Slade PD, Stanley IM, et al. The prediction of chronicity in patients with an acute attack of low back pain in a general practice setting. *Spine* 1995;20:478–484.

38. Lancourt J, Kettelhut M. Predicting return to work for lower back pain patients receiving worker's compensation. *Spine* 1992;17:629–640.

39. Lehmann TR, Spratt KF, Lehmann KK. Predicting long-term disability in low back injured workers presenting to a spine consultant. *Spine* 1993;18:1103–1112.

40. Leino P, Hänninen V. Psychosocial factors at work in relation to back and limb disorders. *Scand J Work Environ Health* 1995;21:134–142.

41. Leino P, Magni G. Depressive and distress symptoms as predictors of low back pain, neck-shoulder pain, and other musculoskeletal morbidity: a 10 year follow-up of metal industry employees. *Pain* 1993;53:89–94.

42. Lethem J, Slade PD, Troup JDG, et al. Outline of a fear-avoidance model of exaggerated pain perceptions. *Behav Res Ther* 1983;21:401–408.

43. Linton SJ. *Smärtans psykologi [the psychology of pain].* Stockholm: Folksam Förlag, 1992.

44. Linton SJ. The role of psychological factors in back pain and its remediation. *Pain Rev* 1994;1:231–243.

45. Linton SJ. A population-based study of the relationship between sexual abuse and back pain: establishing a link. *Pain* 1997;73:47–53.

46. Linton SJ, Bradley LA. Strategies for the prevention of chronic pain. In: Gatchel RJ, Turk DC, eds. *Psychological approaches to pain management: a practitioner's handbook.* New York: Guilford Press, 1996.

47. Linton SJ, Buer N, Vlaeyen J, et al. Are fear-avoidance beliefs related to a new episode of back pain? A prospective study. *Psychol Health* 1999;14:1051–1059.

48. Linton SJ, Halldén K. Risk factors and the natural course of acute and recurrent musculoskeletal pain: developing a screening instrument. In: Jensen TS, Turner JA, Wiesenfeld-Hallin Z, eds. *Proceedings of the 8th World Congress on Pain, vol 8.* Seattle: IASP Press, 1997.

49. Linton SJ, Halldén K. Can we screen for problematic back pain? A screening questionnaire for predicting outcome in acute and subacute back pain. *Clin J Pain* 1998;14:209–215.

50. Linton SJ, Lardén M, Gillow AM. Sexual abuse and chronic musculoskeletal pain: prevalence and psychological factors. *Clin J Pain* 1996;12:215–221.

51. Magni G, Marchitti M, Moreschi C, et al. Chronic musculoskeletal pain and depressive symptoms in the National Health and Nutrition Examination. I. Epidemiological follow-up study. *Pain* 1993;53:161–168.

52. Magni G, Moreschi C, Rigatti-Luchini S, et al. Prospective study on the relationship between depressive symptoms and chronic musculoskeletal pain. *Pain* 1994;56:289–297.

53. Main CJ, Wood PLR, Hollis S, et al. The distress and risk assessment method: a simple patient classification to identify distress and evaluate the risk of poor outcome. *Spine* 1992;17:42–52.

54. Mannion AF, Dolan P, Adams MA. Psychological questionnaires: do "abnormal" scores precede or follow first-time low back pain? *Spine* 1996;21:2603–2611.

55. Melzack R, Wall PD. *The challenge of pain.* New York: Basic Books, 1982.

56. Öhlund C, Eek C, Palmbald S, et al. Quantified pain drawing in subacute low back pain: validation in a nonselected outpatient industrial sample. *Spine* 1996;21:1021–1030.

57. Papageorgiou AC, Macfarlane GJ, Thomas E, et al. Psychosocial factors in the workplace: do they predict new episodes of low back pain? *Spine* 1997;22:1137–1142.

58. Philips HC, Grant L. The evolution of chronic back pain problems. *Behav Res Ther* 1991;29:435–441.

59. Pietri-Taleb F, Riihimäki H, Viikari-Juntura E, et al. Longitudinal study on the role of personality characteristics and psychological distress in neck trouble among working men. *Pain* 1994;58:261–267.
60. Potter RG, Jones JM. The evolution of chronic pain among patients with musculoskeletal problems: a pilot study in primary care. *Br J Gen Pract* 1992;42:462–464.
61. Radanov BP, Sturzenegger M, De Stefano G, et al. Relationship between early somatic, radiological, cognitive and psychosocial findings and outcome during a one-year follow-up in 117 patients suffering from common whiplash. *Br J Rheumatol* 1994;33:442–448.
62. Radanov P, Sturzenegger M, Di Stefano G. Prediction of recovery from dislocation of the cervical vertebrae (whiplash injury of the cervical vertebrae) with initial assessment of psychosocial variables. *Orthopade* 1994;23:282–286.
63. Rosen M. *Clinical Standards Advisory Group: back pain report of a committee on back pain.* London: Her Majesty's Stationery Office, 1994.
64. Sackett DL, Richardson WS, Rosenberg W, et al. *Evidence-based medicine: how to practice and teach EBM.* New York: Churchill Livingstone, 1997.
65. Simmonds MJ, Kumar S, Lechelt E. Psychosocial factors in disabling low back pain: causes or consequences? *Disabil Rehabil* 1996;18:161–168.
66. Skevington SM. *Psychology of pain.* London: Wiley, 1995.
67. Talo S, Rytökoski U, Puukka P, et al. An empirical investigation of the "biopsychosocial disease consequence model": psychological impairment, disability and handicap in chronic pain patients. *Disabil Rehabil* 1995;17:281–292.
68. Turk DC. Biopsychosocial perspective on chronic pain. In: Gatchel RJ, Turk DC, eds. *Psychological approaches to pain management: a practitioner's handbook,* vol 1. New York: Guilford Press, 1996.
69. Turk DC. The role of demographic and psychosocial factors in transition from acute to chronic pain. In: Jensen TS, Turner JA, Wiesenfeld-Hallin Z, eds. *Proceedings of the 8th World Congress on Pain,* vol 8. Seattle: IASP Press, 1997.
70. Turk DC, Flor H. Etiological theories and treatments for chronic back pain. II. Psychological models and interventions. *Pain* 1984;19:209–233.
71. Turk DC, Melzack R. *Handbook of pain assessment.* New York: Guilford Press, 1992.
72. van Tulder MW, Assendelft WJJ, Koes BW, et al. Methodologic guidelines for systematic reviews in the Cochrane Collaboration Back Review Group for spinal disorders. *Spine* 1997;22:2323–2330.
73. Viikari-Juntura EJ, Vuori J, Silverstein BA, et al. A life-long prospective study on the role of psychosocial factors in neck-shoulder and low back pain. *Spine* 1991;16:1056–1061.
74. Vlaeyen JWS, Kole. The role of fear of movement/(re) injury in pain disability. *J Occup Rehabil* 1995;5:235–252.
75. von Korff M, LeResche L, Dworkin SF. First onset of common pain syndromes: a prospective study of depression as a risk factor. *Pain* 1993;55:251–258.
76. Waddell G. Biopsychosocial analysis of low back pain. *Baillieres Clin Rheumatol* 1992;6:523–557.
77. Waddell G, Newton M, Henderson I, et al. A fear-avoidance beliefs questionnaire (FABQ) and the role of fear-avoidance beliefs in chronic low back pain and disability. *Pain* 1993;52:157–168.
78. Weiser S, Cedraschi C. Psychosocial issues in the prevention of chronic low back pain: a literature review. *Baillieres Clin Rheumatol* 1992;6:657–684.
79. Werneke MW, Harris DE, Lichter RL. Clinical effectiveness of behavioral signs for screening chronic low-back pain patients in a work-oriented physical rehabilitation program. *Spine* 1993;18:2412–2418.
80. Wurtele SK, Kaplan GM, Keairnes M. Childhood sexual abuse among chronic pain patients. *Clin J Pain* 1990;6:110–113.

Neck and Back Pain: The Scientific Evidence
of Causes, Diagnosis, and Treatment, edited
by Alf Nachemson and Egon Jonsson.
Published by Lippincott Williams & Wilkins,
Philadelphia 2000.

4

Influences of Individual Factors and Smoking on Neck and Low Back Pain

Alf Nachemson* and Eva Vingård

*Department of Orthopaedics, Sahlgrenska University Hospital, Göteborg, Sweden
†Section of Personal Injury Prevention, Karolinska Institutet, Stockholm, Sweden

OVERVIEW OF INDIVIDUAL FACTORS

This overview is mostly based on several reviews published on the topic in the 1990s (1,19,20,21,43,54,62,66,94,125,153). In addition, a limited MEDLINE search was performed for 1986 to 1997 for age, sex, and anthropometric measurements.

All previous reviews of individual risk factors for future low back pain listed many studies attempting to identify such factors. Unfortunately, these studies are rarely comparable, mainly because the outcome variable differed; some of these studies used insurance data in considering future absence resulting from back pain, whereas others used various types of telephone interviews or postal questionnaires. Dempsey et al. (43) stated that most epidemiologic studies cannot adequately evaluate the possible effect of individual factors.

There are few long-term prospective cohort studies (4,9,64,86,90,126,130,154), and even fewer of these studies have lasted longer than 5 years. Most studies are cross-sectional, and some are disease-specific case series compared with general population morbidity. Some studies look at low back pain alone, and others consider sciatica resulting from disc hernia, but most lump all back syndromes together. Few studies have investigated predictors for neck pain, all with negative results (45,70,77,135,159).

As seen in Table 4.1, structured following the outlines of Andersson (1), Bigos and Battié (19), Bigos et al. (22), and Burdorf et al. (32), many studies, most of them collected from the foregoing reviews with some added from the literature search up to 1998, have tried to find associations of individual factors with lumbar pain syndromes. Few have studied sciatica resulting from disc hernia alone (62,81,83,125,141,156).

Few studies have touched on neck pain. Therefore, in Table 4.1, the studies quoted cover only low back pain syndromes. Given the uncertainties and striking variabilities of results, it is only fair to state that none of the risk factors covered in this overview are strong predictors of future back or neck pain.

From the various reports in the literature, it has thus been impossible to differentiate between individual risk factors for first-time occurrence of low back pain and risk factors for recurrence and chronicity. The associations between mechanical work factors and back pain are detailed in Chapter 5, whereas in Chapters 2 and 3, the

TABLE 4.1. *Findings of association of some commonly examined individual risk factors for low back pain and sciatica[a]*

	Positive association	No/negative association
Age	4,13,24,25,26,28,72,92, 94,118,125,132,136,146	9,11,12,14,15,19,25,28, 32,33,46,67,70,71,76, 77,91,102,121,125,145, 157,158
Gender	16,18,21,141	22,62,91,92,118,132,157
Height	7,61,74,81,82,86,88,138	15,24,26,32,33,62,91,102, 118,132
Weight	7,18,31,61,80	4,24,26,28,32,33,62,70, 86,91,101,102,112,118, 132,157,158
Strength	39,59,90,98,105	14,57,86,106,107,109,117, 152
Flexibility	73,86,116,120	3,8,142,149
Exercise fitness	35,36,37,102,125	2,5,13,27,59,70,72,86,90, 101,107,121,122,124, 132,138,152
Leg length discrepancy <2, 5 cm	40,52,53,56,76,128,129,150	47,50,58,63,76,101,120, 123,140
Shape, posture, Scheuermann's disease	85,139 (Lumbar)	3,10,32,34,41,69,70,71, 76,77,100,108,110,127, 139 (Thoracic)
Congenital anomalies	71,76,87,95,113,137,160	62,68,69,77,87,122,137, 141,160
Spondylolisthesis	21,23,49,71,77,84,131, 160	51,62,69,70,87,137
Low eduation (low IQ)	9,14,27,72,91	21,74,118,124,132

[a] Numbers are from the general reference list.

social and psychologic factors influencing back pain and, in particular, disability from back pain have been described.

The best evidence comes from longitudinal studies of persons without back pain who were followed for longer periods. Bergenudd's study is the longest, with a nearly 50-year follow-up of 575 50-year-old residents of Malmö, Sweden. He analyzed predisposing factors and found that persons with back pain later in life (29%) were less successful in childhood intelligence tests, had less education, and worked at physically more strenuous jobs. Bergenudd specifically delineated body posture, lordosis and kyphosis, and height as nonpredictive factors, whereas some weak association was found for weight increase in men and physical fitness in women but not in men. Overall physical fitness (measured at age 18 to 19 years in men) was not associated with future low back pain.

The findings from the prospective studies can be categorized as applying to (a) subsequent experiences of low back pain or trouble, (b) work-related back pain reports, and (c) hospitalization for diagnosed herniated discs. These categories appear to represent different entities in terms of incidence. Although low back pain or trouble is common, as demonstrated by the 1-year incidence (47%) (114), filing a back pain report at the workplace is much less common (5% per year). Much rarer are diagnoses of herniated discs requiring hospitalization. As the incidence of these entities is different, so may be their risk factors.

In their review, Bigos et al. (22) stressed that reliable evidence demands that sample groups be similar (randomized or cohort) and that outcome criteria be similarly evaluated in all subjects. Prospective studies provide fewer opportunities for undetectable bias or errors than do cross-sectional population studies.

The review by Burdorf et al. (32) mainly dealt with work-related back disorders, but nevertheless, it clearly showed that gender, height, weight, exercise, and marital status were consistently not associated with back disorders in occupational populations.

The insecurity that pertains to many factors in the back pain complex, of course, results from the problem that back pain is rarely objectively verifiable, unlike disorders characterized by a specific anatomic or pathologic lesion. We only know that the patient reports pain, and most epidemiologic studies rely on self-reports of pain from survey responses with demonstrated recall bias (17,143,144). We do not know exactly what this means, but nevertheless the way people respond seems to be changing. Reports from Saskatchewan in Canada (38), as well as from the middle of Sweden (65,93), indicate that 90% of middle-aged people have had back pain at some point and that back pain often recurs (20). Moreover, as noted in several studies (97,115) such as one from the Seattle, Washington, group (161), many patients in primary care and who have acute pain continue to have pain for 1 to 2 years even though they may not necessarily be disabled.

Thus, the variations in incidence and prevalence of neck and back pain in different studies probably depend largely on how questions are asked, on the social and psychologic settings in the particular study area, and on whether the study is concentrated in worksites or whether data are taken from the general population. That the results then differ among various studies regarding individual risk factors should not come as a surprise.

In 1989, Heliövaara (62) reviewed studies up to the late 1980s and found 8 prospective (shorter periods) and 50 cross-sectional or retrospective studies pertaining to risk factors for back pain syndromes. Some of his results are also reported in the Chapter 5. His review centered on low back pain and sciatica, and he found from the literature that age was a significant factor. The peak age in all studies of sciatica resulting from herniated discs is around 40 to 45 years. Men are affected more often than women, in his review 1.5 to 3 times more often, although this figure was questioned in later studies (1,32). Low back pain alone, conversely, affects women as frequently as men. Body height has also been quoted in several other studies with a relative risk for tall men (more than 180 cm tall) of 2.3 to 3.7. Those studies were based on United States army recruits (74) and a Finnish study (78). Gyntelberg (59), however, also reported such an association for low back pain alone in Denmark.

In Heliövaara's review (62), obesity was also found predictive of sciatica resulting from herniated lumbar discs, but only when patients were considerably overweight. In summary, Heliövaara (62) proposed some, in his view relevant, risk factors for low back diseases (Table 4.2).

In another prospective cohort study over 4 years in healthy workers in an airplane manufacturing plant, Battié et al. (4–8) found no relationship of back pain lasting 1 day or more with spinal flexibility, isometric strength, maximal aerobic capacity, sex, or age. This, one of the largest studies, which included 3,020 employees, did not find these factors important by univariate or multivariate analysis. The most important and highly significant predictor in this study was a previous history of back pain, either treated or untreated. In addition, the report of back pain resulting from a straight leg raise was found to be predictive of subsequent low back pain in these healthy volunteers.

TABLE 4.2. *Risk factors for low back disease*

Factor	Low back pain	Sciatica
Male sex	0	+ +
Age 30–50 yr	+	+ +
Age >50 yr	−	−
Body height	0	+ +
Obesity	0	+
Sports	−	− +
Pregnancies	+ +	+

−, negative; 0, no; +, positive; + +, strongly positive.
Adapted from Heliövaara M. Body height, obesity, and risk of herniated lumbar disc. *Spine* 1987;12: 449–472, with permission.

Age and gender as factors have been studied by many investigators (Table 4.1). The highest incidence of disabling back pain occurs between 35 and 55 years of age. Biering-Sörensen's (13,14) data indicate a difference in age pattern between women and men, with increasing incidence and lifetime prevalence in women after 55 years of age. Svensson and Andersson (146), in their study of women in Göteborg, did not, however, find such an effect, whereas Battié et al. (5), in the previously mentioned study at Boeing, found a significantly higher risk of sickness absence in younger workers of both sexes when these investigators used univariate analysis. These are some examples of conflicting results in studies, each of which can be criticized for some aspect or detail. Although sex seems of little difference with respect to low back symptoms, operations for disc herniations are performed more often in men than in women (1,78,141,156).

In 1987, Troup and coworkers (152) reported on a prospective study of the predictive value of preemployment screening tests. Nearly 3,000 British men and women were questioned about their perception of physical exertion at work and about prior experiences of low back pain. They also underwent a battery of tests that included anthropometric measurements, back flexibility, maximal lifting strength, respiratory function, and psychophysical tests. The authors stated that "none of the tests were of any value in predicting new cases of low back pain." Prior history of back problems was the strongest predictor of subsequent back problems. Respiratory function tests were reportedly at least as accurate as strength and mobility tests in predicting low back pain; the association was rarely predictive, however.

MacDonald et al. (96) reported on a prospective study of industrial back pain reports and spinal canal diameter among miners. Spinal canal measurements were obtained by ultrasound on 204 of 373 miners solicited, with a subsequent follow-up of 3 years. The medical and work attendance records for the 3 years before the ultrasound examinations also were reviewed. Miners who left the industry with records indicating prior back problems or related time loss had significantly narrower spinal canal than did other miners. Unfortunately, a reduction in the labor force caused more than half of the miners to leave the industry within the follow-up period, a situation that limited the analyses and conclusions of this study.

A few prospective studies of risk factors for herniated lumbar discs included anthropometric measurements. The first study obtained these measurements at the time of induction in 1,095 United States military recruits who later were hospitalized with the diagnosis of herniated disc (74). When compared with control subjects matched for age and period of military service, the hospitalized patients were determined to be significantly taller and heavier. Another prospective study (81), which considered height, weight, and relative weight as risk factors in 332 patients with herniated discs, found that taller men and women were more likely to be hospitalized with the diagnosis of disc herniation during an 11-year follow-up period than were matched controls. Relative weight (wt/ht^2), when classified by intervals, revealed some predictive significance in men, but not in women.

In a prospective cohort study in patients with low back pain who had consulted general practitioners, van den Hoogen et al. (155) studied 443 patients from general practices around Amsterdam, Netherlands, with questionnaires and follow-up for 12 months and looked for factors that were associated with prolonged back pain. These investigators could not find any individual factors explaining the rate of recovery. In a nonsystematic review from France, Valat et al. (153) also investigated the risk factors for chronicity in low back pain and found that most factors known to be associated with chronicity are work related or psychosocial, and only a few were patient related. The patient's sex was not found significant, and although the rate of occurrence of low back pain declined with age after 50 years, patients older than 45 years were more likely to develop chronic pain. Neither weight nor height influenced the risk of chronicity.

In an epidemiologic study of back pain care, Shekelle et al. (133) found no relation among body mass index, physical activity, general health status, and back pain care in 3,000 adults in a health insurance study. In a search for predictive factors in a 1-year study of patients with back and neck, Skargren and Öberg (135) found age, sex, and smoking noncontributory to prediction of outcome.

Older studies quoted by Hildebrandt (66) in his review of epidemiologic research on risk factors of low back pain depicted no fewer than 55 different individual factors; among them were constitution, age, gender, weight, back muscle strength (absolute and relative), fitness, back mobility, genetic factors, postural with severe scoliosis, leg length discrepancy, and radiographic factors. Factors unrelated to risk in this review were body build, height and weight indices, kyphosis, lordosis, and radiographic changes. Riihimäki (125) in essence confirmed these findings.

When considering obesity and low back pain, Deyo and Bass (44) found some differences: a 1.7 higher prevalence when comparing the highest quintile (body mass index) with the lowest quintile. This finding was also supported by Garzillo and Garzillo (55) in their review.

In a population-based study, Michel et al. (104) found that the severity of back pain was only partly based on clinical findings of a physical examination, which, among other things, included body mass index, kyphosis, lordosis, scoliosis, and mobility. These findings were only weak predictors of pain and disability compared with healthy persons.

One of the first longitudinal studies was presented by Valkenburg and his group (154), whose initial survey included 1,167 women 45 to 64 years of age. Nine years later, 1,000 women were invited to participate in a follow-up survey, and 742 also underwent radiographic study again. In these elderly women, the investigators found that radiologic disc degeneration measured by two independent observers was more common in patients with back pain than in those without, but again with a moderate relative risk of 1.44 (confidence interval [CI], 1.09–1.75) for future back pain. In this study, vertebral fractures were not predictive, nor was the growth of osteophytes. The best predictor for the deterioration of disc degeneration on x-ray studies was the presence of preexisting degeneration noted on the first radiograph.

PHYSICAL FITNESS

Physical activity at leisure time and muscle strength have been the subjects of many studies of all pain syndromes including sciatica. A divergence of results is published. The Copenhagen study (59) found short isometric endurance of back muscles significant for first-time occurrence of pain over a 1-year period in a prospective study, but no negative association between physical activity and the occurrence of low back pain.

Finnish studies (89,90) found no association between muscle function at baseline and later development of low back symptoms. Kelsey (81) and Weber (156) found that physical activity during leisure time prevented or reduced the severity of an attack of sciatica, whereas Hurme (78) found no difference in leisure time physical activity in patients who were subsequently operated on for herniated discs in the general population in Finland.

The Boeing study (5) could not demonstrate an association, although Cady et al. (37) in 1979 presented their findings from a prospective study of physical fitness in relation to subsequent back pain reports among 1,652 firefighters. An overall fitness score was derived from several measures of isometric strength, flexibility, and cardiovascular endurance. These investigators found an association between back pain reporting and fitness level and concluded that "physical fitness and conditioning are preventive of back injuries" (36).

Mostardi et al. (106) measured the isokinetic back strength of 171 nurses and followed them for 2 years. Sixteen injuries occurred during that period, whereupon the authors concluded that isokinetic back strength was not predictive of injury in such a high-risk population. Other studies demonstrated a lack of association between strength measurement and the prediction of future back pain (Table 4.1).

In a 5-year prospective study, Kujala et al. (86) investigated muscle strength, aerobic power, and leisure time physical loading in a cohort of 456 adults free of back pain at age 25 to 45 years, half of whom completed and returned the questionnaire. These investigators found that tallness, but not body mass or muscle strength, leisure time physical activity, or aerobic power predicted future back pain. The aim of these authors was to investigate predictors of back problems in previously healthy asymptomatic adults.

Mundt et al. (107) investigated the association between participation in several specific sports, including free weight lifting, and herniated lumbar and cervical discs in a case-control epidemiologic study and found the relative risk estimates nonpredictive for most common sports, including the use of weight lifting equipment. These results confirmed the thesis of Granhed (57), who found radiologic disc degeneration more prevalent in persons who lifted heavy weights in competition but who did not have back pain complaints. There was, however, a small increase in relative risk (but not significant) with the use of free weights and cervical disc herniation in the study by Mundt et al. (167).

Butterfield et al. (35) found that lower physical fitness in patients with back pain who were receiving compensation was related to longer absence; in other words, continuation of physical fitness activities during the recovery process was found to be a significant predictor for reduction of absenteeism. No premorbid data existed, however.

Huang et al. (75) considered vertebral fractures, mostly osteoporotic, in older women and a possible prediction of back pain in a group of 600 postmenopausal Japanese-American women in Hawaii. These investigators found that a history of a single recent fracture was associated with a threefold increase in back pain risk, a history of 2 recent fractures was associated with an eightfold increase in back pain, and a history of 3 recent fractures was associated with 21 times more back pain. Strangely enough, however, spine bone mineral density was not significantly associated with back pain.

BACK PAIN IN CHILDREN AND ADOLESCENTS

Several studies from Europe (3,29,30,45,60,111,130) investigated the incidence of back pain in cohorts of schoolchildren and then followed these study subjects prospectively for up to 10 years, again in terms of the predictiveness of various individual factors. No strong association was found. Few factors have been found to be moderately predictive. A family history of back pain (i.e., mother and father with such complaints) seems to be more closely associated with back pain in children than anthropometry and fitness (3). Social, psychologic, and emotional factors are more important than height and weight (3,30,130). Brattberg (29,30), in a longitudinal study of 3,000 7-year-old children with many anthropologic measurements in addition to family history, found that more girls than boys reported long-lasting back pain. There was no relationship between physical activities at any age and the prevalence of back pain.

Salminen et al. (130), in their 3-year prospective follow-up study, observed 15-year-old students with and without pain and found that a low frequency of physical activity related to increased frequency of back pain. In their matched-pair case-control study, these investigators noted more back complaints related to reduced flexibility and endurance strength of both abdominal and back muscles. These authors also looked at the magnetic resonance images of a few young patients (62 subjects). Degenerative changes seen early by independent magnetic resonance imaging actually predicted more future problems, but again, those reporting back pain at age 15 also reported back pain more at age 18; that is, previous history is important. This study pertains to the moderate symptoms that usually seem to exist in young people. In addition, these investigators found that Scheuermann-type changes in the lumbar vertebrae predicted future longer-lasting chronic low back pain (at age 18), a finding confirming the much larger and longer-observed cohort in Sörensen's (139) thesis. In conclusion, Salminen et al. said that their results favored the hypothesis of a causal relationship between the early evolution of degenerative processes of lower lumbar discs and frequent low back pain in some young persons. Only 8% of the original 1,500 target population followed had x-ray studies, however.

In contrast, using ordinary radiographs, Harreby et al. (60), who followed another prospective cohort of young patients until age 25 years, found that of the 13% of patients who had radiologic abnormalities in adolescence, mainly Scheuermann's disease anywhere in the spine, no positive correlation with low back pain in the next 25 years could be seen. These investigators could not confirm a positive correlation between x-ray changes in the lower spine in adolescence and the higher prevalence of low back pain in adults. Stepwise logistic regression analysis of this material showed that low back pain in the growth period and familial occurrence of back disease are important risk factors for low back pain later in life, with an observed probability of 88% if both factors are present. This study thus confirmed the results of Brattberg's studies (29,30), that familial and genetic factors are important. In a study by Harreby et al. (60), radiologic abnormalities were relatively few, found only in some 70 people or 15% of the total cohort. The "genetic" familial low back disease factor had an odds ratio (OR) of 2.8, and low back pain previously in school as a predictor of later back pain had an OR of 2.2, with wide confidence limits for both factors.

In another Finnish study, by Nissinen et al. (111), a cohort of 850 adolescents was followed for 2 years to consider the influence of anthropometric measurements on the risk of future back pain. These investigators found sitting height in both sexes predictive, and in boys also standing height, but the OR was fairly low, 1.24. These children were around 14 years of age. Body mass index, kyphosis, lordosis, and pelvic tilt were not significant. Dieck et al. (45) also found that postural asymmetry in teens was not predictive for either neck pain or low back pain later in life.

In a 10-year follow-up study of military conscripts, Hellsing (64) found no significant association with earlier back pain and later reports of work absence resulting from back pain. Her study (63) also from the same cohort found no predictive value of leg length discrepancy of 1 to 2 cm. As seen in Table 4.1, most studies on this topic support her finding.

COMORBIDITY

Back pain is the third most common bodily symptom, after headache and tiredness, so it is not surprising that people with back pain often report other complaints. *The Nuprin Pain Report* (151) found that 90% of persons with frequent back pain had multiple pains, but 50% of them said back pain was the "most troublesome" of their various pains. Other clinical and epidemiologic studies show that up to 60% of people with low back pain also report some neck symptoms (45,70,77,135). Mäkele (99) found that many chronic musculoskeletal pains go together, with a particularly strong association among back pain, neck pain, and osteoarthritis of the hips and knees, although inflammatory joint disorders were distinct.

Bergenudd (9) found that back pain was the most common musculoskeletal complaint in 55-year-old men and women, but it was often associated with other pains (Table 4.3).

Hurwitz and Morgenstern (79) analyzed the 1989 United States National Health Interview Survey and found that a disabling nonback comorbidity produced an OR of 2.21 (2.09–2.34) for a disabling back condition. Yelin (162) analyzed the 1992 United States Health and Retirement Survey of persons aged 51 to 61 years. Fifty-nine percent had one or more musculoskeletal condition, and 38% of these persons had at least one other nonmusculoskeletal comorbid condition. From an epidemiologic and social

TABLE 4.3. *Association of back pain and other pains*

	Men (%)	Women (%)
Back pain	28	30
Shoulder pain	13	15
Knee pain	8	13
Hip pain	4	4

of those with back pain:

	Men and Women (%)
Back pain alone	14
Back pain and shoulder pain	7
Back pain and knee pain	5
Back pain and hip pain	3

Data from Bergenudd H. *Talent, occupation and locomotor discomfort.* Thesis, Lund University, Sweden, 1989.

perspective, neck pain and back pain are not discrete clinical problems, but they are often associated with other pains, comorbidities, psychologic and stress-related symptoms, and work-related or other social problems (42,147) (see Chapters 2 to 5).

Multiple pregnancies as risk factors have shown different results in different studies (1,48,62,83,103). In the Manchester study (134), this factor was also predictive for men.

In conclusion, we have not found any high-quality long-term prospective studies with convincing evidence for any individual factor to predict neck or low back pain syndromes. Some weak evidence supports the concept that tall men suffer sciatica more often, whereas no evidence supports the idea that moderate obesity is associated with any back syndromes. Age is a factor for disability in both neck and back pain, with some small gender difference. For sciatica resulting from disc hernia, age between 40 and 45 years is strongly associated. From the young adolescent to the elderly person, the strongest predictor is a previous history of back pain.

SMOKING AND LOW BACK PAIN (REFERENCE NUMBERS IN THIS SECTION CORRESPOND TO SEPARATE REFERENCE LIST FOR SMOKING)

Smoking as a risk factor for low back pain and sciatica has been extensively discussed (6,18,20). Experimental studies have given support to the hypothesis that blood flow and nutrition to the disc are diminished in smokers (5,11), the pH of the disc is lowered (7), the mineral content of the lumbar vertebrae is decreased (3,8), the fibrinolytic activity is altered (14), and degenerative changes of the lumbar spine are increased (1).

In epidemiologic studies in working or more general populations, with potential confounders acceptably controlled for, the results have been more conflicting (Table 4.4). Kelsey and coworkers reported in 1984 that smoking was more prevalent among patients with prolapsed lumbar discs then among hospital-based control subjects (14). In a large retrospective cohort from the United States, Deyo and Bass found a slightly increased risk (OR, 1.36) for persons who smoked more then 60 cigarettes per day (4). Persons who smoked fewer cigarettes also had a trend toward increased risks. However, the risk elevation is low, and extremely heavy smokers probably have a different risk profile in many aspects. In the Mini-Finland Health Survey (10), no elevated risk was found for sciatica, but a moderate risk was noted for low back pain (OR, 1.5; CI, 1.1–2.1). Leboeuf-Yde found a similar result in a Danish population (15), but in Holland (2), there was no difference between smokers and nonsmokers in reporting low back pain in 13 different occupations. In a prospective industrial cohort from Finland (16), followed for 10 years, no significant differences in low back problems were shown between smokers and nonsmokers. One prospective study of Finnish farmers (17), followed for 12 years, showed an inverse picture, with an increased risk of sciatica but not of low back pain. This study included few cases, however.

A study from the United States (12) compared smoking and nonsmoking patients with back pain and found that smokers showed higher levels of emotional stress, they tended to be inactive, and they relied on medication more often than did nonsmoking patients. Furthermore, patients with pain are at risk of increasing smoking behavior when they experience periods of heightened pain intensity. This factor must be taken into account when cross-sectional studies are interpreted.

In conclusion, experimental studies give some evidence to a relationship between smoking and changes in anatomic structures in the low back. In epidemiologic studies on men and women, there is some evidence for a weak relationship between heavy

TABLE 4.4. *Smoking and low back pain*

Study (ref.)[a]	Design	Population and gender studied	Outcome	Exposure	Confounders adjusted for	Results (OR, RR, p value)
Kelsey et al., 1984 (14), USA	Case-control study	Men and women with prolapsed disc and hospital controls without any disorder from the spine	Prolapsed disc	Smoking in past yr	Lifting, car driving	1.2 (1.0–1.4) for every 10 cigarettes smoked
Ryden et al., 1989 (19), USA	Case-control, study	84 cases of occupational back injury and 168 controls	Occupational injury of LBP	1. Cigarette smoking or not 2. Cigarette smoking in increasing doses		1. 0.82 (0.04–1.70) 2. No trends
Deyo and Bass, 1989 (4), USA	Retrospective cohort study	10,404 men and women >25 yr of age	Pain in the low back >2 wk last yr	Pack-years of smoking in seven categories: 0, 0.1–10, 10.1–20, 20.1–30, 30.1–40, 40.1–50, >50	BMI, chronic cough, age, currently employed or not, education, usual daily activity	OR 1.05 for each pack-year category OR = 1.36 for nonsmokers versus 50 pack-years
Heliövaara et al., 1991 (10), Finland	Cross-Sectional (Mini-Finland Health Survey)	Randomized sample of Finnish men and women 30–64 yr old 3,156 men and 2,946 women	1. Sciatica 2. Low back symptoms	Smoking >20 cigarettes/d	Sex, age, BMI, trauma, occupational physical and mental stress, vehicle driving, alcohol consumption, number of births of women	1. 1.1 (0.7–1.6) 2. 1.5 (1.1–2.1)
Battié et al., 1991 (1), Finland	Matched twin study	20 pair of matched twins	Disc degeneration on MRI, disc signal intensity, disc height	One twin smoker, the other nonsmoker	Occupational exposure, leisure time activities, chronic bronchitis, blood pressure, blood lipids, weight	$p = <.02$
Boshuizen et al., 1993 (2), Holland	Cross-sectional health survey	4,054 men 25–55 yr old in 13 occupations (at least 100 persons in each occupation)	Regular pain or stiffness in the back	Nonsmokers, ex-smokers, current smokers	Working conditions, physical exercise, mental health, age	No significant difference between smokers and nonsmokers in the 13 occupational groups

Reference	Study type	Population	Outcome	Smoking definition	Adjustment factors	Results
Leino, 1993 (16), Finland	Prospective study industrial cohort	607 men and women from metal factories followed at year 0, 5, and 10	Low back morbidity in clinical examination 4-grade scale	Average number of cigarettes each day	Exercise, low back findings at year 0, age occupational class, BMI, stress symptoms	NS for men and women
Riihimäki et al., 1994 (18), Finland	Prospective cohort study		3-year incidence of sciatic pain	Nonsmokers versus smokers and ex-smokers	Age, occupation, car driving, physical exercise, occupational exposures, history of low back problems	$p > .06$
Leboeuf, 1995 (15), Denmark	Cross-sectional study	30–50-yr-old men and women from the Danish population	1. LBP > 30 d last yr 2. LBP < 30 d	Nonsmokers, smokers (Q)	Age, BMI, sex, marital status, physical activity at work	1. 2.3 (1.6–3.3) unclear if adjusted 2. 1.0 (0.7–1.3)
Manninen et al., 1995 (17), Finland	Prospective cohort study	366 farmers followed for 12 yr	1-yr prevalence of: 1. Sciatic pain 2. LBP	Current smokers versus never smokers	Age, height, BMI, type of farm production, mental stress score, pain in the joints	1. 9.6 (1.7–53.0) 2. 0.71 (0.24–2.11)
Toroptsova et al., 1995 (21), Russia	Cross-sectional study	339 men and 362 women from a machine building factory	LBP (Q)	Smoking >10 cigarettes/d		$p < .05$
Harreby et al., 1996 (9), Denmark	Cross-sectional study	578 38-yr-old men and women investigated 24 yr earlier	Severe LBP (Q)	Smoking 16 cigarettes/d for men and 13 cigarettes/d for women		Tendency of increased risk for those who smoke more than 16 cigarettes/d among men for severe LBP

[a] Reference numbers are those from the separate "smoking" list.
BMI, body mass index; LBP, low back pain; MRI, magnetic resonance imaging; NS, not significant; OR, odds ratio; RR, relative risk.

smoking and low back pain but no clear evidence for a relationship between sciatica and smoking.

GENERAL REFERENCES

1. Andersson GBJ. The epidemiology of spinal disorders. In: Frymoyer JW, ed. *The adult spine: principles and practice,* 2nd ed. Philadelphia: Lippincott—Raven, 1997:93–141.
2. Arad D, Ryan MD. The incidence and prevalence in nurses of low back pain. *Aust Nurs J* 1986;16:44–48.
3. Balagué F, Skovron M-L, Nordin M, et al. Low back pain in schoolchildren: a study of familial and psychological factors. *Spine* 1995;20:1265–1270.
4. Battié MC. *The reliability of physical factors as predictors of the occurrence of back pain reports: a prospective study within industry.* Thesis, Göteborg University, Sweden 1989.
5. Battié MC, Bigos SJ, Fisher LD, et al. A prospective study of the role of cardiovascular risk factors and fitness in industrial back pain complaints. *Spine* 1989;14:141–147.
6. Battié MC, Bigos SJ, Fisher LD, et al. Isometric lifting strength as a predictor of industrial back pain. *Spine* 1989;14:851–856.
7. Battié MC, Bigos SJ, Fisher LD, et al. Anthropometric and clinical measurements as predictors of industrial back pain complaints: a prospective study. *J Spinal Disord* 1990;3:195–204.
8. Battié MC, Bigos SJ, Fisher LD, et al. The role of spinal flexibility in back pain complaints within industry: a prospective study. *Spine* 1990;15:768–773.
9. Bergenudd H. *Talent, occupation and locomotor discomfort.* Thesis, Lund University, Sweden 1989.
10. Bergenudd H, Nilsson B. Back pain in middle age: occupational workload and psychologic factors: an epidemiological survey. *Spine* 1988;13:58–60.
11. Bergquist-Ullman M, Larsson U. Acute low back pain in industry. *Acta Orthop Scand Suppl* 1977; 170:1–117.
12. Biering-Sörensen F. Low back trouble in a general population of 30-, 40-, 50- and 60-year old men and women: study design, representativeness and basic results. *Dan Med Bull* 1982;29:289.
13. Biering-Sörensen F. *The prognostic value of the low back history and physical measurements.* Thesis, University of Copenhagen, 1983.
14. Biering-Sörensen F. A prospective study of low back pain in a general population. I. Occurrence, recurrence and aetiology. *Scand J Rehabil Med* 1983;15:71–79.
15. Biering-Sörensen F. Physical measurements as risk indicators for low-back trouble over a one-year period. *Spine* 1984;9:106–119.
16. Biering-Sörensen F. Risk of back trouble in individual occupations in Denmark. *Ergonomics* 1985; 28:51–60.
17. Biering-Sörensen F, Hilden J. Reproducibility of the history of low-back trouble. *Spine* 1984;9:280–286.
18. Biering-Sörensen F, Thomsen CE, Hilden J. Risk indicators for low back trouble. *Scand J Rehabil Med* 1989;21:151–159.
19. Bigos SJ, Battié MC. Surveillance of back problems in industry. In: Hadler N, ed. *Clinical concepts in the regional musculoskeletal diseases.* Orlando, NM: Grune & Stratton, 1987:299–315.
20. Bigos SJ, Battié MC, Spengler DM, et al. A prospective study of work perceptions and psychosocial factors affecting the report of back injury. *Spine* 1991;16:1–6.
21. Bigos SJ, Spengler DM, Martin NA, et al. Back injuries in industry: a retrospective study. III. Employee-related factors. *Spine* 1986;11:252–256.
22. Bigos SJ, Wilson Mr, Davis GE. Reliable science about avoiding low back problems at work. In: Wolter D, Seide K, eds. *Berufsbedingte Erkrankungen der Lendenwirbelsäule.* Berlin: Springer-Verlag, 1998;415–425.
23. Bistrom O. Need degenerative changes in the spinal column entail back pain? *Ann Chir Gynaecol Fenn* 1954;43:29–44.
24. Bongers PM, Hulshof CTJ, Dijkstra L, et al. Back pain and exposure to whole body vibration in helicopter pilots. *Ergonomics* 1990;33:1007–1026.
25. Boshuizen HC, Bongers PM, Hulshof CTJ. Self-reported back pain in tractor drivers exposed to whole-body vibration. *Int Arch Occup Environ Health* 1990;62:109–115.
26. Boshuizen HC, Hulshof CTJ, Bongers P. Long-term sick leave and disability pensioning due to back disorders of tractor drivers exposed to whole-body vibration. *Int Arch Occup Environ Health* 1990;62:117–122.
27. Bovenzi M, Betta A. Low-back disorders in agricultural tractor drivers exposed to whole-body vibration and postural stress. *Appl Ergon* 1994;25:231–241.
28. Bovenzi M, Zadini A. Self-reported low back symptoms in urban bus drivers exposed to whole-body vibration. *Spine* 1992;17:1048–1059.
29. Brattberg G. Back pain and headache in Swedish schoolchildren: a longitudinal study. *Pain Clin* 1993;6:157–162.

30. Brattberg G. The incidence of back pain and headache among Swedish school children. *Qual Life Res* 1994;3:S27–S31.
31. Brown JR. *Manual lifting and handling: an annotated bibliography.* Toronto: Labour Safety Council of Ontario Ministry of Labour, 1972.
32. Burdorf A, Sorock G. Positive and negative evidence of risk factors for back disorders. *Scand J Work Environ Health* 1997;23:243–256.
33. Burdorf A, Govaert G, Elders L. Postural load and back pain of workers in the manufacturing of prefabricated concrete elements. *Ergonomics* 1991;34:909–918.
34. Burdorf A, Naaktgeboren, de Groot HCWM. Occupational risk factors for low back pain among sedentary workers. *J Occup Med* 1993;35:1213–1220.
35. Butterfield PG, Spencer PS, Redmond N, et al. Low back pain: predictors of absenteeism, residual symptoms, functional impairment, and medical costs in Oregon workers' compensation recipients. *Am J Ind Med* 1998;34:559–567.
36. Cady LD, Thomas PC, Karwasky RJ. Program for increasing health and physical fitness of firefighters. *J Occup Med* 1985;2:111–114.
37. Cady LD, Bischoff DP, O'Connell ER, et al. Strength and fitness and subsequent back injuries in firefighters. *J Occup Med* 1979;21:269–272.
38. Cassidy JD, Carroll LJ, Cote P. The Saskatchewan health and back pain survey: the prevalence of low back pain and related disability in Saskatchewan adults. *Spine* 1998;23:1860–1866.
39. Chaffin DB, Herrin GD, Keyserling WM. Preemployment strength testing: an updated position. *J Occup Med* 1978;20:403–408.
40. Clarke GR. Unequal leg length: an accurate method of detection and some clinical results. *Rheum Phys Med* 1972;11:385–390.
41. Collis DK, Ponseti IV. Long term follow-up of patients with idiopathic scoliosis not treated surgically. *J Bone Joint Surg Am* 1969;51:425–455.
42. Coste J, Delecoeuillerie G, Cohen de Lara R, et al. Clinical course and prognostic factors in acute low back pain: an inception cohort study in primary care practice. *BMJ* 1994;308:577–580.
43. Dempsey PG, Burdorf A, Webster BS. The influence of personal variables on work-related low-back disorders and implications for future research. *J Occup Environ Med* 1997;39:8.
44. Deyo RA, Bass JE. Lifestyle and low-back pain. *Spine* 1989;14:501–506.
45. Dieck GS, Kelsey JL, Goel VK, et al. An epidemiologic study of the relationship between postural asymmetry in the teen years and subsequent back and neck pain. *Spine* 1985;10:872–877.
46. Estryn-Behar M, Kaminski M, Peigne E, et al. Strenuous working conditions and musculo-skeletal disorders among female hospital workers. *Int Arch Occup Environ Health* 1990;62:47–57.
47. Fairbank JC, Pynsent PB, Van Poortvliet JA, et al. Influence of anthropometric factors and joint laxity in the incidence of adolescent back pain. *Spine* 1984;9:461–464.
48. Fast A, Shapiro D, Ducommon EJ, et al. Low-back pain in pregnancy. *Spine* 1987;12:368–371.
49. Fischer FJ, Friedman MM, Denmark RE Van. Roentgenographic abnormalities in soldiers with low back pain: a comparative study. *AJR Am J Roentgenol* 1958;79:673–676.
50. Fisk JW, Baigent ML. Clinical and radiological assessment of leg length. *N Z Med J* 1975;81:477–480.
51. Frennered K. *Symptomatic lumbar spondylolisthesis in young patients: a clinical and radiological follow-up after non-operative and operative treatment.* Thesis, Göteborg University, Sweden 1991.
52. Friberg O. Clinical symptoms and biomechanics of lumbar spine and hip joint in leg length inequality. *Spine* 1983;8:643–651.
53. Friberg O. Results of radiologic measurements of leg-length inequality. *Spine* 1992;17:458–460.
54. Frymoyer JW, Pope MH, Clements JH, et al. Risk factors in low back pain. *J Bone Joint Surg Am* 1983;65:213.
55. Garzillo MJD, Garzillo TAF. Does obesity cause low back pain? *J Manipulative Physiol Ther* 1994;17:601–604.
56. Giles LGF, Taylor JR. Low-back pain associated with leg length inequality. *Spine* 1981;6:510–521.
57. Granhed H. *Extreme spinal loadings: effects on the vertebral bone mineral content and strength, and the risks for future low back pain in man.* Thesis, Göteborg University, Sweden, 1988.
58. Grundy PF, Roberts CJ. Does unequal leg length cause back pain? A case-control study. *Lancet* 1984;2:256–258.
59. Gyntelberg F. One Year incidence of low back pain among male residents of Copenhagen aged 40–59. *Dan Med Bull* 1974;21:30–36.
60. Harreby M, Neergaard K, Hesselsoe G, et al. Are radiologic changes in the thoracic and lumbar spine of adolescents risk factors for low back pain in adults? A 25-year prospective cohort study of 640 school children. *Spine* 1995;20:2298–2302.
61. Heliövaara M. Body height, obesity, and risk of herniated lumbar intervertebral disc. *Spine* 1987;12:469–472.
62. Heliövaara M. Risk factors for low back pain and sciatica. *Ann Med* 1989;21:257–264.
63. Hellsing AL. Leg length inequality: a prospective study of young men during their military service. *Upps J Med Sci* 1988;93:245–253.

64. Hellsing AL. Work absence in a cohort with benign back pain: prospective study with 10 year follow-up. *J Occup Rehabil* 1994;4:3:153.
65. Hellsing AL, Linton SJ, Kalvemark M. A prospective study of patients with acute back and neck pain in Sweden. *Phys Ther* 1994;74:116–124.
66. Hildebrandt VH. A review of epidemiological research on risk factors of low back pain. In: Buckle PW, ed. *Musculo-skeletal disorders at work*. London: Taylor & Francis 1987:9–16.
67. Hirsch C, Jonsson B, Lewin T. Low back symptoms in a Swedish female population. *Clin Orthop* 1969;63:171–176.
68. Hodges FJ, Peck WS. Clinical and roentgenological study of low back pain with sciatic radiation. B. Roentgenological aspects. *AJR Am J Roentgenol* 1937;37:461–466.
69. Hodgson S, Shannon HS, Troup JDG. *The prevention of spinal disorders in dock workers. Report to National Dock Labour Board, London, 1974.*
70. Holmstrom EB, Lindell L, Moritz U. Low back and neck/shoulder pain in construction workers:occupational workload and psychosocial risk factors. *Spine* 1992;17:663–671.
71. Horal J. The clinical appearance of low back disorders in the city of Gothenburg, Sweden. *Acta Orthop Scand Suppl* 1969;118:1–109.
72. Houtman ILD, Bongers PM, Smulders PGW, et al. Psychosocial stressors at work and musculoskeletal problems. *Scand J Work Environ Health* 1994;20:139–145.
73. Howell DW. Musculoskeletal profile and incidence of musculoskeletal injuries in lightweight women rowers. *Am J Sports Med* 1984;12:278–282.
74. Hrubec A, Nashbold BS Jr. Epidemiology of lumbar disc lesions in the military in World War II. *Am J Epidemiol* 1975;102:366–376.
75. Huang C, Ross PD, Wasnich RD. Vertebral fractures and other predictors of back pain among older women. *J Bone Miner Res* 1996;11:1026–1032.
76. Hult L. The Munkfors investigation. *Acta Orthop Scand Suppl* 1954;16:1.
77. Hult L. Cervical, dorsal, and lumbar spinal syndromes. *Acta Orthop Scand Suppl* 1954;17:1–102.
78. Hurme M. *Factors predicting the results of surgery for lumbar intervertebral disc herniation*. Turku, Finland: Publications of the Social Insurance Institution, 1985;AL:26 [in Finnish with English summary].
79. Hurwitz EL, Morgenstern H. Correlates of back problems and back-related disability in the United States. *J Clin Epidemiol* 1997;50:669–681.
80. Ikata T. Statistical and dynamic studies of lesions due to overloading on the spine. *Shikoku Acta Med* 1965;40:262–286.
81. Kelsey JL. An epidemiological study of acute herniated lumbar intervertebral discs. *Rheumatol Rehabil* 1975;14:144–159.
82. Kelsey JL. An epidemiological study of the relationship between occupations and acute herniated lumbar intervertebral discs. *Int J Epidemiol* 1975;4:197–204.
83. Kelsey JL, Greenberg RA, Hardy JR, et al. Pregnancy and the syndrome of herniated lumbar intervertebral disc: an epidemiological study. *Yale J Biol Med* 1975;48:361–368.
84. Kettelkamp DB, Wright DG. Spondylolisthesis in the Alaskan Eskimo. *J Bone Joint Surg Am* 1971;53:563–566.
85. Kostuik JP, Bentivoglio J. The incidence of low-back pain in adult scoliosis. *Spine* 1981;6:268–273.
86. Kujala U, Taimela S, Viljanen T, et al. Physical loading and performance as predictors of back pain in healthy adults: a 5-year prospective study. *Eur J Appl Physiol* 1996;73:452–458.
87. LaRocca H, MacNab I. Value of pre-employment radiographic assessment of the lumbar spine. *Can Med Assoc J* 1969;101:49–54.
88. Lawrence JS. Rheumatism in coal miners. III. Occupational factors. *Br J Ind Med* 1955;12:249–261.
89. Leino P. Does leisure time physical activity prevent low back disorders? A prospective study of metal industry Employees. *Spine* 1993;18:863–871.
90. Leino P, Aro S, Hasan J. Trunk muscle function and low back disorders: a ten-year follow-up study. *J Chronic Dis* 1987;40:289–96.
91. Leigh JP, Sheetz RM. Prevalence of back pain among full-time United States workers. *Br J Ind Med* 1989;46:651–657.
92. Liira JP, Shannon HS, Chambers LW, et al. Long-term back problems and physical work exposures in the 1990 Ontario Health Survey. *Am J Public Health* 1996;86:382–387.
93. Linton SJ, Hellsing AL, Halldén K. A population based study of spinal pain among 35–45 year old individuals: prevalence, sick leave, and health care use. *Spine* 1998;23:1457–1463.
94. Loeser JD, Volinn E. Epidemiology of low back pain. *Neurosurg Clin North Am* 1991;2:4;713–718.
95. Lokander S. Sick absence in a Swedish company: a sociomedical study. *Acta Med Scand Suppl* 1962;377:1–172.
96. MacDonald EB, Porter R, Hibbert C, et al. The relationship between spinal canal diameter and back pain in coal miners: ultrasonic measurement as a screening test? *J Occup Med* 1984;26:23–28.
97. Macfarlane GJ, Thomas E, Croft PR, et al. Predictors of early improvement in low back pain amongst consulters to general practice: the influence of pre-morbid and episode-related factors. *Pain* 1999;80:113–119.

98. McNeill T, Warwick D, Andersson G, et al. Trunk strengths in attempted flexion, extension, and lateral bending in healthy subjects and patients with low-back disorders. *Spine* 1980;5:529–538.
99. Makele M. *Common musculoskeletal syndromes: prevalence, risk indicators and disability in Finland.* Helsinki, Finland: Publications of the Social Insurance Institution, 1993;ML123:1–162.
100. Magora A. Investigation of the relation between low back pain and occupation: neurologic and orthopaedic conditions. *Scand J Rehabil Med* 1975;7:146–151.
101. Magnusson ML, Pope MH, Wilder DG, et al. Are occupational drivers at an increased risk for developing musculoskeletal disorders? *Spine* 1996;21:710–717.
102. Mandel JH, Lohman W. Low back pain in nurses: the relative importance of medical history, work factors, exercise and demographics. *Res Nurs Health* 1987;10:165–170.
103. Mantle MJ, Greenwood RM, Currey HLF. Backache in pregnancy. *Rheumatol Rehabil* 1977;16:95–101.
104. Michel A, Kohlmann T, Raspe H. The association between clinical findings on physical examination and self-reported severity in back pain: results of a population-based study. *Spine* 1997;22:296–304.
105. Moreland J, Finch E, Stratford P, et al. Interrater reliability of six tests of trunk muscle function and endurance. *J Orthop Sports Phys Ther* 1997;26:200–208.
106. Mostardi RA, Noe DA, Kovacic MW, et al. Isokinetic lifting strength and occupational injury: a prospective study. *Spine* 1991;17:189–193.
107. Mundt DJ, Kelsey JL, Golden AL, et al. An epidemiological study of sports and weight lifting as possible risk factors for herniated lumbar and cervical discs. *Am J Sports Med* 1993;21:854–860.
108. Nachemson AL. Back problems in childhood and adolescence. *Lakartidningen* 1968;65:2831–2843.
109. Nachemson AL, Lindh M. Measurement of abdominal and back muscle strength with and without low back pain. *Scand J Rehabil Med* 1969;1:60–65.
110. Nilsonne U, Lundgren KD. Long-term prognosis in idiopathic scoliosis. *Acta Orthop Scand* 1968;39:456–465.
111. Nissinen M, Heliövaara M, Seitsamo J, et al. Anthropometric measurements and the incidence of low back pain in a cohort of pubertal children. *Spine* 1994;12:1367–1370.
112. Nuwayhid IA, Stewart W, Johnson JV. Work activities and the onset of first-time low back pain among New York City fire fighters. *Am J Epidemiol* 1993;137:539–548.
113. Paillas JE, Winninger J, Louis R. Role des malformations lobosacrées dans les sciatiques et les lombalgies: étude de 1.500 dossiers radiocliniques dont 500 hernies discales verifiées. *Presse Med* 1969;77:853–855.
114. Papageorgiou AC, Croft PR, Ferry S, et al. Estimating the prevalence of low back pain in the general population: evidence from the South Manchester Back Pain Survey. *Spine* 1995;20:1889–1894.
115. Papageorgiou AC, Croft PR, Thomas E, et al. Influence of previous pain experience on the episode incidence of low back pain: results from the South Manchester Back Pain Study. *Pain* 1996;66:181–185.
116. Pearcy M, Portek I, Shepherd J. The effect of low-back pain on lumbar spinal movements measured by three dimensional x-ray analysis. *Spine* 1985;10:150–153.
117. Pedersen OF, Petersen R, Staffeldt ES. Back pain and isometric back muscle strength of workers in a Danish factory. *Scand J Rehabil Med* 1975;7:125–128.
118. Pietri F, Leclerc A, Boitel L, et al. Low-back pain in commercial travelers. *Scand J Work Environ Health* 1992;18:52–58.
119. Pope M. Risk indicators in low back pain. *Ann Med* 1989;21:387.
120. Pope M, Bevins T, Wilder DG, et al. The relationship between anthropometric, postural, muscular, and mobility characteristics of males, ages 18–55. *Spine* 1985;10:644–648.
121. Punnett L, Fine LJ, Keyserling WM, et al. Back disorders and nonneutral trunk postures of automobile assembly workers. *Scand J Work Environ Health* 1991;17:337–346.
122. Redfield JT. The low back x-rays as a pre-employment screening tool in the forest products industry. *J Occup Med* 1972;13:219–226.
123. Rhodes DW, Mansfield ER, Bishop PA, et al. The validity of the prone leg check as an estimate of standing leg length inequality measured by x-ray. *J Manipulative Physiol Ther* 1995;18:343–346.
124. Riihimäki H, Tola S, Videman T, et al. Low-back pain and occupation. *Spine* 1989;14:204–209.
125. Riihimäki H. Low-back pain: its origin and risk indicators. *Scand J Work Environ Health* 1991;17:81–90.
126. Rohrer MH, Santos-Eggimann B, Paccaud F, et al. Epidemiologic study of low back pain in 1398 Swiss conscripts between 1985 and 1992. *Eur Spine J* 1994;3:2–7.
127. Rowe ML. Preliminary statistical study of low back pain. *J Occup Med* 1963;5:336–341.
128. Rowe ML. Low back disability in industry: updated position. *J Occup Med* 1971;13:476–478.
129. Rush WA, Steiner HA. A study of lower extremity length inequality. *AJR Am J Roentgenol* 1946;56:616–623.
130. Salminen JJ, Erkintalo M, Laine M, et al. Low back pain in the young: a prospective three-year follow-up study of subjects with and without low back Pain. *Spine* 1995;20:2101–2108.
131. Saraste H. *Spondylolysis and spondylolisthesis: clinical and radiographic relationships, and prognostic signs.* Thesis, Karolinska Hospital, Stockholm, 1984.
132. Saraste H, Hultman G. Life conditions of persons with and without low-back pain. *Scand J Rehabil Med* 1987;19:109–113.

133. Shekelle PG, Markovich M, Louie R. An epidemiologic study of episodes of back pain care. *Spine* 1995;20:1668–1673.
134. Silman AJ, Ferry S, Papageorgiou AC, et al. Number of children as a risk factor for low back pain in men and women. *Arthritis Rheum* 1995;38:1232–1235.
135. Skargren EI, Öberg BE. Predictive factors for 1-year outcome of low-back and neck pain in patients treated in primary care: comparison between the treatment strategies chiropractic and physiotherapy. *Pain* 1998;77:201–207.
136. Skovron ML, Szpalski M, Nordin M, et al. Sociocultural factors and back pain: a population-based study in Belgian adults. *Spine* 1994;19:129–137.
137. Slithoff CA. Lumbosacral junction: roentgenographic comparison of patients with and without backaches. *JAMA* 1953;152:1610–1613.
138. Smedley J, Egger P, Cooper C, et al. Manual handling activities and risk of low back pain in nurses. *Occup Environ Med* 1995;52:160–163.
139. Sörensen KH. *Scheuermann's juvenile kyphosis.* Thesis, Munksgaard, Copenhagen, 1964.
140. Soukka A, Alaranta H, Tallroth K, et al. Leg-length inequality in people of working age: the association between mild inequality and low-back pain is questionable. *Spine* 1991;16:429–431.
141. Spangfort EV. The lumbar disc herniation. *Acta Orthop Scand Suppl* 1972;142:1–95.
142. Sweetman BJ, Anderson JAD, Dalton ER. The relationships between little-finger mobility, lumbar mobility, straight-leg raising, and low-back pain. *Rheumatol Rehabil* 1974;13:161–166.
143. Svensson HO. *Low back pain in forty to forty-seven year old men: a retrospective cross-sectional study.* Thesis, Göteborg University, Sweden, 1981.
144. Svensson HO. Low-back pain in 40–47 year old men: some socioeconomic factors and previous sickness absence. *Scand J Rehabil Med* 1982;14:54–59.
145. Svensson HO, Andersson GBJ. Low back pain in forty to forty-seven year old men: work history and work environment factors. *Spine* 1983;8:272–276.
146. Svensson HO, Andersson GB. The relationship of low-back pain, work history, work environment, and stress: a retrospective cross-sectional study of 38- to 64-year old women. *Spine* 1989;14:517–522.
147. Svensson HO, Vedin A, Wilhelmsson C, et al. Low back pain in relation to other diseases and cardiovascular risk factors. *Spine* 1983;8:277–285.
148. Symmons DPM, van Hemert AM, Vandenbroucke JP, et al. A longitudinal study of back pain and radiological changes in the lumbar spines of middle aged women. II. Radiographic findings. *Ann Rheum Dis* 1991;50:162–166.
149. Tanz SS. Motion of the lumbar spine: a roentgenologic study. *AJR Am J Roentgenol* 1953;9:399–412.
150. ten Brinke Albert, van der Aa HE, van der Palen J, et al. Is leg discrepancy associated with the side of radiating pain in patients with a lumbar herniated disc? *Spine* 1999;24:684–686.
151. Taylor H, Curran NM. *The Nuprin pain report.* New York: Louis Harris and Associates, 1985:1–233.
152. Troup JDG, Martin JW, Lloyd DCEF. Back pain in industry: a prospective study. *Spine* 1981;6:61–69.
153. Valat J-P, Goupille P, Védere V. Low back pain: risk factors for chronicity. *Rev Rhum Engl Ed* 1997;64:189–194.
154. Valkenburg HA, Haanen HCM. The epidemiology of low back pain. In: White A, Gordon S, eds. *Symposium on idiopathic low back pain.* Miami: CV Mosby, 1980:9–22.
155. van den Hoogen HJ, Koes BW, Deville W, et al. The prognosis of low back pain in general practice. *Spine* 1997;22:1515–1521.
156. Weber H. Lumbar disc herniation: a prospective study of prognostic factors including a controlled trial. I. *J Oslo City Hosp* 1978;28:33–64.
157. Venning PJ, Walter SD, Stitt LW. Personal and job-related factors as determinants of incidence of back injuries among nursing personnel. *J Occup Med* 1987;29:820–825.
158. Wells J, Zipp JF, Schuette PT, et al. Musculoskeletal disorders among letter carriers. *J Occup Med* 1983;25:814–820.
159. Viikari-Juntura E, Riihimäki H, Tola S, et al. Neck trouble in machine operating, dynamic physical work and sedentary work: a prospective study on occupational and individual risk factors. *J Clin Epidemiol* 1994;47:1411–1422.
160. Wiltse LL. Lumbosacral strain and instability. In: *Proceedings of the American Academy of Orthopaedic Surgeons symposium on the spine.* Chicago: American Academy of Orthopaedic Surgeons, 1969;54–83.
161. von Korff M. The cause of back pain in primary care. *Spine* 1996;21:2833–2837.
162. Yelin E. The earnings, income, and assets of persons aged 51–61 with and without musculoskeletal conditions. *J Rheumatol* 1997;24:2024–2030.

REFERENCES: SMOKING AND LOW BACK PAIN

1. Battié MC, Videman T, Gill K, et al. Smoking and lumbar intervertebral disc degeneration. *Spine* 1991;16:1015–1021.
2. Boshuizen HC, Verbeek JHAM, Broersen JPJ, et al. Do smokers get more back pain? *Spine* 1993; 18:35–40.

3. Daniell HW. Osteoporosis of the slender smoker. *Arch Intern Med* 1976;136:298–304.
4. Deyo RA, Bass EJ. Lifestyle and low back pain: the influence of smoking and obesity. *Spine* 1989; 14:501–506.
5. Ernst E. Smoking a cause of back trouble? *Br J Rheumatol* 1993;32:239–242.
6. Frymoyer JW. Back pain and sciatica. *N Engl J Med* 1988;318:291–300.
7. Hambly MF, Mooney V. Effects of smoking and pulsed electromagnetic fields on intradiscal pH in rabbits. *Spine* 1992;17:83–85.
8. Hansson T, Roos B. Microcalluses of the trabeculae in lumbar vertebrae and their relation to the bone mineral content. *Spine* 1981;6:375–380.
9. Harreby M, Kjer J, Hesselsöe G, et al. Epidemiological aspects and risk factors for low back pain in 38-year-old men and women: a 25-year prospective cohort study of 640 school children. *Eur Spine J* 1996;5:312–318.
10. Heliövaara M, Mäkelä M, Knekt P, et al. Determinants of sciatica and low back pain. *Spine* 1991; 16:608–614.
11. Holm S, Nachemson A. Nutrition of the intervertebral disc: acute effect of cigarette smoking. An experimental study. *Upps J Med Sci* 1988;93:91–99.
12. Jamison RN, Stetson BA, Parris WCV. The relationship between cigarette smoking and chronic low back pain. *Addict Behav* 1991;16:103–110.
13. Jayson MIV, Keegan A, Million R, et al. A firinolytic defect in chronic back pain syndromes. *Lancet* 1984;2:1186–1187.
14. Kelsey JL, Githens PG, O'Connor T, et al. Acute prolapsed lumbar intervertebral disc: an epidemiologic study with special reference to driving automobiles and cigarette smoking. *Spine* 1984;9:608–613.
15. Leboeuf-Yde C. *Low back pain in two Danish populations.* Thesis, Odense University, Denmark, 1995.
16. Leino PI. Does leisure time physical activity prevent low back disorders? A prospective study of metal industry employees. *Spine* 1993;18:863–871.
17. Manninen P, Riihimäki H, Heliövaara M. Incidence and risk factors of low back pain in middle-aged farmers. *Occup Med* 1995;45:141–146.
18. Riihimäki H, Viikari-Juntura E, Moneta G, et al. Incidence of sciatic pain among men in machine operating, dynamic work, and sedentary work. *Spine* 1994;19:138–142.
19. Ryden AL, Molgaard CA, Bobbitt S, et al. Occupational low back injury in a hospital employee population: an epidemiologic analysis of multiple risk factors of a high risk occupational group. *Spine* 1989;14:315–320.
20. Saraste H, Hultman G. Life conditions of persons with and without low-back pain. *Scand J Rehabil Med* 1987;19:109–113.
21. Toroptsova NT, Benevolenskaya LI, Karyakin AN, et al. "Cross sectional" study of low back pain among workers at an industrial enterprise in Russia. *Spine* 1995;20:328–332.

Neck and Back Pain: The Scientific Evidence of Causes, Diagnosis, and Treatment, edited by Alf Nachemson and Egon Jonsson. Published by Lippincott Williams & Wilkins, Philadelphia 2000.

5

Work-Related Influences on Neck and Low Back Pain

Eva Vingård* and Alf Nachemson†

*Section of Personal Injury Prevention, Karolinska Institutet, Stockholm, Sweden
†Department of Orthopaedics, Sahlgrenska University Hospital, Göteborg, Sweden

BACKGROUND

The origin of pain and disorders of both the low back and the neck are complex, and their causes are multifactorial. Many potentially causal and associated factors at the workplace have been discussed, from heavy work to psychosocial strain. In the later 1980s and 1990s, many reviews and oversight articles were published (9,11–13,20, 29,30,32–34,51,79,81,83–86,91,97,110,111).

AIM OF THE CHAPTER

The aim of this chapter is to

1. Investigate whether different exposures at work have any relationship with low back pain and neck pain.
2. Investigate which kind of load–physical, psychosocial, or combined–causes or contributes to low back and neck pain.
3. Investigate the degree of evidence for eventual relationships.
4. Suggest future research needs in this field.

To answer the foregoing questions, a search of MEDLINE from 1966 to 1997 and of NIOSTIC from 1970 to 1998 was made. The reviews and oversight articles mentioned earlier were studied, and references not found in the search process were added. The conclusiveness of most studies, including those discussed here, have been hampered by design problems, statistical shortcomings, varying outcome variables, and limited exposure assessments.

DESIGN

Randomized controlled trials cannot be performed in occupational life because of differences in individual factors, selection, interaction, and modification, as well as ethical considerations. Besides, in an occupation, workers are exposed to entities that they may not be aware of and cannot control.

Intervention studies can have a design similar to that of randomized trials, but other factors in society during the intervention period, such as economic growth or recession, industrial policy, lack of identical base populations, and input from or influence of other factors, may distort the results and their interpretability.

Cross-sectional studies are widely used, but they are less informative because of the difficulty in distinguishing between cause and effect. These studies give a "snapshot" of a specific situation at a given time, with no control over, for example, "healthy worker selection" (115).

Longitudinal studies, in which persons with different exposures are followed for a certain time period, are more valid, especially if the study subjects can be followed prospectively and with continuous exposure assessments. For most disorders, however, the latency period between exposure and clinical disorder is long or is not known, and many disorders are not prevalent in the general population. Those studies are therefore resource and time consuming. Usually, one has to make a retrospective study in which all information on exposures is collected after the disorder under study is reported. This approach can hamper the validity by introducing recall bias or misclassification of exposure and disease.

Two different types of epidemiologic longitudinal studies are most common and informative. In a *cohort study,* exposed persons are compared with unexposed persons in a certain population according to the outcome under study. In a *case-referent study,* all persons in the study base (study population during a special time period) with a special outcome are investigated and form the case group. Randomly chosen persons from the same study base are used as referents. Exposure frequencies are then compared between cases and referents.

STATISTICAL METHOD

The results are presented as an odds ratio, relative risk, prevalence rate ratio, or *p*-value. These values all differ in their construction and underlying theory and cannot be directly compared. For a proper statistical interpretation of these values, textbooks of epidemiology and statistics are recommended. Care is recommended in the interpretation of causality and association between an exposure and an outcome from a weak statistical relationship.

OUTCOME

Low back and neck problems are usually nonspecific disorders without distinct diagnostic criteria. Most patients complain of pain and associated loss of function. Pain is always a private experience and can hardly be measured objectively. The progression from pain to disorder to disability is probably also influenced by cultural and economic factors.

In epidemiologic and other studies of musculoskeletal disorders, outcome definitions differ. In most studies, the outcome is self-reported low back pain of different durations (i.e., ongoing, last 12 months, lifetime), or it may consist of self-reported episodes of sciatica. Some studies also include a clinical examination, but the protocol is rarely published and validated.

The outcome chosen may reflect the risk factors found. Severe sciatica with a slipped disc probably has a different risk profile compared with claiming compensation because of low back pain lasting for 1 day or more. The vague classification of these disorders is a great problem and makes comparisons between studies and conclusions of causes hazardous.

EXPOSURE

The exposure assessments are usually limited and are collected in a way that makes misclassifications common (19). Only external exposures can easily be measured, not the individual dose. The shape of the dose-response curve is also seldom clear. A model for exposure, dose, response, and capacity has been suggested (6) and is presented here in a slightly modified version divided into exposure and effect.

Classification

External exposure refers to external factors that produce a change in the internal state of the individual. External exposure is independent of the individual and can be physical or social.

Internal exposure is the change in the internal state of the individual caused by the external exposure. Internal exposure is by definition dependent on the individual and can be mechanical (e.g., muscle force); physiologic (e.g., blood pressure); or psychologic (e.g., perceived demands). These entities are not mutually exclusive.

Dose refers to those internal exposures that affect the target tissue. Thus, dose is the whole or part of the internal exposure.

Effect

The dose gives a *response* that is a reversible or irreversible reaction in the target tissue or a change in the vulnerability of the target tissue. This change in the target tissue, and perhaps also in other tissues within the individual, that is caused by the external exposure alters the capacity of the individual.

Mechanical (e.g., muscle strength), physiologic, or psychologic *capacity* refers to the ability of the individual to cope with different internal exposures. The capacity can be both reduced and enhanced by earlier exposures. Capacity can be regarded as an effect modifier.

GRADING OF STUDIES

Common Reversible Disorders With a Short Induction Period

1. *Intervention studies with one or more population in which intervention measures are performed and one or more similar control population without any interventions performed.* The interventions performed must be on an individual level, well defined, and adequately described, and the intervention period must be long enough. Other exposures must be similar and well controlled, the society and industrial setting must be stable, and the aim of the intervention must be blinded to the populations under study and in the best case also to the evaluator of the intervention at the field. The statistical procedure must be well accomplished and described. However, this type of intervention is more an ideal model than a practical reality.

2. *Intervention studies with one population investigated before and after an intervention is accomplished.* The same criteria as mentioned earlier are needed. The need for

a period between evaluation before and after an intervention can cause problems in view of the dynamic changes occurring in society and populations. The statistical procedure must be well accomplished and described. This type of intervention can take place, but it is difficult to conduct.

3. *Longitudinal prospective studies in which the study population is big enough and is followed for an appropriate time period for exposure, as well as for outcome.* The exposures and potential confounders must be well defined and assessed with valid and reliable methods. The statistical procedure must be well accomplished and described.

4. *Case-referent studies in which the study population is big enough and is followed for an appropriate time period.* The exposures and potential confounders must be well defined and assessed with valid and reliable methods in which potential recall bias is under control. The case definition must be distinct, and the referents appropriately chosen. The statistical procedure must be well accomplished and described.

5. *Cross-sectional studies in which the study population is well defined and big enough.* The exposures and potential confounders must be well defined and assessed with valid and reliable methods in which potential recall bias is under control. The case definition must be distinct, and the referents appropriately matched. Selection factors must be well controlled. The statistical procedure must be well accomplished and described.

Less Common Disorders With Short or Long Induction Times and Those That Are Not Always Reversible

Longitudinal prospective study, case-referent studies, and cross-sectional studies (with the same criteria as described earlier) have the same grading as for more common reversible disorders. Intervention studies are usually not possible to perform with this type of disorder.

Grading of Evidence

A. Support from metaanalysis or systematic review of good quality of two or more studies.
B. Support from one or more good observational studies.
C. Insufficient or inconclusive evidence (no good observational study).
D. Lack of study or support in scientific studies.

LOW BACK PAIN

Whole-Body Vibrations

Definition of Exposure

Whole-body vibrations (WBVs) are mechanical energy oscillations transferred to the body. In occupational life, this happens usually through a seat or a platform. Exposed occupational groups are truck and automobile drivers, and ship pilots, and certain aircraft personnel. However, in the 1990s, ergonomic efforts were made to improve the working environment for drivers and thus to reduce exposure to WBVs.

Experimental Studies

Laboratory studies have shown that WBVs can cause fatigue of paraspinal muscles and ligaments, lumbar disc flattening, disc fiber strain, intradiscal pressure increase, disc herniation, and microfractures in the vertebral end plate (108, 109). The vertebral end plate seems to be the structure most vulnerable to acute effects (105). Electromyographic experiments have also shown that exhaustion of low back muscles increases during WBV exposure (105).

Occupational Studies

WBV has been investigated in different studies since the mid-1970s. Almost all the studies reported here, in which the design of the study offered a more generalized possibility to conclusion, showed a positive association between WBVs and low back pain. Some studies were longitudinal and had acceptable exposure assessments (15,35,52–54,78). In some studies, hours spent in driving vehicles were used as a proxy for exposure to WBVs (18,35,36,52,53,64,78). Confounding factors were sometimes taken into account, and some studies also indicated a dose-response relationship (53,64). The relative risks differed between 1.5 and 5.7. In the studies by Kelsey (52,53), Heliövaara (35), and Bongers (14), one of the outcomes was herniated lumbar disc and sciatica, and for this more distinct diagnosis, the relationship with WBVs was also positive. A few of the studies did not show any association (36) (Table 5.1).

Bending and Twisting

Flexion or lateral bending of the trunk and bending and rotation of the trunk are considered potential risk factors for low back pain and disorders. In a "semiexperimental" biomechanical study in an occupational setting, different aspects of bending, lifting, and twisting were shown as risk factors for low back pain (69,70). Many occupations involve awkward postures for longer or shorter periods and may also involve other physically demanding tasks, such as lifting. To distinguish among the effects of two or more simultaneous exposures in a work task is difficult, and exposure assessments must be accurate to make conclusions possible. However, most of the studies of acceptable design show an association with forward bending and/or twisting and low back pain (17,21,38,53,60,82,87). A dose-response relationship was observed in certain studies (38,53,82). The studies by Kelsey et al. (53) and Riihimäki et al. (87) noted an association with herniated lumbar disc and sciatica (Table 5.2).

Manual Handling of Materials

Manual handling of materials comprises carrying and/or lifting burdens, as well as pushing and pulling objects. To assess such a complex exposure in questionnaires, interviews, and direct measurements is difficult, and misclassifications are probably substantial. Manual handling of materials also has a relation between time and force, that is, a low force for a long period, a high force for a short period, or a high force for a long period. Which one is most harmful is difficult to determine from most studies. Accidents and near-accidents associated with high forces for a short time can also happen when one handles materials. Many studies have found a relationship between manual handling, mainly lifting and handling of patients in health care workers, and reports of low back pain (5,26,31,60,64,67,68,74,95,96,98,103,104) (Table 5.3).

TABLE 5.1. *Whole body vibrations and low back pain and disorders*

Study (ref.)	Design	Population and gender studied	Outcome	Exposure	Confounders adjusted for	Results given in odds ratio (OR) if nothing else indicated
Kelsey and Hardy, 1975, USA (52)	Case-referent matched study	Male and female 20–64 yr of age	Cases with herniated lumbar disc (clinical examination); referents from hospitals	>50% of working time in a vehicle	Age, race, education, place of residence, BMI	2.75, $p < .02$ in males
Kelsey et al., 1984, USA (53)	Case-referent matched study	Male and female	Herniated lumbar disc	Hours spent in cars	Age, race, education, weight, height	OR for each individual 5 hr/wk exposure 1.2 (1.1–1.5)
Heliövaara, 1987, Finland (35)	Case-referent	592 men and women discharged from hospitals and 2,140 referents	Herniated lumbar disc leading to hospitalization	Job title (motor vehicle drivers) vs white collar workers	Workload, smoking, chronic cough, psychologic distress, use of analgesics	RR = 2.9 p > .05 in males
Bongers et al., 1990, Netherlands (14)	Cross-sectional cohort	133 male helicopter pilots and 228 male nonflying air force officers	1. Low back pain >2 wk last yr (Q) 2. Sciatica	Helicopter pilots vs nonflying officers	Age, height, weight, climate, bending forward, mental stress	1. 3.0 (1.4–6.4) 2. 3.3 (1.3–8.5)
Boshuizen et al., 1990, Netherlands (15)	Longitudinal cohort	450 male tractor drivers and 110 male agricultural workers	Low back pain (Q)	Vibration magnitude 0.3–0.55	Duration of exposure, age, height, weight, smoking, twisted positions, lifting, mental stress	1.98 (0.97–4.09) EF = 39%
Heliövaara et al., 1991, Finland (36)	Cross-sectional population cohort	2,946 women and 2,727 men	1. Low back pain (clinical examination) 2. Sciatica (clinical examination)	Occupational vehicle driving	Sex, age, BMI, previous trauma, physical stress, mental stress, smoking, alcohol, no. of births for women	1. 1.1 (0.7–1.6) 2. 0.7 (0.4–1.2)
Burdorf et al., 1991, Netherlands (21)	Cross-sectional cohort	114 male concrete workers and 52 male maintenance workers	Low back pain previous 12 mo (Q)	Vibration table yes/no	Age	3.06 (1.26–7.45)

102

Reference	Study design	Population	Outcome measure	Exposure	Confounders	RR (95% CI)
Johanning, 1991, USA (42)	Cross-sectional (low response rate)	Male and female: 492 subway train operators and 92 tower operators	Self-reported sciatic pain previous 12 mo (Q)	Vibration magnitude >0.55	Age, gender, job title earlier, duration of employment	3.9 (1.7–8.6)
Pietri et al., 1992, Italy (78)	Longitudinal cohort	Commercial drivers: 893 men and 225 women	1-yr cumulative incidence (I)	≥20 hrs of occupational driving/wk compared to <10 (I)	None	3.6 (1.1–11.5)
Boshuizen et al., 1992, Netherlands (16)	Cross-sectional cohort	Male(?): 242 drivers and 210 blue collar workers	Back pain 1-yr prevalence (Q)	Vibration level 0.8–1.0 m/sec² over a representative working period	1. Age 2. Age, mental stress, lifting, prolonged sitting, looking backward, smoking	1. 1.73 (1.06–2.81) 2. 1.28 (0.62–2.6)
Bovenzi et al., 1992, Italy (18)	Cross-sectional cohort	Male: 234 bus drivers and 125 maintenance workers	Low back pain previous 12 mo (Q)	1. Job title 2. Total vibration dose 2.5–4.5 (yr and vibration magnitude)	1. None 2. Age, BMI, awkward postures, mental stress, smoking, education, sports activities, previous jobs with whole-body vibration	1. 2.54 (1.54–4.21) 2. 3.52 (1.71–7.25)
Bovenzi and Betta, 1994, Italy (17)	Cross-sectional cohort	Male: 1,155 tractor drivers and 220 office workers	1. Self-reported low back pain previous 12 mo (Q) 2. Self-reported sciatica previous 12 mo (Q)	Vibration magnitude 0.5–1.0 m/sec²	Age, BMI, education, sports activities, car driving, marital status, climate, back trauma, postural load	1. 2.39 (1.52–3.76) 2. 3.15 (1.36–7.28)
Liira et al., 1996, Canada (60)	Cross-sectional population cohort (1990 Ontario Health Survey)	8,020 men and women in blue collar occupations	Serious problems with back pain (I)	Operating vibrating vehicle or equipment yes/no	Age, sex, smoking	1.84 (1.25–2.72)
Magnusson et al., 1996, USA and Sweden (64)	Cross-sectional cohort	Male: 228 drivers and 137 sedentary workers	Low back pain previous 12 mo (Q)	1. Being a driver 2. Long-term (?) exposure to vibration	None	1. 1.79 (1.16–2.75) 2. 2.0 (0.98–4.1)

BMI, body mass index; EF, etiological fraction; RR, relative risk.

TABLE 5.2. *Awkward postures (bending and twisting) and low back pain and disorders*

Study (ref.)	Design	Population and gender studied	Outcome	Exposure	Confounders adjusted for	Results given in odds ratio (OR) if nothing else indicated
Kelsey et al., 1984, USA (53)	Case-referent matched study	Male and female	Herniated lumbar disc	Lifting objects >11,3 kg >25 times/d plus body twisted: 1. Knees not bent 2. Knees bent	Age, race, education, weight, and height	1. 7.2 (2.0–25.8) 2. 1.9 (0.8–4.8)
Riihimäki et al., 1989, Finland (87)	Cross-sectional cohort	Male: 852 machine operators, 696 carpenters, 674 office workers	Sciatica in previous 12 mo (Q)	Bending and twisting rather much compared with rather little	Age	1.5 (1.2–1.9)
Burdorf et al., 1991, Netherlands (21)	Cross-sectional cohort	114 male concrete workers and 52 male maintenance workers	LBP previous 12 mo (Q)	Time spent in different bent and twisted postures objectively measured by OWAS system (37% for concrete workers and 27% for maintenance workers)	Age	2.80 (1.31–6.08)
Punnett et al., 1991, USA (82)	Case-referent study in car assembly workers	Male car assembly workers	95 cases with LBP and 124 without	1. Mild flexion 21–45 degrees 2. Severe flexion >45 degrees 3. Twist or lateral bending >20 degrees (videotaped)	Age	1. 4.9 (1.4–17.4) 2. 5.7 (1.6–20.4) 3. 5.9 (1.6–21.4)
Holmström et al., 1992, Sweden (38)	Cross-sectional cohort	1,772 male construction workers	1. LBP last 12 mo (Q) 2. Severe LBP last 12 mo (Q)	Forward bending >4 hr/d compared with never/seldom (Q)	Age	1. pRR 1.29 (1.1–1.59) 2. pRR 2.61 (1.7–3.8)
Bovenzi and Zadini, 1992, Italy (18)	Cross-sectional cohort	Male: 234 bus drivers and 125 maintenance workers	Low back pain previous 12 mo (Q)	Awkward postures frequent compared with rare (Q)	None	2.29 (1.22–4.29)
Burdorf et al., 1993, Netherlands (22)	Cross-sectional	Male: 94 crane operators and 86 office workers	LBP last 12 mo (Q)	Nonneutral trunk positions and sitting (observation)	Age	3.29 (1.52–7.12)
Bovenzi and Betta, 1994, Italy (17)	Cross-sectional cohort	Male: 1,155 tractor drivers and 220 office workers	1. Transient LBP last 12 mo (Q) 2. Chronic LBP last 12 mo (Q)	Postural load (time and frequency) hard versus mild	Age	1. 2.95 (1.79–4.84) 2. 2.19 (1.19–4.03)
Liira and Shannon, 1996, Canada (60)	Cross-sectional population cohort (1990 Ontario Health Survey)	8,020 men and women in blue collar occupations	Serious problems with back pain (I)	Working with back in awkward positions (I)	Age, sex, smoking	2.33 (1.72–3.15)

LBP, low back pain; OWAS, Ovako Working Posture Analysis System; RR, relative risk.

104

TABLE 5.3. *Manual materials handling (lifting, carrying, pushing and pulling) and low back pain and disorders*

Study (ref.)	Design	Population and gender studied	Outcome	Exposure	Confounders adjusted for	Results given in odds ratio (OR) if nothing else indicated
Magora, 1972, Israel (67)	Cross-sectional	3,316 persons, from 8 pre-selected occupations	LBP (more information not given)	Lifting 5 kg often vs rarely or never	None	0.5 (0.4–0.6) (calculations made by Vingård after numbers in article)
Svensson and Andersson, 1983, Sweden (98)	Cross-sectional population cohort	940 men 40–47 yr of age	Lifetime LBP (I, Q)	Heavy lifting	Psychosocial factors, other physical factors	$p < .001$
Wells et al., 1983, USA (103)	Cross-sectional cohort	Male letter carriers, meter readers, and postal clerks	Serious back probls (index constructed by interview)	Job title letter carrier vs all others	Age, distance walked, number of years in the job, previous jobs, body size	$p < .05$
Arad and Ryan, 1986, Australia (5)	Cross-sectional	831 female nurses	LBP last month	>20 lifts vs 0 lifts per shift	None	2.87 (16–5.1) (calculations made by Vingård after numbers in article)
Gilad and Kirschenbaum, 1986, Israel (31)	Cross-sectional	250 male miners	Severe and sporadic LBP	All tasks involving lifting	None	3.2 (2.0–5.4) (calculations made by Vingård after numbers in article)
Venning et al., 1987, USA (104)	Prospective, (12 mo) cohort	4,306 nurses	Back injury	Daily lifts	None	2.19 $p < .05$
Mandel and Lohman, 1987, USA (68)	Cross-sectional	428 female nurses who had worked >5 yr	LBP > 48 hr last 12 mo (Q)	Lifting >10 patients/wk (Q)	Age, LBP before study period, aerobic exercises	1.39 (1.05–1.84)
Stobbe et al., 1988, USA (96)	Longitudinal cohort	415 female nurses	Self-reported back injuries	Lifting >5 patients every shift vs lifting <2 patients every shift vs lifting <2 patients every shift	None	2.5 (1.2–5.0) (calculations made by Vingård after numbers in article)
Estryn-Behar et al., 1990, France (26)	Cross-sectional cohort	1,505 female hospital workers	LBP last 12 mo	Manual materials handling high versus low	Forward bending, previous attacks of back pain	$p < .001$
Nuwayhid et al., 1993, USA (74)	Case-referent	Male fire fighters 115 cases and 109 referents	First time of LBP resulting in >1 d off work (I)	1. Lifting >18 kg (I) 2. Open structure to look for open fire 3. Break any window	Rank, previous occupation, steps climbed, off-duty activities, second job	1. 3.07 (1.19–7.88) 2. 4.32 (1.66–11.29) 3. 4.45 (1.90–10.42)
Smedley et al., 1995, England (95)	Cross-sectional	1,616 female nurses	LBP previous 12 mo	Manually moving a patient around in the bed >10 times per working shift	Age, height, nonmusculo-skeletal symptoms	1.7 (1.2–2.4)
Magnusson et al., 1996, USA and Sweden (64)	Cross-sectional cohort	Male 228 drivers and 137 sedentary workers	Low back pain previous 12 mo (Q)	1. Frequent lifting (lift "every often") 2. Heavy (>10 kg) lifting 3. Frequent and heavy lifting	None	1. 1.55 (1.0–2.39) 2. 1.86 (1.2–2.8) 3. 2.06 (1.3–3.3)
Liira et al., 1996, Canada (60)	Cross-sectional population cohort (1990 Ontario Health Survey)	8,020 men and women in the collar occupations	Serious problems with back pain (I)	Frequent lifting of things >50 lb (I)	Age, sex, smoking	1.28 (0.91–1.81)

LBP, low back pain.

105

Psychosocial Exposures

Psychologic and social environments as risk or health factors for reporting low back pain have been investigated in epidemiologic studies. Those factors are even more complex to assess than are physical factors (25,50,56). Both facts and value statements are included and mixed, and few assessments and methods are tested for validity and reliability. Another problem is that jobs with high physical demands often also include a poor psychosocial environment. If these factors are not assessed and adjusted for in the analysis, the interpretation will be uncertain.

In cross-sectional studies, it is also difficult to evaluate whether poor psychosocial conditions that are reported preceded the disorder under study or whether the impaired health status gave rise to a poor psychosocial situation, especially when value statements are used in questionnaires.

Job dissatisfaction is the exposure with the most consistent evidence for an association with reports of low back pain (8,12,23,28,55,65–67,77,80).

Exposures often investigated are high job demands and low control over the work process. Put together, this entity is called *job strain,* and the model, also known as the demand-control or decision latitude model, was introduced by Karasek and Theorell (49,50). The model is based on the degree of demands from the job situation related to the degree of control or decision latitude (i.e., influence and stimulation). Job strain as an entity and especially the high-demand variable have been associated with reports of low back pain (1,23,28,38,39,41,55,58). Whether that low back pain is caused by psychosocial exposure alone or in combination with physical load is uncertain, however.

Another important factor is *social support* from supervisors and coworkers (46). Low social support is supposed to be associated with different disorders, among them low back pain (1,23,50,55,58,61,63,93,101).

Factors such as monotony at work, a combination of repetitive work and negative psychologic factors, and more diffuse exposures such as "job stress" have also been investigated. Some studies have noted an association, albeit weaker, with reports of low back pain (7,36,38,89,95,98,99).

For all the foregoing psychosocial exposures, there are also negative studies published with no associations found between one or more of the psychosocial factors at work and reports of low back pain (27,28,38,40,41,58,59,77,89) (Tables 5.4 and 5.5). Whether these findings result from lack of association, from selection, or from misclassification of exposure is impossible to tell.

NECK AND SHOULDER PAIN

If the diagnostic criteria are diffuse for low back pain and low back disorders, they are even more so for neck and shoulder disorders. In scientific studies, the anatomic regions comprising the neck and shoulders are put together and are examined as one health outcome. The reason for this is that most muscles in these regions interact, and it is difficult to distinguish between pure neck disorders and combined disorders involving both the neck and shoulder. Disorders affecting only the shoulder, from the tendons of the shoulder muscles, mainly the rotator cuff and biceps longus and the acromioclavicular joint, are better defined, but they are outside the scoop of this review.

Some patients with neck and shoulder pain problems complain of pain in the neck region with stiffness, sometimes decreased range of motion in the neck, and headache.

Other patients have more widespread problems with pain in the neck-shoulder-arm-hand region, sometimes with impaired function in the whole region, decreased range of motion in the neck and the shoulder, and often decreased endurance in arm and hand function.

Radiating pain can have a distinct anatomic origin in patients with a disc disorder in the neck region or irritation of one or more of the cervical roots. However, such a cause of pain is rare, and usually, the pain is diffuse, with many anatomic structures involved in the process. The pain often becomes chronic and makes the patient's clinical status disabling. The terminology of this indistinct pain disorder is unsatisfactory. Terms such as repetitive strain injury, occupational cervicobrachial disorder, and so on, ought not to be used. These terms suggest a causal relationship that is too simplistic and not scientifically proven. As long as a distinct diagnosis cannot be made, the term *cervicobrachial pain* is preferred.

Exposures Investigated

As occupational risk factors for neck and shoulder disorders, repetitive work, static load on the neck region, force or dynamic loads at the neck region, and different psychologic and social factors have been suggested. Few prospective studies with more than one potential risk factor investigated have been published (24,44,90,102) (Table 5.6).

Repetitive Work

Can refer to neck movements themselves or to repeated arm and shoulder motions that generate loads to the neck. These factors are not easily measured and assessed and are seldom distinguished from other potentially harmful exposures such as static load or monotony, which also implies poor psychosocial conditions. Two Swedish studies, one cross-sectional (75) and one prospective (47), both had extensive exposure measurements for repetitiveness and controlled for other potential hazards to the region. The first study showed an OR of 4.6 (1.9–12) for neck shoulder pain, and the second study allocated workers to "healthy status" when they changed to more varied work tasks without extreme static and repetitive neck and arm movements. Many other studies used questionnaire information on both outcome and exposure, and the assessments are often superficial, with potential misclassification. The cross-sectional design also makes temporal relations uncertain (2–4,57,73,75,76,92) (Table 5.7).

Static Load in the Neck Region

Static load in the neck region is common in many work tasks, especially in the assembly line industry. In many factories, women perform these work tasks. Many studies have been conducted. However, for studies of this exposure, the design is also mainly cross-sectional, although the exposure assessments are better (10,48, 57,61,72,73,93,100). Most of the studies show increased risks, and improvement in working conditions lowered the risk estimates (47,90) (Tables 5.6 and 5.8).

Visual display unit work is characterized by working in a static position with hands fixed, often in a stressful environment. Studies of visual display unit operators are numerous. A review of musculoskeletal health effects of this type of work found an increased risk for persons heavily exposed to those work tasks (81).

TABLE 5.4. *Psychosocial work factors and low back pain and disorders*

Study (ref.)	Design	Population and gender studied	Outcome	Exposure	Confounders adjusted for	Results given in odds ratio (OR) if nothing else indicated
Magora, 1973, Israel (65)	Cross-sectional	3,316 persons from 8 preselected occupations	LBP (more information not given)	1. Not satisfied with place of employment 2. Continuous degree of mental concentration 3. Unsatisfied with present social status 4. High degree of fatigue after work 5. High degree of nervousness after work	None	1. 4.3 (3.2–5.8) 2. 3.7 (2.8–4.9) 3. 2.4 (1.8–3.0) 4. 5.3 (3.9–7.3) 5. 2.2 (1.8–2.8) (calculations made by El Vingård after numbers in article)
Dehlin et al., 1977, Sweden (23)	Cross-sectional	233 nursing aides	Lifetime LBP	1. Relations with supervisors and workmates 2. Overall satisfaction with the job 3. Perceived demand of psychologic and physical strength	None	1. $p < .05$ 2. $p < .01$ 3. $p < .05$
Svensson and Andersson, 1983, Sweden (98)	Cross-sectional population cohort	940 men 40–47 yr of age	Lifetime LBP (Q, I)	Monotonous work	Physical load, other psychosocial factors	$p < .001$
Riihimäki et al., 1989, Finland (89)	Longitudinal prospective cohort	167 concrete workers and 161 house painters	Sciatic pain during follow-up	Job stress (frequent versus very rare	Age	1.2 (0.6–2.1)
Heliövaara et al., 1991, Finland (36)	Cross-sectional population cohort	2,946 women and 2,727 men	1. LBP (clinical examination) 2. Sciatica (clinical examination)	Occupational mental stress (sum index 3–6 versus 0)	Sex, age, BMI, previous trauma, physical stress, vehicle driving, smoking, alcohol, no. of births	1. 1.4 (1.1–1.9) 2. 2.0 (1.4–2.9)
Bigos et al., 1991, USA (12)	Longitudinal prospective cohort (follow-up time 1 d to 4.5 yr)	3,020 men and women 21–67 yr old (46 refusals)	Reported LBP	Modified work: Apgar scale for "Enjoying job"	MMPI scale on hysteria and prior back pain	1.70 (1.31–2.21)

Source	Study design	Population	Outcome measure	Psychosocial factor	Controlled variables	Results
Holmström et al., 1992, Sweden (38)	Cross-sectional cohort	1,772 male construction workers	1. LBP last 12 mo (Q) 2. Severe LBP last 12 mo (Q)	A. Mental stress index B. Social support at work C. Low decision latitude D. Quantitative demands E. Job satisfaction	Age	1A. 1.6 (1.4–1.8) 2A. 3.1 (2.3–4.0) 1B. 1.0 (0.9–1.3) 2B. 0.9 (0.7–1.4) 1C. 0.8 (0.7–0.9) 2C. 1.0 (0.7–1.4) 1D. 1.3 (1.2–1.6) 2D. 2.0 (1.2–3.2) 1E. 0.7 (0.7–0.9) 2E. 0.6 (0.4–1.0)
Feyer et al., 1992, Australia (27)	Cross-sectional cohorts	257 nurses (most female and 256 postal workers (most male)	Prevalence and severity of LBP last 12 mo (Q)	1. 28-item GHQ 2. Job satisfaction	None	1. NS 2. NS
Bergenudd and Nilsson, 1994, Sweden (8)	Cross-sectional	575 men and women	LBP (pain drawing)	Job satisfaction	Smoking, income, alcohol, physical workload, body weight, social background	p < .05
Riihimäki et al., 1994, Finland (88)	Longitudinal cohort 3-year follow-up	591 office workers	Sciatic pain 3-yr incidence	Problem with workmates and superiors	Physical exercise, smoking, other LBP	RR = 1.92 (1.12–3.28)
Houtman et al., 1994, Netherlands (39)	Cross-sectional population cohort	5,865 men and women	A. LBP complaints (Q) B. Chronic LBP (Q)	1. High work pace 2. Intellectual discretion (index)	Age, gender, education, physical load (index)	1A. 1.25 (1.09–1.43) 2A. 1.47 (1.08–1.99) 1B. 1.21 (0.94–1.50) 2B. 2.10 (1.24–3.58)
Skovron et al., 1994, Belgium (94)	Cross-sectional population survey	1,865 currently working men and women	1. Ever had LBP 2. Daily LBP	Satisfaction with work	Sex, age, language	1. 2.49 (1.03–6.03) 2. 3.85 (1.42–10.43)
Lagerström et al., 1995, Sweden (58)	Cross-sectional cohort	688 female nurses	Moderate LBP (Q)	1. Low work commitment 2. Low support from superiors 3. High work demand 4. Lack of stimulation 5. Low work control	Age, BMI, physical fitness, smoking, type of ward, work category	1. NS 2. 1.80 (1.13–2.83) 3. NS 4. NS 5. NS
Leino and Hänninen, 1995, Finland (59)	Prospective cohort 10-yr follow-up	902 men and women	LBP (clinical examination)	1. Work content 2. Work control 3. Social relations	Age, gender, social class, social relations	Men white collar 1–3 p < .01 Men blue collar 1–3 p < .05 Women white collar 1–3 p < .01 Women blue collar 1. NS 2. p < 0.05 3. NS

continued

109

TABLE 5.4. Continued

Study (ref.)	Design	Population and gender studied	Outcome	Exposure	Confounders adjusted for	Results given in odds ratio (OR) if nothing else indicated
Ahlberg-Hulthén et al., 1995, Sweden (1)	Cross-sectional cohort	90 nurses	LBP last mo	High demands and low decision latitude	Social support at work	$p < .03$
Smedley et al., 1995, England (95)	Cross-sectional cohort	1,616 female nurses	LBP previous 12 mo (Q)	1. Stress frequent 2. Low mood 3. Fatigue 4. Headache		1. 1.3 (1.0–1.8) 2. 2.0 (1.2–3.1) 3. 1.4 (1.1–1.99 1.7 (1.3–2.3
Hultman et al., 1995, Sweden (41)	Retrospective cohort	148 men; 36 back healthy, 91 with intermittent LBP, 21 with chronic LBP	Intermittent chronic LBP	1. High demands (Q) 2. Low control (Q) 3. Social support (Q)	Physical load	1. <0.01 2. <0.01 between healthy chronic trend between healthy and intermittent 3. NS
Skov et al., 1996, Denmark (93)	Cross-sectional	1,306 sales persons	12-mo prevalence of LBP (Q)	1. Poor social contact with colleagues 2. Tendency to feel overworked	Age, height, smoking, sedentary work, annual driving distance	1. 1.81 (1.25–2.63) 2. 2.04 (1.39–3.00)
Foppa and Noack, 1996, Switzerland (28)	Cross-sectional cohort	850 men and women at 2 work places	1-mo prevalence of LBP	1. Socioeconomic factors 2. Low job discretion 3. High job demands 4. Low job satisfaction 5. Dissatisfaction with salary 6. Psychosomatic complaints	Age, gender, smoking, physical load (logistic regression)	1. NS 2. 1.56 (1.00–2.45) for men NS for women 3. 1.52 (0.98–2.37) for men NS for women 4. 1.48 (0.95–2.28) for men NS for women 5. 3.30 (1.63–6.67) for women NS for men 6. 5.87 (2.88–11.96) for men and 2.95 (1.90–4.58) for women
Papageorgiou et al., 1997, England (77)	Prospective population-based cohort analyzed as a case referent study	1,412 male and female employed persons, 310 with LBP and 537 without LBP	New episodes of LBP: A. 247 had not consulted a physician B. 63 had consulted a physician	1. Dissatisfaction with job 2. Perceived inadequacy with income 3. Social class 4. Severe problems with relationship at work	Age	1A. 2.0 (1.2–3.3) 1B. 0.8 (0.2–2.4) 2A. 1.3 (0.8–2.1) 2B. 3.6 (1.8–7.2) 3A. 0.8 (0.5–1.3) 3B. 4.8 (2.0–11.5) 4A. 0.9 (0.3–3.0)

110

Study	Design	Population	Outcome	Risk factor	Results
Hemingway et al., 1997, England (37)	Longitudinal cohort	6,894 men and 3,414 women 35–55 yr old, all office workers	1. Sick leave ≤7 d for LBP 2. Sick leave >7 d for LBP	A. Employment grade high versus low (6-grade scale) B. Control, low versus high C. Job satisfaction	A and B. Age, gender C. Age, gender, education, housing, BMI, exercise, smoking, earlier back pain, car-owner	1A. p for linear trend <.001 2A. p for linear trend <.001 1B. 1.76 (1.54–2.01) 2B. 1.64 (1.25–2.14) 1C. 1.15 (0.83–1.58) 2C. 1.19 (0.73–1.95)
Huges et al., 1997, USA (40)	Cross-sectional	104 male iron smelter workers	"Worked-related LBP"	1. Low social support 2. Low job satisfaction	Age, decision latitude, job demands, years working in awkward positions	1. 5.3 (1.3–22) 2. 0.17 (0.039–0.70)
Toomingas et al., 1997, Sweden (101)	Cross-sectional	358 in 3 groups (furniture movers, medical secretaries, and population group)	1-yr prevalence of LBP (Q, examination)	1. Social support 2. Job strain	Age, gender, physical load	1. 1.6 (1.2–2.2) 2. 1.2 (0.94–1.6)
Krause et al., 1997, USA (55)	Cross-sectional	1,449 transit vehicle operators	Neck or back pain (Q and clinical examination)	1. Job strain 2. Job dissatisfaction low 3. Coworker support low 4. Supervisor support low 5. Frequency of job problems high	Age, gender, height, weight, vehicle type, physical workload	1. 1.50 (0.98–2.30) 2. 1.62 (1.11–2.67) 3. 1.10 (0.80–1.51) 4. 1.67 (1.22–3.63) 5. 2.30 (1.67–3.18)
Masset et al., 1998, Belgium (71)	Longitudinal cohort	215 male steel workers	Incidence 2-yr of LBP	Lifting requirements high	Other psychosocial and physical factors	2.26 (1.12–4.55)
van Poppel et al., 1998, Netherlands (80)	Longitudinal cohort	238 male workers involved in heavy physical work	1. New episodes of LBP (Q) 2. Sick leave from back pain	Poor job satisfaction	Earlier back pain, age, riding forklift,	1. 1.2 (1.01–1.4) 2. 1.2 (1.05–1.7)
Barnekow-Bergkvist et al., 1998, Sweden (7)	Longitudinal cohort	238 men and women investigated at age 16 and 34 yr	12 mo prevalence of LBP (Q)	1. Monotonous work 2. Vibration 3. Job satisfaction	Logistic regression with age, physical load, sociodemografic factors, physical performance	1 for men. 5.45 (1.07–27.92) 1 for women. 6.39 (1.25–32.73) 2 for men. 5.06 (1.36–18.8) 3 for men. NS 3 for women. NS

BMI, body mass index; GHQ, general health questionnaire; LBP, low back pain; MMPI, Minnesota Multiphasic Personality Inventory; NS, not significant.

111

TABLE 5.5. *Other exposures and combined exposures and low back pain and disorders*

Study (ref.)	Design	Population and gender studied	Outcome	Exposure	Confounders adjusted for	Results given in odds ratio (OR) if nothing else indicated
Magora, 1972, Israel (67)	Cross-sectional	3,316 persons from 8 preselected occupations	LBP	Standing >4 hr/d	None	0.5 (0.4–0.6) (calculations made by Vingård after numbers in article)
Linton, 1990, Sweden (61)	Cross-sectional	22,180 men and women	12-mo prevalence of LBP (Q)	1. Monotonous work plus poor psychosocial environment (index Q) 2. Heavy lifting plus poor psychosocial environment 3. Awkward posture plus poor psychosocial environment		1. 2.58 (1.94–3.43) 2. 2.42 (1.78–3.30) 3. 3.36 (2.56–4.40)
Marras et al., 1993, USA (69)	Biomechanical semiexperimental in occupational setting	403 repetitive industrial jobs	High and low risk of LBP according to external evaluation	Load moment plus lifting frequency plus lateral trunk velocity plus twisting trunk velocity plus saggital flexion		10.7 (4.9–23.69)
Riihimäki et al., 1994, Finland (88)	Longitudinal prospective cohort	1,149 men, carpenters, machine operators and office workers 25–49 yr	Cumulative 3-yr incidence of sciatic pain	1. Machine operators vs office workers 2. Carpenters vs office workers	Physical exercise, smoking, history of other LBP	1. 1.36 (0.99–1.87) 2. 1.50 (1.09–2.07)
Liira et al., 1996, Canada (60)	Cross-sectional population cohort (1990 Ontario Health Survey)	8,020 men and women in blue collar occupations	Serious problems with back pain (I)	1. Frequent lifting plus forward bending 2. Frequent lifting plus forward bending plus whole body vibrations (I)	Age, sex, smoking	1. 1.65 (1.25–1.81) 2. 3.30 (1.82–5.96)

LBP, low back pain.

112

TABLE 5.6. *Prospective studies on neck pain with both physical and psychosocial exposures*

Study (ref.)	Design	Population and gender studied	Outcome	Exposure	Confounders adjusted for	Results given in odds ratio (OR) if nothing else indicated
Jonsson et al., 1988, Sweden (47)	Prospective cohort	69 female workers studied for 2 yr	4-grade scale of severity of symptoms from neck and neck/shoulder angle	Working postures movements of head shoulder and upper arm		1. Deterioration of status over 2 yr 2. More persons remaining healthy
Veierstad and Westgaard, 1994, Norway (102)	Longitudinal cohort 1 yr	30 female workers	Trapezius myalgia (and clinical examination)	1. Working with shoulder elevated 2. Job satisfaction 1. Strenuous postures 2. Perceived stress (including bad relations with colleagues and superiors) All exposures assessed before onset		1. 7.2 (2.1–25.3) 2. 3.3 (0.8–14.2)
Schibye et al., 1995, Denmark (90)	Prospective cohort 1985 and 1991	327 female sewing machine operators (mainly piecework salary)	12-mo. and 7-d, prevalence for neck pain and discomfort and long-lasting pain (>30 d in 1991) Improvement of status for those going from exposed to unexposed cohort	Sewing machine operators 1985 and 1991 (exposed cohort) Sewing machine operators 1985 but not 1991 (unexposed cohort)	1. Stress 2. Strenuous postures	Chance in improvement in 12-mo sign when put in unexposed cohort; OR = 3.26 (1.38–7.72)

113

TABLE 5.7. *Repetitive workload alone or in combination with other exposures and neck pain*

Study (ref.)	Design	Population and gender studied	Outcome	Exposure	Confounders adjusted for	Results given in odds ratio (OR) if nothing else indicated
Kuorinka and Koskinen, 1979, Finland (57)	Cross-sectional	90 female and 3 male scissor makers (exposed cohort); 133 female shop assistants (unexposed cohort)	Tension neck (clinical examination and I)	Job titles	None	OR = 4.1 (2.3–7.2)
Silverstein, 1985, USA (92)	Cross-sectional	1,212 male workers exposed to repetitive work tasks and high force vs 75 male nonexposed workers; 2,226 female exposed workers vs 61 nonexposed female workers	Tension neck (clinical examination and I)	Repetitive movements and high force		1. OR = 1.1 (0.1–10) 2. OR = 0.9 (0.4–2.4)
Amano et al., 1988, Japan (2)	Cross-sectional	102 female matched pairs: assembly line vs non assembly line	Shoulder muscle pain (levator, trapezius, infraspinatus, scalenius)	Assembly line work production of 3,400 shoes/d (repetitive, monotonous)	Matched pairs	p < .01
Mäkelä et al., 1991, Finland (73)	Cross-sectional cohort	5,673 men and women from the Mini-Finland Health Survey, 30–64 yr old	Chronic neck pain (Q and clinical examination)	1. Index for physical stress at work 2. Index for mental stress at work	Age, sex, smoking, obesity, parity and 1 and 2, respectively	1. OR = 1.26 (1.18–1.37) for each additional stress item 2. OR = 1.20 (1.12–1.28) for each additional stress item
Andersen and Gaardboe, 1993, Denmark (4)	Cross-sectional	90 garment workers (exposed cohort); 30 auxillary nurses (unexposed cohort)	1. Cervical syndrome (self-reported chronic neck pain, decreased range of motion, palpatory tenderness or radiating symptoms) 2. Cervical fibromyalgia (tension neck and shoulder tendinitis)	Job title and years employed for exposed cohort		1. p < 0.001 ×2 for trend in garment workers 11.14 2. p ≪ 0.001 ×2 for trend in garment workers 25.15

Reference	Study design	Study population	Outcome definition	Exposure/comparison	Adjustment factors	Results (OR/RR, 95% CI)
Andersen and Gaardboe, 1993, Denmark (3)	Longitudinal cohort	424 female sewing machine operators (exposed cohort); 781 women from general population (control cohort)	Neck pain >30 d last yr (Q)	Job title and employment time 1. 0–7 yr 2. 8–15 yr 3. >15 yr	Age, having children, not doing exercise, socioeconomic status, current n/s exposure	1. 1.9 (1.3–2.9) 2. 3.8 (2.3–6.4) 3. 5.0 (2.9–8.7)
Viikari-Juntura, et al., 1994, Finland (106)	Prospective cohort (1984 and 1987)	688 machine operators; 553 carpenters; 591 office workers	Neck trouble change from 1984 to 1987 (measured as trouble the preceding yr): Not any trouble moderate (1–30 d) Severe >30 d persistently severe = daily (Q)	1. Carpenters vs office workers 2. Machine operators vs office workers 3. Machine operators vs carpenters	Age, smoking, physical exercise	None to moderate 1. 1.6 (1.0–2.5) 2. 1.8 (1.1–2.8) 3. 1.1 (0.7–1.8) None to severe 1. 1.6 (0.8–3.0) 2. 3.9 (2.3–6.9) 3. 2.5 (1.4–4.4) None to persistently severe 1. 3.0 (1.4–6.4) 2. 4.2 (2.0–9.0) 3. 1.4 (0.8–2.6)
Ekberg et al., 1994, Sweden (24)	Case-control	109 new patients with musculoskeletal complaints (no sick leave last month) 327 randomly selected controls from the study base	Neck and shoulder complaints in Q and clinical examination	Q 1. Repetitive work 2. Lifting 3. High work pace 4. Uncomfortable sitting 5. High ambiguity of work role 6. High demands on attention 7. Low work content	Sex, immigrant status, smoking, exercise, age	1. 7.5 (2.4–23) 2. 13.6 (4.8–39) 3. 3.5 (1.3–9.4) 4. 3.6 (1.4–9.3) 5. 16.5 (6.0–46) 6. 3.8 (1.4–9.4) 7. 2.6 (0.7–9.4)
Ohlsson et al., 1995, Sweden (75, 76)	Cross-sectional	82 female industrial workers with repetitive tasks (exposed cohort); 64 female workers without repetitive work tasks (unexposed cohort)	Neck/shoulder diagnosis mainly tension neck	1. Repetitive work 2. Age (54 vs 37 yr) 3. Muscular tension tendency 4. Stress/work tendency	Logistic regression with age and 1, 2, 3, and 4 in the model	1. 4.6 (1.9–12) 2. 1.9 (1.0–3.5) 3. 2.3 (1.3–4.9) 4. 1.9 (1.1–3.5)

TABLE 5.8. *Static exposures alone or in combination with other exposures and neck pain*

Study (ref.)	Design	Population and gender studied	Outcome	Exposure	Confounders adjusted for	Results given in odds ratio (OR) if nothing else indicated
Kuorinka and Koskinen, 1979, Finland (57)	Cross-sectional	90 female and 3 male scissors makers (exposed cohort); 133 female shop assistants (unexposed cohort)	Tension neck (clinical examination and I)	Job titles	None	OR = 4.1 (2.3–7.2)
Tola et al., 1988, Finland (100)	Cross-sectional	852 machine operators; 696 carpenters; 674 office workers	12-mo prevalence of neck/shoulder pain	1. Job title 1a. Machine operators vs office workers 1b. Carpenters vs office workers 1c. Machine operators vs carpenters 2. Twisted and bent positions often 3. Moderate or poor job satisfaction	Age, draft, and 1, 2 and 3, respectively, in a logistic regression	1a. 1.7 (1.5–2.0) 1b. 1.4 (1.1–1.6) 1c. 1.3 (1.1–1.4) 2. 1.8 (1.5–2.2) 3. 1.2 (1.1–1.4)
Milerad and Ekenvall, 1990, Sweden (72)	Cross-sectional	99 dentists and 100 pharmacists 35–55 yr old	Lifetime prevalence of neck symptoms	Job title	?	RR = 2.1 (1.4–3.1)
Linton, 1990, Sweden (61)	Cross-sectional	22,180 men and women, full-time working during day time	Seeking care because of neck pain last 12 mo (Q)	1. Heavy lifting 2. Monotonous work 3. Sitting 4. Uncomfortable postures 5. Vibration 6. Psychosocial factors (work content, social support, and workload)		OR for different age groups <30–39, 40, 49 and >50 yr 1. 1.4, 1.7, 1.6, 1.8 2. 2.3, 2.4, 2.5, 3.0 3. 1.3, 1.1, 1.0, 0.9 4. 1.6, 2.0, 2.0, 2.4 5. 1.0, 1.5, 1.3, 1.8 6. 2.6, 1.9, 2.5, 2.3
Kamvendo et al., 1991, Sweden (48)	Cross-sectional	420 female medical secretaries	Neck pain previous yr	1. Working with office machines >5 hours/day 2. Poor psychosocial working environment versus good (index 10 Q)	1 and 2, age	1. OR = 1.65 (1.02–2.67) 2. p = 0.04

116

Reference	Study design	Population	Outcome	Comparison	Adjustments	Results
Mäkelä et al., 1991, Finland (73)	Cross-sectional cohort	5,673 men and women from the Mini-Finland Health Survey 30–64 yr old	Chronic neck pain (q+clinical exam)	1. Index for physical stress at work 2. Index for mental stress at work	Age, sex, smoking, obesity, parity and 1 and 2, respectively	1. OR = 1.26 (1.18–1.37) for each additional stress item 2. OR = 1.20 (1.12–1.28) for each additional stress item
Viikari-Juntura et al., 1994, Finland (106)	Prospective cohort (1984 and 1987)	688 machine operators; 553 carpenters; 591 office workers	Neck trouble change from 1984 to 1987 (measured as trouble the preceding year): Not any trouble Moderate (1–30 d) Severe >30 d Persistently severe = daily (Q)	1. Carpenters vs office workers 2. Machine operators vs office workers 3. Machine operators vs versus carpenters	Age, smoking, physical exercise	None to moderate 1. 1.6 (1.0–2.5) 2. 1.8 (1.1–2.8) 3. 1.1 (0.7–1.8) None to severe 1. 1.6 (0.8–3.0) 2. 3.9 (2.3–6.9) 3. 2.5 (1.4–4.4) None to persistently severe 1. 3.0 (1.4–6.4) 2. 4.2 (2.0–9.0) 3. 1.4 (0.8–2.6) 1. 1.4 (1.0–1.8) 2. 1.7 (1.4–3.0) 3. 1.7 (1.2–2.5)
Bernard et al., 1994, USA (10)	Cross-sectional	973 randomly selected persons from a newspaper publishing house; case-control study within the cohort	(Q) Pain, stiffness burning in the neck region >once a mo or 7 d continuously during the last yr	1. 4–6 hr in telephone work vs 0–2 hr 2. Number of hr spent with deadline per wk (>30 vs <10) 3. Workload changes (occasionally vs often) (Q)	Age, weight, height, gender psychosocial conditions, health status	
Skov et al., 1996, Denmark (93)	Cross-sectional cohort	1,306 sales people	Neck pain any time last year (Q)	1. Manual driving >50,000 km/yr 2. Sedentary work 3. High demands 4. Low control over time	Logistic regression with age, gender perceived competition, variation in work and 1, 2, 3, and 4 in the model	1. 2.43 (1.36–4.34) 2. 2.80 (1.40–5.59) 3. 1.43 (0.99–2.06) 4. 1.44 (1.07–1.93)
Punnett and Bergqvist, 1997 (81)	Review of mostly cross-sectional studies		Neck/shoulder disorders	VDU work		OR around 2 for VDU work and exposures connected to VDU use, often wide confidence limits

RR, relative risk; VDU, video display unit.

117

Force or Dynamic Load

Forceful movements have been discussed as a risk factor for neck and shoulder disorders. The force usually results from work tasks requiring forceful movements of the arm but not of the neck. Many studies are small and are therefore difficult to judge. Some studies are well performed and show a positive association with reports of neck and shoulder pain (47,106,107) (Table 5.9).

Psychosocial Exposures

The most common exposure with an association of reports of neck pain is high demand (10,43,50,55,58,93,101). The increased risks are moderate. Other exposures investigated have included job satisfaction, perceived stress, poor relations with colleagues and superiors, monotony, poor work content, low control, stress, and tendencies to worry (10,23,24,43–45,48,55,61,62,75,76,81,93,100,107). All these risk factors have been associated with negative outcome from the neck region, with increased pain and sometimes also muscle tension. Work tasks involving these factors often also are associated with a poor physical environment, with repetitive work and static postures, for example. Some studies have controlled for that variable (10,24,55,73,75,76,93,100).

As for low back pain, many studies found no association between different psychosocial conditions and reports of neck pain. Whether this finding results from lack of association, from selection, or from misclassification of exposure is unknown.

As mentioned in Chapter 3, one of the problems in assessing psychosocial factors is the subjective origin of these factors. Some assessment methods include both actual job exposures and the individual's perception of these conditions. Which is most important is difficult to tell, as is the temporality of perceived stress versus pain. Does stress cause pain, or does pain increase stress? However, most studies give evidence of a moderate association between poor psychosocial factors and neck complaints, even if the evidence is weaker than for low back pain (Table 5.10).

SUMMARY AND CONCLUSION

Most studies of the association of occupational factors and low back pain and neck pain are cross-sectional and thereby give insufficient or inconclusive evidence. The outcome also usually consists of reports of pain. The dose and time required to report back pain are not possible to judge from the most studies. However, there seems to be a constant but weak relationship between workload factors and reports of back pain. The impact of occupation on low back and neck pain exists but is modest, except for extreme working situations for a prolonged period without the possibility of changing work tasks.

For low back pain, most published investigations report an association between some types of WBV for prolonged periods (evidence grade B), frequent bending and twisting of the trunk (evidence grade B), frequent heavy lifting (evidence grade C), and different aspects of poor psychosocial conditions including poor job satisfaction (evidence grade B) and low back pain. For persons in extreme working environments such as helicopter pilots (WBV) and firefighters (manual handling of materials), the risk estimates are the highest, and these findings may indicate a dose-response relationship that strengthens the association. In population-based studies in workers with low exposures in general and few heavily exposed workers, the risk estimates are much lower.

TABLE 5.9. *Forceful work tasks alone or in combination with other exposures and neck pain*

Study (ref.)	Design	Population and gender studied	Outcome	Exposure	Confounders adjusted for	Results given in odds ratio (OR) if nothing else indicated
Tola et al., 1988, Finland (100)	Cross-sectional	852 machine operators; 696 carpenters; 674 office workers	12-mo prevalence of neck/shoulder pain	1. Job title 1a. Machine operators vs office workers 1b. Carpenters vs office workers 1c. Machine operators vs carpenters 2. Twisted and bent positions often 3. Moderate or poor job satisfaction	Age, draft, and 1, 2 and 3, respectively, in a logistic regression	1a. 1.7 (1.5–2.0) 1b. 1.4 (1.1–1.6) 1c. 1.3 (1.1–1.4) 2. 1.8 (1.5–2.2) 3. 1.2 (1.1–1.4)
Silverstein, 1985, USA (92)	Cross-sectional	1,212 male workers exposed to repetitive work tasks and high force vs 75 male nonexposed workers 2,226 female exposed workers vs 61 nonexposed female workers	Tension neck (clinical examination and I)	Repetitive movements and high force		1. OR = 1.1 (0.1–10) 2. OR = 0.9 (0.4–2.4)
Linton, 1990, Sweden (61)	Cross-sectional	22,180 men and women full time working during day time	Seeking care because of neck pain last 12 mo (Q)	1. Heavy lifting 2. Monotonous work 3. Sitting 4. Uncomfortable postures 5. Vibration 6. Psychosocial factors (work content social support and workload)		OR for different age groups <30, 30–39, 40, 49 and >50 yr 1. 1.4, 1.7, 1.6, 1.8 2. 2.3, 2.4, 2.5, 3.0 3. 1.3, 1.1, 1.0, 0.9 4. 1.6, 2.0, 2.0, 2.4 5. 1.0, 1.5, 1.3, 1.8 6. 2.6, 1.9, 2.5, 2.3
Ekberg et al., 1994, Sweden (24)	Case-control	109 new patients with musculoskeletal complaints (no sick leave last mo); 327 randomly selected controls from the study base	Neck and shoulder complaints in Q and clinical examination	Q 1. Repetitive work 2. Lifting 3. High work pace 4. Uncomfortable sitting 5. High ambiguity of work role 6. High demands on attention 7. Low work content	Sex, immigrant status, smoking, exercise, age	1. 7.5 (2.4–23) 2. 13.6 (4.8–39) 3. 3.5 (1.3–9.4) 4. 3.6 (1.4–9.3) 5. 16.5 (6.0–46) 6. 3.8 (1.4–9.4) 7. 2.6 (0.7–9.4)
Viikari-Juntura et al., 1994, Finland (106)	Prospective cohort (1984 and 1987)	688 machine operators; 553 carpenters; 591 office workers	Neck trouble change from 1984 to 1987 (measured as trouble the preceding yr): Not any trouble Moderate (1–30 d) Severe >30 d Persistently severe = daily (Q)	1. Carpenters vs office workers 2. Machine operators vs office workers 3. Machine operators vs carpenters	Age, smoking, physical exercise	None to moderate 1. 1.6 (1.0–2.5) 2. 1.8 (1.1–2.8) 3. 1.1 (0.7–1.8) None to severe 1. 1.6 (0.8–3.0) 2. 3.9 (2.3–6.9) 3. 2.5 (1.4–4.4) None to persistently severe 1. 3.0 (1.4–6.4) 2. 4.2 (2.0–9.0) 3. 1.4 (0.8–2.6)

TABLE 5.10. *Psychosocial exposures alone or in combination with other exposures and neck pain*

Study (ref.)	Design	Population and gender studied	Outcome	Exposure	Confounders adjusted for	Results given in odds ratio (OR) if nothing else indicated
Dehlin and Berg, 1977, Sweden (23)	Cross-sectional	233 nursing aides	Neck pain	1. Relations with supervisors and workmates 2. Overall satisfaction with the job 3. Perceived demand of psychologic and physical strength	None	1. NS 2. NS 3. NS
Tola et al., 1988, Finland (100)	Cross-sectional	852 machine operators; 696 carpenters; 674 office workers	12-mo prevalence of neck/shoulder pain	1. Job title 1a. Machine operator vs office workers 1b. Carpenters vs office workers 1c. Machine operators vs carpenters 2. Twisted and bent positions often 3. Moderate or poor job satisfaction	Age, draft, and 1, 2 and 3, respectively, in a logistic regression	1a. 1.7 (1.5–2.0) 1b. 1.4 (1.1–1.6) 1c. 1.3 (1.1–1.4) 2. 1.8 (1.5–2.2) 3. 1.2 (1.1–1.4)
Linton, 1990, Sweden (61)	Cross-sectional	22,180 men and women full time working during daytime	Seeking care because of neck pain last 12 mo (Q)	1. Heavy lifting 2. Monotonous work 3. Sitting 4. Uncomfortable postures 5. Vibration 6. Psychosocial factors (work content social support and workload)		OR for different age groups <30, 30–39, 40, 49 and >50 yr 1. 1.4, 1.7, 1.6, 1.8 2. 2.3, 2.4, 2.5, 3.0 3. 1.3, 1.1, 1.0, 0.9 4. 1.6, 2.0, 2.0, 2.4 5. 1.0, 1.5, 1.3, 1.8 6. 2.6, 1.9, 2.5, 2.3
Kamvendo et al., 1991, Sweden (48)	Cross-sectional	420 female medical secretaries	Neck pain previous yr	1. Working with office machines >5 hr/d 2. Poor psychosocial working environment versus good (index 10 Q)	1 and age	1. OR = 1.65 (1.02–2.67) 2. p = 0.04
Mäkelä et al., 1991, Finland (73)	Cross-sectional cohort	5,673 men and women from the mini-Finland health survey, 30–64 yr old	Chronic neck pain (Q and clinical examination)	1. Index for physical stress at work 2. Index for mental stress at work	Age, sex, smoking, obesity, parity, and 1 and 2, respectively	1. OR = 1.26 (1.18–1.37) for each additional stress item 2. OR = 1.20 (1.12–1.28) for each additional stress item
Johansson, 1994, Sweden (43, 45)	Cross-sectional	305 home care workers; 694 municipal employees	Neck complaint (Q)	Poor psychosocial index and high physical load index		RR = 2.57 (1.66–3.97)

Reference	Study design	Study population	Outcome	Risk factor(s)	Adjustments	RR (95% CI)
Johansson, 1994, Sweden (43, 44)	Cross-sectional	755 male and female employees	Neck symptoms (Q)	Job strain (high demands and low decision latitude)	Age, sex, social support	RR = 2.25 (1.56–3.24)
Ekberg et al., 1994, Sweden (24)	Case-control	109 new patients with musculoskeletal complaints (no sick leave last mo) 327 randomly selected controls from the study base	Neck and shoulder complaints in Q and clinical examination	Q 1. Repetitive work 2. Lifting 3. High work pace 4. Uncomfortable sitting 5. High ambiguity of work role 6. High demands on attention 7. Low work content	Sex, immigrant status, smoking, exercise, age	1. 7.5 (2.4–23) 2. 13.6 (4.8–39) 3. 3.5 (1.3–9.4) 4. 3.6 (1.4–9.3) 5. 16.5 (6.0–46) 6. 3.8 (1.4–9.4) 7. 2.6 (0.7–9.4)
Bernard et al., 1994, USA (10)	Cross-sectional	973 randomly selected persons from a newspaper publishing house; case-control study within the cohort	(Q) Pain, stiffness burning in the neck region >once a mo or 7 d continuously during the last yr	1. 4–6 hr in telephone work vs 0–2 hr 2. Number of hr spent with deadline per wk (>30 vs <10) 3. Workload changes (occasionally versus often)	Age, weight, height, gender psychosocial conditions, health status	1. 1.4 (1.0–1.8) 2. 1.7 (1.4–3.0) 3. 1.7 (1.2–2.5)
Ohlsson et al., 1995, Sweden (75, 76)	Cross-sectional	82 female industrial workers with repetitive tasks (exposed cohort); 64 female workers without repetitive work tasks (unexposed cohort)	Neck/shoulder diagnosis mainly tension neck	1. Repetitive work 2. Age (54 vs 37 yr) 3. Muscular tension tendency 4. Stress/worry tendency	Logistic regression with age and 1, 2, 3, and 4 in the model	1. 4.6 (1.9–12) 2. 1.9 (1.0–3.5) 3. 2.3 (1.3–4.9) 4. 1.9 (1.1–3.5)
Skov et al., 1996, Denmark (93)	Cross-sectional cohort	1,306 sales people	Neck pain any time last year (Q)	(Q) 1. Manual driving >50,000 km/yr 2. Sedentary work 3. High demands 4. Low control over time VDU work	Logistic regression with age, gender, perceived competition, variation in work and 1, 2, 3, and 4 in the model	1. 2.43 (1.36–4.34) 2. 2.80 (1.40–5.59) 3. 1.43 (0.99–2.06) 4. 1.44 (1.07–1.93)
Punnett and Bergqvist, 1997 (81)	Review of mostly cross sectional studies		Neck/shoulder disorders			OR around 2 for VDU work and exposures connected to VDU use, often wide confidence limits
Krause et al., 1997, USA (55)	Cross-sectional	1,449 transit vehicle operators	Neck or back pain (Q and clinical examination)	1. Job strain 2. Job dissatisfaction low 3. Coworker support low 4. Supervisor support low 5. Frequency of job problems high	Age, gender, height, weight, vehicle type, physical workload	1. 1.50 (0.98–2.30) 2. 1.62 (1.11–2.67) 3. 1.10 (0.80–1.51) 4. 1.67 (1.22–3.63) 5. 2.30 (1.67–3.18)

NS, not significant; RR, relative role; VDU, video display unit.

The impact on low back disability of modern working life is probably limited, but there are still special working environments with elevated risks. Improved work organization with better job satisfaction, good social support at work, less exposure to WBVs, better conditions for manual handling of materials, and restricted time spent working in awkward postures are suggested preventive measures to reduce low back pain. However, evidence of the preventive potential is weak or nonexistent (evidence grade D).

For neck pain, repetitive work tasks have been studied in different settings and almost always show an association with acute and more chronic neck complaints (evidence grade B). In addition, prospective studies with good exposure assessments have been performed, and they show a similar association with an OR of 2 and higher. Static load to the neck region has been shown to be a risk factor for acute and chronic pain (evidence grade C). There is also weak evidence for a certain association between forceful work tasks involving the neck and arm region and neck pain (evidence grade C).

Psychosocial factors such as poor job satisfaction, perceived stress, poor relations with colleagues and superiors, monotony, poor work content, high demands, and low control (job strain) have also, in certain studies that adjusted for physical loads, been associated with an increased risk of reporting of neck complaints. However, the adverse effect are mostly seen in cross-sectional studies and not in longitudinal studies (evidence grade C).

The impact of modern working life on neck disorders is greater for women than for men. It is not possible, from any of the better studies of various risk factors, to determine the magnitude of pain or time needed for a person to develop pain.

Theoretically, perhaps a decrease in repetitive and static workload, as well as improvements in the psychosocial working environment could have preventive potential. However, at the moment, there is weak if any scientific evidence to support this hypothesis (evidence grade D). For more information on various psychologic risk factors and prevention of neck and low back pain, see Chapters 3 and 6.

Future Research Goals in the Field of Causality

Goals include the following:

1. To study the effect of combined exposures.
2. To study the eventual interaction between exposures and individual factors such as age and sex.
3. To clarify the shape of the dose-response curve.
4. To clarify the magnitude and time needed for an exposure to cause harm.

Future Research Goals in the Field of Prevention

Goals include studies of the effect on health and capacity (and productivity) of intervention measures on physical, psychosocial, and organizational work factors.

REFERENCES

1. Ahlberg-Hulthén G, Theorell T, Sigala F. Social support, job strain and musculoskeletal pain among female health care personnel. *Scand J Work Environ Health* 1995;21:435–439.
2. Amano M, Umeda G, Nakajima H, et al. Charateristics of work actions of shoe manufacturing assembly

line workers and a cross-sectional factor-control study on occupational cervicobrachial disorders. *Jpn J Ind Health* 1988;30:3–12.

3. Andersen JH, Gaardboe O. Musculoskeletal disorders of the neck and upper limb among sewing machine operators: a clinical investigation. *Am J Ind Med* 1993;24:689–700.
4. Andersen JH, Gaardboe O. Prevalence of persistent neck and upper limb pain in a historical cohort of sewing machine operators. *Am J Ind Med* 1993;24:677–687.
5. Arad D, Ryan MD. The incidence and prevalence in nurses of low back pain. *Austr Nurs J* 1986;16:44–48.
6. Armstrong TJ, Buckle P, Fine LJ, et al. A conceptual model for work related neck and upper-limb musculoskeletal disorders. *Scand J Work Environ Health* 1993;19:73–84.
7. Barnekow-Bergkvist M, Hedberg G, Janlert U, et al. Determinants of self-reported neck-shoulder and low back symptoms in a general population. *Spine* 1998;23:235–243.
8. Bergenudd H, Nilsson B. The prevalence of locomotor complaints in middle age and their relationship to health and socioeconomic factors. *Clin Orthop* 1994;308:264–270.
9. Bernard B, ed. *Musculoskeletal disorders and workplace factors.* Washington, DC: National Institute of Occupational Safety and Health, United States Department of Health and Human Services, 1997.
10. Bernard B, Sauter S, Fine LJ, et al. Job task and psychosocial risk factors for work related musculoskeletal disorders among news paper employees. *Scand J Work Environ Health* 1994;20:419–426.
11. Bigos SJ, Battié MC. Industrial low back pain. In: *The lumbar spine,* vol 2. Philadelphia: WB Saunders, 1996.
12. Bigos SJ, Battié MC, Spengler DM, et al. A prospective study of work perceptions and psychosocial factors affecting the report of back injury. *Spine* 1991;16:1–6.
13. Bongers PM, de Winter CR, Kompier MAJ, et al. Psychosocial factors at work and musculoskeletal disease. *Scand J Work Environ Health* 1993;19:297–312.
14. Bongers PM, Hulshof CTJ, Dijkstra L, et al. Back pain and exposures to whole body vibration in helicopter pilots. *Ergonomics* 1990;33:1007–1026.
15. Boshuizen HC, Bongers PM, Hulshof CTJ. Self-reported back pain in tractor drivers exposed to whole body vibration. *Int Arch Occup Environ Health* 1990;62:109–115.
16. Boshuizen HC, Bongers PM, Hulshof CTJ. Self-reported back pain in fork lift truck and freight container tractor drivers exposed to whole body vibration. *Spine* 1992;17:59–65.
17. Bovenzi M, Betta A. Low back disorders in agricultural tractor drivers exposed to whole body vibration and postural stress. *Appl Ergon* 1994;25:231–241.
18. Bovenzi M, Zadini A. Self reported low back symptoms in urban bus drivers exposed to whole body vibration. *Spine* 1992;17:1048–1059.
19. Burdorf A. Exposure assessment of risk factors of the back in occupational epidemiology. *Scand J Work Environ Health* 1992;18:1–9.
20. Burdorf A, Sorock G. Positive and negative evidence on risk factors for low back disorders. *Scand J Work Environ Health* 1997;23:243–256.
21. Burdorf A, Govaert G, Elders L. Postural load and back pain in workers in the manufactoring of prefabricated concrete elements. *Ergonomics* 1991;34:909–918.
22. Burdorf A, Naaktgeboren HB, de Groot HCWM. Occupational risk factors for low back pain among sedentary workers. *J Occup Med* 1993;35:1213–1220.
23. Dehlin O, Berg S. Back symptoms and psychosocial perception of work among nursing aides in a geriatric hospital. *Scand J Rehabil Med* 1977;9:61–65.
24. Ekberg K, Björkqvist B, Malm P, et al. Case-control study of risk factors for disease in the neck and shoulder area. *Occup Environ Med* 1994;51:262–266.
25. Elsass PM, Veiga JF. Job control and job strain: a test of three models. *J Occup Health Psychol* 1997;2:195–211.
26. Estryn-Behar M, Kaminski M, Peigne E, et al. Strenous working conditions and musculo-skeletal disorders among female hospital workers. *Int Arch Occup Environ Health* 1990;62:47–57.
27. Feyer AM, Williamson A, Mandryk J, et al. Role of psychosocial factors in work-related low-back pain. *Scand J Work Environ Health* 1992;18:368–375.
28. Foppa I, Noack RH. The relation of self-reported back pain to psychosocial, behavioral, and health related factors in a working population in Switzerland. *Soc Sci Med* 1996;43:1119–1126.
29. Frank JW, Pulcins IR, Kerr MS, et al. Occupational back pain: an unhelpful polemic. *Scand J Work Environ Health* 1995;21:3–14.
30. Gerr F, Letz R, Landrigan PJ. Upper-extremity musculoskeletal disorders of occupational origin. *Annu Rev Public Health* 1991;12:543–566.
31. Gilad I, Kirschenbaum A. About the risks of low back pain and work environment. *Int J Ind Ergon* 1986;1:65–74.
32. Hadler NM. Repetitive upper-extremity motions in the workplace are not hazardous. *J Hand Surg [Am]* 1997;22:19–29.
33. Hagberg M. *Neck and shoulder: to prevent work related disorders [in Swedish].* Stockholm: Rådet för arbetslivsforskning, 1996.
34. Hagberg M, Wegman D. Prevalence rates and odds ratios of shoulder-neck diseases in different occupational groups. *Br J Ind Med* 1987;44:602–610.

35. Heliövaara M. Occupation and risk of herniated lumbar intervertebral disc or sciatica leading to hospitalization. *J Chronic Dis* 1987;40:259–264.
36. Heliövaara M, Mäkelä M, Knekt P, et al. Determinants of sciatica and low back pain. *Spine* 1991; 16:608–614.
37. Hemingway H, Shipley MJ, Stansfeld S, et al. Sickness absence from back pain, psychosocial work characteristics and employment grade among office workers. *Scand J Work Environ Health* 1997; 23:121–129.
38. Holmström EB, Lindell J, Moritz U. Low back and neck/shoulder pain in construction workers: occupational work load and psychosocial risk factors. *Spine* 1992;17:663–671.
39. Houtman ILD, Bongers PM, Smulders PGW, et al. Psychosocial stressors at work and musculoskeletal problems. *Scand J Work Environ Health* 1994;20:139–145.
40. Hughes RE, Silverstein BA, Evanoff BA. Risk factors for work-related musculoskeletal disorders in an aluminium smelter. *Am J Ind Med* 1997;32:66–75.
41. Hultman G, Nordin M, Saraste H. Physical and psychological workload in men with and without low back pain. *Scand J Rehabil Med* 1995;27:11–17.
42. Johanning E. Back disorders and health problems among subway train operators exposed to whole body vibration. *Scand J Work Environ Health* 1991;17:414–419.
43. Johansson JÅ. *Psychosocial factors at work and their relation to musculoskeletal symtoms.* Thesis, Department of Psychology, Göteborg University, Sweden, 1994.
44. Johansson JÅ. Risk indicators in the psychosocial and physical work environment for work-related neck, shoulder and low back symptoms: a study among blue- and white-collar workers in eight companies. *Scand J Rehabil Med* 1994;26:131–142.
45. Johansson JÅ. Psychosocial work factors, physical work load and associated musculoskeletal symtoms among home care workers. *Scand J Psychol* 1995;36:113–129.
46. Johnson JV, Hall EM. Job strain, workplace social support and cardiovascular disease: a cross-sectional study of a random sample of the Swedish working population. *Am J Public Health* 1988;78:1336–1342.
47. Jonsson BG. Persson J, Kilbom Å. Disorders of the cervicobrachial region among female workers in the electronics industry. *Int J Ind Ergon* 1988;3:1–12.
48. Kamvendo K, Linton SJ, Moritz U. Neck and shoulder disorders in medical secretaries. *Scand J Rehabil Med* 1991;23:127–133.
49. Karasek RA. Job demands, job decision latitude, and mental strain: implications for job redesign. *Admin Sci Q* 1979;24:285–308.
50. Karasek R, Theorell T. *Healthy work.* New York: Basic Books, 1990.
51. Kelsey JL, Golden AL. Occupational and workplace factors associated with low back pain. In: Deyo RA, ed. *Back pain in workers.* Philadelphia: Hanley and Belfus, 1988:7–16.
52. Kelsey JL, Hardy RL. Driving of motor vehicles as a risk factors for acute herniated lumbar intervertebral disc. *Am J Epidemiol* 1975;102:63–73.
53. Kelsey JL, Githens PB, O'Connor T, et al. Acute prolapsed lumbar intervertebral disc: an epidemiological study with special references to driving automobiles and cigarette smoking. *Spine* 1984;9:608–613.
54. Krause N, Ragland DR, Greider BA, et al. Physical workload and ergonomic factors associated with prevalence of back and neck pain in urban transit operators. *Spine* 1997;22:2117–2126.
55. Krause N, Ragland DR, Greiner BA, et al. Psychosocial factors associated with back and neck pain in public transit operators. *Scand J Work Environ Health* 1997;23:179–186.
56. Kristensen TS. The demand-control-support model: methodological challenges for future research. *Stress Med* 1995;11:17–26.
57. Kuorinka I, Koskinen P. Occupational rheumatic diseases and upper limb strain in manual jobs in a light mechanical industry. *Scand J Work Environ Health* 1979;5 [Suppl 3]:39–47.
58. Lagerström M, Wenemark M, Hagberg M, et al. Occupational and individual factors related to musculoskeletal symptoms in five body regions among Swedish nursing personnel. *Int Arch Occup Environ Health* 1995;68:27–35.
59. Leino I, Hänninen V. Psychosocial factors at work in relation to back and limb disorders. *Scand J Work Environ Health* 1995;21:134–142.
60. Liira JP, Shannon HS, Chambers LW, et al. Long-term back problems and physical work exposures in the 1990 Ontario Health Survey. *Am J Public Health* 1996; 86:382–387.
61. Linton SJ. Risk factors for neck and back pain in a working population in Sweden. *Work Stress* 1990;4:41–49.
62. Linton SJ, Kamvendo K. Risk factors in the psychosocial environment for neck and shoulder pain in secretaries. *J Occup Med* 1989;31:609–613.
63. Linton SJ, Warg LE. Attributions (beliefs) and job satisfaction associated with back pain in an industrial setting. *Percept Mot Skills* 1993;76:51–62.
64. Magnusson ML, Pope MH, Wilder DG, et al. Are occupational drivers at an increased risk for developing musculoskeletal disorders? *Spine* 1996;21:710–717.
65. Magora A. Investigation of the relation between low back apin and occupation V. Psychological aspects. *Scand J Rehabil Med* 1973;5:191–196.

66. Magora A. Investigation of the relation between low back pain and occupation. *Ind Med* 1970; 39:504–510.
67. Magora A. Investigation of the relation between low back pain and occupation. Physical requirements: sitting, standing and weight lifting. *Ind Med* 1972;41:5–9.
68. Mandel JH, Lohman W. Low back pain in nurses: the relative importance of medical history, work factors, exercise and demographics. *Res Nurs Health* 1987;10:165–170.
69. Marras WS, Lavender SA, Leurgans SE, et al. The role of dynamic three-dimensional trunk motion in occupationally-related back disorders: the effects of workplace factors trunk position, and trunk motion characteristics on risk of injury. *Spine* 1993;18:617–628.
70. Marras WS, Lavender SA, Leurgans SE, et al. Biomechanical risk factors for occupationally related low back disorders. *Ergonomics* 1995;38:377–410.
71. Masset DF, Piette AG, Malchaire JB. Relations between functional characteristics of the trunk and occurence of low back pain. *Spine* 1998;23:359–365.
72. Milerad E, Ekenvall L. Symptoms of the neck and upper extremities in dentists. *Scand J Work Environ Health* 1990;16:129–134.
73. Mäkelä M, Heliövaara M, Sievers K, et al. Prevalence, determinants, and consequences of chronic neck pain in Finland. *Am J Epidemiol* 1991;134:1356–1367.
74. Nuwayhid IA, Stewart W, Johnson JV. Work activities and the onset of first-time low back pain among New York City fire fighters. *Am J Epidemiol* 1993;137:539–548.
75. Ohlsson K. *Neck and upper limb disorders in female workers performing repetitive industrial tasks.* Thesis, Lund University, Sweden, 1995.
76. Ohlsson K, Attewall RG, Palsson B, et al. Repetetive industrial work and neck and upper limb disorders in females. *Am J Ind Med* 1995;27:731–747.
77. Papageorgiou AC, Macfarlane GJ, Thomas E, et al. Psychosocial factors in the workplace: do they predict new episodes of low back pain? Evidence from the south Manchester back pain study. *Spine* 1997;22:1137–1142.
78. Pietri F, Leclerc A, Boitel L, et al. Low back pain in commercial travelers. *Scand J Work Environ Health* 1992;18:52–58.
79. Pope MH. Risk indicators in low back pain. *Ann Med* 1989;21:387–392.
80. Poppel MNW van, Koes BW, Devillé W, et al. Risk factors for back pain incidence in industry: a prospective study. *Pain* 1998;77:81–86.
81. Punnett L, Bergqvist U. Visual display unit work and upper extremity musculoskeletal disorders: a review of epidemiological findings. *Arbete och Halsa* 1997;16:1–161.
82. Punnett L, Fine LJ, Keyserling WM, et al. Back disorders and nonneutral trunk postures of automobile assembly workers. *Scand J Work Environ Health* 1991;17:337–346.
83. Rempel DM, Harrison RJ, Barnhart S. Work-related cumulative trauma disorders of the upper extremity. *JAMA* 1992;267:838–842.
84. Riihimäki H. Low back pain, its origin and risk indicators. *Scand J Work Environ Health* 1991;17:81–90.
85. Riihimäki H. Back and limb disorders. In: McDonald C, ed. *Epidemiology of work related diseases.* London: BMJ Publishing Group, 1995.
86. Riihimäki H. Hands up or back to work: future challages in epidemiologic research on musculoskeletal diseases. *Scand J Work Environ Health* 1995;21:401–403.
87. Riihimäki H, Tola S, Videman T, et al. Low-back pain and occupation: a cross sectional questionnaire study of men in machine operating, dynamic physical work, and sedentary work. *Spine* 1989;14:204–209.
88. Riihimäki H, Viikari-Juntura E, Moneta G, et al. Incidence of sciatic pain among men in machine operating, dynamic work, and sedentary work. *Spine* 1994;19:138–142.
89. Riihimäki H, Wickström G, Hänninen K, et al. Predictors of sciatic pain among concrete reinforcement workers and house painters: a five-year follow-up. *Scand J Work Environ Health* 1989;15:415–423.
90. Schibye B, Skov T, Ekner D, et al. Musculoskeletal symtoms among sewing machine operators. *Scand J Work Environ Health* 1995;21:427–434.
91. Shelerud R. Epidemiology of occupational low back pain. *Occup Med* 1998;13:1–22.
92. Silverstein BA. *The prevalence of upper extremity cumulative trauma disorders in industry.* Thesis, University of Michigan, Ann Arbor, 1985.
93. Skov T, Borg W, Örhede E. Psychosocial and physical risk factors for musculoskeletal disorders of the neck, shoulders and lower back in salespeople. *Occup Environ Med* 1996;53:351–356.
94. Skovron ML, Szpalski M, Nordin M, et al. Sociocultural factors and back pain: a population based study in Belgian adults. *Spine* 1994;19:129–137.
95. Smedley J, Egger P, Cooper C, et al. Manual handling activities and risk of low back pain in nurses. *Occup Environ Med* 1995;52:160–163.
96. Stobbe TJ, Plummer RW, Jensen RC, et al. Incidence of low back injuries among nursing personnel as a function of patient lifting frequency. *J Safety Res* 1988;19:21–28.
97. Stock SR. Workplace ergonomic factors and the development of musculoskeletal disorders of the neck and upper limb: a meta-analysis. *Am J Ind Med* 1991;19:87–107.
98. Svensson HO, Andersson GBJ. Low-back pain in 40 to 47 year old men: work history and work environment factors. *Spine* 1983;8:272–276.

99. Svensson HO, Andersson GBJ. The relation of low-back pain, work history, work environment, and stress. *Spine* 1989;14:517–522.
100. Tola S, Riihimäki H, Videman T, et al. Neck and shoulder symptoms among men in machine operating, dynamic physical work and sedentary work. *Scand J Work Environ Health* 1988;14:299–305.
101. Toomingas A, Theorell T, Michélsen H, et al. Associations between self-rated psychosocial work conditions and musculoskeletal symptoms and signs. *Scand J Work Environ Health* 1997;23:130–139.
102. Veierstad KB, Westgaard RH. Subjectively assessed occupational and individual parameters as risk factors for trapezius myalgia. *Int J Ind Ergon* 1994;13:235–245.
103. Wells J, Zipp JF, Schuette PT, et al. Musculoskeletal disorders among letter carriers. *J Occup Med* 1983;25:814–820.
104. Venning PJ, Walter SD, Stitt LW. Personal and job-related factors as determinants of incidence of back injuries among nursing personnel. *J Occup Med* 1987;29:820–825.
105. Wickström BO, Kjellberg A, Landström U. Health effects of long-term occupational exposures to whole body vibrations: a review. *Int J Ind Ergon* 1994;14:273–292.
106. Viikari-Juntura E, Riihimäki H, Tola S, et al. Neck trouble in machine operating, dynamic physical work and sedentary work: a prospective study on occupational and individual risk factors. *J Clin Epidemiol* 1994;47:1411–1422.
107. Viikari-Juntura E, Vuori J, Silverstein B, et al. A life-long prospective study on the role of psychosocial factors in neck-shoulder and low back pain. *Spine* 1991;16:1056–1061.
108. Wilder DG, Pope MH. Epidemiological and aetiological aspects of low back pain in vibration environments: an update. *Clin Biomechanics* 1996;11:61–73.
109. Wilder DG, Woodworth BB, Frymoyer JW, et al. Vibration and the human *Spine.* 1982;7:243–254.
110. Winkel J, Westgaard R. Occupational and individual risk factors for shoulder-neck complaints. II. the scientific basis (literature review) for the guide. *Int J Ind Ergon* 1992;10:85–104.
111. *Work related musculoskeletal disorders (WMSDs): a reference book for prevention.* Kuorinka I, Forcier L, eds. London: Taylor & Francis, 1995.
112. Östlin P. Negative health selection into physically light occupations. *J Epidemiol Commun Health* 1988;42:152–156.

Neck and Back Pain: The Scientific Evidence of Causes, Diagnosis, and Treatment, edited by Alf Nachemson and Egon Jonsson. Published by Lippincott Williams & Wilkins, Philadelphia 2000.

6

Preventive Interventions for Back and Neck Pain

Steven J. Linton* and Maurits W. van Tulder†

*Program for Behavioral Medicine, Department of Occupational and Environmental Medicine, Örebro Medical Center, Örebro, Sweden
†Institute for Research in Extramural Medicine, Vrije Universiteit, Amsterdam, The Netherlands

Prevention offers an alternative to the enormous suffering and colossal expenditures associated with back and neck pain documented in other chapters. The basic idea is to use the limited resources available at an early point to prevent the development of unnecessary suffering and related costs. Consequently, prevention is an appealing proposition and an important challenge for the 21st century that has already been recognized by various agencies and task forces around the world (1,13,14,22,26, 33,36,42).

AIM OF THE CHAPTER

The purpose of this chapter is to review empiric studies investigating the effects of prevention on back and neck pain problems. Because it is difficult to distinguish clearly between primary and secondary interventions, we include studies designed to prevent the development of long-term neck or back pain problems delivered in non-health care settings. Because the programs vary greatly in approach, as well as in content, we have evaluated the literature systematically in an attempt to answer the following specific questions:

1. Which interventions are used in an attempt to prevent back and neck pain?
2. Which interventions are effective in preventing the occurrence of back and neck pain?
3. Which interventions are effective in preventing the development of long-term back and neck pain?

Before delving into the review of the outcome studies, let us consider the concepts associated with prevention.

WHAT IS PREVENTION?

Although *prevention* appears to be a straight forward term, several aspects are important in defining and understanding preventive programs for back and neck pain.

First, an important distinct is often made between *primary prevention* and *secondary prevention*. Usually, primary prevention is provided to healthy people with the aim of preventing the onset of a given disease, whereas secondary prevention is restricted to attempts to halt the further development of a disease. However, back pain and neck pain are not single diseases, but rather a collection of several problems mostly defined by symptoms, and it is normal for people to suffer these symptoms. Such pain, moreover, is not necessarily associated with disease, and thus most forms of it do not require medical attention. Because most people at some point suffer from neck or back pain, the difference between primary and secondary prevention becomes hazy for these health problems. As a result, we do not make a distinction between primary and secondary prevention. Instead, we focus on programs provided to people not seeking medical treatment, and these are usually provided in workplace settings or to the general public.

In light of this approach, we may wish to consider *what* is being prevented. It is not wise to advocate the total prevention of back and neck pain, because pain serves the useful purpose of being a warning signal. Further, because pain is a subjective experience, it is not possible to establish an objective definition without adding other dimensions. One can consider certain variables when assessing the outcome of the prevention of back and neck pain. Examples are pain perception, an injury report, sick leave or absenteeism, physical findings, health care utilization, or dysfunction. These fall into the categories of perceived health, behavior, disease, and economical aspects. Consequently, vastly different outcome measures may be employed, thus making comparisons between studies difficult. Moreover, these various measures may not correspond well to one another. A given program may, for instance, have an effect on pain perception, but not on sick leave. One strategy is to employ multiple outcome variables that reflect various aspects, for example, function, pain experience, and sick leave.

PROBLEMS IN EVALUATING THE EFFECTS OF PREVENTION

Another aspect is the special difficulties associated with evaluating the effectiveness of prevention. Contrary to ordinary outcome studies, prevention trials normally need extremely large groups to have enough statistical power to evaluate the effectiveness of the intervention. This is because only relatively few people will develop the defined back and neck pain problem. In addition, because it is normal to have an occasional bout of back or neck pain, there are problems in objectively determining who has developed a "problem." To separate "normal" bouts clearly from "problem" ones or, in other words, to define an episode of back and neck pain clearly is not an easy task. The recurrent nature of back and neck pain also creates difficulty for measuring and defining effects. Moreover, because the origin of back and neck pain is not entirely clear, it is difficult to alter causal variables, and many programs opt for interventions generated from either experience or theory. Prevention studies also need long follow-up periods to observe adequately the possible benefits of the program because the expected benefits are oriented to the future.

A further methodologic problem involves having sensitive techniques to detect a problem that does *not* develop. Most assessment procedures to date have been developed for clinical trials in which disease and symptom levels are the focus. However, in prevention, the focus may be on low levels of symptoms (e.g., pain or function) or on the absence of these symptoms. Because few people report these problems, the analysis will have little statistical power (7). In short, this may affect sensitivity to detect effects.

Because participants in prevention studies are often from a population-based sample, there may also be obstacles in achieving randomization and in avoiding contamination of the intervention. For example, offering an educational program may be restricted by geographic location (e.g., long distances for participants to travel), this complication may possibly compromise randomization. Moreover, "control" subjects may receive similar interventions from friends in the study or from other sources, such as at work or through the media. Thus, it may be laborious to prevent contamination of the interventions.

Consequently, evaluations of prevention programs may need special assessment techniques and research designs, large numbers of participants, long follow-up periods, and carefully defined and relevant outcome variables. Naturally, these requirements make such studies expensive and arduous to organize and may limit their sensitivity for detecting the effects of the intervention, thereby potentially underestimating the size of the effect. This possibility should be kept in mind when reviewing the literature. Despite the foregoing factors, many attempts at prevention have been reported.

METHODS

Literature Search

To identify as many relevant articles as possible, three databases were searched. These were MEDLINE (1985 to September 1998), PsychInfo (1967 to September 1998), and ArbLine. The MEDLINE search strategy was to include articles about prevention in general, as well as those about specific preventive interventions such as exercise, back schools, and education for back pain, neck pain, or musculoskeletal pain. The search was restricted to include randomized controlled trials (RCTs), nonrandomized controlled trials (CCTs), review articles, comparative studies, follow-up studies, prospective studies, and evaluation studies. This search was conducted by a trained and experienced librarian (Mrs. Viveka Alton, Swedish Council on Technology Assessment in Health Care) and resulted in 407 citations in MEDLINE, 138 citations in PsychInfo, and 14 citations in ArbLine. Finally, articles and reviews were perused to identify additional relevant citations that may not have been included in these database searches. In all, more than 900 articles were identified.

Studies were included in this chapter if they fulfilled three criteria: (a) the study reported on subjects not seeking treatment, (b) the intervention was specifically designed to prevent some form of back or neck problem, and (c) the intervention was specifically designed to prevent the development of long-term back or neck problems. Because interventions directed toward treatment of acute and subacute problems are addressed in previous chapters, studies on various forms of early treatment in health care settings were excluded.

Review Procedure

The review was conducted first by examining critical and systematic review articles in the literature and then by reviewing key studies, as well as studies published after the period covered in these reviews. Finally, a table of key studies (employing RCT or CCT designs) was constructed to provide an overview of the current data specific to prevention of back and neck pain. Classification of the studies was based on the reported outcomes on key variables. The key variables employed were report of pain, report of injury, dysfunction, time lost from work, health care utilization, and cost. A study was classified as positive if the preventive intervention was demonstrated to be more effective (statistically significant) as compared with a control intervention on at least one key variable. If the preventive intervention was less effective than the control or if the prevention was not more effective than no intervention at all, it was rated as negative. A neutral rating was given to studies in which the preventive intervention and control did not differ on any key variables. These tables were employed to summarize the best current information.

RESULTS

Back Schools and Education

Back and neck schools are undoubtedly among the most frequently employed preventive measures in use today. These schools make the assumption that people have higher risk and suffer more than need be because they lack knowledge about a variety of topics as diverse as body mechanics and stress. Therefore, the programs aim to reduce the risk of problems by increasing the participant's knowledge, which, in turn, will alter the person's behavior in such ways as lift technique. Back schools usually contain a series of discussions about anatomy, biomechanics, lifting, and postural changes related to work, as well as a program of exercises. They vary from a single session of less than an hour to several sessions (31,38). In addition, back schools have been incorporated into more elaborate treatment programs (11,24).

Back schools are attractive because they use educational principles, may be done with groups, and involve no expensive or complicated technology. In addition, the method appears to have face validity, and patients may enjoy attending the sessions. Thus, these schools represent a concrete and inexpensive preventive intervention.

However, the utility of back schools has been debated. This is in part because investigations have been conducted in vastly different settings with different types of back schools and populations ranging from healthy workers to patients with chronic pain. The following section is a summary of controlled trials and reviews of the literature concerning back schools. To be included, a review had to deal with studies of "nonpatients," that is, trials conducted outside a medical setting.

Controlled Trials

Nine RCTs and five CCTs on back and neck schools were identified. The characteristics of these studies are summarized in Tables 6.1 and 6.2. Six of the nine RCTs did not find any significant differences on any of the outcome variables compared between the back school intervention and usual care or no intervention (6,9,19,29) or among different types of back or neck schools (6,19,40). Only one RCT reported a significant positive effect on initial sick leave and duration of symptoms (5). In contrast to the consistent negative results found in RCTs, three of the five CCTs reported positive results on at least one variable. One study specifically examined the effects of information oriented toward preventing fear-avoidance and promoting coping (43) and found that the information was effective as compared with no intervention. However, because these studies were not randomized and thus constitute a lower level of evidence,

TABLE 6.1. *Randomized controlled trials on the effectiveness of preventive interventions for back pain*

Study (ref.)	Study population	Interventions (no. analyzed)	Outcome measures	Results (+, −, 0)	Conclusions[a]
Lumbar Support					
Alexander, 1995 (2)	60 health care workers, 12 male, 48 female; excluded: individuals who had back surgery, current workers' compensation claims, pregnant workers and cardiovascular problems; RCT with 3-mo follow-up	Preventive intervention: Back belts at work for 3 mo (n = 30) Control intervention: No intervention (n = 30)	Work-related back injuries Perception of physical pain	0 0	Negative
Reddell et al., 1992 (35)	896 fleet service clerks from 4 international airports; RCT with 8-mo follow-up	Preventive intervention: Back belt (n = 145) Back belt plus 1-hr training session on spine anatomy and body mechanics (n = 127) 1-hr training session on spine anatomy and body mechanics (n = 122) Control intervention: No intervention (n = 248)	Back injury incidence rate Lost work days Workers' compensation rates	0 0 0	Negative (58% stopped using the belt before the end of 8 mo)
Van Poppel et al., 1998 (47)	312 workers at the cargo department of an airline company, mean age (SD) 35.1 (7.8) yr; Workers with work disability were excluded; RCT with 12-mo follow-up	Preventive intervention: Lumbar support during working hours for 6 mo (n = 83) Lumbar support plus education/ lifting instructions (n = 70) Control intervention: Education/lifting instructions (n = 82) No intervention (n = 77)	Back pain incidence Sick leave from back pain	0 0	Neutral; positive for subgroup with back pain at baseline (compliance with wearing lumbar support more than half of the time was 43%)
Walsh and Schwartz, 1990 (50)	90 male warehouse workers, aged 20–46 yr; excluded: individuals currently treated for back pain; RCT with 6-mo follow-up	Preventive intervention: Lumbosacral orthosis during working hours plus 1-hr training on back pain prevention and body mechanics (n = 27) 1-hr training on back pain prevention and body mechanics (n = 27) Control intervention: No intervention (n = 27)	Abdominal strength Cognitive data Work injury incidence Productivity Use of health care services Days lost from work	0 0 0 0 0 + (1 vs 3)	Positive (1 vs 3) Neutral (1 vs 2)
				0 (1 vs 2)	

continued

TABLE 6.1. Continued

Study (ref.)	Study population	Interventions (no. analyzed)	Outcome measures	Results (+, −, 0)	Conclusions[a]
Back School and Education					
Berquist-Ullman and Larsson, 1977 (5)	217 autoworkers, 13% women, $\overline{X}$ age = 35 yr; back pain <3 mo, pain-free 12 mo before current episode; occupational health care setting; RCT	Preventive intervention: Back school: 4 sessions, 45 min (n = 55) Manual physical therapy (n = 61) Control intervention: Placebo: short-wave heat (n = 66)	Initial sick leave Pain Duration of symptoms Recurrence	+ 0 + 0	Positive
Berwick et al., 1989 (6)	222 insurees with >2 wk LBP; $\overline{X}$ age = 33 yr; 60% female; setting = health maintenance organization	Preventive intervention: Back school: one session, 4 hr (n = 72) Back school plus compliance package (n = 76) Control intervention: Usual care control (n = 74)	Pain Function Health care utilization	0 0 0	Neutral
Daltroy et al., 1997 (9)	4,000 US postal workers, 34% women, 33 yr old	Preventive intervention: Back school education: 2 sessions, 1½ hr, plus 4 follow-up sessions (n = 2,534) Control intervention: No intervention control (n = 1,894)	Back injuries Other injuries Time off from work Cost	0 0 0 0	Negative
Donchin et al., 1990 (10)	142 hospital workers (clinical, administrative and technical professions); inclusion criteria: at least 3 annual episodes of LBP; RCT with 12-mo follow-up	Preventive intervention: Back school, 90 min., 4 sessions, 2 wk, plus a 5th session after 2 mo, groups of 10–12 participants, instruction in body mechanics and exercises (n = 46) Exercise program: calisthenics, flexion, pelvic tilt, strengthening abdominal muscles (Williams), 45 min biweekly for 3 mo, groups of 10–12 participants (n = 46) Control intervention: Waiting list controls (n = 50)	Low back pain episodes in the last mo Trunk forward flexion Isometric strength Endurance of back muscles	− (1 vs 2) − (1 vs 2) 0 0	Negative

Study	Population/setting	Intervention	Outcomes	Result	Overall
Kamwendo and Linton, 1991 (19)	79 female hospital secretaries, 39 yr old; inclusion criteria: neck, shoulder pain, sit >5 hr daily, not seeking care	Preventive intervention: Neck school, 4 sessions, 1 hr (n = 25); Neck school plus compliance enhancement, 4 sessions, 1 hr (n = 28). Control intervention: No intervention (n = 26)	Fatigue Pain Sick leave	0 0 0	Negative
Leclaire et al., 1996 (28)	168 off from work for LBP; 42% women, $\overline{X}$ age 32 yr old; Quebec workplace intervention	Preventive intervention: Back school: 90 min, 3 sessions plus daily physical therapy (n = 82). Control intervention: Physical therapy only (n = 86)	Work loss recurrence Time to return Pain Function	0 0 0 0	Neutral
Lindequist et al., 1984 (29)	56 primary care patients seeking care for acute LBP; $\overline{X}$ age 38 yr, 57% female; nonstandard randomization (birthdate, unequal group size)	Preventive intervention: Back school plus physical therapy (n = 24). Control intervention: Usual treatment control (n = 32)	Recurrences Health care utilization Sick leave Pain	0 0 0 0	Neutral
Sirles et al., 1991 (40)	74 city employees with back injury; city fitness center; 11% women, 805 > 30; RCT	Preventive intervention: Back school plus exercise (n = 74); Back school plus exercise plus counseling (n = not stated)	Pain Physical dysfunction Well-being	0 0 0	Neutral (no significant between group differences, within group improvements significant)
Stankovic and Johnell, 1995 (41)	89 LBP, 25% female, $\overline{X}$ age 40 yr; setting? criteria? RCT with 5-yr follow-up	Preventive intervention: Mini back school (n = 49). Control intervention: McKenzie method of treatment (n = 46)	Recurrence Need for care Sick leave	− 0 −	Negative
Exercises Dochin et al., 1990 (10)	142 hospital workers (clinical, administrative and technical professions); inclusion criteria: at least 3 annual episodes of LBP; RCT with 12-mo follow-up	Preventive intervention: Exercise program: calisthenics, pelvic tilt, strengthening abdominal muscles (Williams), 45 min biweekly for 3 mo, groups of 10–12 participants (n = 46); Back school, 90 min, 4 sessions, 2 wk, plus a 5th session after 2 mo, groups of 10–12 participants, instruction in body mechanics and exercises (n = 46). Control intervention: Waiting list controls (n = 50)	Low back pain episodes in the last mo Trunk forward flexion Isometric strength Endurance of back muscles	+ (1 vs 2) + (1 vs 3) + (1 vs 2) + (1 vs 3) 0 0	Positive for calisthenic exercise program

continued

133

TABLE 6.1. Continued

Study (ref.)	Study population	Interventions (no. analyzed)	Outcome measures	Results (+, −, 0)	Conclusions[a]
Gundewall et al., 1993 (17)	69 nurses and nurse's aides at a geriatric hospital with and without back pain, 68 female, aged 18–58 yr; RCT with 13-mo follow-up	Preventive intervention: Dynamic endurance, isometric strength and functional coordination exercises during working hours, 20 min, average 6 sessions/mo (n = 28) Control intervention: No intervention (n = 32)	Days with low back pain Work absenteeism (d) Pain intensity (graphic rating scale) Isometric back muscle strength	+ + + +	Positive (poor presentation of data)
Kellett et al., 1991 (21)	125 employees of a producer of kitchen units; inclusion criteria: self-reported current or previous back pain, willingness to exercise at least once a wk outside working hours; exclusion criteria: sick leave longer than 50 d during 1.5 yr before the study, medical inability to participate; RCT, 18-mo follow-up	Preventive intervention: Exercise program: warming-up, stretching, strengthening and cardiovascular fitness exercises, relaxation conducted to music; 40–45 min once a wk during working hours, plus 30 min weekly at home; program changed every 6 mo (n = 58) Control intervention: No intervention (n = 53)	No. of days of sick leave No. of episodes Cardiovascular fitness	+ + 0	Positive (dropout rate 36% in exercise group)
Takala et al., 1994 (44)	45 women employed in a printing company with light sedentary work; inclusion criteria: frequent neck symptoms, age 20–55 yr; exclusion criteria, signs of nerve root compression or tendinitis	Preventive intervention: Group gymnastics at work, 45 min, once per wk for 10 wk; sessions contained aerobic dynamic exercises, relaxation, and stretching (n = 22) Control intervention: No intervention (n = 22); cross-over design	Pressure pain threshold Pain rating (VAS) Handicap Interference with work	0 0 + +	Positive

Study	Population/inclusion criteria	Intervention	Key variables		Overall rating
Gerdle et al., 1995 (16)	97 women employed as home care service personnel; inclusion criteria: working at least half-time; employed at least 6 mo; not on long-term sick leave	Preventive intervention 1 hr or exercise per wk during 1 yr; exercises included warm-up, muscle strength, and aerobics (n = 46) Control intervention: No intervention (n = 49)	Pain Sick leave Physical fitness Physical examination Perceived work situation	0 0 + + −	Inconsistent findings (however, no between group differences for key variables)
Linton et al., 1996 (30)	48 employees (20 women) working at a company (tobacco or distributor of goods); inclusion criteria: back pain during past year, not currently exercising, no other illnesses	Preventive intervention: An individually designed exercise program using psychologic principles to enhance compliance; graded activity (n = 25) Control intervention: Advice to exercise, information, professional assistance, and a free membership to a health club (n = 23)	Pain	0	Negative
Information: Symonds et al., 1995 (43)	3 light industrial companies; responders: 466 = group 1 (29%), 105 = group 2 (18%); randomized companies	Preventive intervention: Informational pamphlet (n = 466) Control intervention: Nonmedical back pain pamphlet (n = 105)	Work absence Initial extended work absence	+ +	Positive (not statistically tested)

[a] Positive: if the preventive intervention is more effective (statistically significant difference) than the control intervention on at least one key variable (report of pain or injury, dysfunction, time off from work, health care utilization, cost), and there are no statistically significant differences on the other key variables.
Negative: if the preventive intervention is less effective (statically significant difference) than a control intervention on at least one key variable, and there are no statistically significant differences on the other key variables or if the preventive intervention is not more effective than no intervention at all.
Neutral: if there is no statistically significant difference between the preventive intervention and control intervention on any of the key variables. Inconsistent findings: if there are statistically significant positive and negative findings within the same study.
LBP, low back pain; RCT, randomized controlled trials; VAS, visual analogue scale.

135

TABLE 6.2. *Nonrandomized controlled trials on the effectiveness of preventive interventions for back pain*

Study (ref.)	Study population	Interventions (no. analyzed)	Outcome measures	Results (+, −, 0)	Conclusions[a]
Lumbar Support					
Anderson et al., 1993 (3)	266 grocery distribution warehouse workers; nonrandomized controlled trial with 12-mo follow-up	Preventive intervention: Back belt (1 work site) Control intervention: No intervention (2 work sites)	Incidence of back injury	+	Positive (not similar at baseline)
Thompson et al., 1994 (45)	60 men and women aged 21–65 yr, patient transport personnel in a hospital; nonrandomized controlled trial with 3-mo follow-up	Preventive intervention: Back belt plus back school (8 hr in 1–3 sessions) and instructions on warming-up exercises (n = 41) Control intervention: Back school (8 hr in 1–3 sessions) and instructions on warming-up exercises (n = 19)	Incidence of back pain	+	Positive (no data presented; small sample size)
Back School and Education					
Brown et al., 1992 (7)	140 (gender age not stated) municipal employees with job-related back pain; nonequivalent design; controls randomly selected workers meeting criteria	Preventive intervention: Back school 120 min, 5 days, 6 weeks (n = 70) Control intervention: No intervention (n = 70)	Number of injuries Lost work time Medical costs	+ 0 +	Positive
Feldstein et al., 1993 (12)	55 nurses, aides, and orderlies, 79% females, 21% males, aged 19–62 yr (mean 42 yr); nonrandomized controlled trial with 1-mo follow-up; pilot study	Preventive intervention: 2-hr session on body mechanics, patient-transfer techniques, stretching and strengthening advice, instructional handouts plus 8 hr practical time in 2 wk (n = 30) Control intervention: No intervention (n = 25)	Composite back pain score Composite fatigue score	0 0	Negative (small sample size)

Study	Population/Design	Intervention	Key Variables	Result	Rating[a]
Morrison et al., 1988 (32)	120 referrals from a general practitioner, 63% females, 45 yr old; logically equivalent design (not randomized)	Preventive intervention: Back school: 6 sessions, 3 hours (n = 60) Control intervention: Pseudocontrol, no intervention (n = 60)	Pain	0	Negative
Versloot et al., 1992 (49)	500 bus drivers; nonrandomized controlled trial with 2-yr follow-up	Preventive intervention: Back school program on healthy behavior, information on back care, physical fitness, nutrition, stress and relaxation, 3 sessions with 6-mo intervals (n = 200) Control intervention: No intervention (n = 300)	Incidence of work absenteeism Length of work absenteeism	0 0	Negative; positive only for long-term sick leave of more than 42 d; (108 of 200 drivers attended all 3 sessions)
Weber et al., 1996 (51)	865 adults, general population (53% in pain) 80% females, 70% >40 yr; matched	Preventive intervention: Back school: 8 sessions, 90 min (n = 494) Control intervention: No intervention control (n = 371)	Point prevalence of back pain Current pain intensity Doctor's visits Drug intake Sick leave	0 0 + 0 0	Positive
Multidisciplinary Program Yassi et al., 1995 (53)	Nurses working at an acute and tertiary care teaching hospital; inclusion criteria: compensatable soft tissue back injuries; exclusion criteria: planned departure, pregnancy, previously identified concomitant medical or chiropractic treatment; 1-yr follow-up	Preventive intervention: Workplace-based disability management program, multidisciplinary (n = 250) Control intervention: Usual care (n = 1,395)	No. of back injuries No. of lost-time back injuries Total time lost (sick leave) Costs	+ +	Positive (index group high risk at baseline, control group low risk at baseline)

[a] Positive: if the preventive intervention is more effective (statistically significant difference) than the control intervention on at least one key variable (report of pain or injury, dysfunction, time off from work, health care utilization, cost), and there are no statistically significant differences on the other key variables.
Negative: if the preventive intervention is less effective (statistically significant difference) than a control intervention on at least one key variable, and there are no statistically significant differences on the other key variables or if the preventive intervention is not more effective than no intervention at all.
Neutral: if there is no statistically significant difference between the preventive intervention and control intervention on any of the key variables.
Inconsistent findings: if there are statistically significant positive and negative findings within the same study.

conclusions from the table are based mainly on the RCTs. Thus, we conclude that there is consistent evidence from RCTs that back and neck schools are not effective interventions in preventing back pain.

Reviews

The conclusion drawn from our table is similar to conclusions from previously published reviews, although some reviewers used more conservative statements, such as that there is no clear evidence or no conclusion can be drawn.

Nordin et al., 1992. This review analyzed the theory behind back schools, as well as their content before examining empiric results, and therefore, it provides a much needed framework for understanding back schools (34). These investigators narratively reviewed seven studies concerning "primary" prevention for adults that show inconsistent results, but the authors linked this inconsistency in part to the degree of cooperation between management and employees.

King, 1993. This review did not state the search strategy or the criteria for including studies (23). However, the investigator identified four studies that have employed back schools as a preventive measure in general or work populations. Of these, one study showed a decrease in absenteeism (49). Consequently, the author did not draw any conclusion concerning the effect of back schools as a preventive measure.

Cohen et al., 1994. This review examined RCTs of back schools for both chronic and acute problems (8), but only the results for acute problems are summarized here. A systematic search of the literature was conducted, and 13 studies met their criteria, which included the following: an employed control group, education as a primary intervention, orientation toward low back pain, and publication of the report in English or French. Of the 13 studies, 3 dealt with acute pain and were conducted with employees, but only 2 were judged to be of good quality. Of the 2 high-quality studies, 1 found a significant effect for pain duration and sick leave duration (5), whereas the other study found no significant differences (6). Participants suffered pain in both studies, so the population was selected, and the length of intervention was relatively short, consisting of four sessions of no more than 1 hour.

Lahad et al., 1994. Five RCTs on the effectiveness of education were identified (27). The educational interventions that were varied widely. Only one RCT reported a significant decrease in the incidence of low back pain, but the intervention evaluated in this trial was a combination of education and exercises. The studies had small sample sizes, and the follow-up intervals were all less than 2.5 years. The authors' overall conclusion was that there is minimal support for the use of educational strategies to prevent low back pain.

Scheer and Mital, 1995. This systematic review focused on RCTs published between 1975 and 1993 for acute low back pain that employed a return-to-work measure (37). Four studies met their criteria and employed back schools. Although these investigators concluded that back schools made "inherent sense," only one of the four studies showed a significant positive effect on return to work. Consequently, these investigators concluded that the published evidence did not clearly show a benefit as compared with control groups.

Karas and Conrad, 1996. These authors conducted an "integrative" review and included studies that were worksite based, had an experimental or quasiexperimental design, and were published between 1966 and 1995 (20). Six studies including back schools were found, but only four studies used it as the primary program. All programs included education, and most included biomechanics, coaching or demonstrations, and exercise. Two of the four studies were RCTs, whereas the other two employed nonequivalent control groups. These investigators found that two of these studies (one of which was an RCT) produced theoretically consistent and statistically significant results, whereas two studies (one RCT) did not. These investigators concluded that the studies thus far have not provided clear direction.

van Poppel et al., 1997. This systematic review included all controlled trials in which the intervention was aimed at the prevention of back pain and occurred in an industrial setting (46). These investigators identified six studies, of which four were RCTs, and two were CCTs. The interventions varied considerably, ranging from body mechanics, to relaxation, to exercise, to coping strategies. Five of the six studies showed no effect on the incidence of back pain or absenteeism. Thus, the authors concluded that these programs were not effective in the prevention of back pain.

van Tulder et al., 1997. Four studies were found that met the criteria of this systematic review in which back schools were employed for acute low back pain (48). However, these investigators rated the methodologic quality to be low and concluded that there was no evidence that a back school is effective for acute low back pain because two studies showed a positive result and two did not.

Lumbar Supports

The supposed mechanisms by which lumbar supports may prevent low back pain are as follows:

1. They provide support of the trunk and thus prevent pain-producing events caused by overflexion.
2. They remind the wearers to lift properly.
3. They increase intra-abdominal pressure and decrease intradiscal pressure.

Controlled Trials

Four RCTs and two CCTs were identified on the preventive effect of lumbar supports in various types of working populations (Tables 6.1 and 6.2). The results of three RCTs showed no significant differences on any of the outcome measures when lumbar supports were compared with no intervention. No effect was shown when compared with training or instruction in anatomy and body mechanics or education and lifting instructions (2,35,47). Similarly, the remaining RCT did not find any differences between lumbar supports and training on back prevention versus training only. Lumbar supports in this study only seemed to reduce the number of days lost from work when compared with no intervention (50). In contrast to the consistently negative findings in RCTs, the two CCTs showed positive results for lumbar supports on the incidence of back pain and back injury (3,45). Several studies reported problems with participants in complying with the recommendation to use lumbar supports. Because RCTs are methodologically stronger than CCTs and given the overall results, we conclude that there is consistent evidence from RCTs that lumbar supports are not effective in preventing back pain or back injury.

Reviews

The foregoing conclusion differs from previously published reviews, in which the authors often concluded that the evidence was insufficient or conflicting. Besides the consistent findings, the reported low compliance for workers to properly use lumbar supports is another reason for a negative overall conclusion.

Lahad et al., 1994. This review included two trials evaluating the effectiveness of corsets for the prevention of low back pain (27). The results of these trials were conflicting, and the authors therefore concluded that there was insufficient evidence to make a recommendation about the use of lumbar supports to prevent low back pain. In one of the trials, 58% of the lumbar support group stopped using the supports before the end of the study. Compliance, that is, whether subjects will routinely wear the lumbar supports or back belts, seems to be a major problem.

Barron and Feuerstein, 1994. This article provides a narrative review of the use of back belts to prevent low back pain in terms of theoretic mechanisms, as well as outcome trials (4). These investigators concluded that there was no adequate evidence to demonstrate either the suspected mechanisms of action or the efficacy of these devices.

Hodgson, 1996. This literature review narratively examined the use of occupational back belts from certain outcome parameters (18). The review concluded that the data are inconclusive because of methodologic design problems and small sample sizes. It also underscored that one cannot assume that back belts afford any protection against back injury.

van Poppel et al., 1997. Five studies (three RCTs and two CCTs) were identified in this review on the effectiveness of lumbar supports (46). The methodologic quality of the studies was deemed to be low. Two of the RCTs did not find any differences between lumbar supports and the control group, and the other RCT reported a positive effect of wearing a lumbar support in combination with education. It was concluded that there is conflicting evidence to support the use of lumbar supports in industry.

Exercises

The mechanisms by which exercises may prevent low back pain are believed to be the following:

1. They strengthen the back muscles and increase trunk flexibility.
2. They increase blood supply to the spine muscles and joints and intervertebral discs, thus minimizing injury and enhancing repair.
3. They improve mood and thereby alter the perception of pain.

Controlled Trials

Six RCTs were identified evaluating the effectiveness of an exercise program for various types of workers. The results of four of the five studies comparing exercises to no intervention showed that exercises significantly reduced the back pain experience and reduced work absenteeism (10,17,21,44). One study reported inconsistent findings, but the authors of this study did not perform a between group analysis (16). Therefore, we conclude that there is consistent evidence from RCTs that exercises are effective in the prevention of back pain. Donchin et al. also reported exercises to be more effective than attendance at a back school (10). However, Linton et al. (30) found little support for a preventive effect of exercise on pain when compared with advice to exercise and a free membership to a health club. There is inconsistent evidence on the effectiveness of exercise compared with other interventions.

Reviews

Several reviews of the effect of exercise as a preventive measure have appeared, and, in general, they support our conclusion that exercise seems to be effective.

Lahad et al., 1994. Sixteen studies on the prevention of low back pain were identified in this review, of which 5 were prospective trials and 4 were RCTs (27). The authors identified significant methodologic flaws in 2 RCTs. All 4 of the RCTs included at least some subjects with previous low back pain, and all reported positive short-term effects of exercise. Lahad et al. (27) concluded that exercise may be mildly protective against low back pain. However, these investigators concluded that it was not clear whether one type of exercise was more effective than other type.

Gebhardt, 1994. A metaanalysis of studies that evaluated the effect of training on back pain, conducted with employees and using at least a quasiexperimental design, was calculated (15). Six studies met their inclusion criteria. The combined effect size was .24, indicating a significant but rather weak effect.

van Poppel et al., 1997. In this systematic review, three RCTs were included on the effectiveness of exercise in the prevention of back pain (46). The exercise programs consisted of various types of exercises and varied in length from 3 to 18 months. Despite this heterogeneity, the study population of all three studies consisted of subjects with heavy work, and the outcomes were consistent. All three studies reported a positive effect of exercise on the incidence of back pain episodes and/or days lost from work. Because of the low methodologic quality of the studies, it was concluded that there was limited evidence for the effectiveness of exercise in the prevention of back pain.

Ergonomics

Ergonomics is the scientific discipline concerned with the performance of humans at work and how they cope with the working environment, interact with machines, and negotiate their work surroundings. The main objectives of ergonomic interventions are (a) to prevent work-related disorders and injuries; (b) to decrease work absenteeism; (c) to increase productivity; and (d) to increase safety, efficiency and comfort. Therefore, ergonomics may also play a role in containing the costs of back pain related to absenteeism, medical expenses, and liability insurance. Ergonomic interventions are directed toward occupational risk factors such as lifting, physically heavy work, static work posture, frequent bending and twisting, repetitive work, and exposure to vibration. Ergonomic interventions can be divided into job-related interventions and worker-related interventions and include fitness and stretching exercises, lumbar supports, education on lifting techniques, postural instruction, and workplace redesign. Exercises, education, and lumbar supports are separately evaluated in this review and are not included in the ergonomics section.

Controlled Trials

We did not identify any RCTs or CCTs evaluating the effectiveness of ergonomics.

Reviews

Similar to our critical survey of the literature, other reviewers also concluded that there were no controlled studies on ergonomics and back pain.

Frank et al., 1996. The authors stated that there was a vast amount of evidence from laboratory studies to suggest that ergonomic interventions may reduce low back pain, but only a few scientifically sound intervention studies were conducted (14). The authors concluded that there seemed to be some evidence for the effectiveness and cost-effectiveness of ergonomic or workplace interventions to reduce low back pain incidence. However, this conclusion was based on uncontrolled follow-up studies.

Scheer and Mital, 1997. These authors also concluded that there was no evidence on the effectiveness of lifting techniques and workplace redesign because there were no controlled studies conducted to evaluate these specific ergonomics interventions (37).

Westgaard and Winkel, 1997. A different approach was used in this review because relevant literature was first identified by establishing inclusion criteria (52). Criteria were related to the type of intervention, field studies, and documentation. Subsequently, quality was evaluated. These investigators classified studies as dealing with mechanical exposure (traditional ergonomy), production systems or organization, and modifier interventions. However, modifier interventions included education, relaxation, exercise, and physical therapy and consequently are included in separate categories in this chapter. In this way, the authors identified 20 studies classified as mechanical interventions, 32 regarding production systems and work organization, and 39 dealing with modifier interventions. These investigators concluded that there were no controlled studies of mechanical interventions. Moreover, they find little support for redesigning production systems. For organizational changes, conversely, 7 studies with control groups reporting mainly positive outcomes were found. Overall, the authors concluded that attention needed to be paid to the improvement of the design of studies. They suggested that the best evidence to date pointed to strategies employing organizational changes with high commitment of stakeholders as well as modifier interventions focusing on workers at risk.

Risk Factor Modification

Randomized and Controlled Trials

No RCTs or CCTs were identified on risk factor modification. Only one study evaluated the effects of a 1-year back injury prevention program after an extensive health risk assessment (39). However, this study was excluded from our review because it did not report results of the comparison group.

Reviews

Lahad et al., 1994. Certain behavioral factors may predispose to the development of low back pain (27). Potentially modifiable risk factors are smoking, obesity, and psychologic profile. There was no evidence on the effectiveness of risk factor modification because no intervention studies were identified. However, Lahad et al. concluded that there were other reasons to recommend smoking cessation, weight loss, and psychologic interventions.

Frank et al., 1996. Three categories of risk factors were evaluated in this review: (a) individual risk factors (weight, strength, smoking); (b) biomechanical risk factors (lifting, posture); and (c) psychosocial risk factors (job control, job dissatisfaction) (14). Although the epidemiologic studies provided considerable potential for primary preventive interventions for low back pain, Frank et al. concluded that there was limited empirical evidence from intervention studies to support this conclusion.

Conclusions Based on the Evidence

Overall, the studies reviewed provide the current "best evidence" concerning prevention. Final conclusions were drawn using a grading system consisting of the following four levels of scientific evidence:

Level A was defined as strong evidence provided by generally consistent findings from multiple RCTs.

Level B was defined as moderate evidence provided by one RCT or generally consistent findings from multiple CCTs.

Level C was defined as limited evidence from only one CCT.

Level D was defined as no evidence if there were no RCTs or CCTs.

Based on the studies reviewed in this chapter, the following conclusions were drawn:

• There is consistent evidence that lumbar supports are not effective in preventing neck and back pain: level A evidence.
• There is consistent evidence that back schools are not effective in preventing neck and back pain: level A evidence.
• There is consistent evidence that exercise may be effective in preventing neck and back pain: level A evidence.
• There is no good-quality evidence on the effectiveness of ergonomics: level D evidence.
• There is no good-quality evidence on the effectiveness of risk factor modification: level D evidence.

DISCUSSION

The evidence on the effectiveness of prevention programs in workplaces and in the general population on altering key variables such as the occurrence of future pain, disability, and sick leave is sobering. It demonstrates the difficulties encountered in developing programs for general administration that can demonstrate their effectiveness. Nevertheless, some studies meeting our stringent criteria did report positive effects. Thus, there is still reason to believe that preventive measures can be developed that address the problem of neck and back pain.

Although the methodologic quality of many of the studies in the literature needs to be improved, several RCTs and CCTs were identified that have attempted to evaluate the effects of diverse approaches to prevention. These studies provide the best available information as well as "best evidence" on which to base conclusions. However, although every effort has been made to include all relevant articles and to appraise them in a fair and scientific way, the search may not have identified all articles. Furthermore, because prevention is not strictly defined, authors may have used terms not included in our search strategy. Taken together, the evidence to date suggests that traditional approaches to prevention such as back schools, lumbar supports, and ergonomics have little empiric support. In fact, because the number and quality of studies are in dire need of improvement, only exercise has mustered scientific evidence to support its use.

Certain factors may explain the relatively disappointing results found in most of the prevention studies. The methodologic idiosyncrasies involved in the scientific demonstration of an effect were outlined in the introduction. These may well limit our ability to discriminate positive effects that are actually occurring. Moreover, almost all studies had, from a prevention viewpoint, relatively short follow-up periods, so the full preventive effect may not yet be visible.

A second possibility is that the preventive effect is obliterated by the natural course of spinal pain. Neck pain and back pain are a natural part of life. Therefore, developing an episode does not constitute a major medical problem for the individual or for others. Moreover, the usual course of acute neck and back pain is that the problem remits only to recur in the coming months. Thus, the definition of a "problem case" has considerable influence on judging results. Most of the studies we identified used the report of pain or the occurrence of an episode as a measure of outcome. Because these measures identify cases that are probably not "problematic," it may be difficult to show that a preventive intervention results in better outcome than the usual base rate. In other words, the natural course of occasional pain or of a recurrence that quickly remits makes up a base rate of comparison that is difficult to alter. However, improvements may occur in the patients who develop long-term problems or problems requiring considerable resources that are prevented. The research on early interventions for acute pain seems to suggest that the main benefit of early intervention is reduced disability and sick leave, but other variables such as pain reports are not significantly better than control conditions.

A third possible explanation of the sobering results is that reports meeting our criteria have almost exclusively dealt with single-modal programs rather than multidimensional ones. Various single-modal approaches such as back schools, lumbar supports, and exercise have been empirically evaluated. However, because many factors may be relevant for the occurrence or recurrence of back pain or back injury, a multidimensional approach may be needed. A simple example is that risk factors may be specific to the individual. Thus, a given risk factor such as poor muscle strength may be important for one person, but not for another. Exercise therefore may be a powerful preventive measure for some patients, but not at all effective for others. Similar examples could be given for other factors. Suffice it that multidimensional programs may be more powerful because they presumably would cover a wider range of risk factors. Many workplaces seem to have embraced this reasoning and have employed a program containing several interventions. Although this broader approach has been suggested (52), no reports meeting our criteria have evaluated its effectiveness at this time.

A fourth factor to consider is the administration of preventive methods to everyone in a defined setting, as opposed to altering risk factors or selecting people "at risk." Because a large portion of people in any given general or workplace population will at some point suffer from neck or back pain, some investigators have reasoned that all should receive preventive intervention. However, conducting a risk evaluation could isolate those aspects of work or individual factors most in need of intervention as well as provide a profile of specific risk areas. As a result, the preventive intervention could be tailored to the needs of the workplace and individuals. However, the current literature review produced no study that employed any type of screening or risk analysis profile. However, a proper risk analysis has been identified as one of the basic components of a successful program (25). Again, this may be related to the difficulties of meeting the methodologic demands of evaluating such a program. Frank et al. (14) suggested that, for patients seeking care for acute pain, the recovery curve is so robust that it may be questionable if early interventions will improve on the natural rate of recovery. They argued further that, for patients with longer duration problems, early efforts may be powerful. Consequently, the effect may depend on the time factor as well as on the profile of the factors contributing to the problem.

A fifth consideration is the role of compliance. Most of the programs reviewed were aimed at changing some form of behavior, such as with exercise, relaxation, wearing supports, or attending educational meetings. However, compliance to participate has not always been high, and an underlying question is how long people continue to practice or utilize the procedures after the initial intervention is finished. The exercise literature, for example, shows that most patients fail to continue the recommended exercise program after the termination of the initial program (30). Therefore, compliance may be a factor that mediates the effect of the intervention on outcome.

RECOMMENDATIONS

Various interventions are employed to prevent back and neck pain. The most frequently reported interventions include back schools and other educational efforts, lumbar supports, and exercises. Ergonomic interventions appear to be frequently employed but have not been properly evaluated. The current evidence suggests that exercises seem to be the most effective preventive intervention, although most studies on which this conclusion is based were methodologically flawed, and the effects are only weak. In consideration of these results, we see a real need for future studies employing the highest methodologic standards. These studies should focus more on multidimensional programs, should assess risk and tailor the program to the risk profile of the individual or the workplace, should have longer follow-up periods, and should include much larger study populations. Furthermore, we believe that it is essential to put efforts into increasing the compliance to preventive interventions.

REFERENCES

1. Agency for Health Care Policy and Research. *Clinical practice quidelines number 14: acute low back problems in adults.* Rockville, MD: US Department of Health and Human Services, 1994.
2. Alexander MP. Mild traumatic brain injury: pathophysiology, natural history, and clinical management. *Neurology* 1995;45:1253–1260.
3. Anderson CK, Morris TL, Vechin DC. *The effectiveness of using a lumbar support belt.* Dallas, TX: Advanced Ergonomics, 1993.
4. Barron BA, Feuerstein M. Industrial back belts and low back pain: mechanisms and outcomes. *J Occup Rehabil* 1994;4:125–139.
5. Bergquist-Ullman M, Larsson U. Acute low back pain in industry. *Acta Orthop Scand* 1977;170:1–117.
6. Berwick DM, Budman S, Feldstein M. No clinical effect of back schools in an HMO: a randomized prospective trial. *Spine* 1989;14:338–344.
7. Brown KC, Sirles AT, Hilyer JC, et al. Cost effectiveness of a back school intervention for municipal employees. *Spine* 1992;17:1224–1228.
8. Cohen JE, Goel V, Frank JW, et al. Group education interventions for people with low back pain: an overview of the literature. *Spine* 1994;19:1214–1222.
9. Daltroy LH, Iversen MD, Larson MG, et al. A controlled trial of an educational program to prevent low back injuries. *N Engl J Med* 1997;337:322–328.
10. Donchin M, Woolf O, Kaplan L, et al. Secondary prevention of low-back pain: a clinical trial. *Spine* 1990;15:1317–1320.
11. Fabio RPD. Efficacy of comprehensive rehabilitation programs and back school for patients with low back pain: a meta-analysis. *Phys Ther* 1995;75:865–878.
12. Feldstein A, Valanis B, Vollmer W, et al. The back injury prevention pilot study: assessing the effectiveness of back attack, an injury prevention program among nurses, aides, and orderlies. *J Occup Med* 1993;35:178–183.
13. Fordyce WE. *Back pain in the workplace: management of disability in nonspecific conditions. A report of the Task Force on Pain in the Workplace of the IASP.* Seattle: IASP Press, 1995.
14. Frank JW, Kerr MS, Brooker AS, et al. Disability resulting from occupational low back pain. I. What do we know about primary prevention? *Spine* 1996;21:2908–2917.

15. Gebhardt WA. Effectiveness of training to prevent job-related back pain: a meta-analysis. *Br J Clin Psychol* 1994;33:571–574.
16. Gerdle B, Brulin C, Elert J, et al. Effect of a general fitness program on musculoskeletal symptoms, clinical status, physiological capacity, and perceived work environment among home care service personnel. *J Occup Rehabil* 1995;5:1–16.
17. Gundewall B, Liljeqvist M, Hansson T. Primary prevention of back symptoms and absence from work: a prospective randomized study among hospital employees. *Spine* 1993;18:587–594.
18. Hodgson EA. Occupational back belt use: a literature review. *Am Assoc Occup Health Nurs J* 1996;44:438–443.
19. Kamwendo K, Linton SJ. A controlled study of the effect of neck school in medical secretaries. *Scand J Rehabil Med* 1991;23:143–152.
20. Karas BE, Conrad KM. Back injury prevention interventions in the workplace: an integrative review. *Am Assoc Occup Health Nurs J* 1996;44:189–196.
21. Kellett KM, Kellett DA, Nordholm LA. Effects of an exercise program on sick leave due to back pain. *Phys Ther* 1991;71:283–293.
22. Kendall NAS, Linton SJ, Main CJ. *Guide to assessing psychosocial yellow flags in acute low back pain: risk factors for long-term disability and work loss.* Wellington, New Zealand: Accident Rehabilitation & Compensation Insurance Corporation of New Zealand and the National Health Committee, 1997.
23. King PM. Back injury prevention programs: critical review of the literature. *J Occup Rehabil* 1993;3:145–158.
24. Koes BW, van Tulder MW, van der Windt WM, et al. The efficacy of back schools: a review of randomized clinical trials. *J Clin Epidemiol* 1994;47:851–862.
25. Kompier MAJ, Geurts SAE, Gründemann RWM, et al. Cases in stress prevention: the success of a participative and stepwise approach. *Stress Med* 1998;14:155–168.
26. Kuorinka I, Jonsson B, Jörgensen K, et al. Arbetsrelaterade sjukdomar i rörelseorganen: förekomst, orsaker och förebyggande [Work related musculoskeletal disorders: prevalence, causes and prevention]. Copenhagen: Nordiska Ministerrådet, 1990, report number 6.
27. Lahad A, Malter AD, Berg AO, et al. The effectiveness of four interventions for the prevention of low back pain. *JAMA* 1994;272:1286–1291.
28. Leclaire R, Esdaile JM, Suissa S, et al. Back school in a first episode of compensated acute low back pain: a clinical trial to assess efficacy and prevent relapse. *Arch Phys Med Rehabil* 1996;77:673–679.
29. Lindequist S, Lundberg B, Wikmark R, et al. Information and regime at low back pain. *Scand J Rehabil* 1984;16:113–116.
30. Linton SJ, Hellsing AL, Bergström G. Exercise for workers with musculoskeletal pain: does enhancing compliance decrease pain? *J Occup Rehabil* 1996;6:177–190.
31. Linton SJ, Kamwendo K. Low back schools: a critical review. *Phys Ther* 1987;67:1375–1383.
32. Morrison GEC, Chase W, Young V, et al. Back pain: treatment and prevention in a community hospital. *Arch Phys Med Rehabil* 1988;69:605–609.
33. National Board of Health and Welfare. *Att förebygga sjukdomar i rörelseorganen* [*Preventing musculoskeletal pain*]. Stockholm: Socialstyrelsen, 1987.
34. Nordin M, Cedraschi C, Balague F, et al. Back schools in prevention of chronicity. *Baillieres Clin Rheumatol* 1992;6:685–703.
35. Reddell CR, Congleton JJ, Huchingson RD, et al. An evaluation of a weightlifing belt and back injury prevention training class for airline baggage handlers. *Appl Ergon* 1992;23:319–329.
36. Rosen M. *Clinical Standards Advisory Group: back pain report of a committee on back pain.* London: Her Majesty's Stationery Office, 1994.
37. Scheer SJ, Mital A. Ergonomics. *Arch Phys Med Rehabil* 1997;78 [Suppl]: 36–45.
38. Scheer SJ, Radack KL, O'Brien DR J. Randomized controlled trials in industrial low back pain relating to return to work. I. Acute interventions. *Arch Phys Med Rehabil* 1995;76:966–973.
39. Shi L. A cost-benefit analysis of a California county's back injury prevention program. *Public Health Rep* 1993;108:204–211.
40. Sirles AT, Brown K, Hilyer JC. Effects of back school education and exercise in back injured municipal workers. *Am Assoc Occup Health J* 1991;39:7–12.
41. Stankovic R, Johnell O. Conservative treatment of acute low back pain: a 5-year follow-up study of two methods of treatment. *Spine* 1992;20:469–472.
42. Swedish Council on Technology Assessment in Health Care. *Back pain: causes, diagnostics and treatment.* Stockholm: Swedish Council on Technology Assessment in Health Care, 1991.
43. Symonds TL, Burton AK, Tillotson KM, et al. Absence resulting from low back trouble can be reduced by psychosocial intervention at the work place. *Spine* 1995;20:2738–2745.
44. Takala EP, Viikari-Juntura E, Tynkkynen EM. Does group gymnastics at the workplace help in neck pain? A controlled study. *Scand J Rehabil Med* 1994;26:17–20.
45. Thompson L, Pati AB, Davidson H, et al. Attitudes and back belts in the workplace. *Work* 1994;4:22–27.
46. van Poppel MNM, Koes BW, Smid T, et al. A systematic review of controlled clinical trials on the prevention of back pain in industry. *Occup Environ Med* 1997;54:841–847.

47. van Poppel MNM, Koes BW, van der Ploeg T, et al. Lumbar supports and education for the prevention of low back pain in industry: a randomized controlled trial. *JAMA* 1998;279:1789–1794.
48. van Tulder MW, Koes BW, Bouter LM. Conservative treatment of acute and chronic nonspecific low back pain. *Spine* 1997;22:2128–2156.
49. Versloot JM, Rozeman MA, van Son AM, et al. The cost-effectiveness of a back school program in industry. *Spine* 1992;17:22–27.
50. Walsh NE, Schwartz RK. The influence of prophylactic orthoses on abdominal strength and low back injury in the workplace. *Am J Phys Med Rehabil* 1990;69:245–250.
51. Weber M, Cedraschi C, Roux, E, et al. A prospective controlled study of low back school in the general population. *Br J Rheumatol* 1996;35:178–183.
52. Westgaard RH, Winkel J. Ergonomic intervention research for improved musculoskeletal health: a critical review. *Int J Ind Ergon* 1997;20:463–500.
53. Yassi A, Tate R, Cooper JE, et al. Early intervention for back-injured nurses at a large Canadian tertiary care hospital: an evaluation of the effectiveness and cost benefits of a two-year pilot project. *Occup Med* 1995;45:209–214.

Neck and Back Pain: The Scientific Evidence of Causes, Diagnosis, and Treatment, edited by Alf Nachemson and Egon Jonsson. Published by Lippincott Williams & Wilkins, Philadelphia 2000.

7

Neurophysiology of Back Pain: Current Knowledge

Carl-Axel Carlsson* and Alf Nachemson†

*Department of Neurosurgery, Lund University Hospital, Sweden;
†Department of Orthopaedics, Sahlgrenska University Hospital, Göteborg, Sweden

Clinical experience and experimental studies have revealed that afferent information does not become consciously known as pain through any simple systems or easily defined chains of neurons. Because pain is a complex and poorly understood phenomenon, different therapies have a weak theoretic basis. Treating pain symptomatically implies treating an unexplained phenomenon with methods with uncertain functions. For rational and more effective therapies, a closer collaboration between experimental laboratories and clinical practice is needed (93). Currently, each field has its own terminology, and for the clinician, current articles from the basic science laboratories have become increasingly difficult to understand (18,32). The main difference between pain in laboratory experiments and pain experienced by patients has to do with the circumstance that a patient's pain is an emotional experience, colored also by social circumstances, well described in Chapters 2, 3, and 5. Because all patients are unique, pain varies. In fact, the differences in the emotional component make pain a subjective, personal experience that cannot be shared. For the same reason, pain elicited by identical stimuli is experienced differently, not only by different individuals but also by any one individual at different times. Another consequence of the subjective nature of pain is the lack of objective methods for its measurement. The perception of an experimental pain stimulus can be described in terms of stimulation intensity. However, the link between the perception of pain and its emotional impact cannot be expressed mathematically.

In certain psychiatric conditions, a patient may complain of pain even though there is no noxious signal from the periphery or evidence of a deficiency in central processing. In most pain states, both neurophysiologic and emotional factors are present. It is important to consider clinical pain as an individual emotional experience of a specific afferent pattern (noxious signal or central processing error). In addition, psychoneuroimmunologic factors may contribute to pain in patients with chronic sciatica (42).

TYPES OF PAIN

It is common to distinguish among *nociceptive pain, neurogenic pain,* and *psychogenic pain.* The individual patient may show signs or symptoms of any or all types of pain.

Nociceptive pain is caused by activation of pain receptors (nociceptors) that are present in most tissues such as skin, muscle, fasciae, joints, and blood vessels. *Neurogenic pain* originates in the peripheral and central nervous system. Nociceptive and neurogenic pain mechanisms can be intermingled, such as in soft tissue injuries, in which not only are nociceptors activated, but also nerves are inevitably injured. *Psychogenic pain* is an unusual type of pain that appears in psychotic states, such as deep depression and schizophrenia. Psychogenic pain has to be distinguished from impairments, which can develop secondary to chronic pain states.

NOCICEPTIVE PAIN

Most investigators agree that receptors mediating pain can be distinguished from other receptors as a distinct group. They are described as free nerve endings and are called *nociceptors.* Nociceptors inform the central nervous system of the presence of a noxious (tissue-threatening, subjectively painful) stimulus.

The free nerve endings contain several substances stored in vesicles such as substance P (SP), bradykinins (BKs), and prostaglandins (PGs). The working mechanism of nociceptors is not known, but one hypothesis is as follows (11). Nociceptors are released in response to a particular stimulation. The released agent combines with the external surface of the nerve ending and causes it to depolarize, and action potentials are formed. The action is terminated by an appropriate enzyme. The nociceptors are capable of distinguishing between innocuous and noxious events and of encoding in their discharge the intensity of the noxious stimulus (10).

Nociceptors typically have a high stimulation threshold. These receptors do not respond to everyday stimuli such as weak pressure, muscle stretching or contraction, and joint movements within the physiologic range, but they require noxious intensities of stimulation to be clearly activated (72).

The sensibility of pain receptors is not constant. This phenomenon has been illustrated by means of a burn injury on a volunteer. Under controlled conditions, the temperature on a small area of the volunteer's hand was slowly increased. At 45°C, the volunteer reported discomfort, but no pain. The skin was heated to 50°C, which gave a painful sensation and an erythema. The temperature was lowered to room temperature for 1 minute, and then, slowly was increased. At that point, the pain threshold appeared at 42°C. This phenomenon is called *sensitization* and results from increased sensitivity of the nociceptors (87).

The sensitivity of nociceptors can be increased by endogenous substances such as PGs. In the presence of PGE_2, BK has a stronger action on the receptor. BK, conversely, is known to release PGE_2 from tissues. By this mechanism, BK is capable of potentiating its own action. Other examples of such cascade-like liberation of endogenous substances are the release of PGE_2 from synoviocytes by SP and the release of PGs from sympathetic fibers by norepinephrine (1). These processes are probably involved in arthritic tissue changes.

Tissue changes induced by inflammation are accompanied by the release of endogenous substances (e.g., BKs, PGs, serotonin, histamine, and cytokines), many of which sensitize nociceptors. The cytokines induce the release of nerve growth factor (NGF), which, in turn, may activate PGs. NGF and PGs together increase the sensitivity of nociceptors.

In inflammatory tissue, nociceptors show two main changes: (a) an increase in background activity and (b) a lowering of the mechanical threshold. The background activity during inflammation is likely to cause spontaneous pain. An increased activity in receptors, which are not nociceptive, may cause sensations other than pain, such as dysesthesia (22).

The lowering of the mechanical threshold implies that a higher proportion of nociceptors can be activated by weak mechanical stimulation such as normally innocuous pressure and joint movements within the physiologic range (9). This finding offers an explanation for tenderness of inflamed muscles and joints and also for pain during movements.

Data obtained from nociceptors of muscle-nerve preparations *in vitro* (59) have shown that hypoxia of approximately 20 mm Hg has a sensitizing action on nociceptors. The hypoxia that may be present in muscle hardening (contracted "spasm") in patients with acute back pain may influence nociceptors. Measurements of intradiscal pH *in vivo* have shown a low value, a finding also indicating hypoxia in some patients (30,61,74).

Nociceptive afferent fibers terminate in the dorsal horn of the spinal cord, where they form synapses and activate second-order neurons. Sensitization of nociceptors may be further pronounced by additional alterations in the spinal cord. Thus, considerable hyperexcitability of spinal neurons has been observed during inflammation in peripheral tissues.

Certain branches of the second pain neuron connect with motor nerve cells and the sympathetic nervous system on the same side. The connection with motor neurons is responsible for the withdrawal reflex in acute pain. It may also be responsible for some chronic pain states. Thus, a noxious stimulus from the periphery, such as a joint, activates muscle neurons to a muscle. The muscle increases its tonicity, which, in turn, activates its own nociceptors and forms a circuit leading to persistent pain. Low back and neck pain may sometimes be caused by such a mechanism. This would then explain why this circuit can be broken with a nerve block or a short-lasting analgesic, sometimes with long-lasting effects, affording pain relief for weeks. Similar circuits can be built up by the sympathetic route and thereby can maintain and increase ischemic and causalgic pain. The importance of these mechanisms is subject to controversy. One review questioned the existence of these mechanisms (13), whereas another study in rats found connections between the nerve fibers around the disc and sympathetic communicants to the dorsal root ganglia (106).

In a properly functioning system, noxious mechanical, chemical, or thermal stimuli activate nociceptors. Thermal or mechanical nociceptors or thin myelinated Aδ fibers conduct rapidly and are responsible for sensations of sharp, piercing pain. The afferent signals, elicited in tissue injury or inflammation, travel slowly in unmyelinated C fibers and are responsible for dull, aching pain.

After suprathreshold stimulation, the free sensory nerve endings depolarize and generate an action potential that is transmitted to the cell body of the dorsal root ganglion and the terminals in the dorsal horn. The signals from sensory neurons are mediated by excitatory amino acids including glutamate (sharp, rapid signal) and neuropeptides, such as SP (slow, dull signal). Information from these neurons ascends through spinothalamic, spinoreticular, and spinomecencephalic tracts. These tracts project to various parts of the brainstem or brain.

Descending antinociceptive pathways projecting from several areas of the brainstem, to the dorsal horn of the spinal cord, modify the ascending transmission of signals. These pathways activate local interneurons with endogenous opioids (endorphins) (127). The analgesia evoked by such mechanisms is only partially blocked by naloxone (an opioid antagonist), however, a finding indicating that substances other than endogenous opioids are operating. Several studies indicate that serotonin and norepinephrine contribute to the analgesia (130). In addition, A β fibers from the periphery that form synapses in the dorsal horn can reduce pain by means of the so-called gate-control system (71). Severe stress can induce analgesia both by opioid and nonopioid mechanism. The wounded soldier who runs from the battlefield and who does not feel pain until reaching the hospital is one example.

Currently, there is an explosion of knowledge on the neurobiology and molecular nature of neuroplasticity. Changes can occur at several levels, including regulation of receptor sensitivity (18). In addition to the neurophysiologic aspects of pain, the possible social and psychologic influences depicted in Chapters 2 and 3 are important for the understanding of pain symptoms.

Central Nervous System Determinants of Pain Threshold

In patients with fibromyalgia, as well as in those with chronic low back pain, markedly elevated cerebrospinal fluid (CSF) levels of two pronociceptive peptides, SP and NGF, have been reported (46,96,97). These three studies demonstrated that patients with fibromyalgia had approximately threefold higher concentrations of SP in CSF than normal control subjects. SP is a neuropeptide stored in the secretory granules of sensory nerves and released on axonal stimulation. There is remarkable consistency among the findings of these groups of investigators, and in all cases, there is little overlap in SP levels between the patients with fibromyalgia and normal control subjects.

Regarding NGF, patients with fibromyalgia have a fourfold elevation in CSF levels of this peptide, and again, patients display little overlap with control subjects (46). This neurotropin is released during growth or damage to sympathetic nerves, and perhaps in other pathologic circumstances, and it causes hyperalgesia and allodynia when it is given to animals or humans.

These changes in pronociceptive compounds are not just a marker for the presence of pain. The high levels of SP and NGF in the CSF of patients with widespread chronic pain could conceivably be causing the symptoms these persons are experiencing, or they may be the result of the pain. Russell and coworkers (96) showed that, in patients with fibromyalgia, levels of CSF SP remain stable over several months, despite wide fluctuations in the level of pain. Furthermore, SP levels do not change in response to an acute painful stimulus. The same magnitude in elevation of CSF SP is also found in patients with fibromyalgia with and without psychiatric comorbidities (19). These aggregate data, as well as data from animal studies, suggest that SP and NGF levels in the CSF are not influenced by acute pain or by mood. Instead, these data suggest an abnormality in neural function in individuals with this disorder that is independent of psychologic status. Various neuroendocrine abnormalities occur in patients with fibromyalgia, and many investigators agree that this condition is a model for a "central pain syndrome" (24,25,64,114,123,131,132).

Psychosocial factors also play a prominent role in the transition from acute pain to chronic pain and disability. As pain progresses from the acute phase into chronicity, problems emerge for the individual such as job loss, financial constraints, and distancing of friends. If patients' responses to these problems are maladaptive, such as avoidance of work, friends, financial responsibilities, and physical activity, the patient may become distressed and overwhelmed by the pain and its negative impact on life. Increased stress, learned helplessness, depression, increased anxiety, anger, distrust, entitlement, and somatization can all emerge and can worsen the perception of pain (111–113).

Gatchel et al. (40,41) suggested that preexisting personality or psychosocial characteristics of the individual, as well as socioeconomic factors, largely influence the transition from acute to chronic low back pain. In one study, pain intensity, perceived disability, emotional factors, and compensation status accurately predicted more than 90% of the cases. The same group of investigators suggested that the presence of a personality disorder may not directly cause pain to become chronic, but rather it may make the successful adaptation to persistent pain less likely.

Another simplified way of looking at this problem could be that mechanical factors plus global pain sensitivity plus psychosocial factors equal the degree of functional impairment and pain that our patients are experiencing. Global pain sensitivity, conversely, depends on neurophysiologic factors plus cognitive behavioral factors. In patients with chronic low back pain, a preliminary study showed the same type of pressure sensitivity and increase in SP and NGF (26) as seen in patients with fibromyalgia.

Some population-based studies (28,29,128,129), and studies showing disparate CSF levels of neuromodulators in sensitive individuals, lend credence to the notion of physiologic differences in the way individuals process pain. There are other instructive examples of central pain syndromes, wherein diffuse pain can occur in the absence of any peripheral nociceptive input. The best such example is the diffuse pain state that can result from a cerebrovascular accident involving discrete portions of the spinal cord or brainstem (70,102).

In parallel with a better understanding of these clinical syndromes has been an increased understanding of central pain mechanisms in animal models. Such studies have delineated large genetic differences in pain perception within species, and they have defined a large number of antinociceptive and pronociceptive influences on pain transmission (67,73,79,132). This work has begun to shed light on how pathologic processes such as allodynia can occur without any mechanical or inflammatory process in the periphery that are capable of activating nociceptors.

Psychosocial Influences on Pain Sensitivity

As knowledge regarding physiologic mechanisms in pain has advanced, there has been an equal effort to understand better the psychosocial influences on pain. Psychosocial factors include but are not limited to ethnic and cultural influences, patient beliefs and attitudes toward pain, and emotional or stress responses to pain. These psychosocial factors can influence pain perception in both negative and positive ways. The presence of a psychiatric disorder such as depression, anxiety, or a personality disorder typically only acts to increase pain intensity or distress.

Cultural affiliation has been shown to influence perception and response to both experimental and acute pain in multiple studies (5,68,133). Important ethnic factors include the culture's tendency to be emotionally expressive or stoic, beliefs about the meaning of pain and its controllability, and learned models for illness behaviors that influence how a patient responds to pain (117–119). Although some investigators believe that ethnic differences are diminishing as assimilation produces a blending of cultural influences on pain, one study found that heritage and beliefs in *locus of control* (a belief in the controllability of pain associated with specific ethnic groups) accounted for 20% of the variance in pain sensitivity (47,104).

Cognitive factors such as patients' appraisal of whether a stimulus is harmful or not and patients' beliefs about the nature of pain also influence the experience of pain and its subsequent reporting by patients (126). In experimental forms of pain such as the cold pressor test, subjects' beliefs about the future duration of pain significantly influenced pain reports even when the pain stimulus and actual duration of pain were held constant for all subjects. These studies supporting the impact of beliefs on pain perception were replicated in a second study using an experimental ischemic pain stimulus (107). Fear, anxiety, and worry are dominant emotional factors influencing pain perception in experimental and acute pain (39). These findings are supported by other studies that found anxiety rather than depression to be more influential on acute pain perception (23,45). During the acute phase of pain, the evaluation of whether the pain represents "harm" to the patient may also be critical in the elicitation of an emotional response. Once present, emotional responses such as anxiety can decrease the pain threshold and further influence cortically mediated functions associated with pain, such as cardiovascular and neuroendocrine functioning.

NEUROGENIC PAIN

Pain as a result of injury or dysfunction in the peripheral or central nervous system is called neurogenic or neuropathic pain. Much interest has been devoted to the understanding of the mechanisms underlying this type of pain; a simple approach is transection of a peripheral nerve, which may lead to persistent neurogenic pain. When the transected nerve regenerates, it forms outgrowths, so-called *sprouts*. If the regenerative sprouts find the distal part of the nerve, they will grow into it and may reach their former destination. If not, they will grow into other tissues and will become painful or form a neuroma. A neuroma is sensitive to pressure and can also give rise to spontaneous pain. It follows that peripheral nerves or nerve roots should not be transected to relieve pain. The patient may be free from pain for a couple of weeks or months, but the pain usually returns, sometimes even more intensely than before.

Other experimental approaches toward neurogenic pain include the Bennett and Xie (8) and Nachemson and Bennett (77) model based on loosely constricted ligatures applied around the sciatic nerve and the Seltzer (101) model, in which about half of the sciatic nerve is unilaterally ligated. These models have been used to study neuropeptides in the C fibers (55), for example. Changes in neuropeptide levels have been recorded, a finding that may be relevant in the defense against pain. However, whether such changes exist in clinical conditions is not known.

BACK PAIN PHYSIOLOGY

Investigators have assumed that metabolites evoked by inflammation, mentioned earlier, may reach the cell bodies in the dorsal ganglia by means of the axonal transport mechanism. This may cause hyperactivity of the dorsal ganglion cells with implications for back pain (122).

Our knowledge of the organization of pain fibers in the spinal cord arising from the motion segments is still limited. Some possible theoretic principles have been presented. Various injuries of the peripheral nerve or nerve root may lead to degeneration of the fibers of the primary neuron and its terminals (81). This may induce changes in the second-order neuron leading to an altered, possibly noxious discharge. A previous inactive (silent) synapse may begin to function and possibly deliver a nociceptive message. There are probably many such inactive synapses, which will start to work when some type of balance is disturbed. Another possibility is that remaining synapses increase their activity. Yet another possibility is ingrowth of terminals from other locations. Finally, sensitization of the second-order neuron with increased sensitivity to circulating transmitters may lead to continuous discharge of the nerve cells. An important role is probably played by glutamate and its influences on *N*-methyl-D-aspartate receptors (27,125).

Such a development causes a centralization of the original processes and leads to pain. It follows that pain may persist even when the primary origin of pain has healed. The new, centrally located source of pain may be evoked or amplified by nonnoxious stimuli as well as by mental activity, or it may even appear totally spontaneously. Some clinical evidence exists that pharmacologic treatment, aimed at changing these events, can alleviate such pain states (4,31,34).

Pressure on a nerve or a nerve root such as from disc hernias or spondylotic encroachments is considered a common cause of pain, in particular nerve root pain. However, continuous, stable pressure on a normal nerve causes only a brief discharge of impulses (83). Only when a nerve or nerve root has been injured by demyelinization or inflammation does pressure cause a prolonged discharge (81,84,98). Experimental studies have actually demonstrated more than ten different bioactive substances in herniated disc tissue (48). It is argued that cytokines in particular play an important role in degenerative spine disease through a damaging effect on the nerve root (120). This action would also explain why radiculopathy and pain can develop without signs of nerve root compression.

Neurogenic pain is also present in such diseases as painful peripheral diabetic neuropathy, pain after herpes zoster, which is more common in the elderly, and the late stages of cancer. The causes of cancer-associated pain are varied. Nerves may be injured by the mechanical distortion by the tumor mass, by radiation therapy, and by chemotherapy.

Pain associated with spinal cord injury may be especially complex in that it coexists with nociceptive pain from injuries to the muscles, tendons, and the bone structures of the vertebral column. This pain has become more common because of the increased life expectancy of patients with spinal injury.

As discussed in several chapters in this book, the exact causes of nociceptive or even neurogenic pain in the neck and lumbar region are not known in most of our patients. Studies in the 1990s demonstrated nerve fibers of C type in most structures surrounding the discs, the end plates (20), and the vertebrae (65), even though they were not localized in the nucleus pulposus, the center of the disc (2). Small, unmyelinated C fibers are also abundant in muscles, tendons, ligaments, and joint capsules, except the yellow ligaments (60). In a few samples from severely degenerated discs, these fibers were demonstrated concomitant with ingrowth of vessels into the disc (36), a finding that is not seen in healthy and moderately degenerated discs. Chronic inflammation and fibrosis resulting from vascular damage around the disc have also been proposed as a mechanism for back pain (57). In addition, mechanoreceptors have been found in discs and end plates (94,95).

Some specific, pathoanatomically known diseases are associated with inflammation and C-fiber stimulation, such as infections, neoplastic conditions, and even diseases affecting nerve fibers proper such as diabetes. Specific diseases causing neck and back pain have been extensively tabulated by Borenstein, Wiesel, and Boden (16,17). The previous report of the Swedish Council on Technology Assessment in Health Care report (76) had a translation of the table for possible specific causes for low back pain.

Such causes are rare, however, and account for only approximately 1% for the pain in patients with pain of a few weeks' duration. These conditions occur more frequently (15%), however, in patients who have had pain for 3 months or more. They constitute the important "red flags" of back pain that should be looked for and excluded in all patients with back pain syndromes.

In this book, we do not deal with pain syndromes in the dorsal spine for the obvious reasons that they are uncommon, even though a disc hernia can occur and can cause long tract symptoms. The exception may be some of the rheumatic diseases, in which disorders of the costovertebral joints with inflammation can occur.

It is not unfair to state that all structures in the lumbar motion segment containing vertebrae, disc vertebrae, posterior facets, muscles, ligaments, and so forth, can be sources of pain. They all carry nociceptive fibers, seen also in the pseudoarthrosis tissue in patients with spondylolisthesis (35).

Excluding the specific diseases just mentioned, a few pathoanatomically demonstrable diseases have a clear association with back pain. They include disc herniation, which sometimes causes sciatica, but also may occur in high incidence in asymptomatic individuals (14,15,124). Spondylolisthesis, severe degenerative changes with malpositions, osteoporosis with fractures, spinal stenosis, infections, and rheumatoid diseases such as vankylosing spondylitis (Bechterew's disease) are other supposedly specific causes of back pain. (See Chapter 9 for relevance of findings.)

No pathoanatomic changes have been found in muscles, tendons, and ligaments, and no magnetic resonance imaging (MRI) investigations have demonstrated any significant abnormality in patients with "ordinary" mechanical or idiopathic back pain. One-sided reduction of muscle mass size has been proposed from ultrasound and MRI surface area measurements in some patients with back pain (50,51), but this proposal has been refuted by other studies (44).

Muscles have been implicated in several studies as the cause of both acute and chronic pain syndromes, but little research has been done to elucidate how pain should arise from muscles (33,50,51,52). Interest in muscle pain has been renewed by a few research groups that demonstrated, with the electron microscope, that pain resulting from acute overexertion is related to eccentric loads, which, in particular, cause changes in the muscle fibers. Such pain, however, subsides in 1 to 2 weeks (37,38). Investigators have also postulated that afferent impulses directly increase tension in the paravertebral muscles and affect the blood circulation, with resulting pain caused by the formation of acid metabolites (58).

Such mechanisms could also account for pain in so-called trigger points (43,108,109, 110), although the existence of trigger points has been questioned. Again, the proposed myofascial pain syndromes have not been proven pathoanatomically. A newer theory derived from animal studies demonstrating changes in the γ motor system of the muscle spindles is also based on increased muscle tension (58,86).

In addition to the many studies and unsupported theories of "disc disease," the facet joints have been subjected to pathoanatomic studies, biopsies, and injections, but at present, it is fair to say that those studies have all been inconclusive (60), and as seen in Chapter 9, we are unable to correlate anything in the patient's history or in the examination that could be explained by a "facet joint syndrome." Even the chiropractic theory that back pain could be caused by subluxation of the facet joints has been refuted by chiropractors themselves (88,89,90). In a few scientifically tenable studies on patients with chronic neck pain after whiplash, Lord et al. (69) seemed to implicate the facet joint as the pain generator.

Basic science studies on human tissues have thus far failed to find any specific marker for pathologic changes in the motion segment of patients with back pain, compared with changes found in persons subjects of comparable age. Thus, the term "degenerative disc disease" can be considered a misnomer.

Experimental studies in human patients started with Kjellgren and Lewis (62,63), who demonstrated that disc injections of irritating substances resulted in dull pain with the same localization as injections in other structures of the motion segment. Discography, thought to be a reliable diagnostic technique for back pain, has been demonstrated to be more of a psychologic pain test than anything else (12,21,75).

In studies on patients operated on for sciatica resulting from disc hernia, Smythe and Wright (105) demonstrated sciatic pain only from already had compressed nerve roots but not from any other structures, except in a few cases from the posterior longitudinal ligament and posterior part of the annulus fibrosus in the same patients.

Kuslich et al. (66), during operations on 196 patients with disc hernia and using local anaesthesia and a light microscope, successively probed all the structures in their way to the posterior part of the disc and also inside the disc. These investigators, in essence, confirmed Smythe and Wright's findings from the nerve root, but they also included many additional structures. Little pain or discomfort could be elicited anywhere in these patients, with the possible exception of some patients' reports of pain from the facet joint capsules and parts of the central annulus; this pain was not severe, however. No pain was ever elicited from the nucleus proper, but in some patients, it was elicited from the vertebral end plates. The studies by Kuslich et al. nevertheless made these investigators conclude that the posterior outer annulus or the vertebral end plate or tissues in the anterior epidural space could be the major sites of low back pain.

The biomechanics of the human spine was extensively studied in the 1990s, sadly without providing an explanation of back pain. A few biomechanical studies in young dogs demonstrated that sustained loading for a long time can induce changes similar to those seen in aging discs (54). In the late 1990s, several hundred articles were published on various aspects of disc nutrition, anatomy, and the effects of loading and exercise, and so forth, but none of them could pinpoint the nociceptive process for back pain.

NECK PAIN

Our documented inability to pinpoint the cause of ordinary low back pain, the topic of most studies, extends to the neck, in which essentially the same structures could contribute to nociception and neurogenic pain by similar mechanisms. In addition, the richly parasympathically and sympatically innervated vertebral arteries indirectly could contribute to vicserogenic referred pain, a condition that is even more difficult to understand. Except for biomechanical cadaver studies, few basic science studies exist on the tissues of the cervical column (17). The previously mentioned studies by Lord et al. (69) seemed to implicate facet joints as causes of pain in some specific types of chronic neck pain.

SPONDYLOLISTHESES AND INSTABILITY

If a defect occurs in the pars interarticularis of the lamina, this condition is called *spondylolysis*. If the upper vertebra then slides forward in relation to the vertebra below, this is called *spondylolisthesis*. Investigators have presumed that this anatomic defect can cause instability and can give rise to pain. Systematic studies have, however, cast doubt on the existence of such a mechanism, except in rare cases (78). Eisenstein and colleagues (35) found naked nerve C fibers in the spondylolisthesis defect of some operated patients. Refined measurement techniques (3) failed to link increased mobility between vertebrae with pain, that is, casting doubt on the whole instability hypothesis. The basis for the instability diagnosis remains unproven.

SPINAL STENOSIS

Spinal stenosis is another pathoanatomic diagnosis that has been difficult to prove but is clinically important. In this syndrome, which mainly affects people more than 60 years of age, patients usually complain of severe low back pain in combination with leg pain, usually not in a clear-cut nerve root distribution. The main clinical feature is the inability to walk longer distances without resting in a flexed position.

Animal experiments and human observations support the concept that this syndrome results from a diminution of the transverse area of the dural sac most often caused by osteoarthritic changes around the disc and facet joints. Symptoms seem to occur when the available area for the nerve roots is diminished by 50% (approximately 70 mm^2) (99,100).

This condition can lead to increased CSF pressure and thus can affect the blood supply as well as the nutrition of the nerve roots (91). The pressure increase in the CSF of the dural sac causes venous engorgement, as demonstrated by direct myeloscopy in a few patients with the syndrome (85).

FIBROMYALGIA

The lack of peripheral pathoanatomic changes in this clinically well-defined widespread pain syndrome (132) has been already described. There is some agreement that this condition is a central pain syndrome (25,131).

REPETITIVE STRAIN INJURY

Repetitive strain injury is a label for symptoms linked to workplace tasks, mostly in the upper extremity (7,53). This label is rarely used in conjunction with neck or low back pain; the same uncertainties as for any back pain exist about the true cause of the symptoms (49).

POSSIBILITIES FOR THE NEAR FUTURE

Basic science studies of pain using molecular biology and genetics may open new insights into our understanding of back pain (4,32). Animal studies on the possible mechanisms of sciatic pain are opening the possibilities of new pharmacologic approaches (82).

Investigators have also known for some time that there are hereditary traits in the incidence of disc hernias, and Simmons et al. (103) indicated in a case-control study that there may be a familial predisposition to "degenerative disc disease." Although this predisposition could be explained by the genetically induced increased sensitivity to pain alluded to in this chapter, it could also be caused by genetically induced premature disc aging or degeneration of neck and lumbar spines. In studies (6,115) on monozygotic twins, the MRI changes of "disc degeneration" were explained in 60% of cases by twinship, whereas mechanical and lifestyle factors only accounted for a few percent of cases. In addition, the cross-sectional muscle areas around the spine measured by MRI showed the same association.

The gene associated with familial osteoarthrosis has been localized *(COL 2a1)* (56), and Videman and his group (116) also demonstrated two intragenic polymorphisms of the vitamin D receptor gene that were associated with disc degeneration; that is, the existence of a genetic susceptibility to this progressive, age-related process. Wehling and Reinecke and their group (92,121) and Nishida et al. (80) demonstrated that it is possible to perform gene transfer into the nucleus of bovines, using adenovirus transfer of the transforming growth factor-β-1 encoding gene. The recipient cells produce more proteoglycans. This finding raises the possibility that when we really have defined the gene for premature disc aging genetic transfer of healthy cells into patients susceptible to premature disc aging may keep their discs younger for a longer time.

REFERENCES

1. Andres KH, Düring M, Schmidt RF. Sensory innervation of the Achilles tendon by group III and IV afferent fibres. *Anat Embryol* 1985;172:145.
2. Ashton IK, Roberts S, Jaffray DC, et al. Neuropeptides in the human intervertebral disc. *J Orthop Res* 1994;12:186–192.
3. Axelsson P. *On lumbar spine stabilization: roentgenstereophotogrammetric analysis of motion.* Thesis, Lund University, Sweden, 1996.
4. Basbaum A. New techniques, targets and treatments for pain: what promise does the future hold? *IASP Newslett* 1999:16–18.
5. Bates MS, Edwards WT, Andersson KO. Ethnocultural influences on variation in chronic pain perception. *Pain* 1993;53:101–112.
6. Battié MC, Videman T, Gibbons LE, et al. 1995 Volvo award in clinical sciences. Determinants of lumbar disc degeneration: a study relating lifetime exposures and magnetic resonance imaging findings in identical twins. *Spine* 1995;20:2601–2612.
7. Bell DS. "Repetition strain injury": an iatrogenic epidemic of simulated injury. *Med J Aust* 1989;151:280–284.
8. Bennett GJ, Xie Y-K. A peripheral mononeuropathy in rat that produces disorders of pain sensation like those seen in man. *Pain* 1988;33:87–107.
9. Berberich P, Hobeiset U, Mense S. Effects of carrageenan-induced myositis on the discharge properties of group III and IV muscle receptors in the cat. *J Neurophysiol* 1988;59:1395–1409.
10. Besson JM, Chaouch A. Peripheral and spinal mechanisms of nociception. *Physiol Rev* 1987;67:67–186.
11. Bishop B. Pain: its physiology and rationale for management. I. Neuroanatomical substrate of pain. *J Physiol* 1980;225:589.
12. Block AA, Vanharanta H, Ohnmeiss DD, et al. Discographic pain report: influence of psychological factors. *Spine* 1996;21:334–338.
13. Boas RA. Sympathetic nerve blocks: in search of a role. *Reg Anesth* 1998;23:292–305.
14. Boden SD, Davis DO, Dina TS, et al. Abnormal magnetic resonance scans of the lumbar spine in asymptomatic subjects. *J Bone Joint Surg Am* 1990;72:403–408.
15. Boos N, Rieder R, Schade V, et al. The diagnostic accuracy of magnetic resonance imaging, work perception and psychosocial factors in identifying symptomatic disc herniation. *Spine* 1995;20:2613–2625.
16. Borenstein DG, Wiesel SW. *Low back pain: medical diagnosis and comprehensive management.* Philadelphia: WB Saunders, 1989.
17. Borenstein DG, Wiesel SW, Boden SD. *Neck pain: medical diagnosis and comprehensive management.* Philadelphia: WB Saunders, 1996.
18. Borsook D. Molecular and neurobiology of pain. *Prog Pain Res Manage* 1997;9:179–181.
19. Bradley LA, Alberts KR, Alarcon GS, et al. Abnormal brain regional cerebral blood flow and cerebrospinal fluid levels of substance P in patients and non-patients with fibromyalgia. *Arthritis Rheum* 1996;39:1109.
20. Brown MF, Hukkanen MVJ, McCarthy ID, et al. Sensory and sympathetic innervation of the vertebral endplate in patients with degenerative disc disease. *J Bone Joint Surg Br* 1997;79:147–153.
21. Carragee EJ, Tanner, FJ, Vang B, et al. False-positive findings on Lumbar discography. Reliability of subjective concordance assessment during provocative disc injection. *Spine* 1999;24:2542–2547.

22. Chaplan SR, Bach FW, Pogrel JW, et al. Quantitative assessment of tactile allodynia in the rat paw. *J Neurosci Methods* 1994;53:55–63.
23. Chapman CR, Turner JA. Psychologic disorders and chronic pain. In: Bonica JJ, ed. *The management of pain,* 2nd ed. Philadelphia: Lea & Febiger, 1990.
24. Clauw DJ. The pathogenesis of chronic pain and fatigue syndromes, with special reference to fibromyalgia. *Med Hypotheses* 1995;44:369–378.
25. Clauw DJ, Chrousos GP. Chronic pain and fatigue syndromes: overlapping clinical and neuroendocrine features and potential pathogenic mechanisms. *Neuroimmunomodulation* 1997;4:134–153.
26. Clauw DJ, Williams D, Lauerman W, et al. Pain sensitivity as a correlate of clinical status in individuals with chronic low back pain. *Spine* 1999;24:2035–2041.
27. Collingridge GL, Singer W. Excitatory amino acid receptors and synaptic plasticity. *Trends Pharmacol Sci* 1990;11:290–296.
28. Croft P, Rigby AS, Boswell R, et al. The prevalence of chronic widespread pain in the general population. *J Rheumatol* 1993;20:710–713.
29. Croft P, Schollum J, Silman A. Population study of tender point counts and pain as evidence of fibromylagia. *BMJ* 1994;309:696–699.
30. Diamant B, Karlsson J, Nachemson A. Correlation between lactate levels and pH in discs of patients with lumbar rhizopathies. *Experientia* 1968;24:1195–1196.
31. Dickenson AH, McQuay HJ. 25 years of advances in pain research. *IASP Newslett* 1999:14–15.
32. Dubner R. Neural basis of persistent pain: sensory specialization, sensory modulation, and neuronal plasticity. In: Jensen TS, Turner JA, Wiesenfeld-Hallin Z, eds. *Proceedings of the 8th World Congress on Pain: progress in pain research and management,* vol 8. Seattle: IASP Press, 1997:243–257.
33. Edström L, Conradi S, Henriksson KG, et al. Sjukdomar i den motoriska enheten: en översikt. *Lakartidningen* 1989;86:531–534.
34. Eisenberg E, Pud D. Can patients with chronic neuropathic pain be cured by acute administration of the NMDA receptor antagonist amantadine? *Pain* 1998;74:337–339.
35. Eisenstein SM, Ashton IK, Roberts S, et al. Innervation of the spondylolysis "ligament." *Spine* 1994;19:912–916.
36. Freemont AJ, Peacock TE, Goupille P, et al. Nerve ingrowth into diseased intervertebral disc in chronic back pain. *Lancet* 1997;350:178–181.
37. Fridén J. Changes in human skeletal muscle induced by long term eccentric exercise. *Cell Tissue Res* 1984;236:365–372.
38. Fridén J, Lieber RL. Structual and mechanical basis of exercise-induced muscle injury. *Med Sci Sports Exerc* 1992;24:521–530.
39. Gatchel RJ. Psychological disorders and chronic pain: cause-and-effect relationships. In: Gatchel RJ, Turk DC, eds. *Chronic pain: psychological perspectives on treatment.* New York: Guilford Press, 1996.
40. Gatchel RJ, Polatin PB, Kinney RK. Predicting outcome of chronic low back pain using clinical predictors of psychopathology: a prospective analysis. *Health Psychol* 1995;14:415–420.
41. Gatchel RJ, Polatin PB, Mayer TG. The dominant role of psychosocial risk factors in the development of chronic low back pain disability. *Spine* 1995;20:2702–2709.
42. Geiss A, Varadi E, Steinbach K, et al. Psychoneuroimmunological correlates of persisting sciatic pain in patients who underwent discectomy. *Neurosci Lett* 1997;237:65–68.
43. Gerwin RD, Shannon S, Hong CZ, et al. Interrater reliability in myofascial trigger point examination. *Pain* 1997;69:65–73.
44. Gibbons LE, Videman T, Battié MC, et al. Determinants of paraspinal muscle cross-sectional area in male monozygotic twins. *Phys Ther* 1998;78:602–610.
45. Gil KM. Psychological aspects of acute pain. In: Sinatra RS, Ginsberg B, eds. *Acute pain: mechanisms and management.* St Louis: Mosby–Year Book, 1992.
46. Giovengo SL, Russell IJ, Larsson AA. Increased concentration of nerve growth factor (NGF) in cerebrospinal fluid of patients with fibromyalgia. *J Rheumatol* 1999;26:1564–1569.
47. Greenwald HP. Interethnic differences in pain perception. *Pain* 1991;44:157–163.
48. Grönblad M. Spinal disorders: basic science. *Acta Orthop Scand* 1998;69[Suppl 281]:32–37.
49. Hadler NM: *Occupational musculoskeletal disorders.* New York: Raven Press, 1993.
50. Hides JA, Richardson CA, Jull GA. Magnetic resonance imaging and ultrasonography of the lumbar multifidus muscle: comparison of two different modalities. *Spine* 1995;20:54–58.
51. Hides JA, Richardson CA, Jull GA. Multifidus muscle recovery is not automatic after resolution of acute, first-episode low back pain. *Spine* 1996;21:2763–2769.
52. Hides JA, Stokes MJ, Saide M. Evidence of lumbar multifidus muscle wasting ipsilateral to symptoms in patients with acute/subacute low back pain. *Spine* 1994;19:165–172.
53. Hocking B. Epidemiological aspects of "repetition strain injury" in Telecom Australia. *Med J Aust* 1987;147:218–222.
54. Hutton WC, Toribatake Y, Elmer WA, et al. The effect of compressive force applied to the intervertebral disc *in vivo:* a study of proteoglycans and collagen. *Spine* 1998;23:2524–2537.
55. Hokfeldt T, Xu Zhang, Zhi-Qing Xu, et al. Phenotype regulation in dorsal root ganglion neurons after nerve injury. Focus on peptides and their receptors. *Mol Neurobiol Pain* 1997;9:115.

56. Jaffurs D, Evans CH. The human genome project: implications for the treatment of musculoskeletal disease. *J Am Acad Orthop Surg* 1998;6:1–14.
57. Jayson MIV, Freemont AJ. Fibrosis, chronic inflammation, and vascular damage in mechanical back pain syndromes. In: Wiesel SW, Weinstein JN, Herkowitz H, et al., eds. *The lumbar spine,* 2nd ed, vol 2. Philadelphia: WB Saunders, 1996:812–821.
58. Johansson H, Själander P, Djupsjöbacka M. Influences of joint receptors on the fusimotor system: possible implications for proprioception and control of muscle stiffness. Summaries of lecture during the postgraduate course neuro-muscular systems and muscule pain, Sept 29–Dec 12, 1995. *Arbete och Hälsa vetenskaplig skriftserie Solna: Arbetslivsinstitutet* 1996;4:3–6.
59. Kieschke J, Mense S, Prabhakar NR. Influence of adrenaline and hypoxia on rat muscle receptors *in vitro. Prog Brain Res* 1988;74:91.
60. King AI, Cavanaugh JM. Diagnosis and neuromechanisms: neurophysiologic basis of low back pain. In: Wiesel SW, Weinstein JN, Herkowitz H, et al., eds. *The lumbar spine,* 2nd ed, vol 1. Philadelphia: WB Saunders, 1996:74–85.
61. Kitano T, Zerwekh JE, Usui Y, et al. Biochemical changes associated with the symptomatic human intervertebral disk. *Clin Orthop* 1993;293:372–377.
62. Kjellgren JH. The anatomical source of back pain. *Rheumatol Rehabil* 1977;16:3–12.
63. Kjellgren JH, Lewis T. Observations relating to referred pain, visceromotor reflexes and other associated phenomenon. *Clin Sci* 1939;4:46–71.
64. Kosek E. *Somatosensory dysfunction in fibromyalgia: implications for pathophysiological mechanisms.* Thesis, Department of Rehabilitation Medicine, Karolinska Institute/Hospital, Stockholm, 1998.
65. Kreicbergs A, Ahjmed M. Neuropeptides in bone. *Curr Opin Orthop* 1997;8:71–79.
66. Kuslich SD, Ulström CL, Michael CJ. The tissue origin of low back pain and sciatica: a report of pain response to tissue stimulation during operations on the lumbar spine using local anesthesia. *Orthop Clin North Am* 1991;22:181–187.
67. Light AR. Normal anatomy and physiology of the spinal cord dorsal horn. *Appl Neurophysiol* 1988;51:78–88.
68. Lipton JA, Marbach JJ. Ethnicity and the pain experience. *Soc Sci Med* 1984;19:1279–1298.
69. Lord SM, Barnsley L, Wallis BJ, et al. Chronic cervical zygapophysical joint pain after whiplash: a placebo-controlled prevalence study. *Spine* 1996;21:1737–1744.
70. Markenson JA. Mechanisms of chronic pain. *Am J Med* 1996;101:6S–18S.
71. Melzack R, Wall PD. Pain mechanism: a new theory. *Science* 1965;150:971–978.
72. Mense S, Meyer H. Different types of slowly conducting afferent units in cat skeletal muscle and tendon. *J Physiol* 1985;363:403.
73. Mogil JS, Sternberg WF, Marek P, et al. The genetics of pain and pain inhibition. *Proc Natl Acad Sci U S A* 1996;93:3048–3055.
74. Nachemson A. Intradiscal measurements of pH in patients with lumbar rhizopathies. *Acta Orthop Scand* 1969;40:23–42.
75. Nachemson A. Lumbar discography: where are we today [Editorial]. *Spine* 1989;14:555–557.
76. Nachemson A. *Ont i ryggen orsaker, diagnostik och behandling.* Stockholm: Swedish Council on Technology Assessment in Health Care, Stockholm 1991.
77. Nachemson AK, Bennett GJ. Does pain damage spinal cord neurons? Transsynaptic degeneration in rat following a surgical incision. *Neurosci Lett* 1993;162:78–80.
78. Nachemson AL. Scientific diagnosis or unproved label for back pain patients. In: Szpalski M, Gunzburg R, Pope MH, eds. *Lumbar segmental instability.* Philadelphia: Lippincott William & Wilkins, 1999:297–301.
79. Ness TJ, Gebhart GF. Visceral pain: a review of experimental studies. *Pain* 1990;41:167–234.
80. Nishida K, Kang JD, Gilbertson LG, et al. Modulation of the biological activity of the rabbit intervertebral disc by gene therapy: an in-vivo study of adenovirus-mediated transfer of the human TGF-β-1 encoding gene. Volvo Award winner 1999. *Spine* 1999;24:2419–2425.
81. Olmarker K. The experimental basis of sciatica. *J Orthop Sci* 1996;1:230–242.
82. Olmarker K, Larsson K. Tumor necrosis factor alpha and nucleus-pulposus-induced nerve root injury. *Spine* 1998;23:2538–2544.
83. Olmarker K, Myers RR. Pathogenesis of sciatic pain: role of herniated nucleus pulposus and deformation of spinal nerve root and dorsal root ganglion. *Pain* 1998;78:99–105.
84. Olmarker K, Rydevik B. Single-versus double-level nerve root compression. An experimental study on the porcine cauda equina with analyses of nerve impulse conduction properties. *Clin Orthop* 1992;279:35–39.
85. Ooi Y, Mita F, Satoh Y. Myeloscopic study on lumbar spinal canal stenosis with special reference to intermittent claudication. *Spine* 1990;15:544–549.
86. Pedersen J, Sjölander P, Wenngren BI, et al. Increased intramuscular concentration of bradykinin increases the static fusimotor drive to muscle spindles in neck muscles of the cat. *Pain* 1997;70:83–91.
87. Perl ER. Sensitisation of nociceptors and its relation to sensation. In: Bonica JJ, Albe-Fessard DG, eds. *Advances in pain research and therapy, vol 1.* New York: Raven Press, 1976:17.

88. Phillips RB, Hove JW, Bustin G, et al. Stress x-rays and the low back pain patient. *J Manipulative Physiol Ther* 1990;13:127–133.
89. Phillips RB. Plain film radiology in chiroparctic. *J Manipulative Physiol Ther* 1992;15:47–50.
90. Plaugher G, Cremata EE, Phillips RB. A retrospective consecutive case analysis of pretreatment and comparative static radiologic parameters following chiropractic adjustments. *J Manipulative Physiol Ther* 1990;13:498–506.
91. Porter RW. Pathophysiology of neurogenic claudication. In: Wiesel SW, Weinstein JN, Herkowitz H, et al., eds. *The lumbar spine,* 2nd ed, vol 2. Philadelphia: WB Saunders, 1996:717–723.
92. Reinecke JA, Wehling P, Robbins P, et al. *In vitro* transfer von genen in spinale gewebe. *Z Orthop Ihre Grenzgeb* 1997;135:412–416.
93. *Report of the commission on the evaluation of pain.* Washington, DC: Department of Health and Human Services, United States Government Printing Office, 1987.
94. Roberts S, Eisenstein SM, Menage J. Mechanoreceptors in intervertebral discs: morphology, distribution, and neuropeptides. *Spine* 1995;20:2645–2651.
95. Roberts S, McCall IW, Menage J, et al. Does the thickness of the vertebral subchondral bone reflect the composition of the intervertebral disc? *Eur Spine J* 1997;6:385–389.
96. Russell IJ, Orr MD, Littman B, et al. Elevated cerebrospinal fluid levels of substance P in patients with the fibromyalgia syndrome. *Arthritis Rheum* 1994;37:1593–1601.
97. Russell IJ, Vipraio G, Fletcher EM, et al. Characteristics of spinal fluid substance P and calcitonin related gene peptide in fibromyalgia syndrome. *Arthritis Rheum* 1996;39:1485.
98. Rydevik B, Hasue M, Wehling P. Etiology of sciatic pain and mechanisms of nerve root compression. In: Wiesel SW, Weinstein JN, Herkowitz H, et al., eds. *The lumbar spine,* 2nd ed, vol 1. Philadelphia: WB Saunders, 1996:123–140.
99. Schonström N. *The narrow lumbar spinal canal and the size of the cauda equina in man.* Thesis, Göteborg University, Sweden, 1988.
100. Schonström N, Bolender N, Spengler DM. The pathomorphology of spinal stenosis as seen on CT scans of the lumbar spine. *Spine* 1986;10:806–811.
101. Seltzer Z, Dubner R, Shir Y. A novel behavioural model of neuropathic pain disorders produced in rat by partial sciatic nerve injury. *Pain* 1990;43:205.
102. Siddall PJ, Taylor D, Cousins MJ. Pain associated with spinal cord injury. *Curr Opin Neurol* 1995;8:447–450.
103. Simmons ED Jr, Guntupalli M, Kowalski JM, et al. Familial predisposition for degenerative disc disease: a case-control study. *Spine* 1996;21:1527–1529.
104. Slattery ML, Jacobs DR Jr. The inter-relationships of physical activity, physical fitness and body measurements. *Med Sci Sports Exerc* 1987;19:564–569.
105. Smythe MJ, Wright V. Sciatica and the intervertebral disc. An experimental study. *J Bone Joint Surg Br* 1967;49:502–519.
106. Suseki K, Takahashi Y, Takahashi K, et al. Sensory nerve fibres from lumbar intervertebral discs pass through rami communicantes: a possible pathway for discogenic low back pain. *J Bone Joint Surg Br* 1998;80:737–742.
107. Thorn BE, Williams DA. Goal specification alters perceived pain intensity and tolerance latency. *Cognitive Ther Res* 1989;13:171–183.
108. Travell JG, Simmons DG. *Myofascial pain and dysfunction: the trigger point manual,* vol 1. Baltimore: Williams & Wilkins, 1983.
109. Travell JG, Simmons DG. *Myofascial pain and dysfunction: the trigger point manual,* vol 2. Baltimore: Williams & Wilkins, 1992.
110. Tunks E, McCain GA, Hart LE, et al. The reliability of examination for tenderness in patients with myofascial pain, chronic fibromyalgia and controls. *J Rheumatol* 1995;22:944–952.
111. Turk DC. The role of demographic and psychosocial factors in transition from acute to chronic pain. In: Jensen TS, Turner JA, Wiesenfeld-Hallin Z, eds. *Proceedings of the 8th World Congress on Pain: progress in pain and management,* vol 8. Seattle: IASP Press, 1997:101–112.
112. Turk DC, Meichenbaum D, Genest M. *Pain and behavioural medicine: a cognitive-behavioural perspective.* New York: Guilford Press, 1983.
113. Turner JA, Romano JM. Psychological and psychosocial evaluation. In: Bonica JJ, ed. *The management of pain,* 2nd ed. Philadelphia: Lea & Febiger, 1990.
114. Vaeroy H, Helle R, Forre O, et al. Elevated CSF levels of substance P and high incidence of Raynaud's phenomenon in patients with fibrmyalgia: new features for diagnosis. *Pain* 1988;32:21–26.
115. Videman T, Batti, MC, Gibbons LE, et al. Lifetime exercise and disk degeneration: an MRI study of monozygotic twins. *Med Sci Sports Exerc* 1997;29:1350–1356.
116. Videman T, Leppävuori J, Kaprio J, et al. Intragenic polymorphisms of the vitamin D receptor gene associated with intervertebral disc degeneration. *Spine* 1998;23:2477–2485.
117. Waddell G. Biopsychosocial analysis of low back pain. *Clin Rheumatol* 1992;6:523–557.
118. Waddell G. Low back pain: a twentieth-century health care enigma. In: Jensen TS, Turner JA, Wiesenfeld-Hallin Z, eds. *Proceedings of the 8th World Congress on Pain: progress in pain research and management,* vol 8. Seattle: IASP Press, 1997:101–112.

119. Waddell G, Somerville D, Henderson I, et al. A fear-avoidance beliefs questionnaire (FABQ) and the role of fear-avoidance beliefs in chronic low back pain and disability. *Pain* 1993;52:157–168.
120. Wehling P, Evans CH, Schulitz KP. The interaction between synovial cytokines and peripheral nerve function: a potential element in the develpment of radicular syndrone. *Z Orthop Ihre Grenzgeb* 1990;128:442.
121. Wehling P, Schultz KP, Robbins PD, et al. Transfer of genes to chondrocytic cells of the lumbar spine: proposal for a treatment strategy of spinal disorders by local gene therapy. *Spine* 1997;22:1092–1097.
122. Weinstein J. Mechanisms of spinal pain: the dorsal root ganglion and its role as a mediator of low back pain. *Spine* 1986;11:999–1001.
123. Welin M, Bragee B, Nyberg F, et al. Elevated substance p levels are contrasted by a decrease in met-enkephalin-arg-phe levels in CSF from fibromyalgia patients. *J Musculoskel Pain* 1995;3:4(abst).
124. Wiesel SW, Tsourmas N, Feffer HL, et al. A study of computer-assisted tomography. I. The incidence of positive CAT scans in an asymptomatic group of patients. *Spine* 1984;9:549–551.
125. Wiesenfeld-Hallin Z. Combined opioid-NMDA antagonist therapies: what advantages do they offer for the control of pain syndromes? *Drugs* 1998;55:1–4.
126. Williams DA, Thorn BE. Can research methodology affect treatment outcome? A comparison of two cold test paradigms. *Cognitive Ther Res* 1986;10:539–546.
127. Willis WD. Anatomy and physiology of descending control of nociceptive responses of dorsal horn neurons: comprehensive review. *Prog Brain Res* 1988;77:1–39.
128. Wolfe F, Ross K, Anderson J, et al. Aspects of fibromyalgia in the general population: sex, pain threshold, and fibromyalgia symptoms. *J Rheumatol* 1993;22:151–156.
129. Wolfe F, Ross K, Anderson J, et al. The prevalence and characteristics of fibromyalgia in the general population. *Arthritis Rheum* 1995;38:19–28.
130. Yaksh TJ. Pharmacology of spinal adrenergic systems which modulate spinal nociceptive processing. *Pharmacol Biochem Behav* 1988;22:845–858.
131. Yunus MB. Towards a model of pathophysiology of fibromyalgia: aberrant central pain mechanisms with peripheral modulation [Editorial]. *J Rheumatol* 1992;19:846–850.
132. Yunus MH. Research in fibromyalgia and myofascial pain syndromes: current status, problems and future directions. *J Musculoskelet Pain* 1993;1:23–41.
133. Zboroski M. Cultural components in response to pain. *J Soc Issues* 1952;8:16–30.

*Neck and Back Pain: The Scientific Evidence
of Causes, Diagnosis, and Treatment,* edited
by Alf Nachemson and Egon Jonsson.
Published by Lippincott Williams & Wilkins,
Philadelphia 2000.

8

Epidemiology of Neck and Low Back Pain

Alf Nachemson*, Gordon Waddell†, and Anders I. Norlund‡

*Department of Orthopaedics, Sahlgrenska University Hospital, Göteborg, Sweden
†Department of Orthopaedics, The Glasgow Nuffield Hospital, Glasgow, Scotland;
‡Swedish Council on Technology Assessment in Health Care, Stockholm, Sweden

Epidemiology gives insight critical to understanding the scope of a problem and provides information about its magnitude and the demand on medical and social resources. It can also give information on the natural history of a disorder, important for patient counseling about prognosis. In addition, it can identify risk factors both individual and external. In this book, the evaluation of these risk factors has been allocated to separate chapters (Chapters 3–5).

Most studies in the literature talk about *prevalence,* which is the percentage of people in a known population who have the symptom during a specified period of time. *Point prevalence* is the percentage of those who have pain on the day of the interview. *One-month or 1-year prevalence* is the percentage of those who have pain at some time in the past month or in the past year. *Lifetime prevalence* is the percentage of those who can remember pain at some time in their lives. *Incidence* is the percentage of people in a known population who develop new symptoms during a specified period of time. This term is commonly applied to those who report injuries or who present for health care within a specified period.

Most surveys define *low back pain* as pain occurring between the costal margins and the gluteal folds. Some surveys use a diagram. Back pain has often been defined differently. Should it include any back symptoms, no matter how mild or how brief the duration? Is there a distinction among "symptoms," "trouble," and pain? It is important to distinguish among back pain, back disability, and health care for back pain, because each has different epidemiologic rates.

Another major limitation is that surveys depend entirely on peoples' own reporting of pain and disability, which is open to subjective bias. There may be recall bias: the longer the time asked about, the more unreliable the answers. People with more severe trouble may be more likely to include earlier information within the period of the question (2,7,90). Official statistics may overcome this problem to provide more accurate data about work loss, health care use, sickness certification, and sickness benefits, but these statistics usually give lower rates for each of these entities than self-reports from population surveys (79). There may also be sampling bias. Many surveys study selected groups of workers or patients, who may not be representative of the general population.

Raspe (67), Shekelle (72), and Andersson (2) reviewed altogether several hundred epidemiologic studies of low back pain from North America, Britain, and Europe, in particular the Scandinavian countries. Because many of the surveys did not ask comparable questions, they apparently gave different results. Thus, the definition of morbidity chosen for the survey is of importance for the resulting frequency of pain.

The best available evidence on the epidemiology of low back pain and of neck pain is from large, representative, population surveys (back pain: 2,19,21,24,62,63,73, 74,86,92,97; neck pain: 3,9,14,22,49,54,84). Most surveys used similar wording for their questions, and many asked about pain lasting more than 24 hours, to exclude minor or passing symptoms.

Many international surveys of low back pain reported a point prevalence of 15% to 30%, a 1-month prevalence between 19% and 43%, and a lifetime prevalence of about 60% to 70%. The exact figures in different studies appear to depend mainly on the wording of the question, rather than on any differences in the people studied.

The Nuprin Pain Report (86) found that 56% of American adults said they had at least 1 day of back pain in the last year. Fourteen percent had pain for more than 30 days in the year. Back pain was the second most common pain after headache. Most back pain was mild and short-lived and had little effect on daily life, but recurrences were common.

Von Korff et al. (92) found that 41% of American adults aged 26 to 44 years had back pain in the last 6 months. Most people had occasional short attacks of pain, but these people reported that they had had these attacks over a long period. Their pain was usually mild or moderate and did not limit their activities.

British surveys give comparable figures. Mason (56) found point prevalence around 15%, 1-month prevalance of 40%, and lifetime prevalence of 60%. Walsh et al. (97), Mason (56), and Papageorgiou et al. (62) found an almost identical lifetime prevalence of 60%, the same as in Belgium (74).

Population surveys suggest that the age of onset of back pain is spread fairly evenly from the teens to the early 40s. It is uncommon to develop nonspecific low back pain for the first time after the mid-50s. However, several studies of children showed a higher prevalence of back pain than previously realized. Brattberg (10,11) carried out a longitudinal study of 471 schoolchildren aged 10, 13, and 15 years in the county of Gävleborg in Sweden. In each year's survey, about 26% of children said they had back pain, but only 9% of the children reported back pain in both surveys in 1989 and 1991. Burton et al. (16) prospectively studied 216 adolescents from 11 through 15 years of age. Only 12% of 11-year-old children in the study said they had ever had back pain, but by the age of 15 years, this number rose to 50%. Their back pain was usually recurrent but did not deteriorate with time. Adolescents appear to have about the same prevalence of back pain as adults, but it is rarely disabling, and few seek health care. Burton et al. (16) suggested that most adolescent back trouble should be considered to be a normal life experience and should not have undue significance attached to it. There is no evidence on whether it predicts low back trouble in adult life. The study by Hellsing (38) of 19-year-old conscripts suggests the same when these persons were followed up to 10 years later.

The General Survey on Living Conditions in Sweden (70) found that neck and back problems were among the most common causes of "chronic sickness." About 3% to 5% of the population aged 16 to 44 years and 11% to 12% of those aged 45 to 64 years reported back problems as a "chronic sickness." For those aged 65 to 84 years, the frequency of back pain was reduced, or 9% to 11%, although Brattberg et al. (12,13) reported a higher prevalence of 45%. Back trouble is the most common cause of chronic sickness in both men and women less than 64 years of age and the second most common between age 65 and 74 years. Only in the age group of those older than 65 years do symptoms of the circulatory system become more common than back trouble. There is a slight increase over time of back pain in the general population according to the General Survey on Living Conditions (70). As an average for the population aged 16 to 84 years (men and women), 6.5% reported back pain symptoms in 1985, compared with 8.0% in 1994. Linton et al. (49), in a study covering subjects living in the middle part of Sweden but limited to subjects 35 to 45 years of age, found even higher prevalence figures, probably dependent on how the questions were asked. Other Scandinavian studies (5–7,34) all described point prevalence of around 30%, 1-year prevalence of around 50%, and lifetime prevalence up to 80% or more.

The traditional clinical classification of back pain is into acute, recurrent, and chronic, but epidemiologic studies show that back pain is usually a recurrent, intermittent, and episodic problem. Croft et al. (24) suggested that the most important epidemiologic concept, and possibly also an important clinical concept, is the pattern of back pain over long periods of the individual's life, and the experience of back pain may be better expressed as the total days of pain over 1 year. Von Korff (92) from the United States also described this recurrent trait in back symptoms, as have others (18,68). Tables 8.1 and 8.2 summarize the findings of the larger studies.

WORK LOSS RESULTING FROM BACK PAIN

It is difficult to obtain accurate information on the amount of work loss attributed to back pain. In many countries, including Sweden since 1991, the first days or weeks of sick pay are paid by employers, who hold the data individually and do not return any statistics to any central authority. Social security data contain claims and benefits paid, and these depend on entitlement and are not always exactly the same as actual work loss. Some data relate to a particular section of the system; for example, many authors in the United States quote figures for workers' compensation, but that is a selected and relatively small part of the total picture. These questions are further elaborated in Chapters 20 and 21.

Valkenburg and Haanen reported (88) on the so-called Zoetermeer study of 6,500 men and women in that Dutch city who were 20 years of age and older and reported the data shown in Table 8.3. These authors also performed physical and x-ray examinations on these persons.

Andersson (2) found that back problems were the most common cause of activity limitation in adults less than aged 45 years and the fourth most common in those aged 45 to 64 years. Seven percent of adults reported a disability resulting from their back or from both their back and other joint problems that limited their activities for an average of about 23 days each year. These figures suggest that 7% to 14% of adults in the United States have some disability resulting from back pain for a least 1 day each year, just over 1% of Americans are permanently disabled by back pain, and another 1% of adults in the United States are temporarily disabled by back pain at any one time.

Walsh et al. (97) reported the only population survey to use clinical measures of low back disability, based on eight activities of daily living. The 1-year prevalence of a disability score of 50% or more was 5.4% for men and 4.5% for women, whereas the lifetime prevalence was 16% and 13%, respectively. The 1-year prevalence of time

TABLE 8.1. *Low back pain epidemiology: selected larger population-based studies*

Study (ref.)	Country	Design	Sample	Setting	Method	Results
Cassidy et al. (19)	Canada	Population-based cross-sectional mailed survey	2,184 inhabitants; 55% response rate; adults 20–69 yr old	Saskatchewan Health and Back Pain Survey	Survey by mail; responders and nonresponders compared for bias; pain questionnaire for 6 mo prevalence, other prevalence from simple questions; no medical control	Prevalence rates: Point 28.4% (25.6–31.1 CI 0.95) 6-mo 48.9% (45.9–52.0 CI) Lifetime 84.9% (81.9–86.3 CI) 6-mo high intensity and high disability: 10.7% (8.8–12.5 CI)
Linton et al. (49)	Sweden	Population-based mailed survey	2,300 35–45 yr olds, postal survey; response rate, 79%	Central Sweden Occupational Health Clinic, Örebro	Questionnaire; nonresponders evaluated on a 0–10 pain scale; neck and back care point sickness data checked	1y prevalence: 69.5% women, 63.2% men; 19% absenteeism
Taimela et al. (85)	Finland	Survey by questionnaire, cohort-based	1,171 pupils from 45 public schools, 594 girls	Sampling process of public schools in Finland	Nationwide cohort-based questionnaire survey, self-administered; location and duration of back pain; no medical control	12-mo prevalence: 7 yr old 1% 10 yr old 6% 13–18 yr old 18% No gender difference; of those reporting back pain, recurrent pain 26% of boys and 33% of girls
Hillman et al. (39)	United Kingdom	Two-stage cross-sectional survey	1,437 men and 1,747 women aged 25–64 yr	Purchasing district (Bradford), in the planning of questionnaire services for low back pain	Random selection of the population, postal survey; lifetime 59%; no medical control	Prevalence: Point 19% 12-mo 39% Annual incidence 4.7%; absence from work due to low back pain 6.4%
Burton et al. (16)	United Kingdom	5-yr longitudinal interview and questionnaire survey of back pain	Cohort of 216 children 11 yr old at start	Spinal Research Unit, University of Huddersfield	Cohort followed from 11–15 yr of age using a structured questionnaire annually	Prevalence age 11–12 yr: 12-mo 11.8% Lifetime 11.6% Prevalence age 15 yr: 12-mo 21.5% Lifetime 50.4% Experience of low back pain was often forgotten; few children required health care

168

Source	Country	Study type	Sample	Methods	Results
Leboeuf and Lauritsen (47)	Nordic countries	Cross-sectional postal survey, comparison with methodologically similar studies 1971–1985	In all, 3,513	Prevalence estimates from postal survey, adjusted for age and gender; no medical control	Prevalence, aged 30–50 yr: 12-mo 44–54% Lifetime 66%
Carey et al. (17)	USA	Telephone interview from a random sample	4,437 adults; 79% response rate	Detailed interview re; acute low back pain lasting less than 3 mo and functinally limiting; no medical control	Functionally limiting low back pain among adults: <60 yr 8.5%; >60 yr 5.0%
Papageorgiou et al. (62)	United Kingdom	Population-based cross-sectional mailed survey to 18–75-yr-old inhabitants	7,669 adults; response rate 59%	Questionnaire including pain drawing; no medical control	1-mo prevalence: Males 35% Females 42% All 39%
Heliövaara et al. (37)	Finland	Mini-Finland Health Examination Survey prospective cohort study	Representative sample Finns aged >29 yr; 8,000 sample; 90% response rate	Part of Mini-Finland Health Examination Survey 1978 and 1980 with follow-up until 1991; medical examination	History of low back pain 76%; at standardized clinical examination, 17% were diagnosed as having chronic low back pain; no prediction of mortality from low back pain
Skovron et al. (74)	Belgium	Mailed survey to adults, self-administered	4,000 adults	Structured mailed survey, self-administered; no medical control	Prevalence: Point ("current") 33% Lifetime 59% First time ever 5%; increasing age and female gender were associated with history of low back pain, as also work dissatisfaction

TABLE 8.2. *Low back pain epidemiology in specific groups*

Study (ref.)	Country	Design	Sample	Setting	Method	Results
Thomas et al. (87)	Australia	Cross-sectional survey, self-administered	200 military helicopter pilots; 66% response rate	Center for Clinical Epidemiology and Biostatistics and Australia Air Force	Surveys to helicopter pilots; no medical control	Prevalence: Lifetime 64% Low back pain interfered with concentration while flying: 55%
Brown et al. (15)	Canada	Survey of random sample, questionnaire	1,002 policemen; 80% response rate	Department of Medicine, University of Ottawa and Royal Canadian Mounted Police	Structured mail questionnaire to officers on active duty; no medical control	Prevalence: 12-mo 41.8% Lifetime 54.9%
Hignett (40)	United Kingdom	Summary of 80 studies of back pain among nurses		Nottingham City Hospital	Review of earlier published studies	Prevalence: Point 17% 12-mo 40–50% Lifetime 35–80%
Guo et al (32)	USA	Health survey interview of workers	30,074 employed workers	National Institute for Occupational Safety and Health, Cincinatti	Interviews with workers who had had compensation benefits for >7 d during past yr	Prevalence of back pain with compensation benefits of >7 d: 17.6%
Smedley et al. (75)	United Kingdom	Cross-sectional survey	2,405 nurses; 69% response rate	MRC Environm Epidemiology Unit, Southhamton Hospital	Self-administered questionnaire; no medical control	Prevalence: 12-mo 45% Lifetime 60%

lost from work because of back pain was 11% for men and 7% for women, whereas the lifetime prevalence was 34% and 23%, respectively.

The South Manchester Back Pain Study (63) found that 8% of adults said they had bed rest for back pain at some time in the past 12 months. However, these figures are again self-reports about what people said they did about back pain and are not records of the treatment they received.

The Clinical Standards Advisory Group (20) estimated that work loss from back pain in United Kingdom in 1993 was about 52 million days, whereas 106 million days of sickness and invalidity benefits were paid for back pain. However, there was an overlap of only 7 million days between these two groups. Most of the workers who

TABLE 8.3. *Low back complaints and work disability in the Dutch city of Zoetermeer in the 1970s*

	Men		Women	
	Percentage (%)	Relative percentage (%)	Percentage (%)	Relative percentage (%)
Point prevalence	22.2	—	30.2	—
Lifetime incidence	51.4	—	57.8	—
>3 mo	14.3	28	19.6	34
Unfit for work	24.3	47	19.5	34
Work change	4.2	8	2.4	4

From Valkenburg HA, Haanen HCM. The epidemiology of low back pain. In: White AA, Gordon SL, eds. *Symposium on idiopathic low back pain.* St. Louis: CV Mosby, 1982;9–22, with permission.

lost short periods from work were paid by their employers, did not receive any state sickness benefit, and did not appear in the Department of Social Security statistics, whereas most of the benefits went to people who were not working anyway (50).

Guo et al. (32) provided the best estimate of work loss from back pain in the United States; these investigators used data on 30,074 workers from the National Health Interview Survey. In 1988, about 22.4 million people, or 17.6% of all United States workers, lost an estimated 149 million days from work as a result of back pain.

In most studies, about half the total days lost from work because of back pain are accounted for by the 85% of people who are home from work for short periods, with a median of less than 7 days (57). The other half of days lost is accounted for by the 15% of people who are home from work for more than 1 month. This finding is reflected in the social costs of back pain. It is widely quoted that 80% to 90% of the health care costs of back pain are for the 10% of patients with chronic low back pain and disability (2,44,58,99). Watson et al. (98) showed that the same is true for the social costs. In 1994, back pain in the island of Jersey accounted for 11% of all sickness absence. Only 3% of those who lost work because of back pain were off for more than 6 months, but these workers accounted for 33% of the benefits paid.

Work Loss Resulting From Back and Neck Pain in Göteborg

In the studies just mentioned from the 1970s, Svensson and Andersson indicated that between 2% and 6% suffered work loss from back pain. An interesting finding was that one-fourth of the men who said they never had had back pain actually had lost 1 day or more with that diagnosis when insurance data were checked. This finding illustrates the difficulty in relying on memory in questionnaire surveys.

The city of Göteborg, with its 450,000 inhabitants, continues to be a source of many Swedish epidemiologic data (2,57,58,102). Swedish statistics on sickness absence resulting from back pain or neck pain are not available on the national level. However, there are data collected from the Göteborg region for several years on back pain (57). Although limited in population size, and with an average length of episodes of sickness absence longer than the average for Sweden, the Göteborg data have the advantage of being specified into different subgroups of back pain, including that of neck pain. Based on the data from Göteborg, estimates of the number of individuals with sickness absence resulting from back and neck pain have been calculated for the national level (see Chapter 20). There seems to be a reduction in number of workers on sick leave for any back pain. The relative percentage of days absent resulting from neck pain has increased, however, from 24% in 1987 to 56% in 1997.

SCIATICA

Few surveys use strict criteria for *sciatica*. Several reports give a lifetime prevalence of 14% to 40% for leg pain associated with back problems, but they do not distinguish true radicular pain from the more common referred leg pain. Deyo and Tsui-Wu (28) estimated the lifetime prevalence of "surgically important disc herniation" to be about 2%. Lawrence (46) reported a prevalence of "sciatica suggesting a herniated lumbar disc" of 3.1% in men and 1.3% in women. Neither of these studies gave diagnostic criteria. Heliövaara et al. (37) in Finland reported the only large population survey with clinical criteria of radicular pain. That study noted a lifetime prevalence of back pain of 77% in men and 74% in women, whereas the lifetime prevalence of any associated leg pain was 35% in men and 45% in women. If one applies strict diagnostic criteria for radicular pain, however, the lifetime prevalence of actual "sciatica" was only 5% in men and 4% in women, findings also later confirmed (51). Svensson and Andersson (79–82) performed cross-sectional studies of two groups of subjects, one consisting of 940 men 40 to 46 years old and 1,760 women 38 to 64 years of age. These investigators found prevalence rates for all back pain between 60% and 70%, with a 1-month prevalence of 35%. Sciatica (leg pain) was described by around 30%.

FREQUENCY OF NECK PAIN

Neck pain appears to be less common than low back pain, but fewer data are available on the epidemiology of neck pain, which is often simply included in "all spinal pain." Neck pain is also often not differentiated from shoulder pain, and the two are often measured together.

A MEDLINE search was undertaken on neck pain epidemiology for the period 1966 to 1997 using the Medical Subject Heading terms "neck," "pain," "prevalence," and "epidemiology." The search yielded 113 articles. In addition to the MEDLINE search, published articles appearing during 1998 were included by hand search. Twenty-eight articles on neck pain were chosen for further studies. These studies were divided into the following three groups: population studies (n = 11), studies of specific age groups or professional groups (n = 10), and studies of whiplash (n = 7). The population studies were population surveys, two of which (55,66) also included some kind of physical examination.

Population-Based Surveys

There are 11 population studies included in this analysis, of which 9 are from the Nordic countries (Table 8.4). The point prevalence is estimated in 4 studies with approximately the same age groups, from 20 to 69 years of age, to be between 11.5% (average of men and women) in a Finnish study (55), 13.4% according to a study from the Netherlands (89), and 22.2% in a study from Canada (22).

The period prevalence has most of the estimates, 9 of 11 studies, although there is a variation of the definition of the time period measured for neck pain. As regards the period prevalence up to 6 months, Andersson et al. (3) reported an average of 17% (average of men and women) for more than 3 months' duration, Bovim et al. (9) noted 14% for the past 6 months, and Coté et al. (22) had between 5% and 40%, depending on the grade of pain for 6 months. Mäkele (54) reported 41.1% for last month. There is, thus, a relatively large spread between the estimates of period prevalence up to 6 months.

Five studies reported on the 1-year prevalence. The estimates from population studies were 34% according to Bovim et al. (9), 26% in a Swedish study (14), and between 61% and 40% in a Finnish study (66), depending on whether the individuals had depression. Takala et al. (84), in another study from Finland, reported 17.5% for women and 16.5% for men. For retired women, the estimate of Takala et al. was 23%, and for retired men, it was 30%. Finally, in the study by Westerling and Jonsson (100), the estimate in a Swedish survey was 18% as an average for neck and shoulder pain.

Lifetime prevalence was estimated in only two population studies. Coté et al. (22) from Canada estimated lifetime prevalence as 67%, a finding similar to the 71% found by Mäkele (55) in a study from Finland. Even if well-documented population studies give the most adequate estimates of neck pain, studies of specific groups of employees are also important because these studies can point out health problems connected to different professions (Table 8.5).

As regards point prevalence, Hagberg (34) made an estimate from a metaanalysis of 21 published studies. Thus, the point estimate of cervical spondylosis for dentists was 42% to 50%, that of miners was even higher or 54% to 76%, and finally that of meat carriers was 84%. In a Swedish study, Kamwendo et al. (45) estimated the point prevalence of neck pain for medical secretaries to be 33%. This finding corresponds well with the 34% for hospital employees reported by Marshall et al. (52) from Great Britain.

The period prevalence was also high for dentists: 48% for male dentists and 62% for female dentists (69). From a large survey in France of 4.4 million employees, Weill et al. (99) reported a period prevalence for neck pain of 20.6% for all male employees and 36.6% for all female employees. Health care professionals in France had neck pain prevalence between 12% (male) and 18% (female).

In some of these studies of specific groups of employees, physical workload is not correlated to the presence of neck pain (44,65,101). However, neck pain can be significantly related to poorly experienced psychosocial work environment (45,60,101). A previous period of neck pain also increases the prevalence rate (52,99,101), that is, these are often recurrent symptoms.

Whiplash

The third category included in this MEDLINE search on neck pain concerns the *whiplash syndrome*. This clinical syndrome was first described by Crowe in 1928 (26), and initially attempts were made to relate it to a specific cervical acceleration-deceleration injury, but more recently the term has often been expanded to include any type of neck injury (usually vehicle related). The mechanism that actually constitutes whiplash is not well documented, according to a Norwegian metaanalysis of reports on whiplash 1992 to 1994 (77). It appears that there is only a weak empiric evidence for a causal link (construct validity) between the trauma mechanism and chronic symptoms of whiplash. This can also be interpreted from the study by Schrader et al. (71), of traffic-injured patients versus persons who did not have a traffic-related injury, of a representative sample of the general population in Lithuania (Table 8.6). According to Schrader et al. (71), the period prevalence of neck pain was about the same for those injured in traffic accidents as for the control population, that is, 35% for car occupants versus 33% for the standardized (age, sex) control group. Chronic neck pain for more than 9 days was also about the same, that is, 8% for car occupants versus 7% for the control group. One reason for this lack of significant difference could have been the minimal sickness benefits in Lithuania. Furthermore, no car insurance in Lithuania covers complaints on neck pain resulting from traffic accidents.

Apart from these two critical reports on whiplash by Schrader et al. (71) and by Stovner (77), many studies indicate the importance of the whiplash syndrome. In a Norwegian study, Borchgrevink et al. (8) reported that 58% of whiplash symptoms were linked to an accident. In the report by Deans et al. (27) from Great Britain, 62% of whiplash symptoms occurred after traffic accidents. In Sweden, Nygren et al. (61) reported that whiplash symptoms were increasing over time; for the period 1990 to 1992, these symptoms occurred in 46.9% of all the car occupants after traffic accidents. All the latter reports on whiplash had no control or comparison group corresponding to the general population. A gender difference of prevalence of whiplash was reported

TABLE 8.4. *Population-based surveys of neck pain epidemiology*

Study (ref.)	Definition	Country	Sample	Prevalence Lifetime	Prevalence Period	Prevalence Point	Other aspects
Andersson et al. (3)	Drawing on body diagram; duration >3 mo; pain persistent or recurrent	Sweden	Random sample 25–74 yr old; 1,806 individuals; and 90% response rate		Women 19.1% Men 14.5%		No difference of prevalence blue collar vs. white collar workers; neck pain increases up to 45–54 yr of age, then decreases
Bovim et al. (9)	Neck pain >6 mo during past yr	Norway	Random sample 18–67 yr old; 10,000 individuals; 77% resonse rate		34.4% sometime during 12 mo; 13.8% within past 6 mo		Women have higher frequence of chronic neck pain: Women 40% Men 29%
Brattberg et al. (10)	Neck pain > 6 mo	Sweden	Random sample 18–84 yr old; 1,009 individuals; 71.4% response rate		26.2% sometime during 12 mo; 4.6% last mo; obvious pain: <6 mo 1.3% >6 mo 12.7%		Obvious pain most frequent, 50%, for age group 45–64 yr (obvious pain = to quite a high degree)
Coté et al. (22)	Lifetime experience (Have you ever experienced neck pain in your lifetime?); point prevalence (Do you have neck pain right now?); chronic pain questionnaire (grade 1 to IV)	Canada	Random sample 20–69 yr old; 2,184 individuals; 55% response rate	66.7%	6-mo (grade): I: 39.7% II: 10.1% III and IV: 4.6%	22.2%	More women than men had experienced neck pain past 6 mo, women 58.8% vs men 47.2%
van der Donk et al. (89)	Point prevalence (Currently suffering from neck pain?); medical examination and radiography	Netherlands	Inhabitants 20–65 yr; included were 5,765 inhabitants in the town Zoetermeer			13.4%	Neuroticism a more powerful determinant of neck pain than radiologic signs of disc degeneration or osteoarthritis
Hagen et al. (35)	Period prevalence (1 mo) excluding RA; rating scales of pain; mental distress measurement	Norway	Random sample of inhabitants 20–79 yr old of which 11,780 participated or 58.9%		15.4%		Women 18.4% Men 12.9%
Hasvold and Johnsen (36)	Frequency of neck pain according to questionnaire: seldom/never, monthly	Norway	Part of general health screening, aged 20–56 yr old; 17,650 participated			Men 15.4% Women 24.9%	Neck pain seems to follow the pattern of general body pain and increase with age

174

Reference	Country	Symptom definition	Study population	Prevalence	Prevalence	Prevalence	Comments
Mäkele (54)	Finland	Weekly and daily neck pain	Part of general health survey, 30–64 yr 7,217 out of 8,000 participated, of which 3,403 had findings and were examined by a physician	71% (ever)	41.1% (last month)	Neck syndrome Men 9.5% Women 13.5%	Increase of prevalence of neck pain up to age 55–64 yr, then decrease; neck syndrome correlates positively with history of injury of the back, history of mental and physical stress at work and with low back pain syndrome
Rajala et al. (66)	Finland	Symptoms of ache, pain or discomfort in the neck in the past 12 mo	1,008 individuals born in 1935 (= 55 yr old); 77% participated; postal questionnaire and clinical examination; depressive symptoms measured		Depressed/neck pain: Women 65.4% Men 56.5% Not depressed: Women 45.5% Men 35.2%		Relative risk of neck pain depressed vs. not depressed: Men 2.2 Women 2.1
Takala et al. (84)	Finland	Neck pain indicated on body diagram; pain, ache, or soreness with movement in past year	Part of screening program for age-group 40–64 yr, participation rate 93.3%, total of 2,268		Neck cervical spine: Women <50: 13%, >50: 22% Men <50: 13%, >50: 20% Pensioners: Women 23% Men 30%		No significant difference between blue collar and white collar workers: Women 13% vs 14% Men 15% vs 14%
Westerling and Jonsson (100)	Sweden	Symptoms occurring during past 12 mo; symptoms such as pain, tenderness or stiffness	Random sample individuals 18–65 yr old; 2,537 participated		18% neck-shoulder: 18–25 yr 7% 26–45 yr 15% 46–64 yr 28% Only neck pain 10% of all ages		Neither heavy lifting nor social class increased prevalence of neck pain Women 20% Men 16%

RA, rheumatoid arthritis.

TABLE 8.5. *Neck pain: epidemiology in specific groups*

Study (ref.)	Country	Design	Sample	Setting	Method	Results	
Hagberg and Wegman, (34)	Sweden	Study of references from Medlars 1966–1986	21 studies 9 to 858 patients	21 out of 178 references included a physical or a laboratory examination; different occupational groups	Prevalence rates and odds ratio calculated from each article and the referent group given by each author	*Cervical spondylosis* Point prevalence: Dentists 42–50% Miners 54–76% Meat carriers 84% *Cervical syndrome* Point prevalence: Slaughterhouse workers 5% Civil servants 5% *Tension neck syndrome* Point prevalence Filmroll. workers 100% Lamp assemblers 91% (female workers) Certain jobs are associated with neck disorders	Point prevalence of different occupational groups of limited value (no random sample); not possible to control for age or gender; "healthy worker" effect possible for some groups; low power of some syndromes requires large sample sizes
Isacsson et al. (43)	Sweden	Questionnaire to men 68 yr old re: symptoms from neck and low back; comparisons with social network and social support	Random half of all men born in 1914 and living in Malmö; n = 621; participants were 500	Malmö, Sweden; home visits for interviews and hospital visits	Questionnaire at home visits and medical visits; physical therapist, nutritionist, and physicians participated	Daily neck pain 5%; daily LBP or neck pain 15.6%; daily neck and LBP 3.5%; no differences between social classes; no significant difference re: daily neck and LBP and high workload, job strain, low physical activity, high alcohol consumption, smoking, but significant difference as regards social anchorage, informational support	No ranking of pain; no validation of pain; social network of importance for development of neck pain symptoms
Johansson and Rubenowitz (44)	Sweden	Questionnaire to white and blue collar workers in 8 companies	209 white collar and 241 blue collar workers 90% response rate	8 companies in Sweden	Questionnaire surveys at the workplaces during working hours; anonymous answers; Nordic questionnaire for the analysis of musculoskeletal symptoms (NMQ) was used	Physical workload not correlated to the presence of neck pain Blue collar workers: Neck symptoms 44% Shoulder symptoms 43% White collar workers: Neck symptoms 45% Shoulder symptoms 42% 12-mo prevalence	Metal industry employees only, no consistent randomization of the survey

176

Study	Country	Description	Sample	Setting	Results	Comments
Kamwendo et al. (45)	Sweden	Medical secretaries with previous experience of neck pain; questionnaire including the NMQ comparison group	79 of 420 secretaries corresponded to the inclusion criteria	Regional hospital in Örebro	Inclusion criteria to select those with present neck pain and where pain was considered as work-related; comparison group of typists (n = 333)	Period prevalence 12 mo: neck 63%, shoulder 62%; point prevalence 7 d: neck 33%, shoulder 34%; overlapping pain between neck, shoulder and LBP; pain preventing from daily duties: neck 13%; shoulder pain increased significantly with years at work, but not neck pain; neck and shoulder pain were significantly related to poorly experienced psychosocial work environment	Cross-sectional nature of the study limits its value to draw conclusions of cause-effect; selected groups of employees
Marshall et al. (52)	Great Britain	Questionnaire survey of hospital employees	302 of 328 employees participated	Ancoats Hospital, Manchester	Self-administered questionnaire, divided in 2 groups whether or not neck injury had occurred	No previous neck injury (248 of 302) 34% neck pain incidence, increasing rate with age; previous neck injury had 80% neck pain; no gender difference	Neck pain among employees at a hospital
Niemi et al. (60)	Finland	Questionnaire to high school students re: prevalence of neck pain and psychosocial factors	718 teenagers from 5 high schools in Finland; 87% response rate	University of Oulu	Questionnaire including NMQ; answered in presence of teacher	Neck pain disturbing for women 22%, men 10%, all 17%; stress and depressive symptoms associated with neck pain among female teenagers	Questionnaire without any medical verification
Rundcrantz et al. (69)	Sweden	Self-administered questionnaire to dentists	315 of 359 dentists responded	Questionnaire to all dentists in the Malmöhus county council regarding years 1987 and 1990	Self-administered questionnaire plus specific questions to dentists employed in public dental care	Neck pain period prevalence was 48% for men and 62% for women; no amelioration over time from changed working position; disability to work due to back pain among 27% of the dentists. Concerns a special group of employees, dentists, not representative of the general population	
Viikari-Juntura et al. (91)	Finland	Follow-up of earlier healthy child project 23–25 yr later; questionnaire and medical control plus psychologic interview	162 of 180 persons who 25 yr earlier participated in a health project for children	Inhabitants in Helsinki who once participated in child health project	Original data from earlier study plus questionnaire 23–25 yr later; physician and psychologist participation; regression analysis to test for variables to explain neck pain variance	No socioeconomic variables were significant to explain incidence of neck pain; important for neck pain was bent torso >3 hr/d vs <1 hr/d, and sitting in a forward bent posture 1–3 hr vs <1 hr daily; severe neck pain among 65% of women but 10% of men; mild neck pain 85% among women and 68% men	Higher average income level and higher frequency of graduates than in the general population; small groups

continued

TABLE 8.5. Continued

Study (ref.)	Country	Design	Sample	Setting	Method	Results
Weill et al. (99)	France	Summary of epidemiologic evaluations of back pain in France	ESTEV 21,378 volunteers; GAZEL 4.4 million employees 40–50 yr; CREDES 8,000 families; IMS 2,318 general practitioners representing 153,688 consultations; professional groups at 7 hospitals	Summary made of different epidemiologic evaluations as requested by SBU	(see Setting)	Neck pain prevalence, i.e., period prevalence 12-mo: GAZEL: men 20.6%, women 36.6% ESTEV: age 37–52 yr: men 10–18%, women 20–34% Neck pain incidence: GAZEL: 2.6% men and women aged 35–54 yr Prevalence of neck pain among professionals: Hospital employees 14.4% Storemen 7.5% Office workers 20.6% Airport desk staff 16.9% (period prevalence) professionals, men 12%, women 18.2%, period prevalence neck pain
Westgaard et al. (101)	Norway	Interviews and questionnaires include scales of physical fitness	52 female blue collar workers and 34 office workers	Chocolate manufacturing plant and 2 officies in Norway; neck pain within past 12 mo	Interviews and questionnaires; cross-sectional study; multivariate analysis	Workers 77% neck pain during past 12 mo, office workers 74%; higher score of pain from neck than other body regions; higher prevalence of pain if previous period of neck pain; negative correlation body height and symptoms of pain; age no risk factor; 58% explained variance of neck pain by body height and psychosocial problems among workers but only 14% office workers	Small study of selected groups of workers; limited epidemiologic value; interesting method to compare risks of neck pain

LBP, low back pain.

from Canada (78), where 73 of 100,000 male drivers and 131 of 100,000 female drivers suffered from whiplash, compared with the population average of 70 of 100,000 inhabitants.

WORK-RELATED BACK INJURIES

Back injuries make up almost one-third of all work-related injuries in the United States, where there are now about 1 million workers' compensation claims for back injuries per annum; the percentage in Sweden with its general insurance system is considerably lower: 5% to 6% (see Chapter 20). In the United Kingdom in 1990 and 1991, the Health and Safety Executive recorded 34,720 nonfatal back injuries that caused at least 3 days to be lost from work, a number that was approximately 23% of all work-related injuries (94).

Most back injuries are less serious "sprains or strains," but these minor back injuries lead to longer time lost from work and to higher health and compensation costs than do any other minor injuries. The issues of work relatedness are dealt with in greater detail in Chapters 2 to 5.

IS BACK PAIN INCREASING?

A historical review by Allan and Waddell (1) concluded that human beings have had back pain all through history, and it is no more common or severe than it has always been. Epidemiologic studies show no evidence of any convincing change in the prevalence of back pain. Leboeuf-Yde and Lauritsen (47) found no definite trend in 26 Nordic studies from 1954 through 1992, and apparent differences were probably mainly the result of the wording of the questions. Leino and Hanninen (48) in Finland found that the prevalence of back pain remained unchanged from 1978 to 1992 in annual surveys that used identical questions each year. Murphy and Volinn (53) analyzed United States National Health Interview Survey data and found a 22% increase in chronic low back pain (continuous for more that 3 months) and a 35% increase in activity limitation from back pain between 1987 and 1994, but a reduction thereafter. However, that finding must be assessed against a background of increasing self-reports of sickness in the United States since the mid-20th century, despite objective evidence of steadily improving health. Swedish national surveys from 1975 to 1995 did not provide separate data on neck or back pain, but they did show a decrease in subjective reports of problems of the locomotor system, of which neck and back pain form a large part (70). This finding was also supported by the Göteborg data from 1987 presented earlier and recalculated for all of Sweden (see Chapter 20).

Similarly, there is no clear evidence of any increase in the number of work-related back injuries. Data from the United Kingdom (20,21,29) showed no definite trend. Data from the United States are conflicting (53). The National Council on Compensation Insurance (59) reported a gradual rise in the proportion of workers' compensation claims for back injuries from 1981 to 1990. However, Murphy and Volinn (53), also using data from Washington State Department of Labor and Industries and a large workers' compensation provider that covers approximately 10% of the privately insured labor force, estimated that the annual low back pain claim rate actually decreased 34% between 1987 and 1995.

Swedish data detailed until 1991 in the report of the Swedish Council on Technology Assessment in Health Care (57) showed an increase in the incidence and duration of

TABLE 8.6. *Neck pain epidemiology*

Study (ref.)	Country	Design	Sample	Setting	Method	Results	
						Symptoms related to "whiplash"	
Barnsley et al. (4)	Australia	Survey of cervical zygapophysial joint pain after whiplash	50 consecutive patients referred to cervical spine research unit	Mater Misericordiae Hospital, Newcastle, Australia	2 blind controlled diagnostic block plus assessment using VAS and pain questionnaire	Painful joints identified in 54% of patients	Small study but interesting method for assessment of zygapophysial joint pain; almost every second patient had no identifiable pain
Borchgrevink et al. (8)	Norway	Retrospective study of injury after car accidents	426 patients 1985–1990	Emergency clinic of the University Hospital Trondheim	Retrospective follow-up of whiplash injuries from dossiers and social security data	58% reported sustained symptoms linked to the accident; 27% reported sick some period during the follow-up period of 2.5–8.5 yr	Epidemiologic value limited by retrospective study of a limited group of people
Deans et al. (27)	Great Britain	Car occupants already included in multicenter study, follow-up of neck pain 1–2 yr after accident; control group	137 patients, 46% women	Royal Victoria Hospital, Belfast	Questionnaire to patients already included in multicentre study on traffic accidents, after 1–2 yr after accident; MONICA study used as control group	Neck pain: Before accident 7.3% <24 hr from accident 90.6% Following accident 62% >1 yr from accident 26.3% Control group 7.2% Duration of pain: 1 wk 18% 1 mo 18% 3 mo 13% 6 mo 8% 12 mo 1% 12 mo occationally 36% 12 mo constant 6% Rear impacts cause neck pain twice as frequently as frontal collision; sprains of the neck more frequent among unbelted than belted car occupants	Compared to the control group the prevalence of neck pain was 8–9 times higher among car occupants after car accidents, i.e. 62% vs 7.2%
Nygren et al. (61)	Sweden	Diagnosed neck and/or shoulder pain as reason for sick leave registered in Swedish insurance statistics	4 different data bases: SAF 200,000 employees, AMF 2.3 million employees, Folksam Insurance Co., work injury insurance acts; age 16–64 yr	(see Sample)	Review of 4 data bases 1985–1993 re: sickness reported from neck pain or shoulder pain	Car occupants impaired >10% due to neck pain: 1976–1978: 19.2% 1990–1992: 46.9% Neck/cervical spine 29% of all reported occupational diseases in the musculoskeletal system in 1991	Limited to registered sickness absence only; no figures on incidence or prevalence of neck pain

Study	Country	Cohort	Sample	Study design	Source population	Results	Comments
Spitzer et al. (76)	Canada	Compensation claims from the SAAQ followed for 6 yr	All whiplash injuries from car collisions in 1987	Historical cohort study based on the compensation claims to SAAQ	Source population epidemiology study of all persons who sustained a whiplash injury and who submitted a claim for compensation	Whiplash incidence in 70/100,000 inhabitants: Women 84/100,000 Men 54/100,000 Highest incidence for the age group 20–24 yr Whiplash per licenced driver: Men 73/100,000 drivers Women 126/100,000 drivers Whiplash per vehicle: 131/100,000 vehicles	Selected group of inhabitants who submitted a claim for compensation
Schrader et al. (71)	Lithuania	Questionnaire to traffic injured individuals vs not injured individuals	202 accident victims and 202 controls	Records of the traffic police department of Kaunas, Lithuania; controls from population register in the same area	Questionnaire used for interview 1–3 yr after traffic accident; randomly selected control individuals from the local population register	Neck pain frequency: Car occupants 35% Control group 33% Chronic neck pain (>9 d) Car occupants 8.4% Control group 6.9% No significant difference re: neck pain after whiplash in car accident from the average population	In Lithuania, few have personal injury insurance, and the disability compensation is remote, i.e., no economically motivated symptoms are present
Stovner (77)	Norway	Review of empiric studies on whiplash syndrome	Articles on Medline April 1992 to May 1994 on whiplash	Not applicable	Review of published studies from the point of view of epidemiologic methodology	Face validity but not descriptive, constructive or predictive of validity; weak convincing empiric evidence for a causal link (construct validity) between trauma mechanism and chronic symptoms of whiplash	Interesting conclusions in connection to the findings in the study by Schrader concerning whiplash in Lithuania, (see Schrader) i.e., that there was no significant difference of neck pain between those whiplash and those without whiplash in the control group, 35% vs 33%

SAAQ, société de l'assurance automobile du Quebec
VAS, visual analogue scale

sickness absence resulting from back pain in the 1970s and 1980s and a particular increase in the number of workers who went on to long-term disability and early retirement between the mid-1980s and early 1990s. However, since the early 1990s, there has been a definite decrease in sickness absence and early retirement resulting from back pain. Data from the United Kingdom suggest that the annual rate of new Department of Social Security claims for invalidity benefit for back pain have changed little for more than 20 years, but an increasing proportion of people receive the benefit for much longer periods, so the total numbers of workers receiving the benefit and the amount and costs of benefit paid are increasing (29). In most European Union countries, however, the pattern of back pain is little different from that of all other sickness.

Despite popular belief, there is thus no historical or epidemiologic evidence that back pain has changed since the time any recording has been done. There is no evidence of any change in the pathology of low back pain throughout recorded history. The prevalence of low back pain has not changed, at least since 1980. Instead, all the evidence is of an increase in chronic disability attributed to nonspecific neck and low back pain.

WHEN BACK PAIN BECOMES DISABLING

Pain and disability are subjective. Pain itself does not meet the definition of impairment (abnormality), but if activity aggravates pain and the individual avoids or reduces activities, then pain may lead to disability. However, low back pain and disability depend more on psychosocial factors than on the physical condition of the back, and they can best be understood and managed by a biopsychosocial model (93,94), which is more consistent with the latest evidence on the development of chronic pain and disability.

The symptom of back pain arises from a physical process in the back and nociception. The key to chronic pain and disability may be failure to recover as it should, rather than the development of a different syndrome. As pain becomes chronic (lasting longer than 12 weeks), attitudes and beliefs, distress, and illness behavior play an increasing role in the development of chronicity and disability (23,24,30,31,41, 64,93,95,96). This all occurs within the social context, which varies worldwide, and leads to social interactions with others, including in particular family, work, and health care (see Chapter 2).

As described in Chapters 2 and 3, there are close links between physiologic and psychologic events. Nonspecific low back pain seems to be mainly a matter of disturbed function or painful musculoskeletal dysfunction. Disability is reduced function. It is a matter of what the individual does (or does not do) and of altered performance. Pain behavior or illness behavior is also a matter of what the individual does (or does not do).

Disability from back pain involves both physical dysfunction and illness behavior, which, in a sense, are simply two sides of the same coin. Behavior always involves motor and physiologic activity, and physiologic processes always have behavioral expressions.

Low back pain and disability are clearly related, but they are not the same, and the link between them may be much weaker than often assumed. One study (95) found that severity of pain only accounted for about 10% of the variance of low back disability. It is important to make a clear distinction between pain and disability conceptually, in clinical practice, and as the basis for social security and sickness benefits (93,95).

Pain is "an unpleasant sensory and emotional experience associated with actual or potential tissue damage, or described in terms of such damage" (42). Pain is a symptom, not a clinical sign, a diagnosis, or a disease. It is not possible to assess pain directly: Assessment always depends on the individual's report of subjective experience, so the report of pain always depends on how the individual thinks and feels about it and communicates it.

Disability, conversely, is restricted activity. The most comprehensive definition is by the World Health Organization (103): "A disability is any restriction or lack (resulting from an impairment) of ability to perform an activity in the manner or within the range considered normal for a human being." This definition contains certain assumptions. It assumes that the normal state is to have no disability or restriction of any kind, and it does not allow for the range that is normal by gender and age. It assumes that disability is "due to an impairment," a statement that implies a physical basis and a cause-and-effect relationship that may not be an accurate reflection of disability associated with pain. It is often taken to imply that disability is a health problem, which is not always true. Nevertheless, the core of all the definitions is that disability is restricted activity. For the purpose of sickness benefits or compensation, disability is often operationalized as incapacity to work, although the definition and degree of incapacity vary in different jurisdictions. Clinical assessment of disability usually relies on the patient's own report, so again, it is subjective and open to the same influences as the report of pain (83).

Fordyce (30) considered further the nature of impairment and disability associated with low back pain from a biopsychosocial perspective. The problem is that it is not possible to assess back pain, but only the person with the pain. Pain, suffering, and pain behavior all confound questions of impairment and disability. The term disability may mean either loss of capacity or simply reduced activity, but observation of performance cannot distinguish between these two entities. Reduced performance may reflect actual loss of capacity, or the individual may stop before reaching his or her physical limits or may not even attempt the activity. Fordyce (31) further defined a "state of disability . . . is . . . when the person prematurely terminates an activity, underperforms or declines to undertake it." The concept and measure of disability cannot be independent of performance. It is not possible to separate body and mind. Physical defects affect the person's beliefs and expectations about a situation. Conversely, beliefs and expectations help to shape the impact of physical defects on activity. The extent to which psychologic and social processes can influence physical activity should not be underestimated, and vice versa. Concepts of impairment and disability must allow for this dynamic interaction. Disability is not only a question of physical impairment, nor is it only functional capacity: It is a question of behavior and performance. Performance depends on anatomic and physiologic abilities, but also on psychologic and social resources. Performance depends on effort. Testing itself may cause pain and may inhibit performance. Capacity may be set by physiologic limits, but performance is set by psychologic limits (30,31).

ACKNOWLEDGMENTS

Certain sections of this review are adapted and developed with permission from Waddell G. *The back pain revolution.* Edinburgh: Churchill Livingstone, 1998, which provides a more comprehensive review of the biopsychosocial model of low back pain and disability.

REFERENCES

1. Allan DB, Waddell G. An historical perspective on low back pain and disability. *Acta Orthop Scand* 1989;60[Suppl 234]:1–23.
2. Andersson GBJ. The epidemiology of spinal disorders. In: Frymoyer JW, ed. *The adult spine: principles and practice,* 2nd ed, vol 1. New York: Raven Press, 1997:93–141.
3. Andersson HI, Ejlertsson G, Leden I, et al. Chronic pain in a geographically defined general population: studies of differences in age, gender, social class and pain localisation. *Clin J Pain* 1993;9:174–182.
4. Barnsley L, Lord SM, Wallis BJ, et al. The prevalence of chronic cervical zygapophysial joint pain after whiplash. *Spine* 1995;20:20–26.
5. Bergenudd H. *Talent, occupation and locomotor discomfort.* Thesis, Lund University, Sweden, 1989.
6. Bergenudd H, Nilsson B. Back pain in middle age: occupational workload and psychologic factors. An epidemiologic survey. *Spine* 1988;13:58–60.
7. Biering-Sørensen F, Hilden J. Reproducibility of the history of low back trouble. *Spine* 1984;9:280–286.
8. Borchgrevink GE, Lereim I, Röyneland L, et al. National health insurance consumption and chronic symptoms following mild neck sprain injuries in car collisions. *Scand J Soc Med* 1996;24:264–271.
9. Bovim G, Schrader H, Sand T. Neck pain in the general population. *Spine* 1994;19:1307–1309.
10. Brattberg G. Back pain and headache in Swedish schoolchildren: a longitudinal study. *Pain Clin* 1993;6:157–162.
11. Brattberg G. The incidence of back pain and headache among Swedish schoolchildren. *Qual Life Res* 1994;3;S27–S31.
12. Brattberg G, Parker MG, Thorslund M. The prevalence of pain among the oldest old in Sweden. *Pain* 1996;67:29–34.
13. Brattberg G, Parker MG, Thorslund M. A longitudinal study of pain: reported pain from middle age to old age. *Clin J Pain* 1997;13:144–149.
14. Brattberg G, Thorslund M, Wikman A. The prevalence of pain in a general population: the results of a postal survey in a county of Sweden. *Pain* 1989;37:215–222.
15. Brown JJ, Wells GA, Trottier AJ, et al. Back pain in a large Canadian police force. *Spine* 1998;23:821–827.
16. Burton KA, Clarke RD, McClune TD, et al. The natural history of low back pain in adolescents. *Spine* 1996;21:2323–2328.
17. Carey TS, Evans AT, Hadler NM, et al. Acute severe low back pain: a population-based study of prevalence and care-seeking. *Spine* 1996;21:339–344.
18. Carey TS, Garrett JM, Jackman A, et al. Recurrence and care seeking after acute back pain: results of a long-term follow-up study. North Carolina Back Pain Project. *Med Care* 1999;37:157–164.
19. Cassidy JD, Carroll LJ, Côté P. The Saskatchewan Health and Back Pain Survey: the prevalence of low back pain and related disability in Saskatchewan adults. *Spine* 1998;23:1860–1867.
20. *Clinical Standards Advisory Group epidemiology review: the epidemiology and cost of back pain. Annex to the CSAG report on back pain.* London: Her Majesty's Stationery Office, 1994:1–72.
21. *Consumer's Association 1985 Back Pain Survey.* London: Research Surveys of Great Britain, 1985.
22. Coté P, Cassidy JD, Carroll L. The Saskatchewan health and back pain survey: the prevalence of neck pain and related disability in Saskatchewan adults. *Spine* 1998;23:1689–1698.
23. Croft P, Papageorgiou A, McNally R. Low back pain. In: Stevens A, Rafferty J, eds. *Health care needs assessment,* 2nd series. Oxford: Radcliffe Medical Press, 1997:129–182.
24. Croft P, Joseph S, Cosgrove S, et al. *Low back pain in the community and in hospitals: a report to the Clinical Standards Advisory Group of the Department of Health.* Prepared by the Arthritis and Rheumatism Council, Epidemiology Research Unit, University of Manchester, England, 1994.
25. Croft PR, Papageorgiou AC, Ferry S, et al. Psychologica distress and low back pain: evidence from a prospective study in the general population. *Spine* 1995;20:2731–2737.
26. Crowe HE. Injuries to the cervical spine. Paper presented to the Western Orthopaedic Association, San Francisco, 1928.
27. Deans GT, Magalliard JN, Kerr M, et al. Neck sprain: a major cause of disability following car accidents. *Injury* 1987;18:10–12.
28. Deyo RA, Tsui-Wu Y-J. Functional disability due to back pain. *Arthritis Rheum* 1987;30:1247–1253.
29. Erens B, Ghate D. *Invalidity benefit: a longitudinal study of new recipients.* Department of Social Security Research Report Number 20. London: Her Majesty's Stationery Office, 1993:1–127.
30. Fordyce WE, ed. *Back pain in the workplace: management of disability in non-specific conditions.* Seattle: IASP Press, 1995.
31. Fordyce WE. On the nature of illness and disability [Editorial]. *Clin Orthop* 1997;336:47–51.
32. Guo H-R, Tanaka S, Cameron LL, et al. Back pain among workers in the United States: national estimates and workers at high risk. *Am J Ind Med* 1995;28:591–602.
33. Gyntelberg F. One year incidence of low back pain among male residents of Copenhagen aged 40–59. *Dan Med Bull* 1974;21:30–36.
34. Hagberg M, Wegman DH. Prevalence rates and odds ratios of shoulder-neck diseases in different occupational groups. *Br J Ind Med* 1987;44:602–610.

35. Hagen KB, Kvien TK, Björndal A. Musculoskeletal pain and quality of life in patients with non-inflammatory joint pain compared to rheumatoid arthritis: a population survey. *J Rheumatol* 1997;24:1703–1709.

36. Hasvold T, Johnsen R. Headache and neck or shoulder pain: frequent and disabling complaints in the general population. *Scand J Health Care* 1993;11:219–224.

37. Heliövaara M, Impivaara O, Sievers K, et al. Lumbar disc syndrome in Finland. *J Epidemiol Commun Health* 1987;41:251–258.

38. Hellsing AL. Work absence in a cohort with benign back pain: prospective study with 10 year follow-up. *J Occup Rehabil* 1994;3:153.

39. Hillman M, Wright A, Rajaratnam G, et al. Prevalence of low back pain in the community: implications for service provision in Bradford, UK. *J Epidemiol Commun Health* 1996;50:347–352.

40. Hignett S. Work-related back pain in nurses. *J Adv Nurs* 1996;23:1238–1246.

41. Hocking B. Epidemiological aspects of repetitive strain injury in Telecom Australia. *Med J Aust* 1987;147:218–222.

42. International Association for the Study of Pain (Subcommittee on Taxonomy). 1979 pain terms: a list with definitions and notes on usage. *Pain* 1979;6:249–252.

43. Isacsson A, Hansson BS, Ranstam J, et al. Social network, social support and the prevalence of neck and low back pain after retirement: a population study of men born in 1914 in Malmö, Sweden. *Scand J Soc Med* 1995;23:17–22.

44. Johansson JÅ, Rubenowitz S. Risk indicators in the psychosocial and physical work environment for work-related neck, shoulder and low back symptoms: a study among blue- and white-collar workers in eight companies. *Scand J Rehabil Med* 1994;26:131–142.

45. Kamwendo K, Kinton SJ, Moritz U. Neck and shoulder disorders in medical secretaries. I. Pain prevalence and risk factors. *Scand J Rehabil Med* 1991;23:127–133.

46. Lawrence JS. *Rheumatism in populations.* London: Heinemann, 1977.

47. Leboeuf-Yde C, Lauritsen JM. The prevalence of low back pain in the literature: a structured review of 26 Nordic studies from 1954 to 1993. *Spine* 1995;20:2112–2118.

48. Leino PI, Hanninen V. Psychosocial factors at work in relation to back and limb disorders. *Scand J Work Environ Health* 1995;21:134–42.

49. Linton SJ, Hellsing AL, Halldén K. A population-based study of spinal pain among 35-45 year old individuals: prevalence, sick leave, and health care use. *Spine* 1998;23:1457–1463.

50. Macfarlane GF, Thomas E, Papageorgiou AC, et al. Employment and work activities as predictors of future low back pain. *Spine* 1997;22:1143–1149.

51. Manninen P, Riihimäki H, Heliövaara M. Incidence and risk factors of low-back pain in middle-aged farmers. *Occup Med* 1995;45:141–146.

52. Marshall PD, O'Connor M, Hodgkinson JP. The perceived relationship between neck symptoms and precedent injury. *Injury* 1995;26:17–19.

53. Murphy PL, Volinn E. Is occupational low back pain on the rise? *Spine* 1999;24:691–697.

54. Mäkele M. *Common musculoskeletal syndromes: prevalence, risk indicators and disability in Finland.* Publications of the Social Insurance Institution, vol 123. Helsinki: Social Insurance Institution, 1993:1–162.

55. Mäkele M, Heliövaara M, Sievers K, et al. Prevalence, determinants and concequences of chronic neck pain in Finland. *Am J Epidemiol* 1991;134:1356–1367.

56. Mason V. *The prevalence of back pain in Great Britain.* Office of Population Censuses and Surveys, Social Survey Division [now Office of National Statistics]. London: Her Majesty's Stationery Office, 1994:1–2.

57. Nachemson A. *1991 Ont i Ryggen* [*Back pain: causes, diagnosis, treatment*]. *SBU Report.* Stockholm: Swedish Council on Technology Assessment in Health Care, 1992.

58. Nachemson A. Back pain in the workplace: a threat to our welfare states. In: Wolter D, Seide K, eds. *Berufsbedingte Erkrankungen der Lendenwirbelsäule.* Berlin: Springer-Verlag 1998:191–206.

59. National Council on Compensation Insurance. *Report.* Florida: National Council on Compensation Insurance, 1992:1–25.

60. Niemi SM, Levoska S, Rekola KE, et al. Neck and shoulder symptoms of high school students and associated psychosocial factors. *J Adolesc Health* 1997;20:238–242.

61. Nygren Å, Berglund A, von Koch M. Neck-and-shoulder pain, an increasing problem: strategies for using insurance material to follow trends. *Scand J Rehabil Med Suppl* 1995;32:107–112.

62. Papageorgiou AC, Croft PR, Ferry S, et al. Estimating the prevalence of low back pain in the general population: evidence from the South Manchester back pain survey. *Spine* 1995;20:1889–1894.

63. Papageorgiou AC, Croft PR, Thomas E, et al. Influence of previous pain experience on the episode incidence of low back pain: results from the South Manchester Back Pain Study. *Pain* 1996;66:181–185.

64. Papageorgiou AC, Macfarlane GF, Thomas E, et al. Psychosocial factors in the workplace: do they predict new episodes of low back pain? *Spine* 1997;22:1137–1142.

65. Porter RW, Hibbert CS. Back pain and neck pain in four general practices. *Clin Biomechanics* 1986;1:7–10.

66. Rajala U, Keinänen-Kiukkaanniemi S, Uusimäki A, et al. Musculoskeletal pains and depression in a middle-aged Finnish population. *Pain* 1995;61:451–457.

67. Raspe H. Back pain. In: Silman AJ, Hochberg MC, eds. *Epidemiology of the rheumatic diseases.* Oxford: Oxford University Press, 1993:330–374.

68. Rossignol M, Lortie M, Ledoux E. Comparison of spinal health indicators in predicting spinal status in a 1-year longitudinal study. *Spine* 1993;18:54–60.

69. Rundcrantz B-L, Johnsson B, Moritz U. Pain and discomfort in the musculoskeletal system among dentists: a prospective study. *Swed Dent J* 1991;15:219–228.

70. SCB (Statistiska centralbyrån [Statistics Sweden]). *Undersökningar av levnadsförhållanden, ULF [National houshold surveys].* Stockholm: SCB, 1996.

71. Schrader H, Obeliene D, Bovim G, et al. Natural evolution of late whiplash syndrome outside the medicolegal context. *Lancet* 1996;347:1207–1211.

72. Shekelle P. The epidemiology of low back pain. In: Giles LGF, Singer KP, eds. *Clinical anatomy and management of low back pain.* London: Butterworth Heinemann, 1997:18–31.

73. Shekelle PG, Markovich M, Louie R. An epidemiologic study of episodes of back pain care. *Spine* 1995;20:1668–1673.

74. Skovron ML, Szpalski M, Nordin M, et al. Sociocultural factors and back pain: a population-based study in Belgian adults. *Spine* 1994;19:129–137.

75. Smedley J, Egger P, Cooper C, et al. Manual handling activities and risk of low back pain in nurses. *Occup Environ Med* 1995;52:160–163.

76. Spitzer WO, Skovron ML, Salmi LR, et al. Scientific monograph of the Quebec Task Force on whiplash-associated disorders: redefining "whiplash" and its management. *Spine* 1995;20[Suppl 8]:1S–73S.

77. Stovner LJ. The nosologic status of the whiplash syndrome: a critical review based on a methodological approach. *Spine* 1996;21:2735–2746.

78. Suissa S, Harder S, Veilleux M. The Quebec whiplash-associated disorders cohort study: section 2. *Spine* 1995;20:12S–58S.

79. Svensson HO, Andersson GBJ. Low back pain in forty to forty-seven year old men. I. Frequency of occurrence and impact on medical services. *Scand J Rehabil Med* 1982;14:47–53.

80. Svensson HO, Andersson GBJ. Low back pain in forty to forty-seven year old men: work history and work environment factors. *Spine* 1983;8:272–276.

81. Svensson HO, Andersson GBJ. The relationship of low-back pain, work history, work envionment, and stress: a retrospective cross-sectional study of 38- to 64-year-old women. *Spine* 1989;14:517–522.

82. Svensson HO, Andersson GBJ, Johansson S, et al. A retrospective study of low back pain in 38- to 64-year old women: frequency and occurrence and impact on medical services. *Spine* 1988;13:548–552.

83. Swales K, Craig P. *Evaluation of the Incapacity Benefit medical test: in-house report 26.* London: Social Research Branch, Department of Social Security, 1997.

84. Takala J, Sievers K, Kalukka T. Rheumatic symptoms in the middle-aged population in south western Finland. *Scand J Rheumatol Suppl* 1982;47:15–29.

85. Taimela S, Kujala UM, Salminen JJ, et al. The prevalence of low back pain among children and adolescents: a nationwide, cohort-based questionnaire survey in Finland. *Spine* 1997;22:1132–1136.

86. Taylor H, Curran NM. *The Nuprin Pain Report.* New York: Louis Harris and Associates, 1985:1–233.

87. Thomas MK, Porteous JE, Brock JR, et al. Back pain in Australian military helicopter pilots: a preliminary study. *Aviat Space Environ Med* 1998;69:468–473.

88. Valkenburg HA, Haanen HCM. The epidemiology of low back pain. In: White AA, Gordon SL eds. *Symposium on idiopathic low back pain.* St. Louis: CV Mosby, 1982:9–22.

89. van der Donk J, Schouten JSAG, Passchier J, et al. The associations of neck pain with radiological abnormalities of the cervical spine and personality traits in a general population. *J Rheumatol* 1991;18:1884–1889.

90. van Poppel M. *The prevention of low back pain in industry.* Thesis, Amsterdam University, Amsterdam, 1999.

91. Viikari-Juntura E, Vuori J, Silverstein BA, et al. A life-long prospective study on the role of psychosocial factors in neck-shoulder and low-back pain. *Spine* 1991;16:1056–1061.

92. von Korff M, Dworkin SF, Le Resche LA, et al. An epidemiologic comparison of pain complaints. *Pain* 1988;32:173–183.

93. Waddell G. 1987 Volvo award in clinical sciences: a new clinical model for the treatment of low-back pain. *Spine* 1987;12:632–644.

94. Waddell G. The epidemiology of low back pain. In: Waddell G, ed. *The back pain revolution,* vol 5. Edinburgh: Churchill Livingstone, 1998:69–84.

95. Waddell G, Main CJ. Assessment of severity in low-back disorders. *Spine* 1984;9:204–208.

96. Waddell G, Main CJ, Morris EW, et al. Chronic low-back pain, psychologic distress, and illness behavior. *Spine* 1984;9:209–213.

97. Walsh K, Cruddas M, Coggon D. Low back pain in eight areas of Britain. *J Epidemiol Commun Health* 1992;46:227–230.

98. Watson PJ, Main CJ, Waddell G, et al. 1997 Medically certified work loss, recurrence and costs

of wage compensation for back pain: a follow-up study of the working population of Jersey. *Br J Rheumatol* 1998;37:82–86.

99. Weill C, Ghadi V, Nicoulet I, et al. *Back pain in France: epidemiology, present knowledge, current practice and costs.* Paris: CD-Santé, 1998.

100. Westerling D Jonsson BG. Pain from the neck-shoulder region and sick leave. *Scand J Soc Med* 1980;8:131–136.

101. Westgaard RH, Jensen C, Hansen K. Individual and work-related risk factors associated with symptoms of musculoskeletal complaints. *Int Arch Occup Environ Health* 1993;64:405–413.

102. Westrin CG. Low-back sick listing: a nosological and medical insurance investigation. *Acta Soc Med Scand* 1970;2–3:127–134.

103. World Health Organization. *International classification of impairments, disabilities and handicaps.* Geneva: World Health Organization, 1980.

Neck and Back Pain: The Scientific Evidence of Causes, Diagnosis, and Treatment, edited by Alf Nachemson and Egon Jonsson. Published by Lippincott Williams & Wilkins, Philadelphia 2000.

9

Assessment of Patients with Neck and Back Pain: A Best-Evidence Synthesis

Alf Nachemson* and Eva Vingård†

*Department of Orthopaedics, Sahlgrenska University Hospital, Göteborg, Sweden
†Section of Personal Injury Prevention, Karolinska Institutet, Stockholm, Sweden

For the common neck and back pain syndromes, few patients have pathoanatomically well-defined diseases. After 1 month with back symptoms, approximately 15% of patients have a definable disease or injury. In the first few days of an attack of back pain, this percentage is lower, whereas for those who still have pain after 3 months, it is higher (72,73,88,213).

Deyo et al. (94), in a study of primary care patients, found that, at around 4 weeks, 4% to 5% of patients with low back and leg pain had a disc hernia, 4% to 5% had symptoms of spinal stenosis, 4% had compression fracture, and 1% had a primary metastatic tumor or osteomyelitis. Less than 1% could be diagnosed with some visceral disease, aortic aneurysm, or renal or gynecologic disorder. Similar findings were also reported by Udén (351).

Borenstein et al. (46,47), in their monographs on low back pain and neck pain, respectively, tabulated more than 50 definable disease entities that could cause pain in the neck or the lower back, and the examiner must keep these disorders in mind. Fortunately, many of these rarer entities can be elucidated from the patient's history together with some specific questions and examinations. The summary recommendations developed by Deyo et al. (92,94) are helpful in that respect (Tables 9.1 and 9.2).

Anyone with pain is worried. Nociceptive pain influences our brain, as depicted in Chapters 3 and 7. According to Waddell (376), as many as 40% of patients with back pain also fear they have some serious disease.

Our task then is to remove these fears. There is moderate evidence that positive reinforcement can improve treatment results for back pain (346,352). The attitude of the caretaker also influences patients' satisfaction with care (60,69).

This chapter relies basically on the reviews of diagnostic utility performed by Andersson and Deyo (10,11), van Tulder et al. (364), and van den Hoogen et al. (359), as well as the more methodologically based guidelines of the Agency for Health Care Policy and Research (AHCPR) (32) in the United States and those of Health Care Evaluation Unit of Bristol (114) and the Clinical Standards Advisory Group (297), both of Great Britain. In addition, a new MEDLINE search was performed covering 1990 to 1998 (inclusive) that resulted in 510 references, which were checked for diagnostic relevance, compared with previous reviews, and subsequently included if they added new important information. In particular, this refers to the assessment of

TABLE 9.1. *Summary and recommendations of key questions in the patient's history*

1. A few key questions can raise or lower the probability of underlying systemic disease. The most useful items are age, history of cancer, unexplained weight loss, duration of pain, and responsiveness to previous therapy.
2. Intravenous drug use or urinary infection raises the suspicion of spinal infection.
3. Ankylosing spondylitis is suggested by the patient's age and sex (most common in young men), but most clinical findings have limited accuracy.
4. Failure of bed rest to relieve the pain is a sensitive finding for certain systemic conditions, although it is not specific.
5. Neurologic involvement is suggested by symptoms of sciatica or pseduclaudication. Pain radiating distally (below the knee) is more likely to represent a true radiculopathy than pain radiating only to the posterior thigh. A history of numbness or weakness in the legs further increases the likelihood of neurologic involvement.
6. Inquiry should be made concerning symptoms of the cauda equina syndrome: bladder dysfunction (especially urinary retention) and saddle anesthesia in addition to sciatica and weakness.
7. The psychosocial history helps to estimate prognosis and to plan therapy. The most useful items are a history of failed previous treatments, substance abuse, and disability compensation. Brief screening questionnaires for depression and psychosocial problems suggest important therapeutic opportunities. Their use is recommended in the subacute phase of neck and back pain.

Data from Deyo RA, Diehl AK. Cancer as the cause of back pain frequency: clinical presentation and diagnostic strategies. *J Gen Intern Med* 1988;3:230–238; and Deyo RA, Rainville J, Kent DL. What can the history and physical examination tell us about low back pain? *JAMA* 1992;268:760–765.

neck pain, which had not previously been systematically evaluated. A few studies from 1999 were also included, provided they contained new valid and important information.

The Cochrane Collaboration Methods Working Group (163) defined a test as any measurement aimed at identifying individuals who could potentially benefit from intervention. The methodology to evaluate the utility of a test of diagnostic procedures has improved in the last decades (145), and the resulting sensitivities, specificity, and predictive values of these various tests have been presented in metaanalytic reviews (11,94,359).

The term *gold standard* indicates the best available test to diagnose a condition. That means that it is highly sensitive and highly specific; few, if any, patients with the disease have negative test results (*sensitivity*), and all persons who do not have the disease have negative tests (*specificity*). The test itself must also be valid, that is, reproducible with small measurement errors and little intraobserver and interobserver

TABLE 9.2. *Important findings in the physical examination*

1. Fewer findings suggest the possibility of spinal infection, even though most patients with such an infection have no fewer. Intense vertebral tenderness is a sensitive finding for infection, but it is not specific.
2. The search for soft tissue tenderness is unlikely to provide reproducible data or demonstrably valid pathophysiologic inferences.
3. Limited lumbar flexion is neither sensitive nor specific for ankylosing spondylitis or any other diagnoses. However, limited spinal motion may be useful for monitoring response of activation programs.
4. In a patient with sciatica or possible neurogenic claudication, straight leg raising should be assessed bilaterally, preferably using an inclinometer or goniometer.
5. Neurologic examination emphasizes ankle dorsiflexion strength, great toe dorsiflexion strength, ankle reflexes, and the sensory examination. A rapid screening sensory examination tests pinprick sensation in the medial, dorsal, and lateral aspects of the foot.
6. For the patient with subacute and chronic pain, one or more evaluations of distress and cognitive and psychosocial factors should be performed. These tests are helpful in identifying psychologic distress as a result of or as an amplifier of low back symptoms.

Data from references 92 to 94.

variability. In addition, other epidemiologic and statistical parameters should be considered when using a diagnostic test (11,96,357,359,365).

Unfortunately, even today most studies on the value of diagnostic tests that include history taking and physical examination in patients with neck and low back pain show methodologic shortcomings, such as in terms of clear selection criteria, a clear description of the study population, reproducibility of the index (gold standard) and reference test, blinding of interpretation of the index and reference test results, and prevention of workup bias. It was therefore deemed reasonable to make a "best-evidence synthesis" from the available studies. The same conclusion was reached by Spitzer et al. (332) in their review of neck pain resulting from whiplash in 1995.

For low back pain in particular, the new information deals with the utility of magnetic resonance imaging (MRI) in detecting well-defined diseases, as well as attempts at correlating MRI findings with some nonspecific pain syndromes. New information is also emerging from studies covering tests of distress and illness behavior that may be relevant both for treatment and for prediction of prognosis or disability. These investigations have demonstrated clinical utility and have added a new dimension to our diagnostic triage and assessment of patients with back pain.

Specialists come from different training backgrounds and carry with them different doctrines and models. The patient with back pain thus is likely to receive different labels from different specialists, such as a diagnosis of degenerative disc disease, facet syndrome, subluxation, instability, and so forth. There is little scientific evidence for establishment of many of these diagnostic labels. On the contrary, they may be confusing for patients and may even be counterproductive; to give an unproven label may cause a patient to worry if the pain is not immediately relieved. In some patients, that worry may cause abnormal illness behavior, unfortunately possibly leading to chronic pain states with increased disability (1,146,244,352).

In 1994, Cherkin et al. (71) investigated the use of various diagnostic tests for low back pain across eight specialties and found that the diagnostic evaluation and assessment depended heavily on the individual physician and the specialty. These investigators found a lack of consensus and wide variations for the same type of patients among different specialists. Although the low response rate (43%) limits the generalizability of their findings, the authors, nevertheless, stated that they supported the need for guidelines on performing examinations in patients with acute and chronic back pain and sciatica.

To reach maximum benefit from history and physical examination, it is also important to establish a good rapport with the patient and to take time to listen, as well as to ask the proper questions, as described in detail in Chapter 18. Several guidelines, such as those of the Quebec Task Force (249), the AHCPR (32), the Clinical Standards Advisory Group (297), and the Health Care Evaluation Unit of Bristol (114), have emphasized the need for improvement in these areas, particularly at the initial patient visit.

For the clinician, the most important question to answer is whether the examination will help to treat the patient better. Some evidence indicates that a thorough examination in itself has a beneficial effect on patients' worry and pain (69).

To increase the accuracy of excluding specific diseases and to reduce patients' worries, the AHCPR (32) in their recommendations introduced the "*red flag*" categories, and with the increasing knowledge of the importance of psychosocial factors, the New Zealand Guidelines (187) introduced the concept of "*yellow flags.*"

The sensitivity and specificity of the symptoms and signs of spinal malignancy, infection, and compression fracture are seen in Table 9.3. In studies conducted by Deyo et al. in 1992 (92,94) of 2,000 patients with back pain, no malignant disease was found in any patient younger than 50 years old who did not have a history of cancer, weight loss, or failure of conservative therapy. These investigators argued that the sensitivity of this combination of factors is 100% for excluding malignancy as the cause of low back pain.

For the diagnosis of ankylosing spondylitis, Calin et al. (61), in a study of the literature, identified the following questions in a patient's history that had high sensitivity but poor specificity:

• Is there morning stiffness?
• Is there improvement or discomfort with exercise?
• Was the onset of pain before the age of 40 years?
• Did the problem start slowly?
• Has the pain persisted for at least 3 months?

Table 9.4 gives the most common indications from history and examination for red flag disorders pathology that need special attention.

The yellow flags could be thought of as psychosocial risk factors of particular interest in patients with low back pain (187,375,379). Instructions for ascertaining the presence of these risk factors are detailed later in this chapter and also in Chapter 3. In Table 9.5, the observations and examinations for pain and illness behavior that are easier to perform are listed. Waddell et al. (381) originally found their clinical tests to be of predictive value for results after repeat disc surgery, but these tests were later confirmed by several authors also to predict results after nonoperative treatment programs for patients with low back pain, as have the University of Alabama Behavior Scale (UAB) observations (183,200,225,261,308,392).

TABLE 9.3. *Sensitivities and specificities of different elements of the history and examination for some specific causes of low back pain*

Disease or group of diseases	Symptom or sign	Sensitivity	Specificity
Spinal malignancy	Age >50 yr	0.77	0.71
	Previous history of cancer	0.31	0.98
	Unexplained weight loss	0.15	0.94
	Pain unrelieved by bed rest	0.90	0.46
	Pain lasting >1 mo	0.50	0.81
	Failure to improve with 1 mo conservative therapy	0.31	0.90
	Erythrocyte sedimentation rate >20 mm	0.78	0.67
Spinal infection	Intravenous drug abuse, urinary tract infection, skin infection	0.4	
	Fever	0.27–0.83*	0.98
	Vertebral tenderness	"Reasonable"	"Low"
	Age >50 yr	0.84	0.61
Compression fracture	Age >70 yr	0.22	0.96
	Corticosteroid use	0.66	0.99
Herniated intervertebral disc	Sciatica	0.95	0.88

*The sensitivity of "fever" varies depending on the type of infection.
Data from references 32, 92, 114, 358, and 359.

TABLE 9.4. *Most common indications from history and examination for pathologic findings needing special attention and sometimes immediate action including imaging*

Back pain in children <18 yr with considerable pain or onset >55 yr
History of violent trauma
Constant progressive pain at night
History of cancer
Systemic steroids
Drug abuse, human immunodeficiency virus infection
Weight loss
Systemic illness
Persisting severe restriction of motion
Intensed pain or minimal motion
Structural deformity
Difficulty with micturition
Loss of anal sphincter tone or fecal incontinence; saddle anesthesia
Widespread progressive motor weakness or gait disturbance
Inflammatory disorders (ankylosing spondylitis) suspected
Gradual onset <40 yr
Marked morning stiffness
Persisting limitation of motion
Peripheral joint involvement
Iritis, skin rashes, colitis, urethral discharge
Family history

Data from references 32, 61, 244, and 297.

EVIDENCE OF THE UTILITY OF HISTORY AND CLINICAL EXAMINATION

History taking from a patient with back pain should include questions on age, history of malignant disease, unexplained weight loss, intake of immunosuppressive drugs, duration of symptoms, responsiveness to previous therapy, pain that is worse at rest, history of drug use or abuse, and urinary and other infections. Van den Hoogen et al. (359), in their metaanalysis of the diagnostic accuracy of signs and symptoms for diseases of known origin, depicted 19 studies on radiculopathy (nerve root pain), 9 on vertebral cancer and metastases, and 8 on ankylosing spondylitis. In addition, they evaluated 5 studies on reproducibility of history taking and physical examination in patients with low back pain. Their expanded results for the diagnostic accuracy in relation to cancer of the spine also included evaluation of sensitivity and specificity of physical examination, findings including neurologic signs and tenderness in populations of patients with such cancers, sensitivity around 0.50, and specificity 0.70.

Cauda equina syndromes and/or widespread neurologic disorders should also be revealed from a history of difficulty with micturition, loss of anal sphincter tone and fecal incontinence, saddle anesthesia around the anus, perineum, and genitals, and widespread progressive motor weakness in the legs and gait disturbance.

For neck pain, long tract signs, sensory disturbances, and widespread motor weakness both in arms and legs should be investigated. For neck and arm pain alone, there are no studies of sensitivity of specificity for disc hernia or spondylosis. A best-evidence synthesis of important findings in patients with cervical radiculopathy and myelopathy is seen in Table 9.15.

For diagnosis of spinal stenosis and root canal stenosis, the most commonly found signs from the history include reduced walking distance resulting from pseudoclaudication and nonradicular leg pain or sciatica. For fracture, a recent history of trauma,

TABLE 9.5. *Symptoms and signs that should raise suspicion of illness behavior in patients with back pain*[a]

Behavioral symptoms (375, 376, 377)[b]	
Pain at the top of the tailbone	Never pain free
Whole leg pain	Intolerance of treatment
Whole leg numbness	Emergency admission
Whole leg giving away	To hospital with simple backache

Nonorganic signs (376, 381)
Tenderness: superficial, nonanatomic
Increased pain on simulated axial loading and rotation
Positive straight leg raising: negative by distraction
Regional weakness and sensory "stocking" change
(These symptoms not valid in patients with serious spinal pathology, older patients >60 yr or from culturally different ethic minorities)

Overt pain behavior (186, 260)
Guarding, bracing, rubbing, grimacing, sighing

UAB pain behavior scale (261, 287)[a]	
Vocal complaints verbal	Mobility: walking (normal; mild limp or impairment, marked limp or labored walking)
Vocal complaints: nonverbal (moans, groans, gasps, etc.)	Body language (clutching, rubbing site of pain)
Down time because of pain (none; 0–60 min; >60 min/d)	Use of visible physical supports (corset, stick, crutches, leaning on furniture; TENS: none, occasional, dependent, constant use)
Facial grimacing	Stationary movement (sitting or standing still; occasional shift of position; constant movement or shifts of position)
Standing posture (normal, midly impaired, distorted)	Medication (none; nonnarcotic as prescribed, demands for increased dose or frequency, narcotics, analgesic abuse)

[a] Score each item as follows: none, 0; occasional, 0.5; frequent, 1. This gives a total score of 0–10.
[b] Numbers in parentheses are from the reference list.

use of immunosuppressive drugs, and age (osteoporosis) constitute histories that have proven good sensitivity. Other specific causes of back pain such as infections, benign tumors, inflammatory diseases other than ankylosing spondylitis, Reiter's syndrome, Paget's disease, and intrapelvic, abdominal, and retroperineal disease have not been investigated in the same manner depicted, but these conditions are found in fewer than 1% of patients seen in general practice (94).

MOBILITY AND MUSCLE TESTS

From 1992 to 1998, additional studies dealt with these issues, including tests for reliability of different details of the physical examination (221,343,361). McGregor et al. (237), in a study of 138 patients and using a potentiometer, found a lack of relation between the motion measurements and a patient's diagnosis, pain, and symptom severity. The association between physical measurement and assessment of human functions is relatively weak.

Simmonds et al. (321) compared 9 physical performance measures for reliability, validity, and clinical use in 44 patients with back pain and 48 pain-free subjects. Test-retest reliability was adequate, except for trunk flexion measurement in the low back pain group. In addition, self-reported disability was only moderately correlated with the performance tests. A study of lumbar lordosis and lumbar extension was performed by Youdas et al. (401), with good intratester and intertester reliability.

Burton et al. (58) investigated the influence of lumbar sagittal flexibility from intervertebral disc degeneration measured by MRI, which explained only 31% of the variance. Saur et al. (306) tested the reliability of certain physical examinations including flexion and found the Schober test and fingertip-to-floor measurements the most reliable.

The McKenzie (238) methods for evaluating signs of symptom movement to a central location (centralization) have been tested for intraobserver variability, with different results: good results noted by Donelson et al. (99,100,101), but poorer results reported by Riddle and Rothstein (288). Some positive predictive value for recovery has been noted (100,217,393), whereas Karas et al. (183) found a high Waddell score (Table 9.5) better for return to work. Clinical utility of the McKenzie method could not be established by Cherkin et al. (70) in a large, well-controlled study.

Another thorough and statistically correct study on interexaminer reliability in physical examinations in patients with low back pain, by Strender et al. (339), looked at 25 different clinical tests and found the kappa coefficient an acceptable measure of reliability (greater than 0.40), except for sagittal configuration, paravertebral tenderness, springing test, and sacroiliac tests. Again, as in many other studies, the best kappa coefficient was for straight leg raising. This was not a test against any gold standard but an interrater reliability examination in which, in general, the kappa coefficients are low, a finding also found earlier by Maher and Adams (222).

With regard to the sacroiliac pain syndromes, certain tests have been commonly used (102,203,223,233,278,324), and results have indicated poor interrater reliability to the point that most authors agree that it is not possible to diagnose this syndrome. This finding has also been reinforced by the measurements of movements of these "joints" by the roentgenstereophotogrammetric method (193). Other authors (120, 314), however, believe that injection techniques can be used.

Some studies have measured muscle strength and endurance with and without various types of apparatus (97,154). In 1993, Newton and Waddell et al. (254,255) published their results with and review of various "isomachines" to measure muscle strength but found no evidence to support the clinical utility of these techniques. These machines measure performance but not strength or capacity, although they can be used to monitor progress. Simpler methods of strength and endurance exist, however, such as the Biering-Sörensen (31) test or the modification thereof described by Ito et al. (165) with good test-retest correlation. Jorgensen and Nicholaisen (180,257) found lower isometric endurance in patients with severe low back pain, but again the explanation could be pain or psychologic limitation. Evaluating performance of patients with low back pain in a work simulator, psychologic factors predicted strength significantly better than physical findings. Psychologic factors and pain experience influence muscle strength and endurance (76). In a similar study Moreland et al. (242) found large variations in evaluation of trunk extension muscle strength and endurance with acceptable interrater reliability of dynamic endurance tests.

Estlander et al. (112), using an isokinetic dynamometer, found that subjective pain and disability influenced the result of the isokinetic performance and confirmed the results of the review by Newton and Waddell (254). In addition, Gibbons et al. (127) indicated, based on their twin study, that genetics and childhood environment may play a dominant role in determining adult back muscle function. Obviously, many factors influence strength testing for muscle function and mobility, and therefore, it should not come as a surprise that these tests are not reliable for individual assessments of patients. In addition, certain methods have been developed, such as triaxial dynamometry and spinoscopy, for which the inventors have claimed improved diagnostic capability from mobility measurements, claims that have not been substantiated in prospective controlled studies (205,216).

IMAGING OF THE SPINE

Besides the most important history and physical examination of patients with spinal problems, radiologic examinations are frequently used. One Swedish study (142) found that, in a sample of nearly 2,000 people who were listed as being sick for 4 weeks or more as a result of neck and back problems, within 4 weeks of the onset of these pain syndromes, 38% of the patients had undergone x-ray examinations, and within 90 days, the number was 55%. In the United States, even higher numbers of patients are sent for x-ray studies; according to Carey (63,64), the numbers are 46% and 70%, respectively, after 4 weeks and 3 months. Similar figures were published from Belgium by Szpalski et al. (341), who noted cultural differences: more x-ray examinations were ordered for the French-speaking population with back pain than for the Flemish-speaking population.

All the guidelines published in English during the last 15 years, starting with the Quebec report from 1987 (249) and including the British and American guidelines, have stated that ordinary x-ray examinations in the absence of any red flags, that is, suspicion of a specific treatable disease, have no diagnostic or therapeutic value (3,32,50,73,115,118,244,256,300,313,337,368,378). In general, these guidelines support the recommendations made by the Royal College of Radiologists in 1993 (301) and 1995 (302) (Table 9.6). In the 1990s, systematic reviews were published on the subject to find out whether a causal relationship exists between x-ray findings and nonspecific low back pain. The Dutch group (361) searched MEDLINE and EMBASE from 1966 to 1994. Two observers rated all the several hundred articles for quality and calculated the odds ratios for the most prevalent diagnostic labels. The results from the better studies with the highest methodologic scores are summarized in Table 9.7.

These authors (365) also detailed certain biases, particularly in the studies on disc aging or degeneration. Only two studies were of prospective design. Most of the studies were case-control studies in which the low back pain status and x-ray findings were assessed, or radiographs were taken at the time of investigation and were related to past back pain, often subject to recall bias. Nevertheless, the odds ratios for disc degeneration and nonspecific low back pain, which range from 1.2 to 3.3, indicate a positive association, but even so the authors in the discussion of the potential sources of bias concluded that "no firm evidence exists for the presence or absence of an association between x-ray findings and nonspecific low back pain." Larger prospective studies are needed. For x-ray findings of spondylolysis or spondylisthesis, spina bifida, transitional vertebra, spondylosis, and Scheuermann's disease, no association seems to exist with nonspecific low back pain, a finding supported by another review (40).

Andersson and Deyo (10) looked at the sensitivity, specificity, and predictive value for interpretation of diagnostic studies in spinal disorders, and in their thorough review, they refuted the value of preemployment x-ray studies on statistical grounds, a position reinforced in the review by Bigos et al. (33).

TABLE 9.6. *Imaging of the lumbar spine: Royal College of Radiologists recommendations*

Circumstances	Guideline	Exceptions
Back pain	Not recommended routinely Acute back pain is usually due to conditions that cannot be diagnosed by plain film radiography; pain correlates poorly with the severity of degenerative change found on radiology	Symptoms worsening or not resolving Neurologic signs History of trauma
Asymptomatic patients (e.g., preemployment screening)	Not recommended No correlation between radiologic findings and likelihood of future disability	

Clinical problem	X-ray	Guideline	Comment
Chronic back pain with no pointers to infection or tumor	Plain	Not routinely indicated	Degenerative changes common and nonspecific; main value in younger patients (spondylolisthesis), ankylosing spondylitis, etc.) or in older patients with possible vertebral collapse
Back pain with adverse features: sphincter or gait disturbance, saddle anesthesia, severe or progressive motor loss, widespread neurologic deficit, previous cancer, systemic illness, human immunodeficiency virus injection	Imaging	Indicated	Together with URGENT SPECIALIST REFERRAL: MRI usually best; imaging should not delay specialist referral; bone scan also widely used for possible bone destruction; "normal" radiographs may be falsely reassuring
Acute back pain, ? disc herniation, sciatica with not adverse features (see above)	Plain	Not routinely indicated	Acute back pain usually due to conditions that cannot be diagnosed on plain radiography (osteoporotic collapse an exception); "normal" radiographs may be falsely reassuring; demonstration of disc herniation requires MRI or CT and should be considered immediately after failed conservative management; MRI generally preferred (wider field of views, conus, postoperative changes) and avoids irradiation; MRI better than CT for postoperative problems
	MRI/CT	6-wk suggestion	

CT, computed tomography; MRI, magnetic resonance imaging.
Data from Royal College of Radiologists. *Making the best use of a department of radiology.* London: Royal College of Radiologists Publications, 1993; and Royal College of Radiologists. *Making the best use of a department of radiology: guidelines for doctors,* 3rd ed. London: Royal College of Radiologists, 1995:1–96.

Waddell (375) calculated the negative predictive value of a routine x-ray study to 99%, but when the patient's history revealed systemic symptoms, nonmechanical back pain, and a sedimentation rate of more than 25 mm, the positive predictive value increased to 34%. Another older study (210) from 1982 estimated a probability of 0.2% that the person presenting with acute low back pain has a specific treatable cause revealed by x-ray examination. In Göteborg, Sweden, Brolin (55) reviewed 68,000 spinal radiographs obtained over a 10-year period. She found that only 1 in 2,500 patients had a finding of a red flag disease not suspected clinically when the radiographs were ordered. Deyo and Diehl (91), in their prospective study of 620 outpatients with

TABLE 9.7. *Studies on the association between radiographic findings and nonspecific low back pain judged to be valid*

	No. of studies	No. of subjects with low back pain		No. of subjects without low back pain		Odds ratio	Result
		Present	Absent	Present	Absent		
Disc degeneration	12	1,462	1,179	986	1,398	1.2–3.3	Moderately positive (caveats)
Spondylosis	3	400	248	407	501	1.2–2.0	Negative
Spondylolysis and spondylolisthesis	6	204	1,343	206	878	0.82–1	Negative
Spina bifida	2	299	706	253	391	0.5–0.6	Negative
Transitional vertebrae	3	97	768	90	560	0.5–0.8	Negative
Scheuermann' disease	2	40	28	26	326	0.8–3.6	Unclear

Data from van Tulder MW, Assendelft WJJ, Koes BW, et al. Spinal radiographic finding and nonspecific low back pain: a systematic review of observational studies. *Spine* 1997;22:427–434, with permission.

low back pain, reported therapy-dependent findings in 4%, all of whom in patients who were either more than 50 years old or had a recent injury.

The most recent scientific study on observer variations in plain radiography of the lumbosacral spine is by Espeland et al. (109), who reported on 200 consecutive patients in a general practice setting whose radiographs were read by three radiologists independently. There was generally poor interobserver and intraobserver agreement for many of the findings usually reported by radiologists. In particular, kappa statistics showed low values on the evaluation of facet joint arthritis, narrow spinal canal, and degenerative spondylolisthesis and somewhat better agreement for reduced disc height, the presence of osteophytes, and osteoporotic fractures.

Assessment With Magnetic Resonance Imaging

Although the advent of MRI increased our diagnostic capabilities of visualizing abnormalities of spinal structures including red flags (96), there is no evidence that this technique has improved the treatment of common back syndromes (40,90). In a review by Kent and Larson (189) that resulted in 156 studies rated according to methodologic criteria for study design, the authors stated that, for most of abnormalities, the sensitivity of MRI is equal to or better than competing technologies and shows greater contrast and detail than computed tomography (CT) but also more silent abnormalities or incidental findings, as reinforced by Table 9.8. A few studies found a modest impact on therapeutic choices but no impact on quality of life or disability. MRI is less invasive and can be recommended for patients with suspected cervical and lumbar radiculopathy (189,190).

Kent et al. (188) claimed that MRI obviated the need for more than half the CT scans and 90% of the myelograms. In an attempt to analyze cost-effectiveness further, Jarvik et al. (168) even performed a randomized trial comparing low-strength MRI with common radiologic examination performed as the primary imaging investigation; these investigators did not reach any firm conclusion on effectiveness.

In a double-blind prospective study, Brant-Zawadzki et al. (51) measured interob-

TABLE 9.8. *Magnetic resonance imaging studies of structural abnormalities in the cervical and lumbar spine of asymptomatic persons*

Study (ref)	Year	Population size	Modality	Abnormal findings
Powell et al. (279)	1986	n = 302 women	0.15T	Disc degeneration increase from 6% in <20-yr women to 79% >60-yr old women
Weinreb et al. (390)	1989	n = 86 women: 45 pregnant, 41 non-pregnant	1.5T	Disc bulging or herniation in one or more levels 54% in both groups
Boden et al. (35)	1990	n = 57	1.5T	Individuals <50 yr old: 20% disc herniation, 1% spinal stenosis; individuals >60 yr old: 35% disc herniation, 21% spinal stenosis
Boden et al. (36)	1990	n = 63, 20–63 yr old	1.5T	Bulging discs 5%, disc narrowing degeneration 25% <40 yr; 60% in >40 yr Foraminal stenosis 20%
Tertti et al. (344)	1991	n = 39, children matched for sex, age, and school class with low back pain children	0.02T	26% disc degeneration, 3% disc protrusion, 26% spinal muscle atrophy, 8% Scheuermann-type changes, 3% transitional vertebral, 3% narrowed disc space
Parkkola et al. (268)	1993	n = 60, volunteers	0.02T	3% central spinal stenosis, 15% disc bulging, 72 degenerated discs out of 180 analysed discs (40%)
Jensen et al. (171)	1994	n = 98, volunteers	1.5T	52% disc bulging, 27% disc protrusions, 1% disc extrusions, 19% Schmorl's nodes, 14% annular defects, 8% facet arthropathy
Boos et al. (42)	1995	n = 46, asymptomatic persons matched for age, sex, and risk factor matched with patients selected for discectomy	1.5T	76% disc herniations (63% protrusions, 13% extrusions), 85% disc degeneration, 22% neural compromises
Buirski and Silberstein (56)	1993	n = 63, 38 women	1.5T	39% showed disc degeneration with protrusion
Matsumoto et al. (232)	1998	n = 497; 262 women, 235 men; C2-7, 10–70 yr	1.5T 134 0.5T 363	Kappa scores for 3 observers ≈0.6; degeneration, 20 yr old 15%; >60 yr 88%; foramen stenosis, >40 yr 15%; disc protrusion, >40 yr 25%; cord compression, 8%
Battié et al. (26)	1995	n = 115 male twin pairs (21% back pain last 12 mo)	1.5T	Two independent, observers kappa scores ≈0.8 for signal intensity (degeneration), disc bulging, narrowing common, explained by twinship and early shared environment and upbringing more than physical load
Stadnik et al. (336)	1998	n = 36	1.5T, gadolinium enhancement	Bulging discs 81%, disc protrusion 33%, 56% annular tears; of 27 tears,96% contrast enhanced
Lane et al. (202)	1995	n = 30	1.5T, gadolinium enhancement	Radicular enhancement found in 18 of 30
Lehto et al. (206)	1994	n = 89, 9–63 yr old	0.1T	Asympatomatic degeneration in cervical discs, common after 30 yr of age, 57% in subjects >40 yr
Weishaupt et al. (391)	1998	n = 60, 20–50 yr old	1.0T	Disc bulging 62%, protrusion 67%, HIZ 33%; disc extrusion 18%; sequester or nerve root compromise end plate abnormality uncommon

server and intraobserver variability of interpreting lumbar MRI studies of disc abnormalities. These investigators found that experienced readers using standardized nomenclature showed moderate to substantial agreement with interpretation of disc extension beyond the interspace. Kappa statistics were between 0.5 and 0.7, but the most common disagreement was for normal versus bulging discs. In this study, herniation was read in 23% of asymptomatic subjects. The 98 asymptomatic patients in this new study are the same as those tabulated by Jensen et al. (171) in Table 9.8. The methodology itself also has pitfalls, including some artifacts, as described in detail by Taber et al. (342). In a more recent study on MRI as the primary modality for neurologic evaluation of the lumbar spine, Annertz et al. (12) noted a threefold increase in the number of patients examined and a 53% increase in total costs. In a review covering the MRI literature from 1985 to 1995, Boos and Lander (40) could not produce definite evidence that MRI should be used as primary assessment, except in rare instances.

Several studies using MRI have demonstrated a surprisingly high incidence of abnormalities in patients without pain or without radiculopathy in the neck as well as in the lumbar spine (Table 9.8). A look at the findings tabulated clearly shows that a scan that detects an abnormality in the absence of objective neurologic findings in patients may risk initiating a cascade of potentially harmful clinical interventions including surgery. For this reason, Roland and van Tulder recommended that radiologists, in addition to reporting their finding, should also add that "this finding may be unrelated to patients symptoms because it is often seen in asymptomatic subjects" (294). The claim that you can "see" back pain by looking at gadolinium-enhanced MRI (173,372) has also largely been refuted (52,96,202). The presence of a high-intensity zone on MRI claimed by Aprill and Bogduk (13) to be a diagnostic sign of painful internal disc disruption could not be verified by Stadnik et al. (336).

Smith et al. (326), in a study of interobserver and intraobserver error of this high-intensity zone, also compared it with discography in patients with back pain and concluded that the interobserver reliability of this sign for detecting of severely disrupted and painful discs by discography was much lower than previous studies had shown. It had a low positive predictive value, and there was no proof that the high-intensity zone was indicative of painful internal disc disruption.

Saifuddin et al. (304) compared findings of MRI findings and annular tears using discography as a gold standard (although this cannot be considered a gold standard, as explained later in this chapter) and found poor sensitivity even though the specificity was high. Their conclusion was that the usefulness is limited.

Borchgrevink et al. (45) performed MRI examination within 2 days of a motor vehicle accident on 14 patients with neck sprains after whiplash injury. Their MRI findings were correlated to reported symptoms 6 months after the accident and to a control group of 20 volunteers. No difference of the MRI features of brain and neck was revealed between the patients and the control group.

Some correlation of signal intensity, that is, water content in the disc, with symptoms has been demonstrated by Sether et al. (320), among others. However, there have been no studies showing water content or tears in the annulus to have clinical utility (239,240,271,399).

Boos et al. (44) quantitatively evaluated the intervertebral discs and vertebral bodies for diurnal water content and compared degenerative and normal intervertebral discs; these investigators found some, but not "convincing," differences. They attached great hope to this method of quantitative MRI to obtain knowledge of the physiology of discs and development of disc degeneration and back pain, but the limitation of the MRI method made further studies necessary. The same group (41) tried a similar method and concluded that, even though symptomatic and morphologically matched asymptomatic disc herniation differs with regard to matrix composition, this could not explain their earlier reported findings (42) that psychosocial factors are more important for outcome than the size or composition of the herniation in symptomatic patients who undergo operation.

In another study on the relationship among the MRI appearance of the lumbar spine and low back pain, age, and occupation in male patients, Savage et al. (307) studied 149 working men aged 20 to 30 years and 71 men aged 31 to 58 years in five different occupations. One-fourth of the men had never experienced low back pain. Twelve months later, the examination was repeated. As expected, disc degeneration was more prevalent in the older age group (52%) than in the younger (28%), but although low back pain was more prevalent in the older men, there was no relationship between low back pain and disc degeneration. No difference in the MRI appearance on the lumbar spine was observed among the five occupational groups. Forty-seven percent of all the men who had experienced low back pain had normal lumbar spines. During the 12-month follow-up period, 13 of the men experienced low back pain for the first time; however, no change in the MRI appearance of the lumbar spine could account for the onset of this back pain. This study supports the findings of the twin study conducted by Battié et al. (26).

The volunteers who, in the original contributions by Boden et al. (35) and Boos et al. (42), exhibited disc extrusions on their MRI scans, were reexamined 5 and 7 years later, retrospectively. They did not develop sciatica or more than the expected amount of back pain (48,309).

As mentioned earlier, gadolinium-enhanced MRI has been used to evaluate nerve root pain and to assess success or failure after disc surgery (126,128,356,362,372). None of these studies could give definite answers or definite help to improve the diagnostic capability in explaining back pain or failed back surgery syndrome.

In a retrospective examination of 372 patients who had 412 gadolinium-enhanced MRI examinations of the thoracolumbar spine, Stabler et al. (335) looked for the vascularization of Schmorl's nodes and associated bone marrow edema. Thirty-eight percent of patients exhibited Schmorl's node, and there was some indication that the bone marrow edema adjacent to Schmorl's nodes was less frequent in asymptomatic patients than in symptomatic patients.

Grane (131), in his study of 192 patients, of whom 10% were regarded as asymptomatic and served as a control group, evaluated postoperative changes in the symptomatic patients. To visualize the nerve root, MRI was better than CT. Thickened nerve roots were found with equal frequency in asymptomatic and symptomatic patients, and epidural scar tissue diminished with time, showing no difference between asymptomatic and symptomatic patients.

Ross et al. (299) followed sequentially 94 adults who had first-time surgery for herniated discs preoperatively, 3 months, and 6 months after surgery; this study also used gadolinium-enhanced MRI. There was no significant association between disc enhancement and residual symptoms after surgery irrespective of outcome, a finding supporting that postoperative changes are seen frequently in asymptomatic patients after surgery and are not necessarily indicators of infection.

One multicenter study (298) that was randomized and double-blind and that evaluated the effect of a scar-preventing substance in surgery for lumbar disc herniation demonstrated that patients with extensive peridural scar were three times more likely to experience recurrent radicular pain than those with less extensive peridural scarring. This is the first controlled study to demonstrate this finding using gadolinium-enhanced MRI.

In a critical review published in 1999 of the literature on MRI contrast media in neuroimaging, Breslau et al. (52) scrutinized more than 700 articles in English literature until 1997 and found only a single article of good quality, and it was not related to back pain. Of the 6 articles that were rated of moderately good quality by independent interpretation, only 1 article concerned lumbar disc problems (349). The authors of the review concluded that no strong evidence-based guideline exist for the use of contrast material in neuroimaging, a conclusion also depicted in the reviews mentioned earlier. No studies exist to establish valid sensitivity and specificity estimates for their application.

ASSESSMENT OF PSYCHOSOCIAL FACTORS, PAIN, AND PAIN BEHAVIOR

The other area in which new important information is supported by evidence is the studies for evaluation of the so-called yellow flags, the psychosocial enforcers for pain and deterrents of function. In Chapters 3 and 17, the psychologic risk factors and the results of attention to these by different treatment programs demonstrate that the search for such factors should become a natural and necessary part of a comprehensive examination of patients with back pain. These factors are already important in the subacute stage for prognostication and at later stages should be addressed because there is evidence that they should be a part of treatment (350). Randomized controlled trials have demonstrated that, when such factors are dealt with, the results are significantly improved (see Chapters 12 and 17). The most common and scientifically tested methods are seen in the following tables: for evaluating patients pain and pain behavior, Table 9.9; for pain beliefs and coping strategies, Table 9.10; and for pain anxiety and distress, Table 9.11.

Psychologic tests have been used in many clinical settings to predict outcomes of various treatment methods such as surgery (42,143,330,363,380). The Minnesota Multiphasic Personality Inventory was used by Wiltse and Rocchio (397) and Pheasant et al. (272) and since then by Herron et al. (152) and Spengler et al. (331), whereas Main et al. (226) advocated the use of Disease and Risk Assessment Method (DRAM) to predict illness behavior and distress. These studies have demonstrated better predictability than physical findings at examination, clinical radiography, or MRI investigations for the outcome of some treatment modalities, including surgery.

Attempts at assessing pain include the widely used 10-cm visual analog scale (VAS), which has been found reproducible and validated and, in particular, can be recommended in clinical practice as a simple way to follow patients' progression (98,263,286). The VAS has actually been found more reliable than the verbal rating scale (263,319).

Pain drawings (Table 9.9) have also been used for assessment of patients, symptoms and progress, but unfortunately, there is no consensus about how to score the drawings (53,229,230,260,264,267,282,283,291,292,322), even though most studies claim test-retest reliability (260,262,353,354) using the point scale recommended by Ransford et

TABLE 9.9. *Evaluation of pain and pain behavior in patients with back pain*[a]

	Outcome measure	
Undimensional pain assessment	Measures	Validity/reliability
Numeric verbal rating scale	Undimensional rating scale of pain intensity	Varied pain patient populations (191)
Visual analog pain scale (348)	Undimensional measure of pain intensity	Reliability only established for CLBP (220)
	Pain Behaviors Assessment	
Observer rating of pain behaviors (186)	Observers trained to code a live of videotaped observation of pain behaviors based on a symptom checklist (guarding, bracing, grimacing, sighing, rubbing)	Acute LBP (170) CLBP (186)
Pain behaviors checklist (350, 377)	20-item list of common pain behaviors; aims to avoid the need for observational studies of pain behavior	Validated compared to observational methods of pain behavior for CLBP (296)
Waddell's behavioral signs (377)	Short behaviors checklist for clinicians to assess pain behaviors during a patient's LBP consultation	Gold standard pain behavior assessment technique within clinical settings with established reliability and validity for LBP (260)
UAB pain behaviors rating scale (287)	Observers trained to code a live or videotaped observation of pain behaviors based on a symptom checklist	Subacute LBP in Swedish workers (260)
Pain drawings	Patients mark the location and type (e.g., ache, pins and needles) of pain on a graphic representation of the human body	Reliability dependent on the scoring method used (229, 230, 234); validity in terms of measuring psychologic distress (267) or diagnosing specific from nonspecific LBP (267, 377) has not been established
Oswestry Low Back Pain Disability Questionnaire (116)	Daily and social activities and pain rating	Acute LBP (116); acute and subacute LBP and CLBP (158, 348)
	Multidimensional Pain Assessment	
McGill Pain Questionnaire (78, 158)	Sensory, affective, and cognitive components of pain perception	CLP (78, 220, 234)
West Haven-Yale Multidimensional Pain Inventory (192)	Multidimensional pain inventory assessing patient activities, affective distress, social/family/vocational functioning pain severity and other reactions to pain behaviors	Chronic pain (30, 86, 191, 192) and LBP patients

[a] Numbers in parentheses are from the reference list.
CLBP, chronic low back pain; LBP, low back pain.

al. (282). Brismar et al. (53), in a prospective study of 190 patients operated for sciatica resulting from disc hernia, could not correlate properly the pain drawing with a surgical finding in one-third of the cases. Other authors (264,353,354), however, found the pain drawing to be a helpful screening instrument to evaluate psychologic distress as well. Mann et al. (229) found that physician's evaluation was still more diagnostic. Pain drawing at present can only be recommended for general use in patients with sciatica who are in a multidisciplinary chronic pain setting.

TABLE 9.10. *Pain beliefs and coping strategies*[a]

Measure: pain beliefs assessment	Constructs	Reliability and validity	Conclusions
Fear-Avoidance Beliefs Questionnaire (FABQ) (383)	Fear-avoidance beliefs (work-related); fear-avoidance beliefs (physical activity)	Reliable and valid measure for LBP (383)	Fear-avoidance beliefs correlate strongly with self-reported disability, activities of daily living, and work loss; further research required
Pain and Impairment Relationship Scale (PAIRS) (290)	Perceived ability to function in spite of pain	Diagnostically sensitive, valid, and reliable for LBP (323)	Perceived ability function in spite of pain a separate construct from affective distress and cognitive distortions; PAIRS scores associates with patient-rated disease severity, but not physician ratings

[a] Numbers in parentheses are from the reference list.
LBP, low back pain.

Linton and Halldén (214,215) developed a 24-item questionnaire for patients with acute back pain that was compiled from several other questionnaires that had shown validity and reliability, including the Fear-Avoidance Behavior Questionnaire (383). The discriminant analysis demonstrated predictability for chronicity in 73% of patient with a sensitivity of 71% and specificity of 77%.

Another commonly used questionnaire in addition to the inappropriate Waddell signs (379,381) is the Fear-Avoidance Beliefs Questionnaire (383). The main finding from that study on test-retest reproducibility in 26 patients was that it was high and that the fear-avoidance beliefs about work and physical activity had a high internal consistency of around 0.8 and accounted for up to 44% of the total variance. Thus, fear-avoidance beliefs are among the more important factors when examining and investigating patients with back pain. The specific fear-avoidance beliefs about work are strongly related to work loss resulting from low back pain.

TABLE 9.11. *Example of commonly used measures of affective state: depression, anxiety, and psychologic distress*[a]

Measure	Reliability and validity	Conclusions
Beck's Depression Inventory (BDI) (28)	Conflicting evidence; may overestimate major depression (395)	Short, 21-item, self-report test assessing frequency of depression
Distress and Risk Assessment Method (DRAM) (226)	Valid and reliable measure for LBP assessing psychologic distress (226)	Short self-report scales assessing the degree to which someone is perceiving psychologic distress; three-factor structure (no distress, potential psychologic sequelae, and psychologically distressed)
Zung's Self-Rating Depression Scale (ZDS) (403)	Reliable and valid for population surveys; diagnostically sensitive for LBP patients (133, 134)	Short, 20-item, self-report questionnaire designed to identify depression within general populations

[a] Numbers in parentheses are from the reference list.
LBP, low back pain.

TABLE 9.12. *Disability measures for low back pain*[a]

Name of outcome measure	Measures	Test-retest reliability estimates[b]	Reliability[b] Cronbach's alpha coefficients	Validity
Oswestry Low-Back Pain Disability Questionnaire (OLBPDQ) (116)	Daily and social activities and pain rating	0.88 0.99 0.94	0.77 0.92	Acute LBP Acute and subacute LBP and CLBP (22, 27, 116, 348)
Quebec Back Pain Disability Scale (197) (QBPDS) (198)	Functional disability	0.92	0.96	Unspecified mix of LBP (197, 198)
Roland Morris Activity Scale (RMAS) (293)	Shortened version of Sickness Impact Profile, specific for LBP	0.76 0.83 0.91	0.89 0.92	Mixed LBP Acute LBP CLBP (27, 54, 89, 172, 289, 293)

[a] Numbers in parentheses are from the reference list.
[b] Summary of coefficients for OLBPDQ and RMAS taken from Kopec and Esdaile (196,197)
CLBP, chronic low back pain; LBP, low back pain.

OUTCOME MEASURES AND DISABILITY EVALUATIONS

Comprehensive standardized physical examination protocols have been used mostly to predict disability (305,333,371). All these authors included some evidence of sufficient interrater reliability, sufficient repeatability, and predictive validity for comprehensive physical examinations for use in primary care situations (371) as well as in secondary referral centers (305,333).

For assessing the outcome of treatment methods, several questionnaires have been used, tested for rehability and construct validity (Table 9.12). In addition to the VAS, the 36-item short form (SF-36), and the various scales seen in Tables 9-13, Deyo et al. (95) recommended a minimum set of instruments evaluating pain symptoms, back-related function, well-being, and satisfaction with care. These included those recommended by the American Academy of Orthopaedic Surgeons (270) and the North American Spine Society (17,80), the SF-36 and SF-12 (27,385,386), and the EuroQol card (113) and chronic illness inventory (295).

TABLE 9.13. *Multidimensional health status measures*[a]

Outcome measure	Constructs	Validity and reliability
Chronic illness problem	Shortened version of SIP, specific for chronic pain	CLBP (296); further research needed
Low-Back Outcome Score (134)	Disability, LBP, work, social roles, mental health	Acute and CLBP (134); further research needed
Nottingham Health Profile (160)	Pain, emotional state, subjective perception of health	No available evidence
Short form 36-item health survey (124)	Physical and mental health, social roles, pain, general perception of health	Mixed LBP (27, 124, 220)
Sickness Impact Profile (SIP) (29)	Broad generic areas of physical, psychosocial health, daily activities	Acute LBP (89), CLBP (119)

[a] Numbers in parentheses are from reference list.
CLBP, chronic low back pain; LBP, low back pain.

For evaluating changes in health status, Beaton et al. (27) compared the SF-36 to several other generic health status measures and a self-report in two occasions in a sample of workers with musculoskeletal disorders. Their statistically sound study suggested that the SF-36 was the most appropriate questionnaire to measure changes in this population, and it had good test-retest reliability. Grevitt et al. (135) also found that SF-36 valid and internally consistent when it was applied to a group of 120 patients who underwent spinal operations.

In a study (132) of 287 injury-related cases from Australia, recovery from low back pain in surgical cases was considered. The compensation status was most predictive of return to work, followed by some psychometric tests, for which results of the Oswestry Questionnaire and pain drawings were available on the patients before surgery. These psychometric tests were more predictive of patients' own rating of success than the physical examination findings of straight leg raising, neurologic signs, and limited motions, which were also performed preoperatively and at follow-up.

ASSESSING PATIENTS WITH NECK PAIN

Despite the increase in reports of neck syndromes noted in the 1990s and described in Chapter 8, there is a striking lack of studies on the assessment of these patients. Few reviews could be found, with sparse information on the accuracy and utility of either history taking or physical examination (Table 9.14).

Waris et al. (387) proposed a set of clinical examinations, later tested by Kuorinka and Koskinen (201) for reliability. These investigators established good intertester reliability for measurement by a physical therapist of handgrip force, palpable hardenings in the neck and trapezius area, and tender points in the same area, but the study lacked a description of the statistical analysis. The repeatability of measurement of

TABLE 9.14. *Best evidence synthesis for assessment of patients with neck and without arm pain*[a]

	Evidence	Recommendation
History taking	No study exists for evaluation of validity or utility	Ask same questions as for "red flag" exclusion in low back pain (Tables 9.3 and 9.4), in addition to work-related questions
Physical examination	Poor interobserver and intraobserver reliability for motion, palpation (201, 207, 208); better for tests of root involvement and myelopathy (57)	Perform neurologic examination to rule out radiculopathy (Table 9.15)
Plain radiography	Value for ordinary neck pain not established Same as for low back pain (Tables 9.4 and 9.6)	
Magnetic resonance imaging	Value for ordinary neck pain not established	Same as for low back pain (Tables 9.6 and 9.8)
Special examinations	Test for distress and pain behavior of value for prediction of function and disability but not as reliably proven as for low back pain (103, 157, 227, 274, 360)	See Tables 9.9 to 9.11

[a] Numbers in parentheses are from the reference list.

tenderness in the neck shoulder region by a dolorimeter and manual palpation was studied by Levoska et al. (207,208) and showed poor sensitivity and specificity for neck and shoulder symptoms.

Buchbinder et al. (57) performed a critical appraisal of existing classifications of soft tissue disorders of the neck and upper limb utilizing methodologic criteria including appropriateness for purpose, validity, reliability, feasibility, and generalizability. These investigators could find only four studies trying to introduce a classification system for neck pain, and they noted methodologic errors for development in all of them.

One early review article by Wilson (396) dealt with chronic neck pain and cervicogenic headache and contained no valid information on measurements. Another critical review on the same topic of headache and the cervical spine from 1997 by Pollmann et al. (275) quoted the International Headache Society (147), which defined the criteria for headache or facial pain associated with disorder of the neck as a pain localized to neck and occipital region radiating to forehead, orbital region, temples, or ear, precipitated or aggravated by special neck movements or sustained neck posture. In addition, at least one of the following criteria must be fulfilled: resistance to or limitation of passive neck movements; changes in neck muscle contour, texture, and tone; abnormal tenderness of neck muscles; and a "pathologic" finding in radiologic examination. There are no studies to validate these diagnostic criteria. The use of diagnostic blocks of the greater occipital nerve is described by the author (275) as "fairly" accurate. The conclusion was that the term *cervicogenic headache* remains controversial, and the reliability of diagnostic findings according to the International Headache Society criteria is lacking.

Viikari-Juntura et al. (369,370) tested the interrater reliability for the diagnosis of tension neck, general cervical syndrome, and thoracic outlet syndrome. For patients with neck and radicular pain in the arm, the interrater reliability of the palpation of neck and shoulders for presence of tenderness was poor, with a kappa coefficient of around 0.3, and the interrater reliability of muscle tone was similarly low. Unfortunately, the same pertained to the reliability of estimation of range of motion of the cervical spine (kappa coefficient, 0.4–0.5). The diagnostic utility of clinical tests for nerve root compression in cervical disc disease was examined in 69 patients in a neurosurgery clinic (370). These patients were tested for neck compression, axial manual traction, shoulder abduction, neurologic and radiologic signs of disc herniation, and x-ray findings of severe spondylosis. None of these tests were sensitive, and they identified only about half the patients with significant compression on myelography at levels C-6, C-7, and C-8.

The neck compression test, found highly specific by Viikari-Juntura (370), was described in 1944 by Spurling and Scoville (334). The examination is performed by extending the neck and rotating the head to the side of the pain and then applying manual pressure on the head. This maneuver should cause increased arm pain or paresthesia.

Partanen et al. (269) studied, retrospectively and prospectively, 360 patients with suspected nerve root compression of whom 77 underwent both electromyography (EMG) and myelography and subsequent surgery. Of these patients, 26 had sensory impairment, and only 34 had motor weakness. EMG depicted the presence of disease in 57%. No further statistical analysis was done. The clinical usefulness of other electrodiagnostic techniques are unproven.

Ellenberg et al. (108) reviewed the diagnostic assessments of cervical radiculopathy, that is, neck and arm pain in the distribution of one of the nerve roots. These authors gave a thorough description of the examination for nerve root compromise only to state that there is great variation in the clinical findings and a single nerve root level involvement can be diagnosed by clinical means 75% of the time. These investigators also stressed the importance of red flag examinations to detect spinal cord compression: testing of gait and lower extremity reflex and motor and sensory function. They also quoted the confirmatory study by Frykholm (123), who found a 50% overlap between clinical nerve root tests and actual pathologic features at surgery.

The findings of Norlander and Nordgren (258) indicated that, in patients with neck and shoulder pain, reduced mobility in the lower part of the neck explained around 15% of weakness in the hands.

The review on epidemiology, physical examination, and neurodiagnostics by Dvorák (105) did not evaluate the diagnostic procedures in a scientific fashion. His and other authors' findings are tabulated for red flag importance (Table 9.15). In myelopathy, there need not be neck pain or radicular pain but sensory disturbances both in the upper and lower extremities, as well as muscle weakness, clumsiness, and gait disturbance. Current electrodiagnostic techniques (105) showed fair specificity and sensitivity for patients with cervical myelopathy, as did MRI (251). EMG was not regarded of prognostic value, whereas motor-evoked potentials were sensitive but not specific. In particular, there was weak evidence that F-wave tests and evoked potential examinations should be performed in patients with suspected myelopathy. In addition, clinical signs of myelopathy include positive Babinski signs (Table 9.15).

Borghouts et al. (49) performed the first systematic review of the clinical course and prognostic factors of nonspecific neck pain. Six studies reported on such factors, but they were of low methodologic quality, a finding indicating that the localization of pain with radiation to the arms and neurologic signs and the radiologic findings of degenerative changes in the discs and joints were not associated with the worst prognosis. A history of previous neck pain seems to be, however. These investigators found no information on the prediction of attacks of acute neck pain and overall limited scientific evidence regarded prognostic factors for chronic neck pain.

In a longitudinal study of 1,000 working men on the role of personality characteristics and psychologic distress in neck trouble, Pietri-Taleb et al. (274) found that workers who developed neck pain lasting more than 7 days during 1 year showed a weak

TABLE 9.15. *Clinical signs and symptoms of cervical radiculopathy and myelopathy*

Clinical feature	Radiculopathy	Myelopathy
Axial pain	Present	Rarely present
Radicular pain	Present	Not present
Sensory disturbance		
Upper extremities	Present (radicular)	Present
Lower extremities	Not present	Present
Muscle weakness		
Upper extremities	Present	Present
Lower extremities	Not present	Present
Clumsiness	Not present	Present
Gait disturbance	Not present	Present
Axial compression test (Spurling)	Present	Not present
Muscle waisting	Present unilaterally	Present unilaterally
Muscle tone	Normal	Increased
Tendon reflexes	Weak	Hyperactive
Babinski	Negative	Positive

Data from references 47, 105, 108, 161, 269, 370, and 400.

association between neck pain and psychologic variables, but with rather low odds ratios, a finding confirming the studies of Mäkela et al. (227) and Holmstrom et al. (157).

Psychologic factors also seem to influence patients with whiplash, a finding substantiated in a prospective study of Drottning et al. (103), who looked in an acute assessment not only of the clinical findings, but also of the emotional response to the whiplash injury using the Impact of Event Scale. Twice the number of patients with a high Impact of Event Scale score still have pain at 4 weeks, with strong statistical significance. The authors found no predictive value for future chronic pain in the presence or amount of neck pain acutely or in neck stiffness, headache, interscapular pain, or the difference in speed in the cars involved in the accidents causing the injury. Thus, the acute psychologic response to a whiplash incident seems to be a predictor of maintenance of symptoms 4 weeks later.

In an attempt to measure neck pain-related disability, Leak et al. (204) developed the Northwick Park Neck Pain Questionnaire, adapted from the Oswestry Questionnaire for low back pain. It was tested on 44 outpatients with neck pain at 1 week, 1 month, and 3 months. These investigators found good short-term repeatability, with a kappa coefficient of 0.6. At present, the recommended outcome measures for patients with low back pain can also be used for patients with neck pain (Tables 9.12 and 9.13).

The review by Barnsley et al. (24) on whiplash injury is a description of epidemiology, clinical features, possible pathophysiology, and treatment, but it does not evaluate the utlity of various tests in these patients, except to mention that there is reasonable consistency among reports on the manifestation of neck pain. The scientific monograph by Spitzer et al. (332) on the same subject found little of utility in the literature up to 1995.

Radiologic Examinations of the Neck

Gore et al. (129), in a study of ordinary x-ray findings of degenerative changes seen in 200 asymptomatic men and women, demonstrated that by 60 to 65 years of age, 95% of men and 70% of women had at least one disc showing degenerative change on their roentgenograms. Measurement of cervical lordosis did not relate to degenerative changes. In another follow-up study (130) of 205 patients with a minimum of 10 years after onset of neck symptoms, these investigators found no clinical feature other than severe pain on onset that could predict the results 10 years later, results that included severe residual pain in 32%. The presence of severe pain was not related to degenerative changes seen on x-ray studies, including the sagittal diameter of the spinal canal, the degree of cervical lordosis, or any changes in these measurements over the 10-year evaluation period.

In the large Zoetermeer study (360) from Holland, 5,000 inhabitants of that city who were 20 to 65 years old were administered a questionnaire, and then cervical spine radiographs were taken, graded by two independent observers. In addition, personality traits were measured, using the Dutch personality questionnaire. Statistical significant differences between people with and without neck pain were found, with consistently higher odds ratios for psychosocial factors than for x-ray findings in the 14% who reported neck pain compared with the remaining persons who did not. The female-to-male ratio for neck pain was 1.8:1, and it increased particularly after 35 years of age. There was a much stronger association, however, between neck pain and personality traits in both men and women. The radiographs were judged without any knowledge of the subject data such as sex, age, and the presence or absence of pain.

The conclusion of these investigators was that more emphasis should be placed on the psychologic constitution of the patient with neck pain and possible approaches should take these factors into consideration.

The reliability of grading apophysial joint and disc degeneration in the neck was the subject of a study by Coté et al. (77). Three independent examiners assessed 30 lateral cervical spine radiographs. Moderate reliability for the classification of disc degeneration was found, but reliability was not as good for facet joint degeneration.

The review by Ellenberg et al. (108) also contains information on imaging techniques, including ordinary spinal x-ray studies, cervical myelograms, CT, and MRI, which all are often positive in people without pain. Sensitivity may be high, but specificity is low. Ellenberg et al. (108) stressed the importance of correlating the clinical picture, physical findings, and MRI studies.

From China, Li et al. (209) investigated the relationship between the radiographic signs of subluxation in the cervical vertebra and their clinical diagnostic value. In a controlled fashion in a study of 87 patients with neck pain and 21 asymptomatic volunteers, these investigators found little evidence to support that signs of subluxation in the cervical vertebra had diagnostic significance. Table 9.8 gives MRI findings in the cervical spine of nonsymptomatic volunteers.

The assessment of patients with cervical radiculopathy has not been subjected to any rigorous tests, and no correlation exists between findings from history or examination and those at surgery. Our search revealed nothing written about a patient's history that predicted a good result, nor did it show any specific test for that purpose. MRI can visualize nerve and dural sac encroachments and myelopathy (251). In one of the few prospective studies with an independent clinical and radiologic review, Bush et al. (59) followed 13 consecutive patients with cervical radiculopathy who had objective neurologic signs and large posterolateral cervical intervertebral disc herniations detected by MRI. Pain was controlled by periradicular and epidural corticosteroid injections, and the patients were interviewed and rescanned after an interval of 12 months. The scans, reviewed by an independent radiologist, revealed regression of the herniations in 12 of the 13 patients.

Radanow et al. (280), with regression analysis techniques, showed that, with increasing age, whiplash injury disability was related to cognitive impairment. The severity of initial neck pain was predictive of persisting symptoms after 6 months.

The study by Hoffman et al. (156) of 974 patients receiving cervical spine radiography in blunt trauma, of whom 283 had a whiplash injury, suggested that false-positive findings are frequent on radiographs. These investigators therefore concluded that radiographs are not necessary after whiplash injury in patients who are alert and not intoxicated and who have isolated blunt trauma and no neck tenderness on physical examination. Velmahos et al. (366) reached the same conclusion from a similar large study.

ASSESSMENT OF PATIENTS WITH LOW BACK PAIN AND LEG PAIN (SCIATICA)

To find patients with symptoms that may benefit from treatment, the presence of a few diagnostic categories should be established. These include the following:

1. Cauda equina syndrome: emergency measures should be taken.
2. The presence of a disc hernia giving radiculopathy: these patients are possible candidates for surgery.

3. The presence of other specific diseases causing radiculopathy or leg pain (possible red flags).
4. The presence of spinal stenosis or nerve root canal entrapment: surgery may influence symptoms.

Because proven treatment exists for most of categories 1, 2, and 3, it should not come as a surprise that these disease entities have been investigated more frequently than other back pain syndromes including spinal stenosis. A gold standard exists, and the methodologic rigor that is necessary according to Haynes (145) has been followed to a large extent.

Cauda Equina Syndrome

Even if it is not thoroughly supported by evaluation of specificity and sensitivity for this syndrome, as described previously in this chapter, the general recommendation of the AHCPR is that confirmatory tests, especially MRI, if available, should be performed quickly, in view of the serious consequences of neglect in these patients. Acute-onset cauda equina syndrome is unusual, however. A nonsystematic review by Ahn et al. (5) found 322 patients with this syndrome reported in the world literature with a time interval between onset and surgery, but these investigators could find no significant difference in outcome between patients operated on within 24 hours or within 24 to 48 hours of the onset of the syndrome. After 48 hours, however, there seemed to be less chance of resolution of the patients' severe neurologic loss. Urinary incontinence and bowel and sexual function were restored in more than 60% of patients operated on within the above-mentioned time limit.

This finding means that the proper investigations should be performed quickly, to elucidate the true cause of the severe symptoms. When a tumor presses on the spinal cord or a disc hernia presses on the cauda equina, daytime surgery should be performed, all within 48 hours of the onset of this condition.

Radiculopathy: Nerve Root Pain

For patients with suspected disc hernia causing radiculopathy, several studies have demonstrated the importance of the clinical history and the examination to establish the diagnosis. The most important of these studies, with an acceptable interobserver reliability and positive predictive value, are listed in Table 9.16.

The reproducibility of Lasègue's sign or straight leg raising in routine general practice, however, seems to be low, with a kappa coefficient between 0.33 and 0.56. The proportion of positive agreement was 67%, and negative agreement was 91% (357).

Unless a patient has severe neurologic signs indicating the presence of a possible cauda equina syndrome or unless the patient's pain is intolerable, the confirmatory test, usually MRI, should be performed later (in 4 to 5 weeks), according to the recommendations in most guidelines (32,114,297,301,302) (Table 9.6). These guidelines are partly based on the findings of Weber (388,389), who reported that most patients with radiculopathy recover within 1 month without surgical intervention.

The positive predictive value of MRI, CT, and water contrast myelography is good in these patients, but, as seen in the Table 9.8, many disc hernias also occur in persons without symptoms. Thus, the sensitivity is high, but the specificity considerably lower.

The predictors for a good result after surgical intervention have also been investigated by numerous authors (93,199,347,349,373,374,389). These include the absence

TABLE 9.16. *Findings in patients with a history of well-described lumbar nerve root pain of sufficient predictive value for finding a disc hernia at neuroradiographic examination*

Finding	Prediction strength
Crossed straight leg raising (SLR) reproducing pain in the symptomatic leg	+++
SLR <60 degrees (SLR reproduces leg pain)	++
Ankle dorsiflexion weakness	+
Great toe weakness	+
Impaired ankle reflex	+
Sensory loss, pins and needles, paresthesia	+
Patellar reflex weakness	+
Ankle reflex weakness	+
Severe radicular pain	++
Pain causing awakening at night	++
Severe lumbar motion restriction	++
Loss of lordosis and/or sciatic scoliosis	++
Unilateral leg pain worse than back pain	++
Radiation into foot	+
Pain drawing (exact dermatome depicted)	(+)

Data from references 10, 32, 359, and 373.

of psychosocial disturbances (42,43,143,382), more severe pain on a VAS scale (7 or more), pain at night, no previous surgery, and MRI evidence of clear nerve root engagement of the disc hernia (Table 9.17).

Other factors of importance for outcome include insurance systems, social factors, and the patient's working situation. In most studies from the United States, patients with workers' compensation insurance return to work less quickly and receive disability benefits much longer than patients without such insurance (247).

Torvaldsen and Sorensen (347), in a prospective survey of outcome of 130 patients followed for 6 months after lumbar spine surgery, clearly demonstrated that psychologic vulnerability had a relative risk ratio of nearly 2 for persisting pain after such surgery. The association with psychologic vulnerability and employment after surgery was 6.0.

In the study by Vucetic et al. (374), who prospectively followed 160 consecutive patients undergoing primary surgery for suspected disc herniation and considered diagnostic and prognostic factors using stepwise logistic regression analysis, history and pain analysis contained most of the predictive information. Extremely severe pain,

TABLE 9.17. *Assessment of predictors for a good (+) or less good (−) outcome of disc hernia surgery in patients with radiculopathy*

Predictor	Outcome
History and physical examination from Table 9.16 mostly present	++
MRI positive for nerve root involvement	++
MRI bulging disc	−−
Findings at surgery:	
Free fragment	++
Definite protrusion	+
Bulging disc	−
Workers' compensation insurance	−
Presence of psychosocial deterrants or illness behavior signs and symptoms	−−
Absence of any such signs	++

MRI, magnetic resonance imaging.
Data from references 42, 43, 87, 93, 106, 143, 194, 247, 310, 373, and 374.

a crossed Lasègue sign, dislocation of the nerve root on MRI, no comorbidity, no previous surgery, and severe restriction of motion were important predictors in the history and examination for finding a disc hernia at surgery. Pain intensity and pain-related factors (e.g., description of radiation) accounted for 70% of the variability of results in the logistic regression analysis for findings at surgery. Social and behavior factors accounted for approximately 22%. Structural findings on the myelogram, which was the confirmatory test, added only 8%.

Vucetic et al. (374) also found leg pain at night predictive of the presence of a disc hernia, a finding that was corroborated by other authors (2,110,162). In another study, Roach et al. (292) found no factors with extremely high sensitivity to predict the surgical finding. The highest values for sensitivity 87% and for specificity of 50% were obtained by combining the symptoms of difficulty in sleeping, awakening by pain, and pain worsened by walking.

In contrast the relatively poor interobserver and intraobserver reliability of the Lasègue test (straight leg raising) in general practice noted by van den Hoogen et al. (357), Andersson and Deyo (10), in patients in whom the gold standard was disc herniation found at surgery, sensitivity and specificity were considerably better, with prevalence ranging from 60% to 88%, sensitivity ranging from 72% to 97%, and specificity ranging from 11% to 66%; for crossed straight leg raising, the specificity was 85% to 100%.

Wittenberg et al. (398) found no correlation between neurologic deficit and size of the prolapse in 54 consecutive patients operated on and who had undergone preoperative MRI. These investigators concluded that the image of a prolapse on MRI should not be used as an indication for surgery unless there is strong correlation with clinical findings, nor did the clinical follow-up correlate with the MRI images in these patients.

In a large but poorly controlled multicenter longitudinal study (4), approximately 1,000 patients were retrospectively analyzed to determine the association among imaging findings, therapy, and functional outcome (disability days). On the basis of the multivariate analysis, 8 of the 12 baseline potential confounding factors were independently associated with a worse functional outcome. Among these were age older than 40 years, receipt of disability compensation, low level of education, previous lumbar spine surgery, presence of Waddell nonorganic signs, and comorbidity. The strongest confounding factors for poor outcome were involvement in litigation and patients' own reports of inactivity.

The findings at surgery of a ruptured annulus and a sequestered disc were highly predictive of relief of back pain at 2 years. These surgical findings were also considered important by Ackerman et al. (4) and by Deyo et al. (93).

There is no support in the literature that surgery for mild to moderate peripheral muscle weakness in the first month after the onset of sciatica has any significance for the results, nor is that the case for patients with sensory disturbances, as already pointed out by Weber (388) in the first prospective randomized trials performed on these patients. These findings were confirmed by Vucetic et al. (374).

Herron et al. (151,152) and Spengler et al. (331), in large series of patients, demonstrated the value of psychologic questionnaires in predicting outcome in patients operated on for disc herniation.

Boos and collaborators reported on the only known study (42) in which 46 patients with low back pain and sciatica, severe enough to require discectomy, were compared with 46 age-, sex-, and risk factor-matched asymptomatic volunteers (same amount of heavy lifting, twisting, bending, vibration, and sedentary activity). Both groups had a complete clinical and MRI examination and completed a questionnaire to assess differences in psychosocial and work perception profiles. The prevalence, severity, and location of the morphologic alterations (disc herniation, disc degeneration, and neural compromise) were analyzed by two independent radiologists in blinded fashion. MRI findings, work perception, job satisfaction, mental stress, and psychosocial factors (anxiety, depression, self-control, social support, and marital status) were compared between the two groups, using multivariate techniques. Stepwise discriminate analysis was used to identify the best variables within the MRI, work perception, and psychosocial categories in terms of diagnostic accuracy to predict group membership (pain or no-pain group). The surprising finding of 73% MRI-positive disc hernias in the risk factor—matched group of asymptomatic persons is notable. In the operated group, the MRI findings were positive in 96%. The patients had more severe disc herniations and significantly more often laterally located herniations with presence of neural compromise, which constituted a significant difference. The operated group also had significantly more occupational mental stress, less job satisfaction, and abnormal psychologic factors such as anxiety and depression.

Schade et al. (310) further analyzed the general psychologic factors and the psychosocial aspects of work and, with multiple regression, identified the best predictor variables of four different outcome measures (pain relief, reduction of disability in daily activities, return to work, and surgical outcome) on the same material as mentioned earlier. MRI-identified nerve root compromise and social support from the patient's spouse were independent predictors of pain relief 2 years after surgery (patients were reexamined by unbiased observers.) Return to work 2 years after surgery was best predicted by lack of depression and less occupational mental stress, whereas a combination of these two factors was a significant predictor of a good surgical outcome. Return to work was not influenced by any clinical finding or MRI picture, but solely by psychologic factors and psychologic and psychosocial aspects of work.

Factors for good and poor predictors of a positive outcome of lumbar disc surgery are seen in Table 9.17. That spine surgeons need to evaluate the psychosocial factors of their patients has been studied and reinforced (136).

Suspected Spinal Stenosis and/or Root Canal or Foraminal Stenosis

Pain syndromes relating to changes of the aging lumbar spine are increasing because of the shift in population demographics. Increasing bulging of the discs in the neck as well as in the lumbar area combined with osteophytes and arthritic changes of the facet joints can cause narrowing of the spinal canal, encroachment on the content of the dural sack, or localized nerve root canal stenosis. In addition, some patients have congenitally small canals (15,174,367). The clinical presentation of the more common degenerative central spinal stenosis includes back pain, psuedoclaudication, numbness, weakness, and leg pain that is usually diffuse, rarely radicular, and often bilateral. Results of straight leg raising are usually negative (8,140).

There are few scientific evaluations of the sensitivity and specificity of history and physical examinations with correlation to imaging and sometimes to operative findings. Katz et al. (185) used the opinion of two orthopedic surgeons who were "experts" on the presence or absence of spinal stenosis as a gold standard. The investigators study calculated sensitivity, specificity, and likelihood ratios found best for patients aged more than 65 years, pain relief from sitting, and a wide-based gait. In this study, increasing pain in the legs when walking did not reach statistical significance. Other authors, such as Hall et al. (140), found this to be the case, however, in 94% of patients whose findings of stenosis were confirmed by surgery (no mention was made of the measurement method at surgery). Jonsson and Stromqvist (177,178), in their evaluation of symptoms and signs in 100 patients operated on for spinal stenosis and 100 operated on for lateral or root canal stenosis, found in these two categories about 65% of patients with decreased walking ability. Other authors used treadmill walking tests and found this method useful for classification, with high likelihood ratios better than self-reported variables (85,122). Deen et al. (85) tested 50 patients preoperatively and found the walking distance significantly increased at 3-month postoperative follow-up. Szpalski et al. (340) used an isoinertial trunk-testing dynamometric machine to demonstrate decreased extension in patients with clinically suspected stenosis.

Herno et al. (149,150) and Jonsson et al. (179) tried to correlate their results 4 to 5 years postoperatively to various preoperative signs and history, including measurements from radiographs. In these studies, as well as in the study by Atlas et al. (17), which was also uncontrolled, prognosis was poorer for patients with comorbidity such as diabetes, degenerative hip arthritis, and old vertebral fractures, whereas a positive predictor of outcome of surgery was the measured anteroposterior diameter at the narrowest part (less than 6 mm). There has been no proper study to evaluate at what point the radiologic diagnosis of spinal stenosis or root canal stenosis can be ascertained. All follow-up studies lack a correlation between the reported imaging measures and the end result. The figures usually quoted are those of Verbiest (367), who stated that an anteroposterior distance of less than 11 mm constituted stenosis, a measure weakly confirmed by Karantanas et al. (182). For root canal stenosis, Verbiest (367) found that a diameter less than 4 mm indicated stenosis. His measurements were taken during surgery. Karantanas et al. found even 3 mm on measurements from CT unreliable. These investigators evaluated 100 patients with low back pain but not stenosis or leg pain symptoms. As described in the evaluation of the MRI investigations (Table 9.8), radiologists believe that 30% to 40% of nonsymptomatic persons older than 40 years of age have stenosis. Amundsen et al. (8), in their study of 100 patients with clinical stenosis, found the imaging measurements highly variable.

The metaanalysis performed by Kent et al. (188) in their review article on the accuracy of CT, MRI, and myelography in the diagnosis of spinal stenosis concluded that there is a lack of information about the contribution of imaging tests to predict clinical outcomes. Moreover, these investigators could find no studies analyzing the effect of electrophysiologic tests for understanding patients' responses to surgery.

Guigui and collaborators (138) analyzed a series of 61 patients (mean age, 63 years) operated on for spinal stenosis with severe motor deficit and noted complete regression in 22 patients and partial regression in 29. Chances of recovery were better when the deficit was monoradicular and when there was a single-level stenosis.

Schonstrom (312) found symptoms in patients with a transverse area measured on CT myelography of less than 70 mm^2 to be more prevalent, and Hamanishi et al. (141) confirmed this finding. These investigators also confirmed more symptoms in patients who have this finding at two levels, as suggested by Porter and Ward's (276) original observations. Studies have also demonstrated positional variability of surface area measurement, as well as the influence of axial loading and various bodily positions (83,182,394,402). No study was found for proper evaluation of history and imaging findings for the result of surgery for root canal stenosis.

Patients with suspected root canal stenosis usually present with atypical pain patterns in one leg, not like in radiculopathy, in which pain is also present at rest, walking

TABLE 9.18. *Best evidence synthesis for symptoms and findings in patients with possible spinal stenosis who may benefit from treatment*

History or test	Predictor strength
Age >65 yr	Moderate
Bilateral nonradicular leg pain	Moderate
Walking distance <300 m	Weak
Treadmill test total time <5 min	Moderate
Relief from sitting down or squatting	Moderate
MRI/CT diameter <7 mm, area <70 mm^2	Good to Moderate
Neurophysiologic tests	Not demonstrated
Comorbidity	Negative

MRI, magnetic resonance imaging; CT, computed tomography.

usually increases the pain, and there may be some leg weakness. In the prospective study by Jonsson and Stromqvist (178), in which this condition was called lateral stenosis, the most striking difference from patients with disc herniation was the absence of a positive straight leg raising test: 10% in patients with disc hernia and 70% in the stenosis group. Table 9.18 provides a best-evidence synthesis of the foregoing findings.

MISCELLANEOUS ASSESSMENT TOOLS FOR THE PATIENT WITH LOW BACK PAIN AND/OR LEG PAIN

In addition to the more commonly used methods in assessing patients with low back and/or leg pain, other methods have been investigated, in particular for finding additional signs in patients with chronic low back pain that could help to explain and perhaps improve treatment. Rarely, however, have such studies demonstrated clinical utility in scientifically admissible studies and, if so, only in small numbers of patients. In addition, Ramsey et al. (281) found the evaluation of various diagnostic and treatment devices lacking in scientific rigor.

These studies include the following:

1. Facet blocks.
2. Neurophysiologic tests including EMG.
3. Stress radiographs and flexion and extension x-ray studies.
4. Discography.
5. Diagnostic nerve root infiltration.
6. Bone scintigraphy.
7. Thermography.
8. Diagnostic ultrasound.
9. Temporary external fixation.

A short description of the results reported is given here for these assessment modalities in the approximate order of their use in secondary or tertiary referral centers for patients with chronic low back pain.

Facet Blocks

Facet blocks have been used for symptom relief for patients with lumbar, as well as neck pain. Selective blocks have also been used in an attempt to determine some specific symptoms that could characterize such patients (37). These attempts have failed, and clinical utility has not been demonstrated in patients with pain in the lumbar area (23,38,62,166,211,212,231,252,284,315–318) or in patients with common chronic neck pain (25).

In an attempt to improve marginally the efficacy of facet joint injection, Revel et al. (285) tried to determine clinical criteria that could predict significant relief of back pain after injection. By combining certain clinical characteristics, these investigators were able to select patients whose pain was relieved by 70% by the facet joint block. These characteristics were age greater than 65 years, pain not exacerbated by coughing, pain not worsened by hyperextension, pain not worsened by forward flexion, pain not worsened when rising from flexion, pain not worsened by extension-rotation, and pain relieved by recumbency. These criteria distinguished 92% of patients who responded to anesthetic injection and 80% of those who did not respond. This last mentioned study is the first that tried to find possible utility for this test. It should not, according to the authors themselves, be considered as a diagnostic criterion for facet joint syndromes in clinical practice with individual patients, but could help in future randomized studies as a criterion for selecting patients with probable painful facet joints.

The one positive investigation, conducted by Lord et al. (218,219) in patients with chronic whiplash, is described in Chapter 16. These investigators performed two double-blind placebo-controlled local anesthetic cervical facet blocks and found complete relief on two occasions as indicative that the facet was involved. Again in a placebo-controlled prospective randomized trial of electrocauterization of the nerve to this joint, these investigators noted pain relief for 1 year but not longer (219,236). The possible utility of blocks in the cervical region needs to be confirmed for ordinary neck pain.

Neurophysiologic Tests Including Electromyography

Tests especially for nerve root disorders include neurophysiologic examination. Dvorák (105) suggested that electrophysiologic testing may be useful for exclusion of more distal nerve damage (neuropathy or nerve entrapment in the extremities) and for verification of subjective muscle weakness by needle EMG in patients presenting with pain inhibition or lack of cooperation.

Dvorák (104,105) also tabulated all the various neurophysiologic techniques used: somatosensory-evoked potentials, motor-evoked potentials, neurographic F-wave testing, H-reflex testing, and EMG of leg muscles and of paraspinal muscles. He also listed false-negative findings of some of these tests in patients with lumbar radiculopathy: for sensory-evoked potentials, the rate was 65%, and for motor-evoked potentials, it was 75%.

Tullberg (349) prospectively followed 60 patients with single-level disc herniation confirmed on CT for 1 year with evaluation by an unbiased observer. In 20 of these patients, neurophysiologic tests were performed: EMG, sensory-evoked potentials, and F-wave testing. There was discordance between neurophsyiologic and radiologic findings, and the neurophysiologic tests did not predict the success rate. The only positive finding was that when results of ordinary neurophysiologic tests were normal, the outcome was worse than when the test showed abnormality. In Tullberg's study (349), EMG was found to be the most sensitive test, but the sensitivity was only around 45% to predict the exact level of root lesion; for F-wave testing, it was only 34%, and for sensory-evoked potentials, it was 40%. He concluded that neurophysiologic tests are not useful to diagnose the exact level of a nerve root lesion, but they may reveal whether it is present. This testing is recommended only when radiology and clinical findings conflict.

Park et al. (266) also evaluated EMG from the back and from the limbs correlated to the findings at surgery and CT and found it of some confirmatory value but neither sensitive nor specific enough. Arena et al. (14) compared EMG in patients with clinical back pain with EMG in control subjects and found more abnormal readings in the patients with back pain, but again insufficient utility. Date et al. (84) also studied the prevalence of paraspinal lumbar spontaneous activity with EMG in asymptomatic subjects and found it to be positive in approximately 30% of patients older than 40 years.

The result of the literature review of the AHCPR (32) up to 1993 stated equivocal evidence that needle EMG and H-reflex testing of the lower limb may be useful in assessing questionable nerve root dysfunction in patients with leg symptoms lasting longer than 4 weeks, but this report did not recommend electrophysiologic testing if the clinical history and imaging tests were obvious. The AHCPR also found that surface EMG and F-wave testing could not be recommended for assessing patients with acute or chronic back pain, whereas sensory-evoked potentials may be useful in assessing suspected spinal stenosis and spinal cord myelopathy.

Stress Radiography and Flexion and Extension Radiography

The clinical value of these radiographic studies for diagnosis of instability or subluxations in patients without preceding trauma or surgery has not been demonstrated, perhaps because of wide measurement errors from ordinary radiographs (81,82,121, 273,338). Reviews of the literature on the subject (245–248) failed to find any studies showing the clinical utility of any of the methods used to measure instability including roentgenstereophotogrammetric analysis (18–21,82,175,176,184). Roentgenstereophotogrammetric analysis is accurate, but invasive, with good reliability, but no published study exists to demonstrate its utility.

Discography

One of the most controversial diagnostic tests is discography, a method by which fluid with or without contrast media is injected into presumed degenerated and painful discs, as a preoperative test for performing fusion or as a method of choosing the level of fusion (243). When the patient recognizes the pain exactly (pain provocation positive) and the disc also shows signs of degeneration, as the test can demonstrate, this method has been used by many authors as an indication for lumbar or cervical fusion for patients with chronic pain. This test is not generally used to detect disc hernia because studies have demonstrated that MRI or CT is superior in that respect (167).

Clinical utility has not been demonstrated, that is, to determine whether discography helps in the outcome of lumbar fusion, a procedure that in itself has not been proven effective in patients with chronic low back pain or neck pain (see Chapters 13 and 16). The only scientific evaluation performed to assess the specificity and sensitivity of the test is the study by Walsh et al. (384), which used young, healthy volunteers and compared them with patients with chronic back pain. These investigators demonstrated few positive tests in the healthy voluneteers. This study was conducted in response to an older study by Holt (159) using volunteer prisoners, who showed positive responses, and persons without a history of neck pain.

There have been debates on the use of discography in assessment of chronic back pain (39,250). Even though some investigators believe in this approach and others do not, both sides agree with respect to its unproven utility in relation to therapy. In a position statement, the North American Spine Society (139) recommended the use of this technique for further evaluation of abnormal discs to assess the extent of abnormality or correlation of this abnormality with clinical symptoms. Discography has also been recommended as a preoperative test when fusion is considered in a patient with chronic low back pain in whom conservative treatment has failed. However, in the same position statement (139) and in the discussions by proponents of this technique such as Bogduk and Modic (39) and Zdeblick (Nachemson [250]), it has clearly been stated that "in order to determine how a diagnostic test alters the outcome of treatment it is necessary to define the diagnosis, the type of surgery and the outcome evaluation method in ways that have not been done until this day." Until such studies are performed, it will not be possible to endorse or deny the value of a specific test for the surgical outcome.

The response to discography has also been correlated with abnormal pain drawings, a finding showing that psychologic overlay and pain sensitivity are predictive of a positive response (34,264). Colhoun et al. (74) published one of the few studies that prospectively performed discography and then operated on the patients irrespective of the response. These investigators then compared the results in those 137 discography-positive patients that were followed up after fusion, who had an 89% good result, with the 25 patients who had a negative pain provocation test. Only 52% of these patients had a good result. Patients with pseudoarthrosis were excluded, and although the study was consecutive, according to the author, there was no personal follow-up by an unbiased observer. Retrospective studies reported have been negative for discography as a predictor of outcome (153,265).

Knox and Chapman (195) retrospectively evaluated, by objective criteria, 22 patients undergoing anterior lumbar interbody fusion for discography-concordant low back pain and reported the following results for single-level fusion: 35% good, 18% fair, and 47% poor. Moneta et al. (241) analyzed 533 CT discography studies from surgical candidates to correlate discography-positive response with CT findings and concluded that the positive response was significantly correlated with outer annular ruptures only. Their conclusion was that the outer annulus appears to be the origin of pain reproduction. Another similar study, published in 1998 by Ito et al. (164) and consisting of 39 patients, considered the correlation between discogenic lumbar pain by discography-delineated disc morphology and MRI and showed that radial tears commonly were found on MRI but had a low correlation with concordant pain production.

Esses et al. (111), in a small trial of 35 patients with chronic back pain, found external spinal fixation more reliable in predicting the end result than plain radiographs, discograms, or facet blocks. Schellhas et al. (311), in 10 lifelong asymptomatic subjects and in 10 patients with nonchronic neck pain who underwent discography from C-3 to C-7 after MRI demonstrated 20 normal discs by MRI from the asymptomatic volunteers, of whom 17 had painless annular tears discographically. In patients with pain, 11 discs appeared normal at MRI, but 10 had annular tears discographically, and only 2 had pain reproduced at discography. In both groups, normal discs were not made painful by discography.

Carragee, in a series of clinical trials (66–68) in patients and volunteers limited in number to series of six to ten patients or persons without back pain, clearly demonstrated positive responses to pain provocation in 40% to 80% of pain-prone individuals, defined as follows: patients in whom neck surgery failed but who never had low back pain; patients recruited from a psychiatric clinic who have psychologic distress or somatization disorder but no back pain; or patients who had part of their iliac wings resected for transplantation purposes but no history of low back pain. Like Bogduk and Modic (39), Carragee (65) doubts the existence of "internal disc disruption" (79) as a clinical valid concept.

Pain response from discography can be mediated by increased pain sensitivity, perhaps at the spinal cord level or by psychologic disturbances. Discography can depict disc degeneration, but it is less predictive of the presence of disc herniation. Positive discography is rare in normal discs in asymptomatic persons, and the true rate of complications of discography such as infection and bleeding have not been established. Its clinical utility remains unproven.

Nerve Root Infiltration

Investigators have used nerve root injections to attempt to verify the site of suspected clinical foraminal (root canal) compression. Van Akkerveeken (355), in a series of 18 patients, found the positive response predictive of a good outcome, albeit for a short term by personal follow-up. The positive predictive value was 70%.

North et al. (259), in the only scientific study of nerve root infiltrations, did not confirm the value of this technique, whereas Hasue and Kikuchi (144) reported on a series of 129 operated patients in whom false-positive and false-negative results of nerve root injections were determined by operation. These investigators stated a positive predictive value of 93%, but no results of surgery were presented. This diagnostic modality was reviewed in a debate form by Slosar et al. (325). No firm conclusion can be reached for its use at present.

Bone Scintigraphy

In a review, Hendler and Hershkop (148) claimed that bone scintigraphy can determine the age of fracture, can detect spondylolitis, arthritis, and Paget's disease, and can provide a general indicator of malignant versus benign disease. Al-Janabi (6) and Ryan et al. (303) claimed it to be able to confirm metastases before radiographic confirmation. Lack of clinical utility was found by Maigne et al. (224) for sacroiliac syndrome. Claims have also been made of its value in detecting acute spondylolisthesis (75,228).

The exact sensitivity and specificity of bone scintigraphy are unknown, however. This technique demonstrates increased metabolic activity (125). The AHCPR (32) recommended a bone scan to evaluate acute and chronic back problems when spinal tumor, infection, or fracture is suspected from the red flags in the patient's medical history, physical examination, confirmatory laboratory tests, or plain x-ray findings. Bone scans are contraindicated during pregnancy. The summary of the findings of the literature by AHCPR was that bone scan is moderately sensitive for detecting suspected tumors, infection, or recent fractures, but it is not specific. The relative accuracy versus other imaging modalities has not been determined, and a study by Kanmaz et al. (181) retrospectively evaluating 1,400 patients with chronic low back pain could not confirm clinical utility.

Thermography

Thermography as a diagnostic aid for cervical or lumbar root syndrome has not been found a valid investigative tool; its sensitivity is around 50%, and its specificity is 45% (235). The findings in the earlier metaanalytic review by Hoffman et al. (155) confirmed that there is no evidence for its clinical utility. No validation study has surfaced since 1993.

Diagnostic Ultrasound

Porter et al. (277) originally advocated ultrasound lumbar canal measurement as a diagnostic technique, but the method was found unreliable by Asztely et al. (16) and by Anderson et al. (9). In an article by Eisele et al. (107), the claim was made that ultrasound texture analysis of paraspinal lumbar muscles allowed a rapid and easily performed investigation for relating discal disorders on the lumbar spine to the reported pain and disability.

A controlled study by Nazarian et al. (253), however, reached the conclusion that paraspinal ultrasonography is neither accurate nor reproducible in assessing patients with cervical or lumbar back pain. In the same year, 1998, the Therapeutics and Technology Subcommittee of the American Academy of Neurology (345) concluded that no published peer reviewed literature supports the use of diagnostic ultrasound in evaluation of patients with back pain or radicular symptoms. The procedure cannot be recommended for use in the clinical evaluation of such patients. This statement was based on a thorough literature search and is also supported by an earlier similar statement from the American College of Radiology (7).

Temporary External Fixation

Temporary external fixation as a test for predicting success or failure of surgery for back pain and neck pain has been studied by several authors. Axelsson et al. (18) used roentgenstereophotogrammetric analysis to establish whether sagittal intervertebral translation was significantly reduced by the use of an external frame fixed to the iliac wings. The claim was confirmed.

Jeanneret et al. (169) used this technique as an assessment before contemplating fusion in 101 patients with disabling low back pain. In 47 patients whose pain was relieved by stabilization but whose pain returned after destabilization, the result after fusion was available for 34; 76% had acceptable results, compared with fusion performed in 7 of the 52 patients who did not respond positively and who had poor results.

Soini et al. (328,329) had similar experience in a prospective study of 42 patients, and a 2-year follow-up demonstrated that the result of lumbar fusion corresponds to the preoperative fixation test, and this test may be useful in assessment if lumbar fusion is considered. Faraj et al. (117) had significant numbers of complications, as did some other investigators (111,327), and claimed that the test was invasive and its use could not be justified. Grob et al. (137) used this technique as a prospective preoperative test in the cervical spine of 24 patients with neck pain and thought that it could be helpful but stated that the definite clinical value was still lacking.

REFERENCES

1. Abenhaim L, Rossignol M, Gobeille D, et al. The prognostic consequences in the making of the initial medical diagnosis of work-related back injuries. *Spine* 1995;20:791–795.
2. Abramovitz J, Neff S. Lumbar disc surgery: results of the prospective lumbar discectomy study of the joint section on disorders of the spine and peripheral nerves of the American Association of Neurological Surgeons and the Congress of Neurological Surgeons. *Neurosurgery* 1991;29:301–308.
3. Accident Rehabilitation and Compensation Insurance Corporation of New Zealand (ACC) and the National Health Committee. *New Zealand acute low back pain guide.* Wellington, NZ: ACC and the National Health Committee, 1996.
4. Ackerman SJ, Steinberg EP, Bryan RN, et al. Persistent low back pain in patients suspected of having herniated nucleus pulposus: radiologic predictors of functional outcome—implications for treatment selection. *Radiology* 1997;203:815–822.
5. Ahn UM, Ahn NU, Buchowski J, et al. Cauda equina syndrome secondary to lumbar disc herniation: a meta-analysis of surgical outcomes (abst). In: *Abstracts of the ISSLS meeting.* Hawaii: ISSLS, 1999: 40.
6. Al-Janabi MA. Imaging modalities and low back pain: the role of bone scintigraphy. *Nucl Med Commun* 1995;16:317–326.
7. American College of Radiology. *Statement on spinal ultrasound.* Reston, VA: American College of Radiology, 1996.
8. Amundsen T, Weber H, Lilleas F, et al. Lumbar spinal stenosis: clinical and radiologic features. *Spine* 1995;20:1178–1186.
9. Anderson DJ, Adcock DF, Chovil AC, et al. Ultrasound lumbar canal measurment in hospital employees with back pain. *Br J Ind Med* 1988;45:552–555.
10. Andersson GBJ, Deyo RA. History and physical examination in patients with herniated lumbar discs. *Spine* 1996;21;10S–18S.
11. Andersson GBJ, Deyo RA. Sensitivity, specificity, and predictive value: a general issue in screening for disease and in the interpretation of diagnostic studies in spinal disorders. In: Frymoyer JW, ed. *The adult spine: principles and practice,* 2nd ed. Philadelphia: Lippincott–Raven, 1997:305–317.
12. Annertz M, Wingstrand H, Stromqvist B, et al. MR imaging as the primary modality for neuroradiologic evaluation of the lumbar spine: effects on cost and number of examinations. *Acta Radiol* 1996;37:373–380.
13. Aprill C, Bogduk N. High intensity zone: a diagnostic sign of painful lumbar disc on magnetic resonance imaging. *Br J Radiol* 1992;65:361–369.
14. Arena JG, Sherman RA, Bruno GM, et al. Electromyographic recordings of low back pain subjects and non-pain controls in six different positions: effect of pain levels. *Pain* 1991;45:23–28.
15. Arnoldi CC, Brodsky AE, Cauchoix J, et al. Lumbar spinal stenosis and nerve root entrapment syndromes: definition and classification. *Clin Orthop* 1976;115:4.
16. Asztely M, Kadziolka R, Nachemson A. A comparison of sonography and myelography in clinically suspected spinal stenosis. *Spine* 1983;8:885–890.
17. Atlas SJ, Deyto RA, Keller RB, et al. The Maine lumbar spine study. III. One-year outcomes of surgical and nonsurgical management of lumbar spinal stenosis. *Spine* 1996;21:1787–1794.
18. Axelsson P, Johnsson R, Stromqvist B. Diagnostic external fixation of the lumbar spine: a roentgen stereophotogrammetric analysis in the diagnosis of cervical zygapophysial joint pain. *Pain* 1993;55:99–106.
19. Axelsson P. Johnsson R, Stromqvist B. Mechanics of the external fixator test in the lumbar spine: a roentgen stereophotogrammetric analysis. *Spine* 1996;21:330–333.
20. Axelsson P, Johnsson R, Stromqvist B. The spondylytic vertebrae and its adjacent segment: mobility before and after posterolateral fusion. *Spine* 1997;22:414–417.
21. Axelsson P, Johnsson R, Strömqvist B, et al. External pedicular fixation of the lumbar spine: outcome evaluation by functional tests. *J Spinal Disord* 1999;12:148–150.
22. Baker DJ, Pynsent PB, Fairbank JCT. The Oswestry Disability Index revisited: its reliability, repeatability and validity, and a comparison with the St. Thomas's Disability Index. In: Roland MO, Jenner JR, eds. *Back pain: new approaches to rehabilitation and education.* Manchester, UK: Manchester University Press, 1989:174–186.
23. Barnsley L, Lord S, Bogduk N. Comparative local anaesthetic blocks in the diagnosis of cervical zygapophysial joint pain. *Pain* 1993;55:99–106.
24. Barnsley L, Lord S, Bogduk N. Whiplash injury. *Pain* 1994;58:283–307.
25. Barnsley L, Lord SM, Wallis BJ, et al. Lack of effect of intraarticular corticosteroids for chronic pain in the cervial zygapophyseal joints. *N Engl J Med* 1994;330:1047–1050.
26. Battié MC, Videman T, Gibbons LE, et al. Determinants of lumbar disc degeneration: a study relating lifetime exposures and magnetic resonance imaging findings in identical twins. *Spine* 1995;20:2601–2612.

27. Beaton DE, Hogg-Johnson S, Bombardier C. Evaluating changes in health status: reliability and responsiveness of five generic health status measures in workers with muskuloskeletal disorders. *J Clin Epidemiol* 1997;50:79–93.
28. Beck AT, Rush AJ, Shaw BF, et al., eds. *Cognitive therapy of depression.* New York: Guilford Press, 1979.
29. Bergner M, Bobbitt RA, Carter WB, et al. The sickness impact profile: development and final revision of a health status measure. *Med Care* 1981;19:787–805.
30. Bernstein IH, Jaremko ME, Hinkley BS. On the utility of the West Haven-Yale Multidimensional Pain Inventory. *Spine* 1995;20:956–953.
31. Biering-Sörensen F. Physical measurements as risk indicators for low-back trouble over a one-year period. *Spine* 1984;9:106–119.
32. Bigos S, Bowyer O, Braen, et al. *Acute low-back problems in adults: clinical practice guideline no. 14.* AHCPR publication no. 95–0642. Rockville, MD: Agency for Health Care Policy and Research, Public Health Service, United States Department of Health and Human Services, 1994.
33. Bigos SJ, Hansson T, Castillo RN, et al. The value of preemployment roentgenographs for predicting acute back injury claims and chronic back pain disability. *Clin Orthop* 1992;283:124–129.
34. Block AA, Vanharanta H, Ohnmeiss DD, et al. Discographic pain report: influence of psychological factors. *Spine* 1996;21:334–338.
35. Boden SD, Davis DO, Dina TS, et al. Abnormal magnetic-resonance scans of the lumbar spine in asymptomatic subjects: a prospective investigation. *J Bone Joint Surg Am* 1990;72:403–408.
36. Boden SD, McCowin PR, Davis DO, et al. Abnormal magnetic-resonance scans of the cervical spine in asymptomatic subjects: a prospective investigation. *J Bone Joint Surg Am* 1990;72:1178–1184.
37. Bogduk N. Musculoskeletal pain: toward precision diagnosis. In: Jensen TS, Turner JA, Wiesenfeld-Hallin Z, eds. *Proceedings of the 8th World Congress on Pain: progress in pain research and management.* Seattle: IASP Press, 1997:507–525.
38. Bogduk N, Aprill C. On the nature of neck pain, discography and cervical zygapophysical joint blocks. *Pain* 1993;54:213–217.
39. Bogduk N, Modic MT. Lumbar discography. *Spine* 1996;21:402–404.
40. Boos N, Lander PH. Clinical efficacy of imaging modalities in the diagnosis of low-back pain disorders. *Eur Spine J* 1996;5:2–22.
41. Boos N, Dreier D, Hilfiker E, et al. Tissue characterization of symptomatic and asymptomatic disc herniations by quantitative magnetic resonance imaging. *J Orthop Res* 1997;15:141–149.
42. Boos N, Rieder R, Schade V, et al. The diagnostic accuracy of magnetic resonance imaging, work perception, and psychosocial factors in identifying symptomatic disc herniations. *Spine* 1995;20:2613–2625.
43. Boos N, Semmer N, Elfering A, et al. Psychosocial factors and not MRI-based disc abnormalities predict future low-back pain-related medical consultation and work absence (abst). In: *Abstracts of the ISSLS meeting.* Hawaii: ISSLS, 1999:19.
44. Boos N, Wallin A, Gbedegbegnon T, et al. Quantitative MR imaging of lumbar intervertebral disks and vertebral bodies: influence of diurnal water content variations. *Radiology* 1993;188:351–354.
45. Borchgrevink G, Smevik O, Haave I, et al. MRI of cerebrum and cervical columna within two days after whiplash neck sprain injury. *Injury* 1997;28:331–335.
46. Borenstein DG, Wiesel SW, eds. *Low back pain: medical diagnosis and comprehensive management.* Philadelphia: WB Saunders, 1989.
47. Borenstein DG, Wiesel SW, Boden SD, eds. *Neck pain: medical diagnosis and comprehensive management.* Philadelphia: WB Saunders, 1996.
48. Borenstein DG, O'Mara JW, Boden SD, et al. A 7–year follow-up study of the value of lumbar spine MR to predict the development of low back pain in asymptomatic individuals (abst). In: *Abstracts of the ISSLS meeting.* Brussels: ISSLS, 1998:112.
49. Borghouts JAJ, Koes BW, Bouter LM. The clinical course and prognostic factors of non-specific neck pain: a systematic review. *Pain* 1998;77:1–13.
50. Borkan J, Reis S, Ribak J, et al. *Guidelines for the treatment of low back pain in primary care.* Tel Aviv: Israeli Low Back Pain Guidelines Group, 1995.
51. Brant-Zawadzki MN, Jensen MC, Obuchowski N, et al. Interobserver and intraobserver variability in interpretation of lumbar disc abnormalities: a comparison of two nomenclatures. *Spine* 1995;20:1257–1263.
52. Breslau J, Jarvik JG, Haynor DR, et al. MR contrast media in neuroimaging: a critical review of the literature. *AJNR Am J Neuroradiol* 1999;20:670–675.
53. Brismar H, Vucetic N, Svensson O. Pain patterns in lumbar disc hernia: drawings compared to surgical findings in 159 patients. *Acta Orthop Scand* 1996;67:470–472.
54. Brodie D, Burnett JW, Walker JM, et al. Evaluation of low back pain by patient questionnaires and therapist assessment. *J Orthop Sports Phys Ther* 1990;11:519–526.
55. Brolin I. Product control of lumbar radiographs [in Swedish]. *Lakartidningen* 1975;72:1793–1795.
56. Buirski G, Silberstein M. The symptomatic lumbar disc in patients with low-back pain: magnetic

resonance imaging appearances in both a symptomatic and control population. *Spine* 1993;18:1808–1811.

57. Buchbinder R, Goel V, Bombardier C, et al. Classification systems of soft tissue disorders of the neck and upper limb: do they satisfy methodological guidelines? *J Clin Epidemiol* 1996;49:141–149.

58. Burton A, Battié M, Gibbons L, et al. Lumbar disc degeneration and sagittal flexibility. *J Spinal Disord* 1996;9:418–424.

59. Bush K, Chaudhuri R, Hillier S, et al. The pathomorphologic changes that accompany the resolution of cervical radiculopathy: a prospective study with repeat magnetic resonance imaging. *Spine* 1997;22:183–187.

60. Bush T, Cherkin D, Barlow W. The impact of physician attitudes on patients satisfaction with care for low back pain. *Arch Fam Med* 1993;2:301–305.

61. Calin A, Porta J, Fries JF, et al. Clinical history as a screening test for ankylosing spondylitis. *JAMA* 1977;237:2613–2614.

62. Carette S, Marcoux S, Truchon R, et al. A controlled trial of corticosteroid injections into facet joints for chronic low back pain. *N Engl J Med* 1991;325:1002–1007.

63. Carey TS, Garrett J. Patterns of ordering diagnostic tests for patients with acute low back pain: the North Carolina Back Pain Project. *Ann Intern Med* 1996;125:807–814.

64. Carey TS, Evans A, Hadler N, et al. Care-seeking among individuals with chronic low back pain. *Spine* 1995;20:312–317.

65. Carragee E. The prevalence and clinical features of internal disk disruption in patients with low back pain [Letter]. *Spine* 1996;21:776.

66. Carragee EJ, Kim D. A prospective analysis of MRI findings in patients with sciatica and lumbar disk herniation: correlation of outcomes with disk fragment and canal morphology. *Spine* 1997;22:1650–1660.

67. Carragee E, Tanner C, Vittum D, et al. Positive provacative discography as a misleading finding in the evaluation of low back pain. In: *North American Spine Society proceedings.* Chicago, 1997:388.

68. Carragee EJ, Tanner CM, Yang B, et al. False positive lumbar discography: reliability of subjective concordancy assessment during provocative disc injection. *Spine* 1999;24:2542–2547.

69. Cherkin DC, MacCornack FA. Patient evaluations of low back pain care from family physicians and chiropractors. *West J Med* 1989;150:351–355.

70. Cherkin DC, Deyo RA, Battié M, et al. A comparison of physical therapy, chiropractic manipulation and provision of an educational booklet for the treatment of patients with low back pain. *N Engl J Med* 1998;339:1021–1029.

71. Cherkin DC, Deyo RA, Wheeler K, et al. Physician variation in diagnostic testing for low back pain: who you see is what you get. *Arthritis Rheum* 1994;37:15–22.

72. Choler U, Larsson R, Nachemson A, et al. *Ont i ryggen: försök med vårdprogram för patienter med lumbala smärttillstånd.* SPRI report no. 188. 1–100, 1985.

73. Choler U, Larsson R, Nachemson A, et al. A simplified treatment of patients with lumbar pain: relatively simple measures can save a lot of human suffering [in Swedish]. *Lakartidningen* 1989;86:2366–2367.

74. Colhoun E, McCall I, Williams L, et al. Provocation discography as a guide to planning operations on the spine. *J Bone Joint Surg Br* 1988;70:267–271.

75. Collier BD, Johnson RP, Carrera GF, et al. Painful spondylolysis or spondylolisthesis studied by radiography and single-photon emission computed tomography. *Radiology* 1985;154:207–211.

76. Cooke C, Dusik LA, Menard MR, et al. Relationship of performance on the ERGOS work simulator to illness behavior in a workers' compensation population with low back versus limb injury. *J Occup Med* 1994;36:757–762.

77. Coté P, Cassidy D, Yong-Hing K, et al. Apophysial joint degeneration, disc degeneration, and sagittal curve of the cervical spine: can they be measured reliably on radiographs? *Spine* 1997;22:859–864.

78. Coxhead CE, Inskip H, Meade TW, et al. Multicentre trial of physiotherapy in the management is sciatic symptoms. *Lancet* 1981;1(8229):1065–1068.

79. Crock H. Internal disc disruption. *Med J Aust* 1970;1:983–990.

80. Daltroy LH, Cats-Baril WL, Katz JN, et al. The North American Spine Society lumbar spine outcome assessment instrument: reliability and validity tests. *Spine* 1996;21:741–749.

81. Danielson B. *Lumbar isthmic spondylolysis and spondylolisthesis in young and adolescent patients: radiological aspects.* Thesis, Göteborg University, Sweden, 1990.

82. Danielsson B, Frennered K, Irstam L. Roentgenologic assessment of spondylolisthesis. I. A study of measurement variation. *Acta Radiol* 1988;29:345–351.

83. Danielson B, Willén J, Gaulitz A, et al. Axial loading of the spine during CT and MR in patients with suspected lumbar spinal stenosis. *Acta Radiol* 1998;39:604–611.

84. Date ES, Mar EY, Bugola MR, et al. The prevalence of lumpar paraspinal spontaneous acitivty in asymptomatic subjects. *Muscle Nerve* 1996;19:350–354.

85. Deen HG, Zimmerman RS, Lyons MK, et al. Use of the exercise treadmill to measure baseline functional status and surgical outcome in patients with severe lumbar spinal stenosis. *Spine* 1998;23:244–248.

86. De Gagne TA, Mikail SF, D'Eon JL. Confirmatory factor analysis of a 4–factor model of chronic pain evaluation. *Pain* 1995;60:195–202.

87. Deinsberger W, Wollesen I, Jödicke A, et al. Sozioökonomisches Langzeitergebnis nach lumbaler mikrochirurgischer Bandscheibenoperation. *Zentralbl Neurochir* 1997;58:171–176.
88. Deyo RA. Early diagnostic evaluation of low back pain. *J Gen Intern Med* 1986;1:328–338.
89. Deyo RA. Comparative validity of the sickness impact profile and shorter scales for functional assessment in low-back pain. *Spine* 1986;11:951–954.
90. Deyo RA. Magnetic resonance imaging of the lumbar spine: terrific tests or tar baby? *N Engl J Med* 1994;331:115–116.
91. Deyo RA, Diehl AK. Lumbar spine films in primary care: current use and effects of selective ordering criteria. *J Gen Intern Med* 1986;1:20–25.
92. Deyo RA, Diehl AK. Cancer as the cause of back pain frequency, clinical presentation and diagnostic strategies. *J Gen Intern Med* 1988;3:230–238.
93. Deyo R, Loeser J, Bigos S. Herniated lumbar intervertebral disk. *Ann Intern Med* 1990;112:598–603.
94. Deyo RA, Rainville J, Kent DL. What can the history and physical examination tell us about low back pain? *JAMA* 1992;268:760–765.
95. Deyo RA, Battie M, Beurskens AJHM, et al. Outcome measures for low back pain research: a proposal for standardized use. *Spine* 1998;23:2003–2013.
96. Deyo RA, Haselkorn J, Hoffman R, et al. Designing studies of diagnostic tests for low back pain or radiculopathy. *Spine* 1994;19:2057S–2065S.
97. Dillard J, Trafimow J, Andersson GBJ, et al. Motion of the lumbar spine: reliability of two measurements techniques. *Spine* 1991;16:321–324.
98. Dixon JS, Bird HA. Reproducibility along a 10 cm. vertical visual analogue scale. *Ann Rheum Dis* 1981;40:87–89.
99. Donelson R, Silva G, Murphy K. Centralization phenomenon: its usefulness in evaluating and treating referred pain. *Spine* 1990;15:211–213.
100. Donelson R, Aprill C, Medcalf R, et al. A prospective study of centralization of lumbar and referred pain: a predictor of symptomatic discs and annular competence. *Spine* 1999;22:1115–1122.
101. Donelson R, Grant W, Kamps C, et al. Pain response to sagittal end-range spinal motion: a prospective, randomized, multicentered trial. *Spine* 1991;16:S206–S212.
102. Dreyfuss P, Dreyer S, Griffin J, et al. Positive sacroiliac screening tests in asymptomatic adults. *Spine* 1994;19:1138–1143.
103. Drottning M, Staff PH, Levin L, et al. Acute emotional response to common whiplash predicts subsequent pain complaints: a prospective study of 107 subjects sustaining whiplash injury. *Nord J Psychiatry* 1995;49:293–299.
104. Dvorák J. Neurophysiologic tests in diagnosis of nerve root compression caused by disc herniation. *Spine* 1994;21:39S–44S.
105. Dvorák J. Epidemiology, physical examination, and neurodiagnostics. *Spine* 1998;23:2663–2673.
106. Dzobia RB, Doxey NC. A prospective investigation into the orthopaedic and psychological predictors of outcome of first lumbar surgery following industrial injury. *Spine* 1984;9:614–623.
107. Eisele R, Schmid R, Kinzl L, et al. Soft tissue texture analysis by B-mode ultrasound in the evaluation of impairment in chronic low back pain. *Eur J Ultrasound* 1998;8:167–175.
108. Ellenberg MR, Honet JC, Treanor WJ. Cervical radiculopathy. *Arch Phys Med Rehabil* 1994;75:342–352.
109. Espeland A, Korsbrekke K, Albrektsen G, et al. Observer variation in plain radiography of the lumbosacral spine. *Br J Radiol* 1998;71:366–375.
110. Espersen JO, Kosteljanetz M, Halaburt H, et al. Predictive value of radiculography in patients with lumbago-sciatica: a prospective study. II. *Acta Neurochir (Wien)* 1984;73:213–221.
111. Esses SI, Botsford DJ, Kostuik JP. The role of external spinal skeletal fixation in the assessment of low-back disorders. *Spine* 1989;14:594–601.
112. Estlander A-M, Vanharanta H, Moneta GB, et al. Anthropometric variables, self-efficacy beliefs, and pain and disability ratings on the isokinetic performance of low back pain patients. *Spine* 1994;19:941–947.
113. EuroQoL Group. EuroQoL: A new facility for the measurement of health-related quality-of-life. *Health Policy* 1990;16:199–208.
114. Evans G, Richards S. *Low back pain: an evaluation of therapeutic interventions. Health Care Evaluation Unit, Department of Social Medicine, University of Bristol, UK, 1996.*
115. Faas A, Chavannes AW, Koes AW, et al. NHG-practice guideline: low back pain [translation]. *Huisars Bristol Wet* 1996;39:18–31.
116. Fairbank JCT, Couper J, Davies JB, et al. The Oswestry Low Back Pain Disability Questionnaire. *Physiotherapy* 1980;66:271–273.
117. Faraj AA, Akasha K, Mulholland RC. Temporary external fixation for low back pain: is it worth doing? *Eur Spine J* 1997;6:187–190.
118. Feder G, MacIntosh A, Lewis M, et al. *Low back pain evidence review.* London: Royal College of General Practitioners, 1998.
119. Follick MJ, Smith TW, Ahern DK. The sickness impact profile: a global measure of disability in chronic low back pain. *Pain* 1985;21:67–76.

120. Fortin JD, Aprill CN, Ponthieux B, et al. Sacroiliac joint: pain referral maps upon applying a new injection/arthrography technique. II. Clinical evaluation. *Spine* 1994;19:1483–1489.

121. Frennered K. *Symptomatic lumbar spondylolisthesis in young patients: a clinical and radiological follow-up after non-operative and operative treatment.* Thesis, Göteborg University, Sweden, 1991.

122. Fritz JM, Erhard RE, Delitto A, et al. Preliminary results of the use of a two-stage treadmill test as a clinical diagnostic tool in the differential diagnosis of lumbar spinal stenosis. *J Spinal Disord* 1997;10:410–416.

123. Frykholm R. Deformities of dural pouches and strictures of dural sheats in the cervical region producing nerve-root compression: a contribution to the etiology and operative treatment of brachial neuralgia. *J Neurosurg* 1947;4:403–413.

124. Garratt AM, Ruta DA, Abdalla MI, et al. The SF36 health survey questionnaire: an outcome measure suitable for routine use within the NHS? *BMJ* 1993;306:1440–1444.

125. Gates GF. Bone SPECT imaging of the painful back: nuclear medicine atlas. *Clin Nucl Med* 1996;21:560–571.

126. Georgy BA, Hesselink JR, Middleton MS. Fat-suppression contrast-enhanced MRI in the failed back surgery syndrome: a prospective study. *Neuroradiology* 1995;37:51–57.

127. Gibbons L, Videman T, Battié M. Determinants of isokinetic and psychophysical lifting strength and static back muscle endurance: a study of male monozygotic twins. *Spine* 1997;22:2983–2990.

128. Glickstein MF, Sussman SK. Time-dependent scar enhancement in magnetic resonance imaging of the postoperative lumbar spine. *Skeletal Radiol* 1991;20:333–337.

129. Gore D, Sepic S, Gardner G. Roentgenographic findings of the cervical spine in asymptomatic people. *Spine* 1986;11:521–524.

130. Gore D, Sepic S, Gardner G, et al. Neck pain: a long-term follow-up of 205 patients. *Spine* 1987;12:1–5.

131. Grane P. *The post-operative lumbar spine: a radiological investigation of the lumbar spine after discectomy using MR imaging and CT.* Thesis, Karolinska Institute, Stockholm, 1998.

132. Greenough CC. Recovery from low back pain: 1–5 year follow-up of 287 injury-related cases. *Acta Orthop Scand* 1993;64[Suppl] 254;1–34.

133. Greenough CG, Fraser RD. Comparison of eight psychometric instruments in unselected patients with back pain. *Spine* 1991;16:1068–1074.

134. Greenough CG, Fraser RD. Assessment of outcomes in patients with low-back pain. *Spine* 1992;17:36–41.

135. Grevitt M, Khazim R, Webb J, et al. The Short Form-36 Health Survey Questionnaire in spine surgery. *J Bone Joint Surg Br* 1997;79:48–52.

136. Grevitt M, Pande K, O'Dowd J, et al. Do first impressions count? A comparison of subjective and psychologic assessment of spinal patients. *Eur Spine J* 1998;7:218–223.

137. Grob D, Dvorák J, Panjabi MM, et al. Fixateur externe an der Halsworbelsäule: ein neues diagnostisches Mittel. *Unfallchirurg* 1993;96:416–421.

138. Guigui P, Delecourt C, Delhoume J, et al. Severe motor weakness associated with lumbar spinal stenosis: a retrospective study of a series of 61 patients. *Rev Chir Orthop Reparatrice Appar Mot* 1997;83:622–628.

139. Guyer RD, Ohnmeiss DD. Contemporary concepts in spine care: lumbar discography: position statement from the North American Spine Society Diagnostic and Therapeutic Committee. *Spine* 1995;20:2048–2059.

140. Hall S, Bartleson JD, Onofrio BM, et al. Lumbar spinal stenosis: clinical features, diagnostic procedures, and results of surgical treatment in 68 patients. *Ann Intern Med* 1985;103:271–275.

141. Hamanishi C, Matukura N, Fujita M, et al. Cross-sectional area of the stenotic lumbar dural tube measured from the transverse views of magnetic resonance imaging. *J Spinal Disord* 1994;7:388–393.

142. Hansson E, Hansson T. *Medicinska åtgärder för sjukskrivna med rygg- och nackbesvär.* Stockholm: Riksförsäkringsverket, 1999.

143. Hasenbring M, Marienfeld G, Kuhlendahl D, et al. Risk factors of chronicity in lumbar disc patients: a prospective investigation of biologic, psychologic, and social predictors of therapy outcome. *Spine* 1994;19:2759–2765.

144. Hasue M, Kikuchi S. Nerve root injections. In: Frymoyer JW, ed. *The adult spine: principles and practice,* 2nd ed. Philadelphia: Lippincott–Raven, 1997:647–653.

145. Haynes RB. How to read clinical journals. II. To learn about a diagnostic test. *CMA J* 1981;124:703–710.

146. Haynes RB, Sackett DL, Taylor DW, et al. Increased absenteeism from work after detection and labeling of hypertensive patients. *N Engl J Med* 1978;299:741–744.

147. Headache Classification Committee of the International Headache Society. Classification and diagnostic criteria for headache disorders, cranial neuralgias and facial pain. *Cephalalgia* 1988;8[Suppl 7]:1–96.

148. Hendler R, Hershkop M. When to use bone scintigraphy: it can reveal things other studies cannot. *Postgrad Med* 1998;104:59–61.

149. Herno A, Airaksinen O, Saari T, et al. Pre- and postoperative factors associated with return to work following surgery for lumbar spinal stenosis. *Am J Ind Med* 1996;30:473–478.

150. Herno A, Saari T, Suomalainen O, et al. The degree of decompressive relief and its relation to clinical outcome in patients undergoing surgery for lumbar spinal stenosis. *Spine* 1999;24:1010–1014.

151. Herron LD, Turner J. Patient selection for lumbar laminectomy and discectomy with a revised objective rating system. *Clin Orthop* 1985;199:145–152.
152. Herron LD, Turner JA, Weiner P. Lumbar disc herniations: the predictive value of the Health Attribution Test (HAT) and the Minnesota Multiphasic Personality Inventory (MMPI). *J Spinal Disord* 1988;1:2–8.
153. Hess WF, Jackson RP, Ebelke DK, et al. Pain response by discography as a predictor of clinical outcome in patients with solid posterolateral lumbosacrral fusion. In: *Proceedings of the 27th annual meeting of the Scoliosis Research Society.* Kansas City, MO: Scoliosis Research Society, 1992:82.
154. Hirsch G, Beach G, Cooke C, et al. Relationship between performance on lumbar dynamometry and Waddell score in a population with low-back pain. *Spine* 1991;16:1039–1043.
155. Hoffman RM, Kent DL, Deyo RA. Diagnostic accuracy and clinical utlity of thermography for lumbar radiculopathy: a meta-analysis. *Spine* 1991;16:623–628.
156. Hoffman JR, Scriger DL, Mower W, et al. Low-risk criteria for cervical-spine radiography in blunt trauma: a prospective study. *Ann Emerg Med* 1992;21:1454–1460.
157. Holmstrom EB, Lindell J, Moritz U. Low back and neck/shoulder pain in construction workers: occupational workload and psychosocial risk factors. II. Relationship to neck and shoulder pain. *Spine* 1992;17:672–677.
158. Holroyd KA, Holm JE, Keefe FJ, et al. A multi-center evaluation of the McGill Pain Questionnaire: results from more than 1700 chronic pain patients. *Pain* 1992;48:301–311.
159. Holt E. The question of discography. *J Bone Joint Surg Am* 1967;50:720–726.
160. Hunt S, McEven J. Measuring health status: a new tool for clinicians and epidemiologists. *J R Coll Gen Pract* 1985;35:185–188.
161. Hunt WE, Miller CA. Management of cervical radiculopathy. *Clin Neurosurg* 1986;33:485–502.
162. Hurme M, Alaranta H. Factors predicting the result of surgery for lumbar intervertebral disc herniation. *Spine* 1987;12:933–938.
163. Irwig L, Glasziou P. The Cochrane Methods Working Group on systematic review of screening and diagnostic tests: recommended methods. Updated June 6, 1996. Available at http://som.flinders.edu.au/cochrane/
164. Ito M, Incorvaia K, Yu S, et al. Predictive signs of discogenic lumbar pain on magnetic resonance imaging with discography correlation. *Spine* 1998;23:1252–1260.
165. Ito T, Shirado O, Suzuki H, et al. Lumbar trunk muscle endurance testing: an inexpensive alternative to a machine for evaluation. *Arch Phys Med Rehabil* 1996;77:75–79.
166. Jackson RP, Jacobs RR, Montesano PX. Facet joint injection in low-back pain: a prospective statistical study. *Spine* 1988;13:966–971.
167. Jackson RP, Becker GJ, Jacobs RR, et al. The neuroradiographic diagnosis of lumbar herniated nucleus pulposus. I. A comparison of computed tomography (CT), myelography, CT-myelography, discography, and CT-discography. *Spine* 1989;14:1356–1361.
168. Jarvik JG, Maravilla KR, Haynor DR, et al. Rapid MR imaging versus plain radiography in patients with low back pain: initial results of a randomized study. *Radiology* 1997;204:447–454.
169. Jeanneret B, Jovanovic M, Magerl F. Percutaneous diagnostic stabilization for low back pain: correlation with results after fusion operations. *Clin Orthop* 1994;304:130–138.
170. Jensen IB, Bradley LA, Linton SJ. Validation of an observation method of pain assessment in non-chronic back pain. *Pain* 1989;39:267–274.
171. Jensen M, Brant-Zawadzki MN, Obuchowski N, et al. Magnetic resonance imaging of the lumbar spine in people without back pain. *N Engl J Med* 1994;331:69–73.
172. Jensen M, Strom SE, Turner JA, et al. Validity of the sickness impact profile roland scale as a measure of dysfunction in chronic pain patients. *Pain* 1992;50:157–162.
173. Jinkins JR. MR of enhancing nerve roots in the unoperated lumbosacral spine. *AJNR Am J Neuroradiol* 1993;14:193–202.
174. Johnsson K-E. *Lumbar spinal stenosis: a clinical. radiological and neurophysiological investigation.* Thesis, Malmö General Hospital, Lund University, Sweden, 1987.
175. Johnsson R, Axelsson P, Stromqvist B. Mobility provocation of lumbar fusion evaluated by radiostereometric analysis. *Acta Orthop Scand* 1996;67[Suppl 270]:45–46.
176. Johnsson R, Axelsson P, Gunnarsson G, et al. Stability of lumbar fusion with transpedicular fixation determined by roentgenstereophotogrammetric analysis. *Spine* 1999;24:687–690.
177. Jonsson B. *Lumbar nerve root compression syndromes: symptoms, signs and surgical results.* Thesis, Department of Orthopedics, University Hospital, Lund University, Sweden 1995.
178. Jonsson B, Stromqvist B. Symptoms and signs in degeneration of the lumbar spine: a prospective, consecutive study of 300 operated patients. *J Bone Joint Surg Br* 1993:75:381–384.
179. Jonsson B, Annertz M, Sjoberg C, et al. A prospective and consecutive study of surgically treated lumbar spinal stenosis. II. Five-year follow-up by an independent observer. *Spine* 1997;22:2938–2944.
180. Jorgensen K, Nicholaisen T. Trunk extensor endurance: determination and relation to low-back trouble. *Ergonomics* 1987;30:259–267.
181. Kanmaz B, Collier BD, Liu Y, et al. SPET and three-phase planar bone scintigraphy in adult patients with chronic low back pain. *Nucl Med Commun* 1998;19:13–21.

182. Karantanas AH, Zibis AH, Papaliaga M, et al. Dimensions of the lumbar spinal canal: variations and correlations with somatometric parameters using CT. *Eur J Radiol* 1998;8:1581–1585.
183. Karas R, McIntosh G, Hall H, et al. The relationship between nonorganic signs and centralisation of symptoms in the prediction of return to work for patients with low back pain. *Phys Ther* 1997;77:354–360.
184. Karrholm J. Roentgen stereophotogrammetry: review of orthopaedic application. *Acta Orthop Scand* 1989;60:491–503.
185. Katz JN, Dalgas M, Stucki G, et al. Degenerative lumbar spinal stenosis: diagnostic value of the history and physical examination. *Arthritis Rheum* 1995;38:1236–1241.
186. Keefe FJ, Block AR. Development of an observation method for assessing pain behaviour in chronic low-back pain patients. *Behav Ther* 1982;13:363–375.
187. Kendall NAS, Linton SJ, Main CJ. *Guide to assessing psychosocial yellow flags in acute low back pain: risk factors for long-term disability and work loss.* Wellington, NZ: Accident Rehabilitation and Compensation Insurance Corporation of New Zealand and the National Health Committee, 1997.
188. Kent DL, Haynor DR, Larson EB, et al. Diagnosis of lumbar spinal stenosis in adults: a metaanalysis of the accuracy of CT, MR, and myelography. *AJR Am J Roentgenol* 1992;158:1135–1144.
189. Kent DL, Larson EB. Disease, level of impact, and quality of research methods: three dimensions of clinical efficacy assessment applied to magnetic resonance imaging. *Invest Radiol* 1992;27:245–254.
190. Kent DL, Haynor DR, Longstreth WT Jr, et al. The clinical efficacy of magnetic resonance imaging in neuroimaging. *Ann Intern Med* 1994;120:856–871.
191. Kerns RD, Jacob MC, Assessment of the psychosocial context of the experience of chronic pain. In: Melzack R, Turk DC, eds. *Handbook of pain assessment.* New York: Guilford Press, 1992:235–253.
192. Kerns RD, Turk DC, Rudy TE. The West Haven-Yale Multidimensional Pain Inventory (WHYMPI). *Pain* 1985;23:345–356.
193. Kissling RO, Jacob HA. The mobility of the sacroiliac joint in healthy subjects. *Bull Hosp Jt Dis* 1996;54:158–164.
194. Klekamp J, McCarty E, Spengler DM. Results of elective lumbar discectomy for patients involved in the workers' compensation system. *J Spinal Disord* 1998;11:277–282.
195. Knox B, Chapman T. Anterior lumbar interbody fusion for discogram concordant pain. *J Spinal Disord* 1993;6:242–244.
196. Kopec JA, Esdaile JM. *Spine* update: functional disability scales for back pain. *Spine* 1995;20:1943–1949.
197. Kopec JA, Esdaile JM, Abrahamowicz M, et al. The Quebec back pain disability scale: measurement properties. *Spine* 1995;20:341–352.
198. Kopec JA, Esdaile JM, Abrahamowicz M, et al. The Quebeck back pain disability scale: conceptualization and development. *J Clin Epidemiol* 1996;49:151–161.
199. Kosteljanetz M, Espersen JO, Halaburt H, et al. Predictive value of clinical and surgical findings in patients with lumbago-sciatica: a prospective study. I. *Acta Neurochir (Wien)* 1984;73:67–76.
200. Kummel BM. Nonorganic signs of significance in low back pain. *Spine* 1996;21:1077–1081.
201. Kuorinka I, Koskinen P. Occupational rheumatic diseases and upper limb strain in manual jobs in a light mechanical industry. *Scand J Work Environ Health* 1979;5:39–47.
202. Lane Jl, Koeller KK, Atkinson JD. Contrast-enhanced radicular veins on MR of the lumbar spine in an asymptomatic study group. *AJNR Am J Neuroradiol* 1995;16:269–273.
203. Laslett M. The value of the physical examination in diagnosis of painful sacroiliac joint pathologies. *Spine* 1998;23:962–964.
204. Leak AM, Cooper J, Dyer S, et al. The Northwick Park Neck Pain Questionnaire, devised to measure neck pain and disability. *Br J Rheumatol* 1994;33:469–474.
205. Leclaire R, Esdaile JM, Jéquier JC, et al. Diagnostic accuracy of technologies used in low back pain assessment: thermography, triaxial dynamometry, spinoscopy, and clinical examination. *Spine* 1996;21:1325–1331.
206. Lehto IJ, Tertti MO, Komu ME, et al. Age-related MRI changes at 0.1 T in cervical discs in asymptomatic subjects. *Neuroradiology* 1994;36:49–53.
207. Levoska S. Manual palpation and pain threshold in female office employees with and without neck-shoulder symptoms. *Clin J Pain* 1993;9:236–241.
208. Levoska S, Keinänen-Kiukaanniemi S, Bloigu R. Repeatability of measurement of tenderness in the neck-shoulder region by a dolorimeter and manual palpation. *Clin J Pain* 1993;9:229–235.
209. Li YK, Zhang YK, Zhong SZ. Diagnostic value on signs of subluxation of cervical vertebrae with radiological examination. *J Manipulative Physiol Ther* 1998;21:617–620.
210. Liang M, Komaroff AL. Roentgenograms in primary care patients with acute low back pain. *Arch Intern Med* 1982;142:1108–1112.
211. Lilius G, Harilainen A, Laasonen EM, et al. Chronic unilateral low-back pain: predictors of outcome of facet joint injections. *Spine* 1990;15:780–782.
212. Lilius G, Laasonen EM, Myllynen P, et al. Lumbar facet joint syndrome: a randomised clinical trial. *J Bone Joint Surg Br* 1989;71:681–684.
213. Lindstrom I. *A successful intervention program for patients with subacute low back pain: a randomized study using an operant-conditioning behavioral approach with special reference to pain, pain behavior,*

subjective disability, physical performance, physical work demands and sick-leave. Thesis, Göteborg University, Sweden, 1994.

214. Linton SJ, Halldén K. Risk factors and the natural course of acute and recurrent musculoskeletal pain: developing a screening instrument. In: Jensen TS, Turner JA, Wiesenfeld-Hallin Z, eds. *Proceedings of the 8th World Congress on Pain: progress in pain research and management.* Seattle: IASP Press, 1997;8:527–536.

215. Linton SJ, Halldén K. Can we screen for problematic back pain? A screening questionnaire for predicting outcome in acute and subacute back pain. *Clin J Pain* 1998;14:209–215.

216. Loisel P, Poitras S, Lemaine J, et al. Is work status of low back pain patients best described by an automated device or by a questionnaire? *Spine* 1998;23:1588–1595.

217. Long AL. The centralization phenomenon: its usefulness as a predictor or outcome in conservative treatment of chronic low back pain (a pilot study). *Spine* 1995;20:2513–2520.

218. Lord SM, Barnsley L, Bogduk N. The utility of comparative local anesthetic blocks versus placebo-controlled blocks for the diagnosis of cervical zygapophysial joint pain. *Clin J Pain* 1995;11:208–213.

219. Lord SM, Barnsley L, Wallis BJ, et al. Chronic cervical zygapophysial joint pain after whiplash: a placebo-controlled prevalence study. *Spine* 1996;21:1737–1744.

220. Love A, Loeboeuf DC, Crisp TC. Chiropractic chronoc low back pain sufferers and self-report assessment methods. I. A reliability study of the visual analogue scale, the pain drawing and the McGill pain questionnaire. *J Manipulative Physiol Ther* 1989;12:21–25.

221. Lowery WD, Horn TJ, Boden SD, et al. Impairment evaluation based on spinal range of motion in normal subjects. *J Spinal Disord* 1992;5:398–402.

222. Maher C, Adams R. Reliability of pain and stiffness assessments in clinical manual lumbar spine examination. *Phys Ther* 1994;9:801–809.

223. Maigne JY, Aivaliklis A, Pfefer F. Results of sacroiliac joint double block and value of sacroiliac pain provocation tests in 54 patients with low back pain. *Spine* 1996;21:1889–1892.

224. Maigne JY, Boulahdour H, Chatellier G. Value of quantitative radionuclide bone scanning in the diagnosis of sacroiliac joint syndrome in 32 patients with low back pain. *Eur Spine J* 1998;7:328–331.

225. Main CJ, Waddell G. *Spine* update: behavioral responses to examination. A reappraisal of the interpretation of "nonorganic signs." *Spine* 1998;23:2367–2371.

226. Main CJ, Wood PLR, Hollis S, et al. The distress and risk assessment method: a simple patient classification to identify distress and evaluate the risk of poor outcome. *Spine* 1992;17:42–52.

227. Mäkela M, Heliövaara M, Sievers K, et al. Prevalence, determinants, and consequences of chronic neck pain in Finland. *Am J Epidemiol* 1991;134:1356–1367.

228. Mandell GA, Harcke HT. Scintigraphy in spinal disorders in adolescents. *Skeletal Radiology* 1993;22:393–401.

229. Mann NH 3d, Brown MD, Enger I. Expert performance in low-back disorder recognition using patient pain drawings. *J Spinal Disord* 1992;5:254–259.

230. Mann NH III, Brown MD, Hertz DB, et al. Initial-impression diagnosis using low-back pain patient pain drawings. *Spine* 1993;18:41–53.

231. Marks RC, Houston T, Thulbourne T. Facet joint injection and facet nerve block: a randomised comparison in 86 patients with chronic low back pain. *Pain* 1992;49:325–328.

232. Matsumoto M, Yoshikazu F, Nobumasa S, et al. MRI of cervical intervertebral discs in asymptomatic subjects. *J Bone Joint Surg Br* 1998;80:19–24.

233. McCombe PF, Fairbank JCT, Cockersole BC, et al. Reproducibility of physical signs in low-back pain. *Spine* 1989;14:908–918.

234. McCreary C, Turner J, Dawson E. Principal dimensions of pain experience and psychological disturbance in chronic low back pain patients. *Pain* 1981;11:85–92.

235. McCulloch J, Steurer P, Riaz G, et al. Thermography as a diagnostic aid in sciatica. *J Spinal Disord* 1993;6:427–431.

236. McDonald GJ, Lord SM, Bogduk N. Long-term follow-up of patients treated with cervical radiofrequency neurotomy for chronic neck pain. *Neurosurgery* 1999;45:61–67.

237. McGregor AH, Doré CJ, McCarthy ID, et al. Are subjective clinical findings and objective clinical tests related to the motion characteristics of low back pain subjects? *J Orthop Sports Phys Ther* 1998;28:370–377.

238. McKenzie RA. *The lumbar spine: mechanical diagnosis and therapy.* Waikanae, NZ: Spinal Publications, 1981:22–80.

239. Modic MT, Herfken RJ. Intervertebral disk: normal age-related changes in MR signal intensity. *Radiology* 1990;177:332–334.

240. Modic MT, Ross JS, Obuchowski NA, et al. Contrast-enhanced MR imaging in acute lumbar radiculopathy: a pilot study of the natural history. *Radiology* 1995;195:429–435.

241. Moneta GB, Videman T, Kaivanto K, et al. Reported pain during lumbar discography as a function of annular ruptures and disc degeneration: a re-analysis of 833 discograms. *Spine* 1994;19:1968–1974.

242. Moreland J, Finch E, Stratford P, et al. Interrater reliability of six tests of trunk muscle function and endurance. *J Orthop Sports Phys Ther* 1997;26:200–208.

243. Nachemson A. Lumbar discography: where are we today? *Spine* 1989;14:555–557.

244. Nachemson A. *Ont i ryggen, orsaker, diagnostik och behandling.* Stockholm: Statens Beredning för Utvärdering av medicinsk metodik (SBU), 1991.
245. Nachemson AL. Instability of the lumbar spine: pathology, treatment and clinical evaluation. *Neurosurg Clin North Am* 1991;2:785–790.
246. Nachemson AL. Instrumented fusion of the lumbar spine for degenerative disorders: a critical look. In: Szpalski M, Gunzburg R, Spengler DM, Nachemson A, eds. *Instrumented fusion of the degenerative spine: state of the art, questions, and controversies.* Philadelphia: Lippincott–Raven, 1996:307–317.
247. Nachemson A. Failed back surgery syndrome is syndrome of failed back surgeons. *Pain Clin* 1999;11:271–284.
248. Nachemson A. Scientific diagnosis or unproved label for back pain patients? In: Szpalski M, Gunzburg R, Pope M, eds. *Lumbar segmental instability.* Philadelphia: Lippincott–Raven, 1999:297–301.
249. Nachemson A, Spitzer WO, LeBlanc FE, et al. Scientific approach to the assessment and management of activity-related spinal disorders. A monograph for clinicians: report of the Quebec Task Force on Spinal Disorders. *Spine* 12[Suppl 7]:S1–S59, 1987.
250. Nachemson A, Zdeblick TA, O'Brien JP. Controversy Lumbar disc disease with discogenic pain: what surgical treatment is most effective? *Spine* 1996;21:1835–1838.
251. Nagata K, Kanichirou K, Ohashi T, et al. Clinical value of magnetic resonance imaging for cervical myelopathy. *Spine* 1990;15:1088–1096.
252. Nash TP. Facet joints: intra-articular steroids or nerve block? *Pain Clin* 1990;3:77–82.
253. Nazarian LN, Zegel HG, Gilbert KR, et al. Paraspinal ultrasonography: lack of accuracy in evaluations patients with cervical or lumbar back pain. *J Ultrasound Med* 1998;17:117–122.
254. Newton M, Waddell G. Trunk strength testing with iso-machines. I. Review of a decade of scientific evidence. *Spine* 1993;18:801–811.
255. Newton M, Thow M, Somerville D, et al. Trunk strength testing with iso-machines. II. Experimental evaluation of the Cybex II back testing system in normal subjects and patients with chronic low back pain. *Spine* 1993;18:12–24.
256. National Health Service Executive. *Clinical guidelines: using clinical guidelines to improve patient care within the NHS.* London: NHS Executive, 1997.
257. Nicholaisen T, Jorgensen K. Trunk strength, back muscle endurance, and low-back trouble. *Scand J Rehabil Med* 1985;17:121–127.
258. Norlander S, Nordgren B. Clinical symptoms related to musculoskeletal neck-shoulder pain and mobility in the cervico-thoracic spine. *Scand J Rehabil Med* 1998;30:243–251.
259. North RB, Kidd DH, Zahurak M, et al. Specificity of diagnostic nerve blocks: a prospective, randomised study of sciatica due to lumbosacral spine disease. *Pain* 1996;65:77–85.
260. Ohlund C, Eek C, Palmblad S, et al. Quantified pain drawing in subacute low back pain: validation in a nonselected outpatient industrial sample. *Spine* 1996;21:1021–1030.
261. Ohlund C, Lindstrom I, Areskoug B, et al. Pain behavior in industrial subacute low back pain. I. Reliability: concurrent and predictive validity of pain behavior assessments. *Pain* 1994;58:201–209.
262. Ohlund C, Lindstrom I, Eek C, et al. The causality field (extrinsic and intrinsic factors) in industrial subacute low back pain patients. *Scand J Med Sci Sports* 1996;6:98–111.
263. Ohnhaus EE, Adler R. Methodological problems in the measurement of pain: a comparison between the verbal rating scale and the visual analogue scale. *Pain* 1975;1:379–384.
264. Ohnmeiss DD, Vanharanta H, Guyer RD. The association between pain drawings and computed tomographic/discographic pain responses. *Spine* 1995;20:729–733.
265. Pace WT, Castello P, Brugman J, et al. Clinical success of lumbar fusion as predicted by provocative discography. Paper read at Scoliosis Research Society Ottawa 1996. In: *Proceedings from SRS meeting.* Ottawa: SRS, 1996.
266. Park ES, Park C II, Kim A Y, et al. Relationship between electromyography and computed tomography in the evaluation of low back pain. *Yonsei Med J* 1993;34:84–89.
267. Parker H, Wood PLR, Main CJ. The use of the pain drawing as a screening measure to predict psychological distress in chronic low back pain. *Spine* 1995;20:236–243.
268. Parkkola R, Rytokoski U, Kormano M. Magnetic resonance imaging of the discs and trunk muscles in patients with chronic low back pain and healthy control subjects. *Spine* 1993;18:830–836.
269. Partanen J, Partanen K, Oikarinen H, et al. Preoperative electroneuromyography and myelography in cervical root compression. *Electromyogr Clin Neurophysiol* 1991;31:21–26.
270. Patrick DL, Deyo RA, Atlas SJ, et al. Assessing health related quality of life in patients with sciatica. *Spine* 1995;20:1899–909.
271. Pearce RH, Thompson JP, Bebault CM, et al. Magnetic resonance imaging reflects the chemical changes of aging degeneration in the human intervertebral disk. *J Rheumatol* 1991;18[Suppl 27]:42–43.
272. Pheasant HC, Gilbert D, Goldfarb J, et al. The MMPI as a predictor of outcome in low-back surgery. *Spine* 1979;4:78–84.
273. Phillips RB, Howe JW, Bustin G, et al. Stress X-rays and the low back pain patient. *J Manipulative Physiol Ther* 1990;13:127–133.
274. Pietri-Taleb F, Riihimäki H, Viikari-Juntura E, et al. Longitudinal study on the role of personality characteristics and psychological distress in neck trouble among working men. *Pain* 1994;58:261–267.

275. Pollmann W, Keidel M, Pfaffenrath V. Headache and the cervical spine: a critical review. *Cephalalgia* 1997;17:801–816.
276. Porter RW, Ward D. Cauda equina dysfunction: the significance of two level pathology. *Spine* 1992;17:9–15.
277. Porter RW, Wicks M, Ottewell D. Measurement of the spinal canal by diagnostic ultrasound. *J Bone Joint Surg Br* 1978;60:481–484.
278. Potter NA, Rothstein JM. Intertester reliability for selected clinical tests of the sacroiliac joint. *Phys Ther* 1985;65:1671–1675.
279. Powell MC, Wilson M, Szypryt P, et al. Prevalence of lumbar disc degeneration observed by magnetic resonance in symptomless women. *Lancet* 1986;13:1366–1367.
280. Radanow BP, Stefano G, Schnidrig A, et al. Role of psychosocial stress in recovery from common whiplash. *Lancet* 1991;338:712–715.
281. Ramsey SD, Luce BR, Deyo R, et al. The limited state of technology assessment for medical devices: facing the issues. *Am J Managed Care* 1998;4:SP188–199.
282. Ransford AO, Cairns D, Mooney V. The pain drawing as an aid to the psychologic evaluation of patients with low-back pain. *Spine* 1976;1/2:127–134.
283. Reigo T, Tropp H, Timpka T. Pain drawing evaluation: the problem with the clinically biased surgeon. *Acta Orthop Scand* 1998;69:408–411.
284. Revel M, Listrat VM, Chevalier XJ, et al. Facet joint block for low back pain: identifying predictors of a good response. *Arch Phys Med Rehabil* 1992;73:824–828.
285. Revel M, Poiraudeau S, Auleley GR, et al. Capacity of the clinical picture to charecterize low back pain relieved by facet joint anesthesia: proposed criteria to identify patients with painful facet joints. *Spine* 1998;23:1972–1976.
286. Revill SI, Robinson JO, Rosen M, et al. The reliability of a linear analogue for evaluating pain. *Anaesthesia* 1976;31:1191–1198.
287. Richards JS, Nepomuceno C, Riles M, et al. Assessing pain behavior: the UAB pain behavior scale. *Pain* 1982;14:393–398.
288. Riddle DL, Rothstein JM. Intertester reliability of McKenzie's classifications of the syndrome types present in patients with low back pain. *Spine* 1993;18:1333–1344.
289. Riddle DL, Stratford PW, Binkley JM. Sensitivity to change of the Roland-Morris Back Pain Questionnaire. II. *Phys Ther* 1998;78:1197–1207.
290. Riley JF, Ahern DK, Follick MJ. Chronic pain and functional impairment: assessing beliefs about their relationship. *Arch Phys Med Rehabil* 1988;59:579–582.
291. Roach KE, Brown MD, Dunigan KM, et al. Test-retest reliability of patient reports of low back pain. J Orthop Sports *Phys Ther* 1997;26:253–259.
292. Roach KE, Brown M, Ricker E, et al. The use of patient symptoms to screen for serious back problems. *J Orthop Sports Phys Ther* 1995;21:2–6.
293. Roland M, Morris R. 1982 Volvo award in clinical science: a study of the natural history of back pain. I. Development of a reliable and sensitive measure of disability in low-back pain. *Spine* 1983;8:141–144.
294. Roland M, van Tulder M. Should radiologists change the way they report plain radiography of the spine? *Lancet* 1998;352:229–230.
295. Romano JM, Turner JA, Jensen MP. The chronic illness problem inventory as a measure of dysfunction in chronic pain patients. *Pain* 1992;49:71–75.
296. Romano JM, Syrjala KL, Levy RL, et al. Overt pain behaviours: relationship to patient functioning and treatment outcome. *Behav Ther* 1988;19:191–201.
297. Rosen M, Breen A, Hamann W, et al. *Report of a Clinical Standards Advisory Group committee on back pain.* London: Her Majesty's Stationery Office, 1994.
298. Ross JS, Robertson JT, Frederickson RC, et al. Association between peridural scar and recurrent radicular pain after lumbar discectomy: magnetic resonance evaluation. ADCON-L European Study Group. *Neurosurgery* 1996;38:855–861;discussion 861–863.
299. Ross JS, Zepp R, Modic MT. The postoperative lumbar spine: enhanced MR evaluation of the intervertebral disk. *Am J Neuroradiol* 1996;17:323–331.
300. Royal College of General Practitioners. *The development and implementation of clinical guidelines: report of the clinical guidelines working group.* London: Royal College of General Practitioners, 1995.
301. Royal College of Radiologists. *Making the best use of a department of radiology.* London: Royal College of Radiologists Publications, 1993.
302. Royal College of Radiologists. *Making the best use of a department of clinical radiology: guidelines for doctors,* 3rd ed. London: Royal College of Radiologists Publications, 1995:1–96.
303. Ryan PJ, Evans PA. Gibson T, et al. Chronic low back pain: comparison of bone SPECT with radiography and CT. *Radiology* 1992;182:849–854.
304. Saifuddin A, Braithwaite I, White J, et al. The value of lumbar spine magnetic resonance imaging in the demonstration of annular tears. *Spine* 1998;23:453–457.
305. Salén BA, Spangfort EV, Nygren ÅL, et al. The disability rating index: an instrument for the assessment of disability in clinical settings. *J Clin Epidemiol* 1994;47:1423–1434.

306. Saur P, Pfingsten M, Ensink F-B, et al. Interrater-Untersuchungen zur Reliablitätsprüfung somatischer Befunde. *Rehabilitation (Stuttg)* 1996;35:150–160.
307. Savage RA, Whitehouse CH, Roberts N. The relationship between the magnetic resonance imaging appearance of the lumbar spine and low back pain, age and occupation in males. *Eur Spine J* 1997;6:106–114.
308. Scalzitti DA. Screening for psychological factors in patients with low back problems: Waddell's nonorganic signs. *Phys Ther* 1997:77:306–312.
309. Schade V, Semmer N, Main Ch, et al. Prediction of low-back pain in individuals with asymptomatic disc alterations in MRI (abst). In: *Proceedings of the ISSLS meeting.* Brussels: ISSLS, 1998:17.
310. Schade V, Semmer N, Main CJ, et al. The impact of clinical, morphological, psychosocial and work-related factors on the outcome of lumbar discectomy. *Pain* 1999;80:239–249.
311. Schellhas KP, Smith MD, Gundry CR, et al. Cervical discogenic pain: prospective correlation of magnetic resonance imaging and discography in asymptomatic subjects and pain sufferers. *Spine* 1996;21:300–311.
312. Schonstrom N. *The narrow lumbar spinal canal and the size of the cauda equina in man: a clinical and experimental study.* Thesis, Göteborg University, Sweden, 1988.
313. Schott A-M, Nizard R, Mainsonneuve H, et al. Methods used to develop clinical guidelines in France: the example of common lumbosciatic syndrome. *Rev Rhum Engl Ed* 1996;63:830–836.
314. Schwarzer A, Aprill CN, Bogduk N. The sacroiliac joint in chronic low back pain. *Spine* 1995;20:31–37.
315. Schwarzer A, Aprill CN, Derby R, et al. Clinical features of patients with pain stemming from the lumbar zygapophysial joints: is the lumbar facet syndrome a clinical entity? *Spine* 1994;19:1132–1137.
316. Schwarzer A, Aprill CN, Derby R, et al. The false-positive rate of uncontrolled diagnostic blocks of the lumbar zygapophysial joints. *Pain* 1994;58:195–200.
317. Schwarzer A, Aprill CN, Derby R, et al. The relative contributions of the disc and zygapophyseal joint in chronic low back pain. *Spine* 1994;19:801–806.
318. Schwarzer A, Derby R, Aprill CN, et al. Pain from the lumbar zygapophysial joints: a test of two models. *J Spinal Disord* 1994;7:331–336.
319. Scott J, Huskinsson EC. Accuracy of subjective measurements made with or without previous scores: an important source of error in serial measurement of subjective states. *Ann Rheum Dis* 1979;38:558–559.
320. Sether LA, Shiwei Y, Haughton VM, et al. Intervertebral disk: normal age-related changes in MR signal intensity. *Radiology* 1990;177:385–388.
321. Simmonds MJ, Olsson SL, Jones S, et al. Psychometric characteristics and clinical usefulness of physical performance tests in patients with low back pain. *Spine* 1998;23:2412–2421.
322. Sivik T, Gustafsson E, Klinberg Olsson K. Differential diagnosis of low-back pain' patients: a simple quantification of the pain drawing. *Nord J Psychiatry* 1992;46:55–62.
323. Slater MA, Hall HF, Atkinson JH, et al. Pain and impairment beliefs in chronic low back pain: validation of the Pain and Impairment Relationship Scale (PAIRS). *Pain* 1991;44:51–56.
324. Slipman CW, Sterenfeld EB, Chou LH, et al. The predictive value of provocative sacroiliac joint stress maneuvers in the diagnosis of sacroiliac joint syndrome. *Arch Phys Med Rehabil* 1998;79:288–292.
325. Slosar PJ, White AH, Wetzel FT. Controversy. The use of selective nerve root blocks: diagnostic, therapeutic, or placebo? *Spine* 1998;23:2253–2256.
326. Smith BM, Hurqitz EL, Solsberg D, et al. Interobserver reliability of detecting lumbar intervertebral disc high-intensity zone on magnetic resonance imaging and association of high-intensity zone with pain and annular disruption. *Spine* 1998;23:2074–2080.
327. Soini JR, Seitsalo SK. The external fixation test of the lumbar spine: 30 complications in 25 patients of 100 consecutive patients. *Acta Orthop Scand* 1993;64:147–149.
328. Soini JR, Harkonen HI, Alaranta HT, et al. External fixation test in low back pain: function analyzed in 25 patients. *Acta Orthop Scand* 1994;65:87–90.
329. Soini J, Slatis P, Kannisto M, et al. External transpedicular fixation test of the lumbar spine correlates with the outcome of subsequent lumbar fusion. *Clin Orthop* 1993;293:89–96.
330. Sorensen LV. Preoperative psychological testing with the MMPI at first operation for prolapsed lumbar disc: five year follow-up. *Dan Med Bull* 1992;39:186–190.
331. Spengler DM, Ouellette EA, Battié M, et al. Elective discectomy for herniation of a lumbar disc: additional experience with an objective method. *J Bone Joint Surg Am* 1990;72:230–237.
332. Spitzer WO, Skovron ML, Salmi LR, et al. Scientific monograph of the Quebec task force on whiplash-associated disorders: redefining "whiplash" and its management. *Spine* 1995;20;8S.
333. Spratt KF, Lehmann TR, Weinstein JN, et al. A new approach to the low-back physical examination: behavioral assessment of mechanical signs. *Spine* 1990;15:96–102.
334. Spurling RG, Scoville WB. Lateral rupture of the cervical intervertebral discs: a common cause of shoulder and arm pain. *Surg Gynecol Obstet* 1944;78:350–358.
335. Stabler A, Bellan M, Weiss M, et al. MR imaging of enhancing intraosseous disk herniation (Schmorl's nodes). *AJR Am J Roentgenol* 1997;168:933–938.

336. Stadnik TW, Lee RR, Coen HI, et al. Annular tears and disk herniation: prevalence and contrast enhancement on MR images in the absence of low back pain or sciatica. *Radiology* 1998;206:49–55.
337. Steven ID, chairperson. *Guidelines for the management of back-injured employees.* Australia: Work-Cover Corporation, 1993.
338. Stokes IA, Frymoyer JW. Segmental motion and instability. *Spine* 1987;12:688–691.
339. Strender L-E, Sjöblom A, Sundell K, et al. Interexaminer reliability in physical examination of patients with low back pain. *Spine* 1997;22:814–820.
340. Szpalski M, Michel F, Hayez JP. Determination of trunk motion patterns associated with permanent of transient stenosis of the lumbar spine. *Eur Spine J* 1996;5:332–337.
341. Szpalski M, Nordin M, Skovron ML, et al. Health care utilization for low back pain in Belgium. *Spine* 1995;20:431–442.
342. Taber KH, Herrick RC, Wather SW, et al. Pitfalls and artifacts encountered in clinical MR imaging of the spine. *Radiograph* 1998;18:1499–1521.
343. Tallroth K, Alaranta H, Soukka A. Lumbar mobility in asymptomatic individuals. *J Spinal Disord* 1992;5:481–484.
344. Tertti MO, Salminen JJ, Paajanen HE, et al. Low-back pain and disk degeneration in children: a case-control MR imaging study. *Radiology* 1991;180:503–507.
345. Therapeutics and Technology Assessment Subcommittee of the American Academy of Neurology. Review of the literature on spinal ultrasound for the evaluation of back pain and radicular disorders. *Neurology* 1998;51:343–344.
346. Thomas KB. General practice consultations: is there any point in being positive? *BMJ* 1987;294:1200–1202.
347. Thorvaldsen P, Sorensen EB. Psychological vulnerability as a predictor for short-term outcome in lumbar spine surgery: a prospective study. II. *Acta Neurochir (Wien)* 1990;102:58–61.
348. Triano JJ, McGregor M, Cramer GD, et al. A comparison of outcome measures for use wich back pain patients: results of a feasibility study. *J Manipulative Physiol Ther* 1993;16:67–73.
349. Tullberg T. *Lumbar disc herniation: results of micro and standard surgical treatment evaluated by clinical, radiological and neurophysiological methods.* Thesis, St Göran Hospital and Karolinska Hospital, Stockholm, 1993.
350. Turk DC, Wack JT, Kerns RD. An empirical examination of the "pain behaviour" construct. *J Behav Med* 1985;8:119–130.
351. Udén A. Specified diagnosis in 532 cases of back pain. *Qual Life Res* 1994;3[Suppl 1]:S33–S34.
352. Udén A. Choose the words carefully! Information with a positive content may affect the patients with spinal problems so they dare to live a normal life [in Swedish]. *Lakartidningen* 1996;93:3923–3925.
353. Udén A. *Pain* drawing in lumbar disc hernia. *Acta Orthop Scand* 1997;68:182.
354. Udén A, Landin LA. *Pain* drawing and myelography in sciatic pain. *Clin Orthop* 1987;216:124–130.
355. van Akkerveeken PF. *Lateral stenosis of the lumbar spine: a new diagnostic test and its influence on management of patients with pain only.* Thesis, University of Utrecht, Netherlands, 1989.
356. Van de Kelft EJZ, Van Coethem JWM, De la Porte CH, et al. Early postoperative gadolinium-DTPA–enhanced MR imaging after successful lumbar discectomy. *Br J Neurosurg* 1996;10:41–49.
357. van den Hoogen HJM, Koes BW, Devillé W, van Eijk JTHM, et al. The inter-observer reproducibility of Lasègue's sign in patients with low back pain in general practice. *Br J Gen Pract* 1996;46:727–730.
358. van den Hoogen HJ, Koes BW, Deville W, et al. The prognosis of low back pain in general practice. *Spine* 1997;22:1515–1521.
359. van den Hoogen HMM, Koes BW, van Eijk JThM, et al. On the accuracy of history, physical examination, and erythrocyte sedimentation rate in diagnosing low back pain in general practice: a criteria-based review of the literature. *Spine* 1995;20:318–327.
360. van der Donk J, Schouten JS, Passchier J, et al. The associations of neck pain with radiological abnormalities of the cervical spine and personality traits in a general population. *J Rheumatol* 1991;18:1884–1889.
361. van Dillen LR, Sahrmann SA, Norton BJ, et al. Reliability of physical examination items used for classification of patients with low back pain. *Phys Ther* 1998;78:979–987.
362. van Goethem JWM, Parizel PM, van den Hauwe L, et al. Imaging findings in patients with failed back surgery syndrome. *J Belge Radiol-BTR* 1997;80:81–84.
363. van Susante J, van de Schaaf D, Pavlov P. Psychological distress deteriorates the subjective outcome of lumbosacral fusion: a prospective study. *Acta Orthop Belg* 1998;64:371–377.
364. van Tulder MW, Koes BW, Bouter LM. *Low back pain in primary care: effectiveness of diagnostic and therapeutic interventions.* Faculteit der Geneeskunde VU, EMGO-Instituut, Amsterdam, 1996.
365. van Tulder MW, Assendelft WJJ, Koes BW, et al. Spinal radiographic finding and nonspecific low back pain: a systematic review of observational studies. *Spine* 1997;22:427–434.
366. Velmahos GC, Theodorou D, Tatevossian R, et al. Radiographic cervical spine evaluation in the alert asymptomatic blunt trauma victim: much ado about nothing? *J Trauma* 1996;40:768–774.
367. Verbiest H. Neurogenic intermittent claudication in cases with absolute and relative stenosis of the lumbar vertebral canal ASCL and RSLC, in cases with narrow lumbar intervertebral foramina, and in cases with both entitites. *Clin Neurosurg* 1973;20:204.

368. Victorian Workcover Authority. *Guidelines for the management of employees with compensable low back pain.* Melbourne: Victorian Workcover Authority, 1996.
369. Viikari-Juntura E. Interexaminer reliability of observations in physical examinations of the neck. *Phys Ther* 1987;67:1526–1532.
370. Viikari-Juntura E, Prras M, Laasonen EM. Validity of clinical tests in the diagnosis of root compression in cervical disc diseases. *Spine* 1989;14:253–257.
371. Viikari-Juntura E, Takala E-P, Riihimki H, Malmivaara A, et al. Standarized physical examination protocol for low back disorders: feasibility of use and validity of symptoms and signs. *J Clin Epidemiol* 1998;51:245–255.
372. Vroomen PC, Van Hapert SJ, Van Acker RE, et al. The clinical significance of gadolinium enhancement of lumbar disc herniations and nerve roots on preoperative MRI. *Neuroradiology* 1998;40:800–806.
373. Vucetic N. *Clinical diagnosis of lumbar disc herniation outcome predictors for surgical treatment.* Thesis, Department of Orthopaedics, Karolinska Institute, Stockholm, 1998.
374. Vucetic N, Astrand P, Güntner O, et al. Diagnosis and prognosis in lumbar disc herniation. *Clin Orthop* 1999:361:116–122.
375. Waddell G. An approach to backache. Br J Hosp Med 1982;3:187–219.
376. Waddell G. *The back pain revolution.* Edinburgh: Churchill Livingstone, 1998.
377. Waddell G, Turk DC. Clinical assessment of low back pain. In: Melzack R, Turk DC, eds. *Handbook of pain assessment.* New York: Guildford Press, 1992:15–36.
378. Waddell G, Feder G, MacIntosh A, et al. *Low back pain evidence review.* London: Royal College of General Practitioners, 1996.
379. Waddell G, Main CS, Morris EW, et al. Normality and reliability in the clinical assessment of backache. *BMJ* 1982;284:1519–1523.
380. Waddell G, Main CJ, Morris EW, et al. Chronic low-back pain, psychologic distress, and illness behavior. *Spine* 1984;9:209–213.
381. Waddell G, McCulloch JA, Kummel E, et al. Non-organic physical signs in low back pain. *Spine* 1980;5:117–125.
382. Waddell G, Morris EW, DiPaola MP, et al. A concept of illness tested as an improved basis for surgical decisions in low back pain. *Spine* 1986;11:712–719.
383. Waddell G, Newton M, Henderson H, Somerville D, Main CJ. A Fear-Avoidance Beliefs Questionnaire (FABQ) and the role of fear-avoidance in chronic low back pain and disability. *Pain* 1993;52:157–168.
384. Walsh TR, Weinstein JN, Spratt KF, et al. Lumbar discography in normal subjects. *J Bone Joint Surg Am* 1990;72:1081–1088.
385. Ware JE, Sherbourne C. The MOS 36–item short-form-survey (SF-36). I. Conceptual framework and item selection. *Med Care* 1992;30:473–483.
386. Ware JE, Jr, Snow KK, Kosinski M, et al. *SF-36 health survey manual and interpretation guide.* Boston: Health Institute, 1993.
387. Waris P, Kuorinka I, Kurppa K. Epidemiological screening of occupational neck and upper limb disorders. *Scand J Work Environ Health* 1979;6[Suppl]:25–38.
388. Weber H. *Lumbar disc herniation: a prospective study of prognostic factors including a controlled trial.* Thesis, Oslo City Hospital, Oslo, 1978.
389. Weber H. The natural history of disc herniation and the influence of intervention. *Spine* 1994;19:2234–2238.
390. Weinreb JC, Wolbarsht LB, Cohen JM, et al. Prevalence of lumbosacral intervertebral disk abnormalities on MR images in pregnant and asymptomatic nonpregnant women. *Radiology* 1989;170:125–128.
391. Weishaupt D, Zanetti M, Hodler J, et al. MR imaging of the lumbar spine: prevalence of intervertebral disk extrusion and sequestration, nerve root compression, end plate abnormalities, and osteoarthritis of the facet joints in asymptomatic volunteers. *Radiology* 1998;209:661–666.
392. Werneke MW, Harris DE, Lichter RL. Clinical effectiveness of behavioral signs for screening chronic low-back pain: patients in a work-oriented physical rehabilitation program. *Spine* 1993;18:2412–2418.
393. Werneke M, Hart DL, Cook D. A descriptive study of the centralization phenomenon: a prospective analysis. *Spine* 1999;24:676–683.
394. Willén J, Danielsson B, Gaulitz R, et al. Dynamic effects on the lumbar spinal canal: axially loaded CT-myelography and MRI in patients with sciatica and/or neurogenic claudication. *Spine* 1997;22:2968–2976.
395. Williams AC de C, Richardson PH. What does the BDI measure in chronic pain? *Pain* 1993;55:259–266.
396. Wilson P. Chronic neck pain and cervicogenic headache. *Clin J Pain* 1991;7:5–11.
397. Wiltse LL, Rocchio PD. Preoperative psychological tests as predictors of success of chemonucleolysis in the treatment of the low back syndrome. *J Bone Joint Surg Am* 1975;57:478–483.
398. Wittenberg RH, Lutke A, Longwitz D, et al. The correlation between magnetic resonance imaging and the operative and clinical findings after lumbar microdiscectomy. *Int Orthop* 1998;22:241–244.
399. Xu GL, Haughton VM, Carrera GF. Lumbar facet joint capsule: appearance at MR imaging and CT. *Radiology* 1990;177:415–420.

400. Yoss RE, Corbin KB, McCarthy CS,et al. Significance of symptoms and signs in localization of involved root in cervical disc protrusion. *Neurology* 1957:7:673–683.
401. Youdas JW, Garrett TR, Harmsen S, et al. Lumbar lordosis and pelvic inclination of symptomatic adults. *Phys Ther* 1996;76:1066–1081.
402. Zander DR, Lander PH. Positionally dependent spinal stenosis: correlation of upright flexion-extension myelography and computed tomographic myelography. *Can Assoc Radiol J* 1998;49:256–261.
403. Zung WWK. A self-rating depression scale. *Arch Gen Psychiatry* 1965;12:63–70.

Neck and Back Pain: The Scientific Evidence of Causes, Diagnosis, and Treatment, edited by Alf Nachemson and Egon Jonsson. Published by Lippincott Williams & Wilkins, Philadelphia 2000.

10

Introduction to Treatment of Neck and Back Pain

Alf Nachemson

Department of Orthopaedics, Sahlgrenska University Hospital, Göteborg, Sweden

In the landmark review on the importance of placebo effects in pain treatment and research, Turner et al. (15) clearly demonstrated, in a thorough scrutiny of the literature on the subject up to 1993, the important beneficial effects of placebo, in particular in patients with pain resulting from nonspecific diseases that are difficult to understand, such as neck pain and back pain. These patients are likely to improve with any treatment because of the following:

1. Natural history and regression to the mean are factors in this finding. Most acute and some chronic pain problems resolve on their own irrespective of treatment, even though many patients have recurrent episodes. In addition, patients with chronic conditions have fluctuating symptoms and seek medical care when symptoms are at their worst. Thus, the next change is likely to be an improvement. This tendency of extreme symptoms or findings to return to the patient's more normal state is known as *regression to the mean* (17).
2. Improvement may be caused by a specific effect of the treatment given. For example, morphine specifically reduces pain, and antiinflammatory medication reduces inflammation.
3. Nonspecific effects of treatment are attributed to factors other than those of specific active components. These include the following: physician attention; interest and concern in a healing setting; patients' and physicians' expectations of treatment effects; the reputation, expense, and impressiveness of the treatment; and characteristics of the setting that influence patients to report improvement.

The term *placebo effect* is often used synonymously with nonspecific effects. A *placebo* is thus an intervention designed to simulate medical therapy but not believed to by the investigator to be a specific therapy for the target condition. It is used either for its psychologic effect or to eliminate observer bias in an experimental setting.

From several hundred randomized controlled trials specifically dealing with this effect, it can be concluded that the efficacy of any specific treatment for a condition such as back pain must be supported by significant positive results from an admissible randomized controlled trial. A placebo response usually varies around 50% but can reach 70% for a "strong" intervention such as surgery. The effect is not necessarily brief, nor are the persons responding abnormal in any way (5).

There are several explanations for the placebo effect. Treatment can decrease anxiety. It can be effective because of the patient's expectations, previous experience or learning, or family attitudes, or treatment may be effective because the provider is warm, friendly, and empathic, with a positive attitude toward the patient and the treatment. Some studies have suggested that the effect actually may be mediated by endogenous opiate release in the central nervous system that mobilizes endorphins (7).

These findings all have implications for research design. If at all possible, everyone should be unaware of or "blind" to the treatment given if there are two alternatives. Therefore, the control treatment arm in a trial should be as similar as possible to the active treatment arm to create similar expectations. Patients receiving sham therapy should have visit frequency, contacts, and support equivalent to those of the active therapy group. It can be difficult to create placebo controls that appear to be active treatments, but creative placebos have been devised (4,15), such as sham transcutaneous electrical nerve stimulation, the intentional use of misplaced needles as a control for acupuncture, the use of subtherapeutic weight as a control for traction, and the use of soft massage as a control for spinal manipulation. Trials in which control treatments mimic the active intervention typically have found less advantage of the active treatment over the control than have trials with obviously different types of therapy or with inert placebo controls (4,14).

A completely untreated group (e.g., a waiting list) is not the same as a placebo-treated group. A *waiting list condition* controls for the effects of the passage of time, but not for patient expectations. However, inclusion of an untreated group in addition to a placebo group can help to distinguish nonspecific effects from natural history. For chronic conditions, long baselines with multiple measures of the outcome variable before treatment can reveal changes in the absence of treatment and thereby help to estimate the magnitude of regression to the mean as a source of within-patient change (8,9).

Ethical and practical factors make it difficult to conduct surgical trials with sham controls. When it is not possible to have a sham surgery control condition, randomized trials of surgery versus credible alternative minimal or nonsurgical therapies may be feasible, as has been done with coronary artery bypass surgery and discectomy (3,16). Other alternatives have been described by Rudicel and Esdail (12) and by Stirrat et al. 1992 (13).

Uncontrolled but well-executed complete clinical follow-up series, using validated outcome measures (1,2,6,10,11), are useful to prove treatment efficacy *only* if outcomes for most patients are obvious, dramatic, immediate and cannot be explained by any other factors. Such is unfortunately not the case for any of our patients with back pain of unspecific diagnosis.

In Chapters 11 through 17, which discuss various treatment modalities for patients with acute or subacute (0 to 12 weeks' duration) and chronic (more than 3 months' duration) back pain, we have concentrated on evaluating the evidence from randomized or controlled clinical studies. In the latter group, the method of randomization is not blind or is questionable. This evaluation has been made possible because the number of such studies has increased in the past decade, and modern technology has helped in the search of library databases.

REFERENCES

1. Beaton DE, Hogg-Johnson S, Bombardier C. Evaluating changes in health status: reliability and responsiveness of five generic health status measures in workers with musculoskeletal disorders. *J Clin Epidemiol* 1997;50:79–93.
2. Block R. Methodology of clinical back pain trials. *Spine* 1987;12:430–432.
3. CASS Principal Investigators. Coronary Artery Surgery Study (CASS): a randomized trial of coronary artery bypass surgery. *Circulation* 1983;68:939–950.
4. Deyo RA. Clinical research methods in low back pain. *Physiol Med Rehabil* 1991;5:209–222.
5. Fine PG, Roberts WJ, Gillette RG, et al. Slowly developing placebo responses confound tests of intravenous phentolamine to determine mechanisms underlying idiopathic chronic low back pain. *Pain* 1994;56:235–242.
6. Gartland JJ. Orthopaedic clinical research: deficiencies in experimental design and determinations of outcome. *J Bone Joint Surg Am* 1988;70:1357–1364.
7. Levine JD, Gordon NC, Fields HL. The mechanism of placebo analgesia. *Lancet* 1978;61:201–207.
8. McDonald CJ, Mazzuca SA. How much of the placebo "effect" is really statistical regression? *Stat Med* 1983;2:417–427.
9. Miller NE. Placebo factors in treatment: views of a physiologist. In: Shepherd M, Sartorius N, eds. *Nonspecific aspects of treatment.* Toronto: Hans Huber, 1989:39–51.
10. Murray BW, Britton AR, Bulstrode CJK. Loss to follow-up matters. *J Bone Joint Surg Br* 1997;79:254–257.
11. Ohlund C, Lindström, I, Areskoug B, et al. Pain behavior in industrial subacute low back pain. I. Reliability: concurrent and predictive validity of pain behavior assessments. *Pain* 1994;58:201–209.
12. Rudicel S, Esdail J. The randomized clinical trial in orthopaedics: obligation or option? *J Bone Joint Surg Am* 1985;67:1284–1293.
13. Stirrat GM, Farrow SC, Farndon J, et al. The challenge of evaluating surgical procedures. *Ann R Coll Surg Engl* 1992;74:80–84.
14. Thomson R. Side effects and placebo amplification. *Br J Psychiatry* 1982;140:64–68.
15. Turner JA, Deyo RA, Loeser JD, et al. The importance of placebo effects in pain treatment and research. *JAMA* 1994;271:1609–1614.
16. Weber H. Lumbar disc herniation: a controlled prospective study with ten years of observation. *Spine* 1983;8:131–140.
17. Whitney CW, Von Korff M. Regression to the mean in treated versus untreated chronic pain. *Pain* 1992;50:271–285.

Neck and Back Pain: The Scientific Evidence of Causes, Diagnosis, and Treatment, edited by Alf Nachemson and Egon Jonsson. Published by Lippincott Williams & Wilkins, Philadelphia 2000.

11

Conservative Treatment of Acute and Subacute Low Back Pain

Maurits W. van Tulder* and Gordon Waddell†

*Institute for Research in Extramural Medicine, Vrije Universiteit, Amsterdam, The Netherlands
†Department of Orthopaedics, The Glasgow Nuffield Hospital, Glasgow, Scotland

This review is based on two complementary sources: (a) an update of the Agency for Health Care Policy and Research guidelines using other published systematic reviews (106); and, as a supplement, (b) an extensive systematic literature review by the Institute for Research in Extramural Medicine (103). This review combines the advantages of a rigorous methodologic approach with a cross-check of completeness and conclusions against other reviewers.

This chapter should answer the following questions:

Which interventions are the most effective in the treatment of acute low back pain (LBP) with and without radiation?
Are these interventions more effective than placebo, no treatment, or other conservative treatments (including other drugs)?
Are these interventions effective regarding relevant outcome measures, that is, overall improvement, functional status, return to work, pain intensity, or pain behavior?
Are these interventions effective in the short and/or long term?

The information provided in this chapter may be useful in the development of evidence-based guidelines for general practitioners, physical therapists, or other primary health care professionals (112).

METHODS

Selection of Studies

For the guidelines of the Royal College of General Practitioners of the United Kingdom (85), an update of the guidelines of the United States Agency for Health Care Policy and Research (9) was undertaken. Other systematic reviews of treatment for back pain that were published since the Agency for Health Care Policy and Research guidelines and used for this update were as follows:

1. Cohen et al., 1994: back schools, 13 randomized controlled trials (RCTs) included, 3 on acute LBP (18).
2. Koes and van den Hoogen, 1994: bed rest, 5 RCTs included (54).

3. Koes and van den Hoogen, 1994: orthoses, 5 RCTs included (54).
4. Koes et al., 1994: back schools, 16 RCTs included, 6 on acute or recurrent LBP (61).
5. Gam and Johannsen, 1995: ultrasound, 22 RCTs in various musculoskeletal disorders, 2 RCTs on LBP (36).
6. Koes et al., 1995: epidural steroids, 12 RCTs included, 9 RCTs on acute or subacute LBP and sciatica (59).
7. van der Heijden et al., 1995: traction, 14 RCTs included, 3 RCTs on neck pain (101).
8. Faas, 1993: back exercises, 11 RCTs since 1990 included (32).
9. Koes et al., 1995: manipulation, 36 RCTs included (59).
10. Evans and Richards, 1996: conservative treatments (29).
11. Koes et al., 1997: nonsteroidal antiinflammatory drugs (NSAIDs), 26 RCTs included (60).
12. Waddell et al., 1997: bed rest, 9 RCTs included (105).
13. Waddell et al., 1997: advice on activity, 8 RCTs included (105).

A study was included if it met the following criteria:

1. It concerned, exclusively or separately, patients with acute LBP of less than 3 months' duration or recurrent LBP.
2. It was an RCT.
3. It was relevant to primary care.
4. It had at least ten patients in each group.
5. It had patient-centered outcomes.
6. It was published in English.

In the published systematic review, a search was made of the MEDLINE database from 1966 through September 1995, the EMBASE drugs and pharmacology database from 1980 through September 1995, and the PsycLIT database from 1984 through September 1995, using medical subject headings and free text words (102,103). The keywords used were LBP, backache, musculoskeletal diseases, joint diseases, spinal diseases, physical therapy, chiropractic, and osteopathy, as well as the names of specific interventions. Subsequently, the references given in relevant identified publications were examined further. We reviewed the titles and abstracts of the identified articles in order to determine the relevance of the articles for our systematic review. When there was any doubt, the article was retrieved and read. Abstracts and unpublished studies were not selected. For the update of the literature search, we used a highly sensitive search strategy for MEDLINE published by Dickersin et al. (25) and for EMBASE developed by the Cochrane Center in the United Kingdom.

A study was included and considered relevant if it met the following criteria:

1. It concerned, exclusively or separately, patients with acute or subacute nonspecific LBP of less than 3 months' duration.
2. It was a true RCT; trials with quasirandom procedures such as alternate allocation or allocation based on dates of birth were excluded.
3. The treatment regimen consisted of a conservative intervention.
4. At least one of the clinical outcome measures was pain intensity, overall improvement, functional status, or return to work.
5. The article was published in English.

Acute LBP was defined as LBP persisting for 6 weeks or less. Studies were included if they reported on a mix of patients with acute and subacute (6 to 12 weeks' duration) LBP. Studies were excluded if they reported on patients with chronic (12 weeks' duration or more) LBP or on a mix of patients with acute and chronic LBP. Studies also were excluded if they reported on patients with neck pain or a mix of low back and neck pain, unless the results for LBP were separately presented.

Methodologic Quality of the Studies

Some empiric evidence has suggested that dimensions of methodologic quality are associated with biased estimates of treatment effects in controlled trials (91). All trials were scored as described in the published review (102,103). The quality criteria were based on generally accepted principles of intervention research and referred to various aspects of study population, description of interventions, outcome measurements, and data presentation and analysis (54,56–60). We used the same criteria list that was used in previously published systematic reviews of back pain (55,74). A weight was attached to each criterion, resulting in a maximum score of 100 points for each study. The methodologic quality of the RCTs was assessed by two independent reviewers. Disagreements between the two reviewers were resolved by consensus or by consulting a third researcher who acted as referee. The assessments resulted in a hierarchic list in which higher scores indicated studies with a higher methodologic quality. An RCT was (arbitrarily) considered to be of high quality if the methodologic score was 50 points or more and of low quality if the methodologic score was less than 50 points.

Outcome of the Studies

The main results from each study were extracted according to the most important outcome measures, that is, pain intensity, overall improvement, functional status, and return to work. A study was considered positive if the therapeutic intervention was more effective than the reference treatment with regard to at least one of these outcome measures. A study was considered negative if the authors reported no differences between the intervention under study and the reference treatment on these outcome measures or if the reference treatment was reported to be more effective with regard to at least one of these outcome measures. If the therapeutic intervention under study was reported to be more effective on one of the outcome measures, but less effective on another, or if these outcome measures were not assessed in a study, no conclusion was drawn. (Conclusions and results are noted in Tables 11.1 to 11.3.)

Levels of Evidence

The conclusions on the effectiveness of the therapeutic interventions were based on the strength of the scientific evidence. The rating system consisted of four levels of scientific evidence, based on the quality and the outcome of the studies:

A. Strong evidence: provided by generally consistent findings in multiple high-quality RCTs.
B. Moderate evidence: provided by generally consistent findings in one high-quality RCT and one or more low-quality RCTs or generally consistent findings in multiple low-quality RCTs.

TABLE 11.1. *Randomized controlled trials on the effectiveness of drug therapy in acute low back pain in order of methodologic score*

Investigators (ref.)	Scores for methodologic criteria																	Total score	Conclusion[a]
	A 2	B 5	C 4	D 3	E 4	F 12	G 10	H 5	I 5	J 5	K 9	L 8	M 8	N 5	O 5	P 5	Q 5	100	
Analgesics																			
Videman et al. (104)	1	3	—	2	4	—	8	5	—	—	5	7	7	3	—	5	—	50	Negative
Wiesel et al. (110)	2	3	—	3	4	—	6	5	5	—	—	4	—	3	5	5	—	45	Positive
Brown et al. (16)	2	1	—	—	2	—	10	5	5	—	—	7	1	3	—	5	—	41	Negative
Evans et al. (28)	1	1	—	—	4	—	10	5	5	—	5	5	1	3	—	—	—	35	Negative
Hackett et al. (42)	1	2	—	3	4	—	—	5	—	5	5	3	3	3	—	—	—	34	Negative
Nwuga (78)	2	4	—	—	—	—	5	5	—	—	—	4	1	3	—	5	—	29	Negative
Nonsteroidal antiinflammatory drugs																			
Hosie (51)	2	5	—	2	4	12	10	5	5	—	5	8	8	3	5	5	—	79	Negative
Amlie et al. (3)	2	4	—	2	4	12	10	—	5	5	5	7	7	3	—	5	—	71	Positive
Goldie (41)	2	4	4	3	4	—	10	—	5	5	5	5	5	3	5	5	—	65	Negative
Weber et al. (109)	2	3	—	—	4	6	10	5	5	5	5	6	6	3	5	5	5	65	Negative
Bakshi et al. (4)	2	4	—	2	2	6	10	5	—	—	5	7	7	3	5	5	—	63	Negative
Blazek et al. (10)	2	3	—	3	4	—	10	5	5	5	5	6	6	3	5	5	—	62	Negative
Szpalski and Hayez (98)	2	4	—	1	4	12	10	—	5	5	5	6	6	3	—	5	—	56	Positive
Lacey et al. (58)	—	3	—	1	2	12	10	5	—	5	5	6	6	3	—	—	—	53	Positive subgroup
Videman et al. (104)	1	3	—	2	4	—	10	5	—	—	5	7	7	3	—	5	—	52	Negative
Sweetman et al. (96)	2	4	—	—	2	—	8	5	—	—	5	8	8	3	—	5	—	50	Negative
Orava (79)	2	5	—	1	4	6	10	5	5	—	—	8	—	3	—	5	—	49	Negative
Wiesel et al. (110)	2	3	—	3	4	—	8	5	5	—	—	4	—	3	5	5	—	47	Negative
Agrifoglio et al. (2)	1	3	—	2	2	—	10	5	—	—	5	5	5	3	—	5	—	46	Positive
Weber et al. (108)	2	2	—	—	—	—	10	—	—	5	5	6	6	3	—	5	—	44	Positive
Waterworth and Hunter (107)	2	2	—	2	4	—	10	5	5	—	—	8	—	3	—	—	—	41	Negative

	A	B	C	D	E	F	G	H	I	J	K	L	M	N	O	P		Total	
	2	5	4	3	4	17	10	5	5	5	5	10	10	5	5	5			
Brown et al. (16)	2	1	—	—	2	—	10	5	5	5	—	7	1	3	—	5	—	41	Negative
Evans et al. (28)	1	1	—	—	4	—	10	5	5	5	—	5	1	3	—	—	—	35	Positive
Aghababian et al. (1)	2	3	—	1	—	—	10	5	—	—	—	6	—	3	—	5	—	35	Positive
Postacchini et al. (83)	2	—	—	—	2	—	8	5	—	—	—	5	—	5	—	—	—	27	Not clear
Muscle relaxants																			
Berry and Hutchinson (7)	1	3	—	3	4	6	8	5	5	5	5	4	4	3	5	5	—	66	Positive
Baratta (5)	—	3	4	—	4	6	8	—	—	5	5	8	8	3	5	5	—	64	Positive
Casale (17)	1	4	4	3	4	—	8	—	5	5	5	3	3	3	5	5	—	55	Positive
Boyles et al. (15)	2	3	4	3	2	—	8	5	5	—	5	7	7	3	—	—	—	54	Positive
Hindle (49)	—	2	4	—	—	—	8	5	—	5	5	8	8	3	—	5	—	53	Positive
Middleton (73)	2	3	—	3	4	6	8	5	5	—	—	7	—	3	5	—	—	53	Negative
Dapas et al. (21)	1	3	4	—	—	6	8	—	5	5	5	8	8	3	—	5	—	52	Positive
Rollings et al. (86)	2	3	—	3	—	—	8	5	5	5	5	7	7	3	—	—	—	52	Negative
Berry and Hutchinson (8)	1	3	—	3	2	6	8	—	—	—	5	4	4	3	—	—	—	49	Positive
Gold (40)	—	1	—	3	4	—	8	5	—	5	5	4	4	3	5	5	—	44	Positive
Sweetman et al. (96)	1	1	—	—	—	—	8	5	5	—	—	5	5	3	—	—	—	43	Positive
Borenstein et al. (14)	1	2	—	3	4	—	8	5	—	5	5	7	—	3	5	5	—	40	Positive
Hingorani (50)	—	—	—	—	4	—	8	—	—	—	5	2	2	3	5	5	—	39	Negative
Tervo et al. (99)	—	3	4	—	—	—	8	—	—	5	5	2	2	3	—	—	—	27	Positive
	A	B	C	D	E	F	G	H	I	J	K	L	M	N	O	P		Total	
	2	5	4	3	4	17	10	5	5	5	5	10	10	5	5	5		100	
Epidural steroid injections																			
Mathews et al. (70)	1	3	4	3	4	—	10	—	5	5	3	4	4	5	5	5	—	61	Positive
Coomes (19)	2	3	2	3	4	—	5	5	—	—	—	4	—	3	5	—	—	36	Positive

[a] Positive if the therapeutic intervention involved was more effective than the reference treatment(s) with regard to pain intensity, overall improvement, or functional status; negative if there was no difference between the intervention and the reference treatment(s) on these outcome measures or if the reference treatment was more effective.

245

TABLE 11.2. Randomized controlled trials on the effectiveness of other conservative treatments for acute low back pain in order of methodologic score

Investigators (ref.)	A 2	B 5	C 4	D 3	E 4	F 17	G 10	H 5	I 5	J 5	K 5	L 10	M 15	N 5	O 5	P 5	Total score 100	Conclusion[a]
Bed rest																		
Malmivaara et al. (68)	2	5	4	2	2	8	10	5	3	5	—	10	12	3	—	5	76	Negative
Gilbert et al. (37); Evans et al. (27)	2	5	—	2	4	8	10	5	3	—	3	10	12	5	—	5	71	Negative
Deyo et al. (24)	1	5	4	2	2	8	10	5	3	—	—	10	12	3	5	—	70	Negative
Wilkinson (111)	2	4	4	2	2	—	10	5	5	—	—	6	6	3	—	5	54	Negative
Pal et al. (81)	1	2	2	3	4	—	10	—	—	5	—	8	8	5	5	5	53	Negative
Wiesel et al. (110)	2	3	—	—	4	—	—	5	5	—	—	4	—	—	—	—	23	Positive
Postacchini et al. (83)	2	3	—	2	2	—	5	5	—	—	—	6	—	5	—	—	28	Negative
Szpalski and Hayez (97)	2	4	4	2	2	—	10	5	—	—	3	4	6	3	5	—	42	Negative
Coomes (19)	2	3	2	3	4	—	5	5	—	—	—	4	—	3	—	—	36	Negative
Rupert et al. (88)	2	4	—	—	—	—	10	5	—	5	—	2	3	3	—	—	34	Negative
Advice on staying active																		
Malmivaara et al. (68)	2	5	4	2	2	8	10	5	3	5	—	10	12	3	—	5	76	Positive
Lindequist et al. (63)	2	4	2	1	4	—	10	5	3	—	—	6	9	5	—	5	56	Positive
Wilkinson (111)	2	4	4	2	2	—	10	5	5	—	—	6	6	3	—	5	54	Positive
Indahl et al. (53)	2	2	3	—	4	17	5	5	—	—	—	2	6	5	—	5	53	Positive
Fordyce et al. (35)	2	3	2	—	4	—	10	5	3	—	—	8	9	5	—	5	52	Positive
Lindström et al. (64,65)	2	2	4	3	4	8	10	5	—	—	—	4	3	2	—	5	52	Positive
Linton et al. (66)	1	2	—	2	—	—	10	5	3	—	3	6	9	5	—	3	46	Positive
Philips et al. (82)	1	—	—	2	—	—	10	5	—	—	3	2	3	2	—	2	27	Positive

Investigators (ref.)	A 2	B 5	C 4	D 3	E 4	F 17	G 10	H 5	I 5	J 5	K 5	L 10	M 10	N 5	O 5	P 5	Total 100	Conclusion
Exercise therapy																		
Faas et al. (32,33)	2	5	4	—	2	17	10	5	5	5	3	6	—	5	—	5	74	Negative
Gilbert et al. (37); Evans et al. (27)	2	5	—	—	—	8	10	5	—	—	—	10	2	5	—	5	52	Negative
Malmivaara et al. (68)	1	5	4	—	2	8	5	5	—	—	—	10	2	—	—	5	47	Negative
Stankovic and Johnell (94,95)	1	3	4	3	4	—	10	5	—	—	—	2	—	5	5	5	47	Positive
Waterworth and Hunter (107)	2	5	—	3	4	—	5	5	5	—	3	6	—	3	5	—	43	Negative
Nwuga (77)	2	4	2	—	—	—	10	5	—	—	—	2	2	3	—	5	38	Negative
Farrell and Twomey (34)	2	5	—	—	2	—	10	5	—	—	—	8	2	3	—	—	37	Negative
Davies et al. (22)	2	3	—	—	4	—	—	5	—	—	3	6	2	3	—	5	33	Negative

Study														Score	Result[a]
Delitto et al. (23)	1	2	2	—	—	—	10	5	—	—	—	—	—	30	Positive
Nwuga and Nwuga (76)	2	2	2	—	3	—	—	5	—	—	3	2	2	28	Positive
Back schools															
Bergquist-Ullman and Larsson (6)	2	3	2	—	2	2	10	5	—	—	—	—	—	46	Positive
Stankovic and Johnell (94, 95)	2	3	4	—	4	—	10	—	—	5	—	—	—	39	Negative
Lindequist et al. (63)	1	2	—	—	4	—	5	5	—	5	—	—	—	36	Negative
Morrison et al. (75)	—	—	—	—	—	8	—	—	—	—	—	—	—	22	Positive
Manipulation															
MacDonald and Bell (67)	1	4	—	3	4	—	10	5	5	5	—	6	—	51	Overall negative; positive subgroup only
Sanders et al. (89)	—	2	2	3	2	—	10	5	5	5	3	2	2	51	Not clinically relevant
Hadler et al. (43)	1	3	—	—	4	—	10	5	5	5	3	4	—	48	Positive subgroup
Bergquist-Ullman and Larsson (6)	2	1	2	—	4	8	10	5	—	—	2	2	—	46	Positive compared with placebo; negative compared with back school
Mathews et al. (71)	—	2	—	3	2	17	5	5	—	5	—	2	—	46	Positive subgroup
Helliwell and Cunliffe (46)	1	3	—	3	4	—	5	5	5	5	—	2	2	43	Negative
Glover et al. (38)	—	3	4	3	4	—	5	—	5	5	5	2	—	39	Negative
Blomberg et al. (11–13)	1	2	4	—	4	—	—	5	—	5	—	6	2	37	Positive
Rasmussen (84)	1	1	—	—	4	—	—	5	5	5	—	4	—	33	Positive
Delitto et al. (23)	—	1	2	—	4	—	10	5	—	5	—	2	—	32	Positive
Farrell and Twomey (34)	2	4	—	—	2	—	—	5	5	5	—	6	—	32	Positive
Nwuga (77)	2	3	—	3	—	—	10	5	5	5	—	2	2	32	Positive
Waterworth and Hunter (107)	2	3	—	—	4	—	—	5	5	5	—	6	—	31	Negative
Postacchini et al. (83)	—	2	—	—	2	—	10	5	5	5	5	4	—	28	Positive
Wreje et al. (113)	1	2	—	—	2	—	—	—	—	5	5	2	—	25	Positive
Godfrey et al. (39)	1	1	—	—	2	—	—	5	5	5	—	8	2	22	Negative
Transcutaneous electrical nerve stimulation															
Herman et al. (48)	1	3	4	3	—	—	10	—	5	—	3	6	6	56	Negative
Hackett et al. (42)	1	2	—	3	4	—	—	5	—	5	3	4	4	39	Positive
Traction															
Larsson et al. (62)	2	4	—	3	4	—	10	5	—	5	—	2	—	43	Positive
Mathews and Hickling (69)	—	2	3	3	2	8	5	5	—	5	—	2	—	35	Positive subgroup
Behavioral therapy															
Fordyce et al. (35)	2	4	—	—	—	—	—	5	—	—	—	4	—	20	Positive

[a] Positive if the therapeutic intervention involved was more effective than the reference treatment(s) with regard to pain intensity, overall improvement or functional status; negative if there was no difference between the intervention and the reference treatment(s) on these outcome measures or if the reference treatment was more effective.

TABLE 11.3. *Details of randomized controlled trials on the effectiveness of analgesics for acute low back pain*

Investigators (ref.)	Analgesics; dose/frequency/duration (no. of patients)	Reference treatment(s) (no. of patients)	Results
Videman et al. (104)	I: meptazinol 200 mg q.i.d./3 wk (35)	R: diflunisal 250 mg q.i.d./4 wk (35)	Mean change in degree of pain (100-mm VAS) at 3 wk: I, 45, vs. R, 40; similar improvement regarding capacity for daily tasks (data in graphs); no significant differences; side effects similar: I, 19, vs. R, 23 patients
Wiesel et al. (110)	I1: acetaminophen (dosage not given) b.i.d./2 wk (?) I2: codeine 60 mg q.i.d./2 wk (?) I3: oxycodone + aspirin 1 tablet q.i.d. (?)	—	Mean (SD) no. of days before return to full activity: I1, 5.6 (0.6); I2, 5.2 (0.6); I3, 5.6 (0.7); no significant differences; no data on side effects given
Brown et al. (16)	I: acetaminophen 300 mg + codeine 50 mg, 2 capsules; initially, one capsule every 4 hr/15 d (21)	R: diflunisal (capsules) initial dose 1,000 mg; 500 mg every 12 hr/15 d (19)	Pain assessment by patient and investigator on 3-point ordinal scale shows similar improvement curves (data in graphs); no. of patients rating drugs as excellent or very good: I, 9, vs. R, 9; no significant differences; more side effects in I (10) than in R (3)
Evans et al. (28)	I1: dextropropoxyphene 32.5 mg + paracetamol 325 mg, 2 capsules q.i.d./1 wk (30 crossover) I2: paracetamol 500 mg, 2 capsules q.i.d./1 wk (30 crossover)	R1: aspirin 300 mg, 3 capsules q.i.d./1 wk (30 crossover) R2: indomethacin 50 mg t.i.d./1 wk (30 crossover) R3: mefenamic acid 250 mg, 2 capsules t.i.d./1 wk (30 crossover) R4: phenylbutazone 100 mg t.i.d./1 wk (30 crossover)	Mean daily pain index during intervention period (4-point ordinal scale): I1, 1.7; I2, 1.7; R1, 1.4; R2, 1.5; R3, 1.4; R4, 1.4; R3 significantly different from I1 and I2; R1 significantly different from I1; more side effects in R1 (20), R2 (19), and I1 (19) than in R3 (12), I2 (13), and R4 (4)
Hackett et al (42)	I: paracetamol 2 tablets every 4 hr (?)	R: electroacupuncture, 2 treatments in 4 d (?)	Pain scores (VAS) pretreatment and after 1, 2, and 6 wk: I, 54.5, 23.4, 22.0, 13.7, vs. R, 52.7, 23.2, 18.3, 3.3; R significantly less pain after 6 wk.
Nwuga (78)	I: analgesics (unspecified) (?)	R1: ultrasound (?) R2: placebo ultrasound (?)	Proportion of patients pain-free after 4 wk: I, 6.8%; R1, 40.7%; R2, 12%; R1 significanty more improved than I.

I, index treatment; R, reference treatment; SD, standard deviation; VAS, visual analog scale; ?, number of patients not given.

C. Limited or contradictory evidence: provided by one RCT (either high or low-quality) or inconsistent findings in multiple RCTs.
D. No evidence: no RCTs.

RESULTS

Analgesics

Six RCTs were identified, of which only one was considered to be of high methodologic quality (104). The scores ranged from 29 to 50 points. The high-quality RCT (Table 11.3) did not show a better improvement in pain intensity when comparing meptazinol with diflunisal (NSAID). The results of the five low-quality RCTs (16,28,42,78,110) did not show a better improvement in pain intensity with certain analgesics compared with aspirin, mefenamic acid, electroacupuncture, or ultrasound.

There is moderate evidence that analgesics (paracetamol and paracetamol-weak opioid compounds) are not more effective than NSAIDs, electroacupuncture, or ultrasound (level 2). The proportion of adverse effects (constipation and drowsiness) is slightly higher with combinations of paracetamol and weak opioids (20).

Nonsteroidal Antiinflammatory Drugs

Nineteen RCTs (Table 11.4) were identified, of which 10 were considered to be of high quality (3,4,10,41,51,58,96,98,104,109) and nine of low quality (1,2,16,28,79,83,107, 108,110). The scores ranged from 27 to 79 points. Five of the 10 high-quality RCTs compared NSAIDs with a placebo. Three of these RCTs reported a positive outcome for uncomplicated LBP (3,58,104), but only for one of the follow-up moments or for a subgroup only. The two negative high-quality RCTs compared NSAIDs with a placebo for patients with acute LBP with sciatica or acute sciatica with nerve root symptoms (41,109). The high-quality RCT comparing an NSAID to an analgesic did not show a difference in improvement of pain intensity (104). In addition, the three high-quality RCTs comparing different types of NSAIDs did not report any differences (4,10,51).

There is strong evidence (level A) that NSAIDs prescribed at regular intervals provide effective pain relief for simple acute LBP, but they do not affect return to work, natural history, or chronicity. There is limited evidence (level C) that NSAIDs do not provide effective pain relief for nerve root pain. There is strong evidence (level A) that different types of NSAIDs are equally effective. NSAIDs can have serious adverse effects, particularly at high doses and in elderly patients. Ibuprofen has the lowest risk of gastrointestinal complications of the most commonly used NSAIDs, followed by diclofenac, mainly because of the low doses used in clinical practice (47).

Muscle Relaxants and Benzodiazepines

Eight high-quality RCTs (5,7,15,17,21,49,73,86) and six low-quality RCTs (8,14,40,50, 96,99) were identified on the efficacy of muscle relaxants (Table 11.5). The scores ranged from 27 to 66 points. All five high-quality RCTs comparing a muscle relaxant with a placebo (5,7,15,17,21,49,73) reported a better improvement in pain intensity for the muscle relaxant (Table 11.6). The three high-quality RCTs comparing different

TABLE 11.4. Details of randomized controlled trials on the effectiveness of nonsteroidal antiinflammatory drugs for acute low back pain

Investigators (ref.)	NSAIDs dose/frequency/duration (no. of patients)	Reference treatment(s) (no. of patients)	Results
Hosie (51)	I1: ibuprofen capsules 400 mg t.i.d. + placebo foam t.i.d./14 d (147) I2: felbinac (foam 3%) t.i.d. + placebo capsules t.i.d./14 d (140)	—	Patients (%) reporting none or mild severity after 1 and 2 wk: I1, 84, 92; I2, 76, 88; no significant differences; no. of side effects: I1, 22; I2, 26
Amlie et al. (3)	R: piroxicam 20-mg capsules b.i.d. first 2 d, 1/d next 5 d/7 d (140)	R: placebo capsules (142)	I: More pain relief (VAS) than R after 3 d; after 7 d, no significant differences; side effects similar: I 13%; R, 17%
Goldie (41)	I: indomethacin 25-mg capsules t.i.d./course of 50 capsules (25)	R: placebo capsules (25)	No. of patients with complete relief of pain after 7 and 14 d: I, 7, 14; R, 9, 16; no significant differences; side effects similar: I, 8; R, 5
Weber et al. (109)	I: piroxicam 20-mg capsules 40 mg/d first 2 d; 20 mg/d next 12 d/14 d (120)	R: placebo capsules (94)	Reduction of pain in back and leg measured by VAS after 4 wk the same in the two groups (data in graphs); no significant differences; more side effects in I (22) than in R (13)
Bakshi et al. (4)	I1: diclofenac resinate capsules 75 mg b.i.d./14 d (66) I2: piroxicam capsules 20 mg b.i.d. for 2 d + q.d. for 12 d (66)	—	Mean pain intensity scores at rest (VAS) pre- and posttreatment: I1, 70.0, 22.7; I2, 67.1, 21.0; efficacy excellent or good according to patients: I1, 81.8%; I2, 87.7%; no differences; side effects similar: I1, 17; I2, 15
Blazek et al. (10)	I1: diclofenac 25-mg capsules/q.i.d. first 4 d and t.i.d. next 8 d/12 d (14) I2: biarison 300-mg capsules/qid first 4 d and t.i.d. next 8 d/12 d (14)	—	Average improvement on 5-point ordinal scale (0 = no response, 4 = very good response) during and after the intervention period of 12 d according to physician and patient: I1, 2.6 and 2.8; I2, 2.8 and 3; no significant differences in recovery rate; side effects: mild side effects in 3 patients in each group
Szpalski and Hayez (98)	I: tenoxicam 20 mg i.m. injection on day 1 + 20 mg capsules 1 d for day 2 to 14 (+7 d bed rest) (37)	R: placebo injection + placebo capsules (36)	Mean pain intensity (VAS) on days 1, 8, and 15: I, 7.4, 1.9, 0.6; R, 7.1, 2.8, 0.8; I significantly better on day 8; side effects: 1 patient in group I
Lacey et al. (58)	I: piroxicam 10-mg capsules/q.i.d. first 2 d, b.i.d. next 12 d/14 d (168)	R: placebo capsules (169)	Patients (%) improved after 1 wk only in subgroups with initial moderate to severe pain: I, 82%/49%; R, 53%/38%; no differences for subgroup with mild initial pain; results after 2 wk not reported, and no data presented on side effects for subgroup with back pain
Videman et al. (104)	I: diflunisal 250-mg capsules q.i.d./3 wk (35)	R: meptazinol 200-mg capsules q.i.d./3 wk (35)	Mean change in pain (100-mm VAS) at 3 wk: I, 45; R, 40; similar improvement regarding capacity for daily tasks (data in graphs). No significant differences; side effects similar: I, 19; R, 23 patients
Sweetman et al. (96)	I: mefenamic acid 500 mg t.i.d. + placebo b.i.d. (40)	R1: chlormezanone 100 mg and paracetamol 450 mg, 2 capsules tid + placebo t.i.d. (42) R2: ethoheptazine 75 mg and meprobamate 150 mg and aspirin 250 mg, 2 capsules + placebo t.i.d. (40)	No. of patients reporting no pain after 1 and 7 d: I, 7, 21; R1, 12, 23; R2, 10, 20; no. of patients with adverse events: I, 9; R1, 10; R2, 16

Study	Index treatment (I)	Reference treatment (R)	Results
Orava (79)	I1: diflunisal 500-mg capsules b.i.d./7 d (66); I2: indomethacin 50-mg capsules t.i.d./7 d (67)	—	No. of patients (%) assessing therapy as good or excellent after 3 and 7 d: I1, 45%, 64%; I2, 45%, 64%; no significant differences; more side effects in I2 (31%) than in I1 (18%)
Wiesel et al. (110)	I1: aspirin 625-mg capsules q.i.d./2 wk (?); I2: phenylbutazone 100-mg capsules q.i.d. (first 5 d); no further information given (?)	R: acetaminophen (dosage not given) b.i.d. (2 wk) (?)	Mean no. of days before return to full activity: I1, 5.7; I2, 6.5; R, 5.7; no significant differences; no data on side effects given
Agrifoglio et al. (2)	I1: aceclofenac 150 mg i.m. injection b.i.d./2 d + tablet 100 mg b.i.d./5 d (50); I2: diclofenac 75 mg i.m. injection b.i.d. 2 d + tablet 50 mg t.i.d. 5 d (50)	—	No significant difference in pain intensity (VAS) pre- and posttreatment (data in graph); percentage of patients not limited in functional impairment posttreatment: I1, 65.9%; I2, 40.5%; significant; overall assessment of efficacy good/very good: I1, 85%; I2, 76%; significant; side effects: I1, 1; I2, 8
Weber and Aasand (108)	I: phenylbutazone 200 mg, 2 capsules t.i.d./3 d; 1 capsule t.i.d. next 2 d (28)	R: placebo capsules (29)	No. of patients reporting definite positive effect after intervention period: I, 14; R 8; no significant differences; no side effects reported by the patients
Waterworth and Hunter (107)	I: diflunisal 500-mg capsule 1,000 mg immediately; 500 mg b.i.d./10 d (36)	R1: physicaetherapy: local heat, ultrasound, and exercises, 5 × 45-min session weekly (34); R2: spinal manipulation and/or McKenzie therapy, 5 × 45-min sessions weekly (38)	Mean change in pain intensity on 4-point scale after 4 and 12 d: I, −0.9, −1.7; R1, −0.9, −1.6; R2, −1.1, −1.7; no significant differences in pain and mobility
Brown et al. (16)	I: diflunisal capsules, initial dose 1,000 mg; 500 mg every 12 hr/15 d (19)	R: acetaminophen 300 mg with codeine 50 mg, 2 capsules initially; 1 capsule every 4 hr/15 d (21)	Pain assessment by patient and investigator on 3-point ordinal scale show similar improvement curves (data in graphs); no. of patients rating drugs as excellent or very good: I, 9; R, 9; no significant differences; side effects: more side effects in R (10) than in I (3)
Evans et al. (28)	I1: aspirin 300 mg, 3 capsules q.i.d./1 wk (30); I2: indomethacin 50 mg t.i.d./1 wk (30); I3: mefenamic acid 250 mg/2 capsules t.i.d./1 wk (30); I4: phenylbutazone 100 mg t.i.d./1 wk (30)	R1: dextropropoxyphene 32.5 mg + paracetamol 325-mg capsules, 2 capsules q.i.d./1 wk (30); R2: paracetamol 500 mg, 2 capsules q.i.d./1 wk (30)	Mean daily pain index during intervention period (on 4-point ordinal scale): I1, 1.4; I2, 1.5; I3, 1.4; I4, 1.4; R1, 1.7; R2, 1.7; I3 significantly different from R1 and R2; I1 significantly different from R1; side effects: more side effects in I1 (20), I2 (19), R1 (19) than in I3 (12), R2 (13), I4 (4)
Aghababian et al. (1)	I1: diflunisal capsules/1,000 mg initially, 500 mg every 8–12 hr/2 wk (16); I2: naproxen capsules/500 mg initially, 250 mg every 6–8 hr/2 wk (17)	—	No. of patients (%) reporting no pain (4-point ordinal scale) after 2 wk: I1, 81%; I2, 41%; no significance tests reported; no adverse experiences reported by the patients
Postacchini et al. (83)	I: diclofenac "full dosage"/10–14 d (34)	R1: chiropractic manipulation (35); R2: physical therapy (31); R3: bed rest (29); R4: placebo (antiedema gel) (30)	Mean improvement on combined pain, disability, and spinal mobility score (5–32) after 3 wk and 2 and 6 mo: I, 3.0, 10.7, 14.0; R1, 7.5, 9.7, 12.3; R2, 5.0, 8.4, 10.2; R3, 5.4, 7.5, 7.3; R4, 1.8, 7.3, 11.0; R1 significantly better than others after 3 wk; no other differences; no data on side effects reported.

NSAIDs, nonsteroidal antiinflammatory drugs; I, index treatment; R, reference treatment; VAS, visual analog scale; ?, number of patients not given.

TABLE 11.5. *Details of randomized controlled trials on the effectiveness of muscle relaxants for acute low back pain*

Investigators (ref.)	Muscle relaxants dose/frequency/duration (no. of patients)	Reference treatment(s) (no. of patients)	Results
Berry and Hutchinson (8)	I: tizanidine 4 mg + ibuprofen 400 mg t.i.d./7 d (51)	R: placebo plus ibuprofen 400 mg t.i.d./7 d (54)	Mean changes (SD) in pain score (VAS 100 mm) after 3 d: I, pain at night, 20 (32.8), pain at rest, 18 (25.3), and pain on walking, 23 (25.4), vs. R, 22 (34.6), 16 (24.9), and 13 (22.6); after 7 d: I, 32 (39.5), 29 (43.3), and 36 (34.1), vs. R, 33 (39.8), 33 (32.9), and 30 (32.8); percentage of patients improved after 3 d: I, 76%, vs. R, 67%; and after 7 d: I, 85%, vs. R, 81%; no significant differences; I significantly more central nervous system side effects, R significantly more gastrointestinal side effects; significantly fewer patients had moderate or severe pain at rest or pain at night in I than in R
Baratta (5)	I: cyclobenzaprine 10 mg t.i.d.–q.i.d./10 d (58)	R: placebo t.i.d.–q.i.d./10 d (59)	Mean decrease in pain (10-point scale) from day 1 to 9: I, −0.8 to −5.5, vs. R, −0.3 to −4.0; I significantly better; moderate to marked global improvement: I, 71%, vs. R, 25%; significant; significantly more central nervous side effects in I
Casale (17)	I: dantrolene sodium 25 mg, 1 capsule/d/4 d (10)	R: placebo 1 capsule/d/4 d (10)	Pain during maximal voluntary movement (VAS) decreased significantly more in I than in R; muscle spasm significantly more improved in I 85% than in R 30%
Boyles et al. (15)	I1: carisoprodol 350 mg q.i.d./8 d (36)	I2: diazepam 5 mg q.i.d./8 d (35)	Patient's assessment of muscle tension, stiffness, and overall relief significantly more improved in I1 than in I2 after 6 and 7 d; no significant difference in pain; physician's assessment of overall improvement and muscle spasm significantly better in I1 than in I2 after 7 d, but not after 3 d; data in graphs
Hindle (49)	I: carisoprodol 350 mg q.i.d./4 d (16)	R1: placebo q.i.d./4 d (16) R2: butabarbital 15 mg q.i.d./4 d (16)	Pain score (VAS 0–100) at baseline and after 2 and 4 d: I, 86.0, 33.0, and 15.5; R1, 65.5, 58.5, and 64.0; R2, 75.2, 58.7, and 49.1; I significantly more improved; ADLs significantly more improved in I than in R1 and R2; but not muscle spasm
Middleton (73)	I1: methocarbamol 400 mg + acetylsalicylic acid 325 mg, 2 tablets q.i.d./7 d (55)	I2: chlormezanone 100 mg + paracetamol 450 mg, 2 tablets t.i.d./7 d (52)	Percentage of patients with moderate to very severe pain on days 1 and 7 in I1, 87% and 51%, vs. I2, 85% and 52%; percentage of patients with overall improvement posttreatment: I1, 66%, vs. I2, 61%; not significant; significantly more side effects in I2 than in I1
Dapas et al. (21)	I: baclofen 10 mg, 1–2 tablets t.i.d.–q.i.d./10 d (100)	R: placebo 2 tablets q.i.d./ 10 d (100)	For patients with severe symptoms at baseline, I significantly more improved at day 10 in pain, patient's opinion, ADLs, muscle spasm, and spinal mobility; significantly more side effects in I
Rollings et al. (86)	I1: carisoprodol 350 mg q.i.d./7 days (28)	I2: cyclobenzaprine HCL 10 mg q.i.d./7 d (30)	No statistically significant differences between I1 and I2 on pain, muscle stiffness and tension, ADLs, and overall relief; data in graphs

Study	Index treatment (I)	Reference treatment (R)	Results
Berry and Hutchinson (7)	I: tizanidine 4 mg t.i.d./7 d (59)	R: placebo t.i.d./7 d (53)	Mean (SD) pain score (VAS 100 mm) at baseline and after 3 and 7 d: pain at night, I, 51 (31.5), 39 (32.3), and 15 (20.6), vs. R, 52 (33.1), 38 (28.8), and 18 (20.8); pain at rest, I 51 (29.4), 39 (29.6), and 19 (23.2), vs. R, 51 (26.9), 34 (27.9), and 19 (22.9); pain on movement, I 55 (30.0), 46 (30.4), and 18 (22.9), vs. R, 49 (27.8), 36 (25.6), and 18 (23.1); no differences between I and R; overall improvement after 3 and 7 d: I, 17% and 84% of patients; and R, 8% and 82% of patients; not significant; side effects in I, 41%, and R, 21%; I significantly more central nervous system side effects, R significantly more gastrointestinal side effects
Gold (40)	I: orphenadrine citrate 100 mg b.i.d./7 d (20)	R1: placebo b.i.d./7 d (20) R2: phenobarbital 32 mg b.i.d./7 d (20)	No. of patients improved after 2 d: I, 7; R1, 0; R2, 3; I significantly more improved than R1; no. of patients with reduced pain after 2 d: I, 9; R1, 4; R2, 3; I significantly more reduced than R1 and R2; no. of patients with side effects; I, 5; R1, 1; R2, 2
Sweetman et al. (96)	I: chlormezanone 100 mg + paracetamol 450 mg/2 capsules t.i.d./7 d (42)	R1: mefenamic acid 500 mg t.i.d./7 d (40) R2: ethoheptazine 75 mg + meprobamate 150 mg + aspirin 250 mg 2 tablets t.i.d./7d (40)	Number of patients with overall improvement after 7 d: I, 24; R1, 24; R2, 22; not significant; no. of patients reporting side effects on day 7: I, 5; R1, 5; R2, 13; significant
Borenstein et al. (14)	I: cyclobenzaprine 10 mg t.i.d. + naproxen 500 mg initially, 250 mg q.i.d./14 d (20)	R: naproxen 500 mg initially, 250 mg q.i.d./14 d (20)	Treatment outcome significantly better on muscle spasm and tenderness in I than in R; no significant differences on pain and functional capacity; significantly more side effects in I than in R
Hingorani (50)	I: diazepam 10 mg/4 i.m. injections 24 hr + 2 mg oral q.i.d./5 d + aspirin 10 gr t.i.d./5 d (25)	R: placebo 4 injections 24 h + oral q.i.d.5 d plus aspirin 10 gr t.i.d./5 d (25)	No. of patients improved: I, 19, vs. R, 18; side effects: drowsiness in I, 7 patients, vs. 3 in R
Tervo et al. (99)	I: orphenadrine i.m. injection 60 mg/2 mL mg/2 mL + oral orphenadrine citrate 35 mg + paracetamol 450 mg, 2 tablets t.i.d./8 d (25)	R: placebo saline injection 2 mL + oral paracetamol 450 mg, 2 tablets t.i.d./8 d (25)	No significant differences in subjective impression of improvement, muscle spasm, and spinal flexion; walking and sitting ability significantly more improved in I than in R; side effects in I, 2 patients, and in R, 1 patient

ADLs, activities of daily living; I, index treatment; R, reference treatment; SD, standard deviation; VAS, visual analog scale.

TABLE 11.6. *Details of randomized controlled trials on the effectiveness of epidural steroid injections for acute low back pain*

Investigators (ref.)	Epidural steroid injection (no. of patients)	Reference treatment (no. of patients)	Results
Coomes (19)	I: Epidural 50 mL 0.5% procaine injection (20)	R: bed rest at home on fracture boards or admission to hospital and administration of analgesics to ease the pain (20)	Mean no. of days to recovery: I, 11; R, 31; no. of patients recovered on neurologic signs: I, 12; R, 5; median no. of weeks taken for relief of pain: I, 1.5; R, 4.5
Mathews et al. (70)	I: 80 mg (2 mL) methylprednisolone + 20 mL bupivacaine 0.125%, caudal route (23)	R: 2 mL lidocaine s.c. (34)	No. of patients recovered after 1 mo: I, 67%; R, 56%; not significant; after 3 mo, I significantly more pain free than R

I, index treatment; R, reference treatment.

types of muscle relaxants (15,73,86) reported no differences with regard to pain intensity. One of these trials did report a better overall improvement for one type of muscle relaxant (15).

There is strong evidence (level A) that muscle relaxants effectively reduce acute LBP and that the different types of muscle relaxants are equally effective. Muscle relaxants have significant adverse effects including drowsiness and carry a significant risk of habituation and dependency even after relatively short courses (i.e., 1 week) (26,80).

Antidepressants

There is no evidence available on the use of antidepressants in acute LBP (level D) (100).

Colchicine

Three RCTs were identified on the effectiveness of colchicine in the treatment of acute LBP (72,90,92). There is limited and conflicting evidence (level C) that intravenous colchicine has any effect on acute low back problems. Serious potential side effects have been reported (9).

Systemic Steroids

One RCT was identified on the effectiveness of a 1-week course of oral dexamethasone compared with placebo (44). The limited available evidence suggests that oral steroids are not effective for acute low back problems (level C). Serious potential complications are associated with long-term use, but potential complications appear minimal with short-term use (9).

Epidural Steroid Injections

Two RCTs were identified on the efficacy of epidural steroid injections for acute LBP (Table 11.6) (19,70). One trial reported better outcomes for patients treated with epidural injections than with bed rest (19). The other trial reported significantly more pain-free patients after treatment with epidural steroid injections compared with a placebo injection at 3 months' follow-up, but not after 1 month (70).

There is limited evidence (level C) that epidural steroid injections are more effective than placebo or bed rest for acute LBP with nerve root pain. There is no evidence (level 4) that they are effective for acute LBP without nerve root pain.

Trigger Point and Ligamentous Injections

There is no evidence available on the effectiveness of trigger point injections for acute LBP (level D). Ligamentous and sclerosant injections are invasive and can expose patients to serious potential complications (9).

Facet Joint Injections

There is no evidence available on the use of facet joint injections in acute LBP (level D).

Bed Rest

Ten RCTs were included in a systematic review of bed rest (116). Five RCTs were of high quality (24,27,37,65,76,107), and five were of low quality (19,83,88,97,110). The methodologic scores ranged from 34 to 76 points. Seven of the trials, including four high-quality RCTs, reported negative results (Table 11.7).

There is strong evidence (level A) that bed rest is not effective for treating acute LBP. Bed rest is not as effective as the alternative treatments with which it has been compared for any patient outcomes, that is, relief of pain, rate of recovery, return to daily activities, or days lost from work. Despite widespread practice, there is limited evidence (level C) on the effectiveness of bed rest for acute disc prolapse or nerve root pain (20). There is limited evidence that bed rest with traction is not effective (level C). Traction adds the complications of immobilization to the deleterious effects of bed rest, in particular joint stiffness, muscle wasting, loss of bone mineral, pressure sores, and thromboembolism (81).

Advice on Staying Active

Eight RCTs were included in a systematic review of medical advice to stay active for acute LBP (105). All six high-quality studies and the two low-quality studies showed consistently positive findings, although different trials used different outcomes (Table 11.8).

There is strong evidence (level A) that advice to continue ordinary activity as normally as possible can foster equivalent or faster symptomatic recovery from the acute attack and can lead to less chronic disability and less time lost from work than "traditional" medical treatment with analgesics as required and advice to rest and "let pain be your guide" for return to normal activity. There is also strong evidence (level A) that, for patients with subacute LBP, graded reactivation over a short period of days or a few weeks, combined with behavioral management of pain, leads to less chronic disability and work loss, but it makes little difference to the rate of initial recovery

TABLE 11.7. *Details of randomized controlled trials on the effectiveness of bed rest for acute low back pain*

Investigators (ref.)	Treatment with bed rest (no. of patients)	Reference treatment(s) (no. of patients)	Results
Malmivaara et al. (68)	I: complete bed rest for 2 d, routine activities as tolerated thereafter (67)	R: continuation of ordinary activities as tolerated (67)	Differences in adjusted group means (95% CI) of I minus R on pain intensity (11-point scale), functional status (Oswestry), and satisfaction with treatment (11-point scale) after 3 wk: 0.3 (−0.4 to 0.9), 3.9 (−0.2 to 8.0), and −0.7 (−1.8 to 0.4); and after 12 wk: 0.7 (0.03 to 1.4), 3.8 (0.1 to −7.5), and −0.6 (−1.6 to 0.4); pain intensity and functional status significantly better in I after 12 wk
Gilbert et al. (37); Evans et al. (27)	I1: bed rest at least 4 d (instructed) (60); I2: bed rest at least 4 d (instructed) and physical therapy and instruction (65)	R1: exercise and education (62); R2: no intervention (65)	No. of patients reporting no pain after 6 and 12 wk: I1, 34, 37; I2, 33, 46; R1, 36, 44; R2, 33, 43; no significant differences in pain, mobility, or daily activities
Deyo et al. (24)	I1: bed rest (2 d recommended) (101); I2: bed rest (7 d recommended) (102)	—	No differences in functional status, self-rated, and clinician-rated improvement and duration of pain after 3 wk and 3 mo; no. of days absent from work after 3 wk: I1, 3.1; I2, 5.6; significant
Wilkinson (111)	I: complete bed rest for 48 hr (20)	R: no daytime rest and remaining mobile (22)	Mean (SD) functional status (Roland) at days 1, 7, and 28. I, 13.9 (5.4), 9.7 (19.9), 5.9 (5.6); R, 11.0 (11.0), 5.3 (5.7), 3.2 (4.0); I significantly more improved between days 7 and 28; no differences in mobility and time lost from work
Pal et al. (81)	I: bed rest plus continuous traction (24)	R: bed rest plus "sham traction" (15)	Median pain score (VAS 0–100 mm) on admission and after 1, 2, and 3 wk: I, 50, 25, 6, 5; R, 50, 15, 9, 3; not significant; no. returned to work after 6 mo: I, 18/24; R, 9/15; not significant
Wiesel et al. (110)	I: bed rest in hospital for maximal 14 d (?)	R: ambulatory treatment without physical exercise (patients are kept on their feet) (?)	Average (SE) no. of pain points within 2 wk: I, 51.7 (5.3); R, 107.6 (10.1); significant; no. of days (SE) before return to work: I, 6.6 (0.23); R, 11.8 (0.12); significant
Postacchini et al. (83)	I: 20 to 24 hr for the first 4 to 6 d and 15 to 20 hr/d for a further 2 d (29)	R1: manipulation (daily first wk and then twice/wk for 3 wk) (35); R2: NSAIDs, 10 to 14 d (34); R3: Physical therapy: light massage, analgesic currents, and infrared: daily for 2 to 3 wk (31); R4: placebo: antiedema gel to be spread on the lumbar region twice/d for 1–2 wk (30)	Mean improvement on combined pain, disability, and spinal mobility score (range, 5–32) after 3 wk and 2 and 6 mo: in subgroup with acute low back pain only: I, 5.4, 7.5, 7.3; R1, 7.5, 9.7, 12.3; R2, 3.0, 10.7, 14.0; R3, 5.0, 8.4, 10.2; R4, 1.8, 7.3, 11.0; R1 significantly better after 3 wk; no other differences
Szpalski and Hayez (97)	I: 7 d bed rest	R: 3 d bed rest	
Coomes (19)	I: bed rest at home on fracture boards or admission to hospital and administration of analgesics to ease the pain (20)	R: epidural 50 mL 0.5% procaine injection (20)	Mean number of days to recovery: I, 31; R, 11; no. of patients recovered on neurologic signs: I, 5; R, 12; median no. of weeks taken for relief of pain: I, 4.5; R, 1.5
Rupert et al. (88)	I: Bed rest and drugs administered by a team of medical orthopedic specialists (?)	R1: chiropractic adjustments (short-lever manipulation) (?); R2: "sham manipulation": nontherapeutic massage to a site unrelated to the area of pain (?)	Percentage improvement on 100-mm VAS at fourth visit: I, 0; R1, 17; R2, 2; I worse than R1

I, index treatment; CI, confidence interval; NSAIDs, nonsteroidal antiinflammatory drugs; R, reference treatment; SD, standard deviation; SE, standard error; VAS, visual analog scale; ?, number of patients not given.

TABLE 11.8 Details of randomized controlled trials on the effectiveness of advice on staying active for acute low back pain

Investigators (ref.)	Exercise regimen (no. of patients)	Reference treatment (no. of patients)	Results
Malmivaara et al. (68)	I: mobilizing exercises: back extension and lateral bending (52)	R: continuation of ordinary activities as tolerated (67)	Differences in adjusted group means (95% CI) between I and R on pain intensity (11-point scale), functional status (Oswestry), and satisfaction with treatment (11-point scale) after 3 wk: 0.9 (−0.001 to 1.7), 6.6 (2.0 to 11.1), and 0.5 (−0.6 to 1.6); and after 12 wk: 0.2 (−0.5 to 1.0), 2.6 (−1.6 to 6.7), and 0.4 (−0.6 to 1.4).
Lindequist et al. (63)	I: advice not to strain the back and to use analgesics when needed; no physical therapy (32)	R: Postural education "back school type" and training program supervised by a physical therapist (24)	Percentage of patients pain free after 1, 3, and 6 wk: I, 16, 66, 81; R, 21, 75, 83; no significant differences
Wilkinson (111)	I: advice to remain mobile and no daytime rest (22)	R: complete bed rest for 48 hr (20)	Mean (SD) functional status (Rolan) at days 1, 7, and 28: I, 11.0 (11.0), 5.3 (5.7), 3.2 (4.0); and R, 13.9 (5.4), 9.7 (19.9), 5.9 (5.6); R significantly more improved between days 7 and 28; no differences in mobility and time lost from work
Indahl et al. (53)	I: intense personal advice, reduction of fear, activity, normal walking, reduction of sick behavior, setting goals of (463)	R: conventional medical system (512)	I: significantly greater reduction in sick leave; after 200 days, 70% returned to work compared with 40% in R; no. of patients still on sick leave at the end of the study (after 13–19 mo): I 24; R, 64 ($p < 001$)
Fordyce et al. (35)	I: advice to continue exercising on a fixed time interval and time-contingent analgesics (57)	R: traditional management: analgesics and exercise until pain had subsided (50)	Mean (SD) score on pain drawings and claimed impairment after 9–12 mo: I, 1.98 (2.46), 4.84 (3.20), vs. R, 3.06 (2.45), 6.25 (3.25); I significantly better than R after 9–12 mo on pain drawings and claimed impairment; no significant differences after 6 wk
Lindström et al. (64, 65)	I: graded activity: individual, submaximal, gradually increased exercise program: endurance and strength training, lifting, walking, jogging, swimming, fitness (51)	R: traditional medical care by own physician (52)	Proportion of patients returned to work within 6 or 12 wk after randomization: I, 59%, 80%, vs. R, 40%, 58%; significant; mean duration of sick leave from low back pain during second follow-up year: I, 12.1 (18.4) wk, vs. R, 19.6 (20.7) wk; significant; no differences in functional status after 1 yr
Linton et al. (66)	I: early activation, reinforcement of healthy behavior, maintenance of daily activities training (68)	R: treatment as usual, analgesics, rest, and sick leave (38)	Pain and disability not significantly different; I better satisfaction and less 1-yr sick leave
Philips et al. (82)	I: graded reactivation +/− behavioral counseling (60)	R: 'let pain be your guide', return to normal (57)	Pain not significantly different; rate of recovery (return to activities) faster in I

I, index treatment; CI, confidence interval; R, reference treatment; SD, standard deviation.

of pain and disability. Advice to return to normal work within a planned short time may lead to shorter periods of work loss and less time lost from work.

Specific Back Exercises

Ten RCTs were identified on specific back exercises (e.g., flexion, extension, aerobics, or stretching exercises), two high-quality (27,32,33) and eight low-quality RCTs (22,23,34,68,76,77,94,95,107). The methodologic scores ranged from 28 to 74. Seven RCTs (22,27,30,33,34,68,77,107), including the two of high quality, reported negative results, and three RCTs reported positive results (23,76,94,95). In eight trials, exercises were compared with various reference treatments such as usual care by the general practitioner, no intervention, continuation of ordinary activities, bed rest, manipulation, NSAIDs, mini-back school, or short-wave diathermy (Table 11.9). Seven of these eight trials, including the two high-quality RCTs, reported a negative result, whereas only one low-quality RCT reported a positive result.

There is strong evidence (level A) that most types of specific back exercises (e.g., flexion, extension, aerobics, or strengthening exercises) are not more effective than alternative treatments for acute LBP with which they have been compared, including no intervention. There is conflicting evidence that McKenzie exercises may produce some short-term symptomatic improvement in acute LBP (level C).

Back Schools

Four low-quality RCTs (6,63,75,94,95) were identified on the efficacy of some type of back school (Table 11.10). The scores ranged from 22 to 46 points. Two trials reported positive results for a back school, and two reported negative results. There is conflicting evidence on the effectiveness of back schools for acute LBP (level C).

Manual Therapy (Manipulation and Mobilization)

Sixteen RCTs were identified, of which only two were of high quality (67,89) and 14 were of low quality (6,11–33,23,34,38,39,43,46,71,77,83,84,107,113). The methodologic scores ranged from 22 to 51 points. Twelve trials, including the two high-quality RCTs, reported positive results, and 4 trials (38,39,46,107) reported negative results. However, in one of the high-quality trials, a fatal flaw (a follow-up period of only 30 minutes after a single manipulation) was identified, and this trial was not included in our assessment of evidence (89). In four nonpragmatic trials (Table 11.11), manipulation was compared with some type of placebo therapy. Three of the four low-quality RCTs reported a positive result for manipulation compared with placebo. Fourteen pragmatic trials (one high-quality RCT) were identified that compared manipulation with other conservative types of treatment (Table 11.11), such as physical therapy (including short-wave diathermy, massage, exercises), back school, no therapy, and drug therapy. In 10 of these RCTs, the results were positive, and in four RCTs, including one high-quality RCT, the results were negative. The high-quality trial reported overall negative results, but positive results were noted for the subgroup with LBP durations of 14 to 28 days.

There is moderate evidence that manipulation is more effective than a placebo treatment for short-term pain relief of acute LBP (level B). Because of inconsistent findings, it is not possible to judge whether manipulation is more effective than (other) physical therapeutic applications (massage, short-wave diathermy, exercises) or drug

TABLE 11.9. *Details of randomized controlled trials on the effectiveness of exercise therapy for acute low back pain*

Investigators (ref.)	Exercise regimen (no. of patients)	Reference treatment (no. of patients)	Results
Faas et al. (32, 33)	I: stretching, flexion, side movements, and advice (156)	R1: usual care by general practitioner: analgesics, information (155); R2: placebo ultrasound therapy (162)	No significant differences in no. of recurrences, duration of pain, or functional status (NHP) during 1-yr follow-up; only NHP-energy more improved in I than in R1 during first 3 mo
Gilbert et al. (37); Evans et al. (27)	I1: isometric flexion, education, and bed rest (65); I2: isometric flexion and bed rest (162)	R1: bed rest (60); R2: no intervention (65)	No. of patients reporting no pain after 6 and 12 wk: I1, 34, 47; I2, 33, 46; R1, 36, 44: R2, 33, 43; no significant differences in pain, mobility, or daily activities
Malmivaara et al. (68)	I: mobilizing exercises: back extension and lateral bending (52)	R: continuation of ordinary activities as tolerated (67)	Differences in adjusted group means (95% CI) between I and R on pain intensity (11-point scale), functional status (Oswestry), and satisfaction with treatment (11-point scale) after 3 wk: 0.9 (−0.001 to 1.7), 6.6 (2.0 to 11.1), and 0.5 (−0.6 to 1.6); and after 12 wk: 0.2 (−0.5 to 1.0), 2.6 (−1.6 to 6.7), and 0.4 (−0.6 to 1.4)
Stankovic and Johnell (94, 95)	I: McKenzie extension (50)	R: "Mini" back school (50)	Significantly less pain and better spinal mobility in I at 3 wk and after 1 yr (no data); no. of recurrences after 1 and 5 yr significantly less in I, 22/49, 30/47, than in R, 37/49, 37/42
Waterworth and Hunter (107)	I: flexion and extension, short-wave diathermy, and ultrasound (34)	R1: NSAIDs (36); R2: manipulation (38)	Mean change in pain intensity on 4-point scale after 4 and 12 d: I, −0.9, −1.6; R1, −0.9, −1.7; R2, −1.1, −1.7; no significant difference in pain or mobility
Nwuga (77)	I: isometric flexion back and abdominal muscles and microwave diathermy (25)	R: manipulation (26)	Improvement in spinal flexion and straight leg raising: I, 13°, 4°; R, 34°, 39°; manipulation significantly better than exercise
Farrell and Twomey (34)	I: isometric flexion abdominal muscles and microwave diathermy (24)	R: manipulation and mobilization (24)	R: symptom free in significantly fewer days than I
Davies et al. (22)	I1: extension and short-wave diathermy (14); I2: isometric flexion and short-wave diathermy (14)	R: short-wave diathermy (15)	No. of patients showing improvement after 2 and 4 wk: I1, 11, 13; I2, 7, 12; R, 8, 10; not significant
Dellito et al. (23)	I1: McKenzie extension and mobilization (14); I2: Williams flexion (10)	—	I1: significantly more improved on functional status (Oswestry) than I2 after 3 and 5 d (data in graphs)
Nwuga and Nwuga (76)	I1: McKenzie extension (31); I2: Williams flexion (31)	—	Change in 10-point pain rating after 6 wk: I1, −5.3, vs. I2, −2.7; I1, significantly better than I2

I, index treatment; CI, confidence interval; NHP, Nottingham Health Profile; NSAIDs, nonsteroidal antiinflammmatory drugs; R, reference treatment.

TABLE 11.10. *Details of randomized controlled trials on the effectiveness of back schools for acute low back pain*

Investigators (ref.)	Back school program (no. of patients)	Reference treatment(s) (no. of patients)	Results
Bergquist-Ullman and Larsson (6)	I: Swedish back school: 4 × 45 min in 2 wk (lessons include information on anatomy, causes of low back pain, semi-Fowler position, ergonomics, exercises, and advice on physical activity) (70)	R1: combined physical therapy: manual therapy according to Cyriax, Kaltenborn, Lewitt, and Janda (72) R2: "Placebo": short-waves at lowest intensity; a maximum of 10 treatments (75)	Mean no. d until recovery: I, 14.8, R1, 15.8; R2, 28.7; I significantly better than R2, but not R1; no differences in decrease of pain after 3 and 6 wk
Stankovic and Johnell (94, 95)	I: "Mini" back school: 1 lesson of 45 min on back care and education (50)	R: McKenzie method: 20-min exercises and postural instructions to restore or maintain lumbar lordosis (50)	Less pain in R than in I after 3 and 52 wk. (no data)
Lindequist et al. (63)	I: postural education "back school type" and training program supervised by a physical therapist (24)	R: advice not to strain the back and to use analgesics when needed. No physical therapy (32)	Percentage of patients pain-free after 1, 3, and 6 wk. I, 21, 75, 83; R, 16, 66, 81; no significant differences
Morrison et al. (75)	I: outpatient back program including education (body mechanics, causes and remediation, psychologic stress) and exercise (increasing physical strength and mobility): 6 3-hr sessions over 2, 3, or 6 wk. (?)	R: control group (no further information) (?)	Significantly more improvement with regard to body mechanics, physical strength, mobility, and physical ability in I compared with R after the program

I, index treatment; R, reference treatments.

260

TABLE 11.11. *Details of randomized controlled trials on the effectiveness of spinal manipulation for acute low back pain*

Investigators (ref.)	Manipulation (no. of patients)	Reference treatment (no. of patients)	Results
MacDonald and Bell (67)	I: osteopathic (49)	R: exercises and postural advice (46)	All patients: no significant different recovery rates between treatment groups; in subgroup with current attack duration of 2–4 wk: I, 46% and R, 17%, recovered after 1 wk
Sanders et al. (89)	I: chiropractic (6)	R1: no treatment (6) R2: sham manipulation (6)	Mean pain scores (VAS) slightly reduced in I 5 and 30 min after intervention; no changes found in R1 or R2; no statistics on group differences presented
Hadler et al. (43)	I: rotational (26)	R: spinal mobilization (28)	All patients: no difference in functional status (Roland); in subgroup with current attack duration of 2–4 wk, better results in manipulation group I after 1 wk
Bergquist-Ullman and Larsson (6)	I: Cyriax, Kaltenborn, Lewitt, Janda (72)	R1: low-intensity short-wave diathermy (75) R2: back school (70)	Mean no. of days until recovery: I, 15.8; R1, 28.7; R2, 14.8; I and R2 significantly better than R1; no significant differences I and R2
Mathews et al. (71)	I: Cyriax (165)	R: infrared heat (126)	Percentage of patients recovered after 2 wk in subgroup (n = 58) with SLR negative: I, 62%, vs. R, 70%, in subgroup (n = 233) with SLR positive: 80%, vs. R, 67%; manipulation significantly better in SRL = positive subgroup
Helliwell and Cunliffe (46)	I: Cyriax (6)	R: analgesics (8)	Combined symptom score (maximum 28) after 1 wk: I, 2.6 ± 2.6, vs. R, 3.8 ± 3.3; and after 4 wk: I, 6.1 ± 7.2, vs. R, 2.2 ± 2.5; no significant differences
Glover et al. (38)	I: rotational (43)	R: detuned short-wave diathermy (41)	Pain relief on VAS posttreatment and after 3 and 7 d: I, 34%, 50%, 75%, vs. R, 22%, 56%, 80%
Blomberg et al. (11–13)	I: sacroiliac joint mobilization and thrust techniques (48)	R: active, optimal conventional physical therapy (53)	Mean pain score (VAS) after 1, 2, and 4 mo: I, 13.7, 11.4, 8.5; R, 23.9, 19.3, 20.9; I significantly better; average no. of days on sick leave during 8-mo follow-up: I, 25.4, R, 58.5
Rasmussen (84)	I: rotational (12)	R: short-wave diathermy (12)	Percentage of patients with total recovery after 2 wk: I, 92%, vs. R, 25%; manipulation significantly better
Delitto et al. (23)	I: mobilization of the sacroiliac joint (14)	R: flexion exercises (10)	Group I significantly more improved in functional status (Oswestry) after 3 and 5 d compared with group R
Farrell and Twomey (34)	I: Stoddard, Maitland (24)	R: short-wave diathermy and exercises (24)	Group I symptom free in significantly fewer days than group R
Nwuga (77)	I: rotational (26)	R: short-wave diathermy and exercises (25)	Improvement after 6 wk in spinal flexion: I, 34°, vs. R, 13°; and in SLR: 39°, vs. R, 4°; group I significantly better than group R
Waterworth and Hunter (107)	I: at discretion of the therapist (38)	R1: short-wave diathermy, ultrasound, and exercises (34) R2: NSAIDs (36)	Mean change in pain intensity on 4-point scale after 4 and 12 ds: I, −1.1, −1.7; R1, −0.9, −1.6, R2, −0.9, −1.7; no significant differences in pain intensity and mobility
Postacchini et al. (83)	I: chiropractic manipulation (35)	R1: physical therapy (31) R2: NSAIDs (34) R3: bedrest (29) R4: placebo: antiedema gel (30)	Mean improvement on combined pain, disability, and spinal mobility score after 3 wk: I, 7.5, R1, 5.0, R2, 3.0, R3, 5.4, R4, 1.8, after 2 mo: I, 9.7, R1, 8.4, R2, 10.7, R3, 7.5, R4, 7.3, and after 6 mo: I, 12.3, R1, 10.2, R2, 14.0, R3, 7.3, R4, 11.0; manipulation significantly better after 3 wk
Wreje et al. (113)	I: sacroiliac joint mobilization (18)	R: massage (21)	Pain (VAS) after 3 wk not different (data in graphs); sick leave and analgesic consumption significantly less in I than in R
Godfrey et al. (39)	I: rotational (44)	R: massage and electrical stimulation (37)	Percentage of patients with moderate or marked improvement on general symptoms on a 5-point scale after 2 wk: I, 77%, vs. R, 70%, no significant differences on other outcome measures

I, index treatment; R, reference treatment; NSAIDs, nonsteroidal antiinflammatory drugs; SLR, straight leg raising; VAS, visual analog scale.

therapy (analgesics, NSAIDs) for acute LBP (level C). The risks of manipulation are low, provided patients are selected and assessed properly, and treatment is carried out by a trained therapist or practitioner. Manipulation should not be used in patients with severe or progressive neurologic deficit in view of the rare but serious risk of neurologic complications. There is no evidence that manipulation performed while the patient is under general anesthesia is effective. It is associated with an increased risk of serious neurologic damage (45).

Physical Agents and Modalities

There is no evidence on the effectiveness of ice, heat, short-wave diathermy, massage, or ultrasound for the treatment of acute LBP (Level D) (29,36).

Transcutaneous Electrical Nerve Stimulation

Two trials (Table 11.12) studied the effectiveness of transcutaneous electrical nerve stimulation, one of high quality (48) and one of low quality (42). There is conflicting evidence on the effectiveness of this treatment for acute LBP (level C).

Traction

Only two low-quality RCTs (62,69) were identified on acute LBP (Table 11.13). Because of poor methodologic quality and small sample sizes, there is conflicting

TABLE 11.12. *Details of randomized controlled trials on the effectiveness of transcutaneous electrical nerve stimulation for acute low back pain*

Investigators (ref.)	TENS/acupuncture (no. of patients)	Reference treatment(s) (no. of patients)	Results
Herman et al. (48)	I: rehabilitation program (4 hr/d, 5 d/wk, 4 wk) plus TENS (15 min high-frequency, 15 min low-frequency, 5 d/wk, 4 wk) (29)	R: rehabilitation program plus placebo TENS (29)	Mean (SD) scores pretreatment and posttreatment of functional status (RDQ): I, 12.5 (5.1), 8.9 (5.0), vs. R, 14.3 (5.2), 9.9 (6.4); pain (100-mm VAS): I, 42.7 (23.3), 35.8 (27.7), vs. R, 47.9 (21.3), 35.9 (27.0); and lumbar flexion (Schober test mm): I, 50.9 (16.2), 60.2 (10.5), vs. R, 44.8 (15.9), 61.7 (13.9); not significant
Hackett et al. (42)	I: TENS low-amplitude, 15 min, 2 treatments, 4 d (—)	R: paracetamol 2 tablets every 4 hr (—)	Scores for pain (VAS) pretreatment and after 6 wk: I, 52.7, 3.3, vs. R, 54.4, 13.7; significant after 6 wk, but not after 1 and 2 wk; scores for mobility (VAS) pretreatment and after 6 wk: I, 53.4, 1.9, vs. R, 51.2, 15.8; significant after 6 wk, but not after 1 and 2 wk

I, index treatment; R, reference treatment; RDQ, Roland Disability Questionnaire; SD, standard deviation; TENS, transcutaneous electrical nerve stimulation; VAS, visual analog scale.

TABLE 11.13. *Details of trials on the efficacy of traction for acute low back pain*

Investigators (ref.)	Traction (no. of patients)	Reference treatment (no. of patients)	Results
Larsson et al. (62)	I: autotraction plus corset plus bed rest, 1 hr, 1–3 treatments, 1 wk (41)	R: corset plus bed rest (41)	No. of patients improved after 1 wk, 3 wk, and 3 mo. I, 17/41, 20/41, 19/41; R, 2/41, 8/41, 17/41; I, significant better after 1 and 3 wk
Mathews and Hickling (69)	I: continuous motorized traction >45 kg, 30 min, 5 d/5 wk, maximum 3 wk (83)	R: infrared heat 15 min, 3 times/wk, 2–3 wk (60)	Recovery after 2 wk: I, 40/77; R, 27/54; not significant

I, index treatment; R, reference treatment.

evidence (level C) on the effectiveness of traction for acute LBP. It is not possible to make any judgment on the effectiveness of traction for acute LBP (101).

Lumbar Corsets and Supports

There is no evidence available (level D) on the use of lumbar corsets or back belts in acute LBP.

Acupuncture

There is no evidence available (level D) on the use of acupuncture in acute LBP.

Behavioral Therapy

Only one low-quality RCT (35) was identified (Table 11.14), and it indicated that limited evidence (level C) suggested that behavioral therapy may be effective for acute LBP.

TABLE 11.14. *Details of trials on the efficacy of behavioral therapy for acute low back pain*

Investigators (ref.)	Behavioral therapy (no. of patients)	Reference treatment (no. of patients)	Results
Fordyce et al. (35)	I: behavioral management; analgesics, and exercise continued on a fixed time interval (57)	R: traditional management: analgesics and exercise until pain had subsided (50)	Mean (SD) score on pain drawings and claimed impairment after 9–12 mo: I, 1.98 (2.46), 4.84 (3.20), vs. R, 3.06 (2.45), 6.25 (3.25); I, significantly better than R after 9–12 mos on pain drawings and claimed impairment; no significant differences after 6 wk

I, index treatment; R, reference treatment; SD, standard deviation.

CONCLUSIONS

Strong evidence exists for the following:

NSAIDs prescribed at regular intervals are effective in providing pain relief for simple acute LBP.
Different types of NSAIDs are equally effective.
Muscle relaxants effectively reduce acute LBP.
The different types of muscle relaxants are equally effective.
Bed rest is not effective for treating acute LBP.
Advice to continue ordinary activity gives equivalent or faster symptomatic recovery and leads to less chronic disability and less time lost from work.
Specific back exercises are not effective for treating acute LBP.

For the other interventions, the evidence was either moderate, limited, or conflicting, or there was no evidence at all. There seemed to be a lack of evidence for any of the interventions with regard to return to work or prevention of chronic disability. Most evidence only related to symptomatic pain relief.

RECOMMENDATIONS FOR TREATMENT OF ACUTE LOW BACK PAIN

The following recommendations are based on the evidence summarized earlier, on the Royal College of General Practitioners clinical guidelines for the management of acute LBP (106), and on the Dutch general practice guideline for LBP (31).

Bed Rest

Do *not* recommend or use bed rest as a treatment for simple back pain. Some patients may be confined to bed for a few days (a maximum of 2 days is recommended) as a consequence of their pain, but this confinement should not be considered a treatment.

Advice on Staying Active

Advise patients to stay as active as possible and to continue normal daily activities. Advise patients to increase their physical activities progressively over a few days or weeks. If a patient is working, then advising the patient to stay at work or to return to work as soon as possible or after a specified period is probably beneficial.

Drug Therapy for Pain Relief

Prescribe analgesics at regular intervals for a fixed period, if required. Start with paracetamol. If that is inadequate, substitute NSAIDs (e.g., ibuprofen or diclofenac) and then a paracetamol-weak opioid compound (e.g., codydramol or coproxamol). Prescription of muscle relaxants, benzodiazepines, or narcotics is not advisable because of the side effects and the risk of dependency.

Manual Therapy (Manipulation or Mobilization)

Consider manipulative treatment within the first 6 weeks for patients who need additional help with pain relief or those who are failing to return to normal activities.

RECOMMENDATIONS FOR TREATMENT OF SUBACUTE LOW BACK PAIN

Advice on Staying Active

Advise patients to increase their physical activities gradually, both in daily life and at work, in spite of the pain, by using a fixed time quota.

Back Exercises

Patients who have not returned to ordinary activities and work by 6 weeks should be referred for reactivation or rehabilitation. The treatment to improve daily functioning can be given by a physical therapist, exercise therapist, manual therapist, or chiropractor. There is no preference for a particular specialist, but the therapist should be willing to support the treatment plan.

Drug Therapy

If necessary, analgesics are prescribed for a fixed period to enable the patient to increase activities gradually. Analgesics are taken at fixed times regardless of the presence of pain.

REFERENCES

1. Aghababian RV, Volturo GA, Heifetz IN. Comparison of diflunisal and naproxen in the management of acute low back strain. *Clin Ther* 1986;9[Suppl C]:47–51.
2. Agrifoglio E, Benvenuti M, Gatto P, et al. Aceclofenac: a new NSAID in the treatment of acute lumbago. Multicentre single blind study vs diclofenac. *Acta Ther* 1994;20:33–43.
3. Amlie E, Weber H, Holme I. Treatment of acute low-back pain with piroxicam: results of a double-blind placebo-controlled trial. *Spine* 1987;12:473–476.
4. Bakshi R, Thumb N, Bröll H, et al. Treatment of acute lumbosacral back pain with diclofenac resinate: results of a double-blind comparative trial versus piroxicam. *Drug Invest* 1994;8:288–293.
5. Baratta RR. A double-blind study of cyclobenzaprine and placebo in the treatment of acute musculo-skeletal conditions of the low back. *Curr Ther Res* 1982;32:646–652.
6. Bergquist-Ullman M, Larsson U. Acute low-back pain in industry: a controlled prospective study with special reference to therapy and confounding factors. *Acta Orthop Scand* 1977;170[Suppl]:1–117.
7. Berry H, Hutchinson DR. A multicentre placebo-controlled study in general practice to evaluate the efficacy and safety of tizanidine in acute low-back pain. *J Int Med Res* 1988;16:75–82.
8. Berry H, Hutchinson DR. Tizanidine and ibuprofen in acute low-back pain: results of a double-blind multicentre study in general practice. *J Int Med Res* 1988;16:83–91.
9. Bigos S, Bowyer O, Braen G, et al. *Acute low back problems in adults.* Clinical practice guideline no. 14. AHCPR Publication no. 95–0642. Rockville, MD: Agency for Health Care Policy and Research, 1994.
10. Blazek M, Keszthelyi B, Varhelyi M, et al. Comparative study of Blarison and Voltaren in acute lumbar pain and lumbo-ischialgia. *Ther Hung* 1986;34:163–166.
11. Blomberg S, Svardsudd K, Mildenberger F. A controlled multicentre trial of manual therapy in low-back pain. *Scand J Prim Health Care* 1992;10:170–178.
12. Blomberg S, Svardsudd K, Tibblin G. Manual therapy with steroid injections in low-back pain. *Scand J Prim Health Care* 1993;11:83–90.
13. Blomberg S, Hallin G, Grann K, et al. Manual therapy with steroid injections: a new approach to treatment with low-back pain. *Spine* 1994;19:569–577.

14. Borenstein DG, Lacks S, Wiesel SW. Cyclobenzaprine and naproxen versus naproxen alone in the treatment of acute low back pain and muscle spasm. *Clin Ther* 1990;12:125–131.
15. Boyles WF, Glassman JM, Soyka JP. Management of acute musculoskeletal conditions: thoracolumbar strain or sprain. A double-blind evaluation comparing the efficacy and safety of carisoprodol with diazepam. *Today's Ther Trends* 1983;1:1–16.
16. Brown FL, Bodison S, Dixon J, et al. Comparison of diflunisal and acetaminophen with codeine in the treatment of initial or recurrent acute low back pain. *Clin Ther* 1986;9[Suppl C]:52–58.
17. Casale R. Acute low back pain: symptomatic treatment with a muscle relaxant drug. *Clin J Pain* 1988;4:81–88.
18. Cohen JE, Goel V, Frank JW, et al. Group interventions for people with low back pain: an overview of the literature. *Spine* 1994;19:1214–1222.
19. Coomes EN. A comparison between epidural anaesthesia and bed rest in sciatica. *BMJ* 1961;264:20–24.
20. de Craen AJM, Di Giulio G, Lampe-Schoenmaeckers AJEM, et al. Analgesic efficacy and safety of paracetamol-codeine combinations versus paracetamol alone: a systematic review. *BMJ* 1996; 313:321–325.
21. Dapas F, Hartman SF, Martinez L, et al. Baclofen for the treatment of acute low-back syndrome: a double blind comparison with placebo. *Spine* 1985;10:345–349.
22. Davies JR, Gibson T, Tester L. The value of exercises in the treatment of low back pain. *Rheumatol Rehabil* 1979;18:243–247.
23. Delitto A, Cibulka MT, Erhard RE, et al. Evidence for use of an extension-mobilization category in acute low back syndrome: a prescriptive validation pilot study. *Phys Ther* 1993;73:216–228.
24. Deyo RA, Diehl AK, Rosenthal M. How many days of bed rest for acute low-back pain: a randomized clinical trial. *N Engl J Med* 1986;315:1064–1070.
25. Dickersin K. The existence of publication bias and risk factors for its occurrence. *JAMA* 1990;263:1385–1389.
26. Edwards JG, Cantopher T, Olivieri S. Benzodiazepine dependence and the problems of withdrawal. *Postgrad Med J* 1990;66[Suppl 2]:S27–S35.
27. Evans C, Gilbert JR, Taylor W, et al. A randomized controlled trial of flexion exercises, education, and bed rest for patients with acute low-back pain. *Physiother Can* 1987;39:96–101.
28. Evans DP, Burke MS, Newcombe RG. Medicines of choice in low back pain. *Curr Med Res Opin* 1980;6:540–547.
29. Evans G, Richards S. *Low back pain: an evaluation of therapeutic interventions.* Bristol, UK: Health Care Evaluation Unit, University of Bristol, 1996.
30. Faas A. Exercises: which ones are worth trying, for which patients and when. *Spine* 1996;21:2874–2879.
31. Faas A, Chavannes AW, Koes BW, et al. NHG-Standaard "Lage-Rugpijn" [in Dutch]. *Huisarts Wet* 1996;39:18–31.
32. Faas A, Chavannes AW, van Eijk JThM, et al. A randomized, placebo-controlled trial of exercise therapy in patients with acute low back pain. *Spine* 1993;18:1388–1395.
33. Faas A, van Eijk JThM, Chavannes AW, et al. A randomized trial of exercise therapy in patients with acute low back pain. *Spine* 1995;20:941–947.
34. Farrell JP, Twomey LT. Acute low-back pain: comparison of two conservative treatment approaches. *Med J Aust* 1982;1:160–164.
35. Fordyce WE, Brockway JA, Bergman JA, et al. Acute back pain: a control-group comparison of behavioral vs traditional management methods. *J Behav Med* 1986;9:127–140.
36. Gam AN, Johannsen F. Ultrasound therapy in musculoskeletal disorders: a meta-analysis. *Pain* 1995;63:85–91.
37. Gilbert JR, Taylor DW, Hildebrand A, et al. Clinical practice of common treatments for low-back pain. *BMJ* 1985;291:789–792.
38. Glover JR, Morris JG, Khosla T. Back pain: a randomized clinical trial of rotational manipulation of the trunk. *Br J Ind Med* 1974;31:59–64.
39. Godfrey CM, Morgan PP, Schatzker J. A randomized trial of manipulation for low-back pain in a medical setting. *Spine* 1984;9:301–304.
40. Gold RH. Orphenadrine citrate: sedative or muscle relaxant. *Clin Ther* 1978;1:451–453.
41. Goldie I. A clinical trial with indomethacin (Indomee) in low back pain and sciatica. *Acta Orthop Scand* 1968;39:117–128.
42. Hackett GI, Seddon D, Kaminski D. Electroacupuncture compared with paracetamol for acute low back pain. *Practitioner* 1988;232:163–164.
43. Hadler NM, Curtis P, Gillings DB, et al. A benefit of spinal manipulation as adjunctive therapy for acute low-back pain: a stratified controlled trial. *Spine* 1987;12:703–705.
44. Haimovic IC, Beresford HR. Dexamethasone is not superior to placebo for treating lumbosacral radicular pain. *Neurology* 1986;36:1593–1594.
45. Haldeman S, Rubinstein SM. Cauda equina syndrome in patients undergoing manipulation of the lumbar spine. *Spine* 1992;17:1469–1473.
46. Helliwell PS, Cunliffe G. Manipulation in low-back pain. *Physician 1987;April:187–188.*
47. Henry D, Lim LLY, Rodriguez LAG, et al. Variability in risk of gastrointestinal complications with

individual non-steroidal anti-inflammatory drugs: results of a collaborative meta-analysis. *BMJ* 1996;312:1563–1566.

48. Herman E, Williams R, Stratford P, et al. A randomized controlled trial of transcutaneous electrical nerve stimulation (CODETRON) to determine its benefits in a rehabilitation program for acute occupational low back pain. *Spine* 1994;19:561–568.

49. Hindle TH. Comparison of carisoprodol, butabarbital, and placebo in treatment of the low back syndrome. *Calif Med* 1972;117:7–11.

50. Hingorani K. Diazepam in backache: a double-blind controlled trial. *Ann Phys Med* 1965;8:303–306.

51. Hosie GAC. The topical NSAID, felbinac, versus oral ibuprofen: a comparison of efficacy in the treatment of acute lower back injury. *Br J Clin Res* 1993;4:5–17.

52. Hurri H. The Swedish back school in chronic low back pain. Part II. Factors predicting the outcome. *Scand J Rehabil Med* 1989;21:41–44.

53. Indahl A, Velund L, Reikeraas O. Good prognosis for low back pain when left untampered. *Spine* 1995;20:473–477.

54. Koes BW, Hoogen HMM van den. Efficacy of bed rest and orthoses for low back pain: a review of randomized clinical trials. *Eur J Phys Med Rehabil* 1994;4:86–93.

55. Koes BW, Bouter LM, Heijden GJMG van der. Methodological quality of randomized clinical trials on treatment efficacy in low back pain. *Spine* 1995;20:228–235.

56. Koes BW, Assendelft WJJ, van der Heijden GJMG, et al. Spinal manipulation for low back pain: an updated systematic review of randomized clinical trials. *Spine* 1996;21:2860–2873.

57. Koes BW, Bouter LM, Beckerman H, et al. Physiotherapy exercises and back pain: a blinded review. *BMJ* 1991;302:1572–1576.

58. Lacey PH, Dodd GD, Shannon DJ. A double-blind placebo controlled study of piroxicam in the management of acute musculoskeletal disorders. *Eur J Rheumatol Inflamm* 1984;7:95–104.

59. Koes BW, Scholten RJPM, Mens JMA, et al. Efficacy of epidural steroid injections for low-back pain and sciatica: a systematic review of randomized clinical trials. *Pain* 1995;63:279–288.

60. Koes BW, Scholten RJPM, Mens JMA, et al. Efficacy of non-steroidal anti-inflammatory drugs for low back pain: a systematic review of randomised clinical trials. *Ann Rheum Dis* 1997;56:214–223.

61. Koes BW, Tulder MW van, Windt DAWM van der, et al. The efficacy of back schools: a review of randomized clinical trials. *J Clin Epidemiol* 1994;47:851–862.

62. Larsson U, Chöler U, Lidström A, et al. Auto-traction for treatment of lumbago-sciatica. *Acta Orthop Scand* 1980;51:791–798.

63. Lindequist SL, Lundberg B, Wikmark R, et al. Information and regime at low-back pain. *Scand J Rehabil Med* 1984;16:113–116.

64. Lindström I, Öhlund C, Eek C, et al. The effect of graded activity on patients with subacute low back pain: a randomized prospective clinical study with an operant-conditioning behavioral approach. *Phys Ther* 1992;72:279–293.

65. Lindström I, Öhlund C, Eek C, et al. Mobility, strength, and fitness after a graded activity program for patients with subacute low back pain. *Spine* 1992;17:641–652.

66. Linton SJ, Bradley LA, Jensen I, et al. The secondary prevention of low back pain: a controlled study with follow-up. *Pain* 1989;36:197–207.

67. MacDonald RS, Bell CMJ. An open controlled assessment of osteopathic manipulation in nonspecific low-back pain. *Spine* 1990;15:364–370.

68. Malmivaara A, Häkkinen U, Aro T, et al. The treatment of acute low back pain: bed rest, exercises, or ordinary activity. *N Engl J Med* 1995;332:351–355.

69. Mathews JA, Hickling J. Lumbar traction: a double-blind controlled study for sciatica. *Rheumatol Rehabil* 1975;14:222–225.

70. Mathews JA, Mills SB, Jenkins VM, et al. Back pain sciatica: controlled trials of manipulation, traction, sclerosant and epidural injections. *Br J Rheumatol* 1987:26;416–423.

71. Mathews W, Morkel M, Mathews J. Manipulation and traction for lumbago and sciatica: physiotherapeutic techniques used in two controlled trials. *Physiother Pract* 1988;4:201–206.

72. Meek JB, Giudice VW, Enrick NL. Colchicine highly effective in disk disorders: results of a double-blind study. *J Neuro Orthop Med Surg* 1984;5:215–220.

73. Middleton RSW. A comparison of two analgesic muscle relaxant combinations in acute back pain. *Br J Gen Pract* 1984:107–109.

74. Moher D, Jadad AJ, Nichol G, et al. Assessing the quality of randomized controlled trials: an annotated bibliography of scales and checklists. *Control Clin Trials* 1995;16:62–73.

75. Morrison GEC, Chase W, Young V, et al. Back pain: treatment and prevention in a community hospital. *Arch Phys Med Rehabil* 1988;69:605–609.

76. Nwuga G, Nwuga V. Relative therapeutic efficacy of the Williams and McKenzie protocols in back pain management. *Physiother Pract* 1985;1:99–105.

77. Nwuga VCB. Relative therapeutic efficacy of vertebral manipulation and conventional treatment in back pain management. *Am J Phys Med* 1982;61:273–278.

78. Nwuga VCB. Ultrasound in treatment of back pain resulting from prolapsed intervertebral disc. *Arch Phys Med Rehabil* 1983;64:88–89.

79. Orava S. Medical treatment of acute low back pain: diflinisal compared with indomethacin in acute lumbago. *Int J Clin Res* 1986;6:45–51.
80. Owen RT, Tyrer P. Benzodiazepine dependence: a review of the evidence. *Drugs* 1983;25:385–398.
81. Pal P, Mangion P, Hossian MA, et al. A controlled trial of continuous lumbar traction in the treatment of back pain and sciatica. *Br J Rheumatol* 1986;25:1181–1183.
82. Philips HC, Grant L, Berkowitz J. The prevention of chronic pain and disability: a preliminary investigation. *Behav Res Ther* 1991;29:443–450.
83. Postacchini F, Facchini M, Palieri P. Efficacy of various forms of conservative treatment in low back pain: a comparative study. *Neurol Orthop* 1988;6:28–35.
84. Rasmussen GG. Manipulation in treatment of low-back pain: a randomized clinical trial. *Manual Med* 1979;1:8–10.
85. *RCGP Clinical guidelines for the management of acute low back pain.* London: Royal College of General Practitioners, 1996.
86. Rollings HE, Glassman JM, Soyka JP. Management of acute musculoskeletal conditions–thoracolumbar strain or sprain: a double-blind evaluation comparing the efficacy and safety of carisoprodol with cyclobenzaprine hydrochloride. *Curr Ther Res* 1983;34:917–928.
87. Rosen M, Breen A, Hamann W, et al. *Report of a Clinical Standards Advisory Group committee on back pain.* London: Her Majesty's Stationery Office, 1994.
88. Rupert RL, Wagnon R, Thompson P, et al. Chiropractic adjustments: results of a controlled trial in Egypt. *ICA Int Rev Chiropract* 1985:58–60.
89. Sanders GE, Reinert O, Tepe R, et al. Chiropractic adjustive manipulation on subjects with acute low-back pain: visual analog pain scores and plasma beta-endorphin levels. *J Manipulative Physiol Ther* 1990;13:391–395.
90. Schnebel BE, Simmons JW. The use of oral colchicine for low-back pain: a double-blind study. *Spine* 1988;13:354–357.
91. Schulz KF, Chalmers I, Hayes RJ, et al. Empirical evidence of bias: dimensions of methodological quality associated with estimates of treatment effects in controlled trials. *JAMA* 1995;273:408–412.
92. Simmons JW, Harris WP, Koulisis CW, et al. Intravenous Colchicine for low-back pain: a double-blind study. *Spine* 1990;15:716–717.
93. Spitzer WO, LeBlanc Fe, Dupuis M, eds. Scientific approach to the assessment and management of activity-related spinal disorders. *Spine* 1987;7[Suppl]:1–59.
94. Stankovic R, Johnell O. Conservative treatment of acute low-back pain. A prospective randomized trial: McKenzie method of treatment versus patient education in "mini-back school." *Spine* 1990;15:120–123.
95. Stankovic R, Johnell O. Conservative treatment of acute low back pain: a 5-year follow-up study of two methods of treatment. *Spine* 1995;20:469–472.
96. Sweetman BJ, Baig A, Parsons DL. Mefenamic acid, chlormazanone-paracetamol, ethoptazine-aspirin-meprobamate: a comparative study in acute low back pain. *Br J Clin Pract* 1987;41:619–624.
97. Szpalski M, Hayez JP. How many days of bed rest for acute low back pain: objective assessment of trunk function. *Eur Spine J* 1992;1:29–31.
98. Szpalski M, Hayez JP. Objective functional assessment of the efficacy of tenoxicam in the treatment of acute low back pain: a double-blind placebo-controlled study. *Br J Rheumatol* 1994;33:74–78.
99. Tervo T, Petaja L, Lepisto P. A controlled clinical trial of a muscle relaxant analgesic combination in the treatment of acute lumbago. *Br J Clin Pract* 1976;30:62–64.
100. Turner JA, Denny MC. Do antidepressant medications relieve chronic low back pain. *J Fam Pract* 1993;37:545–553.
101. van der Heijden GJMG, Beurskens AJHM, Koes BW, et al. The efficacy of traction for back and neck pain: a systematic, blinded review of randomized clinical trial methods. *Phys Ther* 1995;75:93–103.
102. van Tulder MW, Koes BW, Bouter LM, eds. *Low back pain in primary care: effectiveness of diagnostic and therapeutic interventions.* Amsterdam: Institute for Research in Extramural Medicine, 1996:1–285.
103. van Tulder MW, Koes BW, Bouter LM. Conservative treatment of acute and chronic nonspecific low back pain: a systematic review of randomized controlled trials of the most common interventions. *Spine* 1997;22:2128–2156.
104. Videman T, Heikkila J, Partanen T. Double-blind parallel study of meptazinol versus diflunisal in the treatment of lumbago. *Curr Med Res Opin* 1984;9:246–252.
105. Waddell G, Feder G, Lewis M. Systematic reviews of bedrest and advice to stay active for acute low back pain. *Br J Gen Pract* 1997;47:647–652.
106. Waddell G, Feder G, McIntosh A, et al. *Low back pain evidence review.* London: Royal College of General Practitioners, 1996.
107. Waterworth RF, Hunter IA. An open study of diflunisal, conservative and manipulative therapy in the management of acute mechanical low back pain. *N Z Med J* 1985;98:372–375.
108. Weber H, Aasand G. The effect of phenylbutazone on patients with acute lumbago-sciatica: a double blind trial. *J Oslo City Hosp* 1980;30:69–72.
109. Weber H, Holme I, Amlie E. The natural course of acute sciatica with nerve root symptoms in a double-blind placebo-controlled trial evaluating the effect of piroxicam. *Spine* 1993;18:1433–1438.

110. Wiesel SW, Cuckler JM, Deluca F, et al. Acute low back pain: an objective analysis of conservative therapy. *Spine* 1980;5:324–330.
111. Wilkinson MJB. Does 48 hours' bed rest influence the outcome of acute low back pain. *Br J Gen Pract* 1995;45:481–484.
112. Wilson MC, Hayward RSA, Tunis SR, et al. User's guides to the medical literature. VIII. How to use clinical practice guidelines, B: what are the recommendations and will they help you in caring for your patients. *JAMA* 1995;274:1630–1632.
113. Wreje U, Nordgren B, Aberg H. Treatment of pelvic joint dysfunction in primary care: a controlled study. *Scand J Prim Health Care* 1992;10:310–315.

Neck and Back Pain: The Scientific Evidence
of Causes, Diagnosis, and Treatment, edited
by Alf Nachemson and Egon Jonsson.
Published by Lippincott Williams & Wilkins,
Philadelphia 2000.

12

Conservative Treatment of Chronic Low Back Pain

Maurits W. van Tulder*, Mariëlle Goossens†, Gordon Waddell‡,
and Alf Nachemson§

**Institute for Research in Extramural Medicine, Vrije Universiteit, Amsterdam,
The Netherlands*
†*Institute for Rehabilitation Research, Hoensbroek, The Netherlands*
‡*Department of Orthopaedics, The Glasgow Nuffield Hospital, Glasgow, Scotland*
§*Department of Orthopaedics, Sahlgrenska University Hospital, Göteborg, Sweden*

An extensive systematic literature review of the management of low back pain (LBP), including chronic LBP, was published (98). This review evaluated randomized controlled trials (RCTs) on various therapeutic interventions used in the treatment of chronic LBP, including spinal manipulation, exercise therapy, physical therapy modalities, back school, acupuncture, nonsteroidal antiinflammatory drugs (NSAIDs), antidepressants, injection therapy, electromyographic (EMG) biofeedback, and behavioral therapy. Some of the interventions included in this review, such as spinal manipulation, NSAIDs, back schools, exercise therapy, behavioral therapy, and acupuncture have already been included in protocols for systematic reviews within the framework of the Cochrane Back Review Group for Spinal Disorders. Actualization and incorporation of systematic reviews on the effectiveness of therapeutic interventions for LBP within the Cochrane Collaboration seem to be the most meaningful, considering the best current recommendations. These Cochrane reviews may lead to a better understanding of the effectiveness of various treatments for LBP, including chronic LBP, because more recent developments in the methodology of quality assessment and systematic reviews are included (99).

In this chapter, the effectiveness of the most common therapeutic interventions for chronic LBP are evaluated. We updated the previous systematic review (98) by including all relevant RCTs that were published between September 1995 and July 1998.

This chapter should answer the following questions:

Which interventions are the most effective in the treatment of chronic LBP with and without radiation?

Are these interventions more effective than placebo, no treatment, or other conservative treatments (including other drugs)?

Are these interventions effective regarding relevant outcome measures, that is, overall improvement, functional status, return to work, pain intensity, or pain behavior?

Are these interventions effective in the short and/or long term?

The information provided in this chapter may be useful in the development of evidence-based guidelines for general practitioners, physical therapists, or other primary health care professionals.

METHODS

Selection of Studies

In the published review, a search was made of the MEDLINE database from 1966 through September 1995, the EMBASE drugs and pharmacology database from 1980 through September 1995, and the PsycLIT database from 1984 through September 1995, by using medical subject headings and free text words (91). The keywords used were LBP, backache, musculoskeletal diseases, joint diseases, spinal diseases, physical therapy, chiropractic, and osteopathy, as well as the names of specific interventions. Subsequently, the references given in relevant identified publications were examined further. We reviewed the titles and abstracts of the identified articles to determine the relevance of the articles for our systematic review. When there was any doubt, the article was retrieved and read. Abstracts and unpublished studies were not selected. For the update of the literature search up to July 1998, we used a highly sensitive search strategy for MEDLINE published by Dickersin et al. (22), and for EMBASE, we used a strategy developed by the Cochrane Center in the United Kingdom.

A study was included if the following criteria were met:

1. It concerned a true RCT; trials with quasirandom procedures such as alternate allocation or allocation based on dates of birth were excluded.
2. The treatment regimen consisted of a conservative type of intervention.
3. The results, exclusively or separately, concerned patients with chronic LBP.
4. The article was published in English.

Chronic LBP was defined as LBP persisting for 12 weeks or more. Studies were included if they reported on a mix of patients with subacute (4 to 12 weeks' duration) LBP and chronic LBP. Studies were excluded if they reported on patients with acute (4 weeks' duration or less) LBP, a mix of patients with acute and chronic LBP, cervical back pain, or a mix of low and cervical back pain, unless the results for chronic LBP and LBP were presented separately.

Methodologic Quality of the Studies

All trials were scored according to the criteria listed in Table 12.1. The criteria were based on generally accepted principles of intervention research and referred to various aspects of study population, description of interventions, outcome measurements, and data presentation and analysis. The same criteria list was used in previously published systematic reviews of back pain (48–50,55,93,106). A weight was attached to each criterion, resulting in a maximum score of 100 points for each study. The methodologic quality of the RCTs was assessed by two independent reviewers. The reviewers agreed with each other regarding 78% of the scores. Disagreements between the two reviewers were resolved by consensus. The assessments resulted in a hierarchic list in which higher scores indicated studies with a higher methodologic quality. We used the original scores of our previously published systematic review. All additional RCTs included in the update were assessed by the same two reviewers (M. van Tulder and M. Goossens).

TABLE 12.1. *Criteria for the methodologic assessment of randomized clinical trials of therapeutic interventions for chronic low back pain*

Study population
A   Homogeneity
B   Comparability of relevant baseline characteristics
C   Randomization procedure adequate
D   Dropouts described for each study group separately
E   <20% loss to follow-up
    <10% loss to follow-up
F   >50 subjects in the smallest group
    >100 subjects in the smallest group
Interventions
G   Interventions standardized and described
H   Pragmatic study/control group adequate[a]
I   Cointerventions avoided
J   Placebo controlled
Effect
K   Patients blinded
L   Outcome measures relevant
M   Blinded outcome assessment
N   Follow-up period adequate
Data presentation and analysis
O   Intention-to-treat analysis
P   Frequencies of most important outcomes presented for each treatment group
Only trials of analgesics, muscle relaxants, nonsteroidal antiinflammatory drugs, and antidepressants
Q   Compliance measured and satisfactory in all study groups

[a] Criterion H was defined as pragmatic study for randomized controlled trials (RCTs) of therapeutic interventions for which a placebo treatment was feasible (i.e., drug therapies, manipulation, electromyographic biofeedback, traction, orthoses, transcutaneous electrical nerve stimulation, and acupuncture); criterion H was defined as control group adequate for RTCs of therapeutic interventions for which a placebo treatment was less feasible (i.e., back schools, exercise therapy and behavioral therapy).
Data from references 45, 46, 51, and 52.

Outcome of the Studies

We extracted the main results from each study according to what we considered to be the most important outcome measures, that is, pain intensity, overall improvement, functional status, and return to work (Tables 12.2 to 12.10). A study was considered positive if the therapeutic intervention was more effective than the reference treatment with regard to at least one of these outcome measures. A study was considered negative if the authors reported no differences between the intervention under study and the reference treatment on these outcome measures or if the reference treatment was reported to be more effective with regard to at least one of these outcome measures. If the therapeutic intervention under study was reported to be more effective on one of the outcome measures, but less effective on another, or if these outcome measures were not assessed in a study, no conclusion was drawn (see conclusions sections in Tables 12.11 and 12.12).

Levels of Evidence

Our conclusions on the efficacy of the therapeutic interventions were based on the strength of the scientific evidence. The rating system consisted of four levels of scientific evidence, based on the quality and the outcome of the studies:

A. Strong evidence: provided by generally consistent findings in multiple high-quality RCTs.

TABLE 12.2. *Details of trials on the effectiveness of various drug therapies for chronic low back pain*

Investigators (ref.)	Dose, frequency, and duration (no. of patients)	Reference treatment(s) (no. of patients)	Results
Analgesics			
Hickey (38)	I: paracetamol 1,000 mg q.i.d./4 wk (13)	R: diflunisal 500 mg b.i.d./4 wk (16)	No. of patients with none or mild low back pain after 2 and 4 wk: I, 9, 7; R, 11, 13; significantly more patients in R (10 of 16) considered the therapy good or excellent compared with I (4 of 12); side effects comparable (I, I; R, 2)
Muscle relaxants			
Arbus et al. (4)	I: tetrazepam 50 mg t.i.d./10 d (25)	R: placebo t.i.d./10 d (25)	Overall efficacy significantly better in I (64%) than in R (29%); mean (SD) pain score (5-point scale) at baseline and after 4 and 10 d in I, 3.40 (0.82), 2.50 (0.94), and 1.73 (1.31), vs. R, 3.36 (0.63), 3.10 (0.71), and 2.38 (1.08); I significantly more improved; no difference in side effects
Antidepressants			
Goodkin et al. (30)	I: trazodone 50 mg/1 tablet initially to maximum 12 tablets/6 wk (22)	R: placebo (20)	Mean (SD) pain score (VAS) pre- and posttreatment: I, 6.5, 5.3, vs. R, 6.5, 5.9; physical functioning (SIP): I, 26.7, 24.4, vs. R, 27.7, 22.8; psychosocial functioning (SIP): I, 28.5, 29.0, vs. R, 27.0, 20.8; depression (BDI): I, 16.3, 14.1, vs. R, 15.2, 11.8; pain and depression not significantly different; placebo significantly better physical and psychosocial functioning
Alcoff et al. (2)	I: imipramine 75 mg 1–2 tablets/d/8 wk (28)	R: placebo (22)	I significantly better than R in decreasing limitation of physical functioning; no significant difference in pain severity or depression; no means and SDs presented for any outcome measure
Jenkins et al. (41)	I: imipramine 25 mg/ t.i.d./4 wk (23)	R: placebo (21)	No differences between I and R on improvement of pain, depression, and spinal mobility from pre- to posttreatment; data in graphs; in the 15 most depressed patients, depression decreased in I in 6 of 8 subjects vs. R, in 3 of 7 subjects; not significant
Pheasant et al. (86)	I: amitriptyline 50 mg/ 1–3/tablets/d/6 wk (9)	R: placebo: atropine 0.2 mg/1–3 tablets/d/6 wk (9)	Crossover design; change in functional evaluation: I, 0.00; R, −0.06; not significant; mean no. (SD) of analgesics/wk: I, 4.7 (3.4), vs. R, 8.7 (4.8); significant

Nonsteroidal antiinflammatory drugs

Study	Index treatment	Reference treatment	Results
Hickey (38)	I: diflunisal 500 mg b.i.d./4 wk (16)	R: paracetamol 1,000 mg q.i.d./4 wk (13)	No. of patients with none or mild low back pain after 2 and 4 wk: I, 11, 13; R, 9, 7; significantly more patients in I (10 of 16) considered the therapy good or excellent compared with R (4 of 12); side effects comparable: I, 2; R, 1
Siegmeth and Sieberer (94)	I1: ibuprofen/1,200 mg d/14 d (15); I2: diclofenac/75 mg d/14 d (15)	—	No. of patients reporting to be improved after 1, 3, and 4 wk: I1, 5, 10, 6; I2, 5, 12, 11; no significant differences; side effects comparable; one in each group
Videman and Osterman (104)	I1: piroxicam 20 mg d/6 wk (14); I2: indomethacin 25 mg t.i.d./6 wk (14)	—	Mean improvement on VAS (range, 0–31) after 6 wk: I1, 8, vs. 12, 9; similar improvement rates (data in graphs); comparable side effects: I1, 13, vs. 12, 15
Berry et al. (10)	I1: naproxen sodium 550 mg b.i.d./14 d (37); I2: diflunisal 500 mg b.i.d./14 d (37)	R: placebo (37)	Crossover design; I1, reduction of pain (VAS); I2, no change; R, increase of pain (data in graphs); I1 significantly better than R and somewhat better than I2; side effects comparable in the three groups: I1, 18; I2, 18; R, 16
Matsumo et al. (70)	I1: ketoprofen 150 mg d/duration not given (77); I2: diclofenac 75 mg d/duration not given (78)	—	Patients improved after 1 and 2 wk: I1, 71%, 86%; I2, 62%, 79%; no significant differences; side effects comparable in both groups: I1, 18%; I2, 21%
Postacchini et al. (87)	I: diclofenac "full dosage" 15–20 d (81)	R1: manipulation (87); R2: physical therapy (78); R3: back school (50); R4: antiedema gel (73)	Mean improvement on combined pain, disability, and spinal mobility score after 3 wk and 2 and 6 mo in subgroup with chronic pain: I, 2.6, 2.2, 4.0; R1, 2.2, 2.6, 4.3; R2, 3.9, 4.2, 6.0; R3, 0.5, 4.6, 8.9; R4, 0.7, 1.2, 2.0; group I not significantly better; no data on side effects reported

BDI, Beck Depression Inventory; I, index treatment; R, reference treatment; SD, standard deviation; SIP, Sickness Impact Profile; VAS, visual analog scale.

TABLE 12.3. *Details of trials studying the effectiveness of epidural steroid injections for chronic low back pain*

Investigators (ref.)	Epidural steroid injection (no. of patients)	Reference treatment (no. of patients)	Results
Carette et al. (17)	I: methyl prednisolone acetate 80 mg (2 mL) + 8 mL isotonic saline, 1–3 injections (78)	R: saline 1 mL (80)	Mean VAS (100-mm) of pain at baseline and after 3 wk and 3 mo: I, 65.6, 44.9, 38.9; R, 61.5, 49.1, 39.5; mean Oswestry score: I, 49.6, 41.6, 32.2; R, 50.0, 44.5, 34.6; mean finger-to-floor distance: I, 37.4, 29.5, 26.9; R, 32.8, 33.3, 27.5; significant; % of patients improved after 3 wk and 3 mo: I, 32.9, 55.4; R, 29.5, 55.8; no. of patients (%) returned to work after 3 mo: I, 14 (33%); R, 18 (44%)
Breivik et al. (13)	I: methyl prednisolone 80 mg (2 mL) + 20 mL bupivacaine 0.25%, caudal route, 1–3 injections (16)	R: bupivacaine 20 mL 0.25% + 100 mL saline (19)	Percentage of patients with considerable pain relief and objective neurologic improvement (before crossover): I, 56%; R, 26%; significant.
Bush and Hillier (15)	I: triamcinolone 80 mg + 25 mL procaine 0.5%, caudal route, 2 injections (12)	R: saline 25 mL (11)	Mean VAS (100 mm) of back and leg pain at baseline and at 4 and 52 wk: I, 39, 16, 14; R, 49, 45, 30; mean (SLR, degrees) at baseline and at 4 and 52 wk: I, 44, 73, 80; R, 63, 65, 74; short-term I significantly better results on pain and SLR; long-term I significantly better SLR
Cuckler et al. (20)	I: methyl prednisolone 80 mg (2 mL) + 5 mL procaine 1%, lumbar route, 1–2 injections (42)	R: saline 2 mL + 5 mL procaine 1% (31)	Average subjective improvement after 24 hr: I, 42%; R, 44%; not significant; long-term follow-up (about 20 mos) showed no significant differences
Serrao et al. (92)	I: prednisolone 80 mg + 10 mL saline (epidural) + 3 mL dextrose (intrathecal), lumbar route, 1 injection (14)	R: saline 10 mL (epidural) + 2 mg midazolam + 3 mL dextrose 5% (intrathecal) (14)	No. of patients reporting overall improvement initially and after 2 mo: I, 3, 5; R, 10, 7; R significantly better short-term improvement; no significant differences for pain and activity scores; R significantly less use of self-administered medications
Rocco et al. (90)	I1: triamcinolone 75 mg (10.9 mL) + 50 mg lidocaine, lumbar route (8), 1–3 injections I2: triamcinolone 75 mg + 50 mg lidocaine + 8 mg morphine (10.9 mL), 1–3 injections (7)	R: lidocaine 50 mg + 8 mg morphine (10.9 mL) (7)	Mean improvement on pain (VAS) after 1 and 6 mo: I1, 0.9, 2.2; I2, −0.6, −1.7; R, 0.4, −0.8; no. of patients reporting pain relief after 1 and 6 mo: I1, 5, 1; I2, 6, 0; R, 7, 0; no significant differences
Ridley et al. (88)	I: methyl prednisolone 80 mg + 10 mL saline, lumbar route (19)	R: saline 2 mL, interspinous ligament (16)	Percentage of patients improved after 2 wk: I, 90%; R, 19%; short-term I significantly better than R in relieving pain

I, index treatment; R, reference treatment; VAS, visual analog scale; SLR, straight leg raising.

276

TABLE 12.4. *Details of trials on the effectiveness of manipulation for chronic low back pain*

Investigators (ref.)	Manipulation (no. of patients)	Reference treatment (no. of patients)	Results
Koes et al. (51–54)	I: spinal manipulation and mobilization (65)	R1: physical therapy (66) R2: usual care by GP (61) R3: detuned short-wave diathermy and detuned ultrasound (64)	No differences on pain and functional status; mean improvement for main complaint (10-point scale) after 3 wk: I, 2.3; R1, 2.0; R2, 1.3; R3, 1.7; after 6 wk: I, 3.4; R1, 3.4; R2, 2.0; R3, 2.7; after 12 wk: I, 4.0; R1, 3.8; R2, 3.9; R3, 3.8; global perceived effect (6-point scale) after 3 wk: I, 2.5; R1, 2.6; R2, 1.6; R3, 2.1; after 6 wk: I, 3.4; R1, 3.3; R2, 1.9; R3, 2.8; after 12 wk: I, 3.4; R1, 3.7; R2, 2.2; R3, 3.3; groups I and R1 significantly better than group R2; no differences between groups I and R1; I significantly better global perceived effect than R3
Ongley et al. (85)	I: Bourdillon (40)	R: Nonforceful manipulation (41)	Mean (SEM) pain score (VAS) after 1, 3, and 6 mo: I, 2.1 (0.2), 1.8 (0.2), 1.5 (0.2), vs. R, 3.1 (0.3), 2.9 (0.3), and 3.1 (0.3); all differences significant
Triano et al. (97)	I: high-velocity-low amplitude (48)	R1: back education (46) R2: high-velocity low-force mimic (42)	Mean pain score (VAS) at baseline, after 2 wk, and 2 wk after treatment: I 38.4, 13.9, 13.3; R1, 35.6, 19.6, 15.1; R2, 37.4, 19.8, 21.7, respectively; I significantly more improved on pain score after 2 wk than R1; mean functional status score (Oswestry) at baseline, after 2 wk, and 2 wk after treatment: I, 17.5, 9.5, 10.6; R1, 20.2, 12.3, 11.4; R2, 21.7, 15.5, 14.0, respectively; no significant differences
Gibson et al. (29)	I: osteopathic (41)	R1: short-wave diathermy (34) R2: detuned short-wave diathermy (34)	Percentage of patients free of pain after 4 wk: I, 28%; R1, 28%; R2, 42%; and after 12 wk: I, 42%; R1, 37%; R2, 44%; not significant; median pain scores (VAS) at baseline and after 2, 4, and 12 wk: I, 35, 25, 21, 13; R1, 45, 35, 28, 25; R2, 48, 28, 27, 6; not significant
Herzog et al. (37)	I: chiropractic (16)	R: back school (13)	Group R significantly better improvement on pain and functional status (Oswestry) than I; I significantly better on gait symmetry than R
Evans et al. (27)	I: rotational (15)	R: analgesics (17)	No. of patients assessing treatment as effective after 3 wk: I, 9, vs. 3; R, significant
Waagen et al. (105)	I: chiropractic (9)	R: massage and sham manipulation (10)	Group I significantly better improvement on 10-cm VAS after 2 wk: 2.3, I, vs. 0.6, R
Arkuszewski (5)	I: Lewit (50)	R: bed rest, analgesics, and massage (50)	Mean (SD) pain-intensity (4-point scale) posttreatment and after 6 mo: I, 0.6 (0.5), 0.7 (0.6), vs. R, 1.0 (0.4), 1.0 (0.5); I significantly more improved
Postacchini et al. (87)	I: chiropractic (87)	R1: physical therapy: light massage, analgesic currents, and diathermy daily for 3 wk (78) R2: diclofenac "full dosage" 15–20 d (81) R3: low back school (50) R4: antiedema gel (73)	Mean improvement on combined pain, disability, and spinal mobility score after 3 wk and 2 and 6 mo in subgroup with chronic pain: I, 2.2, 2.6, 4.3; R1, 3.9, 4.2, 6.0; R2, 2.6, 2.2, 4.0; R3, 0.5, 4.6, 8.9; R4, 0.7 1.2, 2.0; I not significantly better

GP, general practitioner; I, index treatment; R, reference treatment; SD, standard deviation; SEM, standard error of the mean; VAS, visual analog scale.

TABLE 12.5. *Details of trials on the effectiveness of back schools for chronic low back pain*

Investigators (ref.)	Back school (no. of patients)	Reference treatment (no. of patients)	Results
Hurri and Julkunen et al. (39,40,43)	I: modified Swedish back school: 60-min education and exercise session, 6 times in 3 wk; refresher course 2 × 60 min after 6 mo; supervised by physical therapist; 11 patients per group (95)	R: Instruction material of the back school in written form; no actual treatment, but free to use health care services (93)	VAS, Pain Index, and Oswestry's Index after 6-mo follow-up: I significantly better than R; after 12 mo no differences (data in graphs)
Lankhorst et al. (56)	I: Swedish back school: 4 sessions of 45 min in the course of 2 wk (anatomy and causes of low back pain, function muscles and posture, ergonomics, advice on physical activity) (21)	R: 4 sessions with detuned short-wave applications in a period of 2 wk (22)	Mean pain on 10-point scale after the intervention and after 3, 6, and 12 mo: I, 6.0, 5.9, 6.2, 5.6; R, 6.8, 6.5, 5.8, 6.5; no significant differences (including functional capacity)
Keijsers et al. (45)	I: Maastricht back school: education and skills program in group setting (10–12 patients); 7 lessons of 2.5 hr, refresher lesson after 6 mo; including postural education, exercises, information on psychologic factors (n.a.)	R: waiting-list control group (n.a.)	Mean pain (VAS) after 2 and 6 mo: I, 5.4, 5.4, vs. R, 5.2, 4.6; no significant differences, including functional status
Donchin et al. (24)	I: 4 90-min sessions during a 2-wk period plus a fifth session after 2 mo; 10–12 patients per group supervised by a physical therapist (education and exercises for back and abdominal muscles) (46)	R1: calisthenics in 45-min sessions biweekly for 3 mo in groups of 10–12 patients (flexion and strengthening exercises) (46) R2: control group (were promised the most effective program in the future) (50)	Incidence of low back pain episodes (mean of painful months during 12 mo follow-up): I, 7.3; R1: 4.5, R2: 7.4; R1 significantly better than I and R2
Postacchini et al. (87)	I: based on Canadian Back Education Unit: four 1-hr sessions in a 1-wk period (including muscle exercises) (50)	R1: manipulation daily first wk, then, twice/wk for 6 wk (52) R2: NSAIDs (15–20 d) (47) R3: physical therapy: light massage, analgesic currents, and diathermy daily for 3 wk (47) R4: antiedema gel twice/d for 2 wk (43)	Mean improvement on combined pain, disability, and spinal mobility scores after 3 wk and 2 and 6 mos: I, 0.5, 4.6, 8.9; R1, 2.2, 2.6, 4.3; R2, 2.6, 2.2, 4.0; R3, 3.9, 4.2, 6.0; R4, 0.7, 1.2, 2.0; back school significantly better after 2 and 6 mo
Herzog et al. (37)	I: back school program (including instruction on how to move and stretching postural exercises) supervised by physical therapist: 10 sessions in a 4-wk period (13)	R: manipulation: 10 treatment sessions in 4 wk (16)	Mean pain score after 4 wk significantly lower in I compared with R (data in graphs); R significantly better in restoring gait symmetry
Klaber et al. (47)	I: Swedish back school: 3 sessions containing education on anatomy and body mechanics, semi-Fowler position, ergonomic counseling, and exercises aiming at strengthening the abdominal muscles (40)	R: exercises only (same as in group I) (38)	Change in mean pain and functional disability scores after 8 and 16 wk significantly larger in I compared with R (data in graphs)
Keijsers et al. (44)	I: Maastricht back school: education and skills program in group setting (10–12 patients); 7 lessons of 2.5 hr and refresher lesson after 8 wk; including postural education, exercises, information on psychologic factors (20)	R: waiting-list control group (20)	VAS for pain after the program: I, 28.9; R, 31.9; no significant differences for most of the outcome measures, including daily activities

I, index treatment; NSAIDs, nonsteroidal antiinflammatory drugs; R, reference treatment; VAS, visual analog scale.

TABLE 12.6. *Details of trials on the effectiveness of electromyographic biofeedback therapy for chronic low back pain*

Investigators (ref.)	Index treatment (no. of patients)	Reference treatment (no. of patients)	Results
Asfour et al. (6)	I: rehabilitation program and progressive extension training in lying position with auditory and visual EMG biofeedback (8 sessions) (15)	R: rehabilitation program (15)	Mean (SD) pain intensity pretreatment and posttreatment (2 wk): I, 6.1 (2.9), 4.7 (2.6); R, 5.6 (2.4), 5.6 (2.4); not significant; ROM not different between groups; I significantly more increase in strength
Bush et al. (14)	I: auditory EMG biofeedback training in sitting position until decrease and increase of 2 uV without feedback was reached with maximum 8 sessions (22)	R1: placebo feedback of back temperature (22) R2: waiting-list control (22)	No significant differences in pain intensity, functional status, or psychosocial status
Nouwen (84)	I: auditory and visual EMG biofeedback training in standing position, 15 sessions in 3 wk (10)	R: waiting-list control, no treatment (10)	Mean (SD) pain level (duration × intensity) pre- and posttreatment: I, 15.8 (9.4), 14.3 (8.6), vs. R, 18.4 (11.8), 19.1 (15.6); not significant.
Newton-John et al. (80)	I: EMG biofeedback: multiple, short, criterion-oriented feedback trials, sitting position, plus psychoeducational session, diaphragmatic session, diaphragmatic breathing exercises, 1 hr, twice/wk, 8 sessions (?)	R1: cognitive-behavioral therapy: education, goal setting, autogenic relaxation, cognitive pain control and restructuring techniques, homework tasks; groups of 4 subjects, 8 sessions of 1 hr, twice/wk (?) R2: waiting-list controls (?)	Mean (SD) pretreatment, posttreatment, and after 6 mo for pain: I, 16.81 (11.66), 8.42 (6.05), 8.40 (7.31); R1, 15.72 (13.97), 10.38 (11.37), 8.68 (10.54); R2, 16.37 (11.47), 17.56 (9.05); for disability: I, 22.56 (9.93), 15.12 (8.38), 23.06 (23.28); R1, 27.25 (19.71), 18.00 (15.19), 16.38 (14.02); R2, 25.17 (13.80), 26.33 (17.09); no significant differences between I and R1 for pain, disability, and several behavioral outcomes posttreatment and after 6 mo
Stuckey et al. (96)	I: relaxation training: progressive relaxation, breathing techniques, autogenic training, visual imagery; 8 45-min sessions (8)	R1: EMG-biofeedback training; 8 45-min sessions (8) R2: placebo EMG: no feedback, no relaxation instructions; 8 45-min sessions (8)	Mean scores of pain intensity during function test (range, 0–100) at first and last treatment session: I, 36.8, 28.0; R1, 26.2, 31.6; R2, 42.4, 44.4, and ADLs (range, 1–7): I, 2.4, 2.9; R1, 2.6, 2.5; R2, 2.2, 2.4; I, significantly more improved on pain intensity than R1 and R2 and significantly more improved on ADLs than R1
Donaldson et al. (23)	I: progressive relaxation training (Lehrer and Woolfolk) 10 35-min sessions (12)	R1: single motor unit biofeedback training (Johnson, Mulder) 10 35-min sessions (12) R2: education on anatomy, exercise, depression, stress, etc., 10 35-min sessions (12)	Mean scores on McGill Pain Questionnaire and pain intensity (VAS) pretreatment: I, 31.08, 2.51; R1, 28.75, 2.23; R2, 34.50, 3.48; posttreatment: I, 27.67, 1.90; R1, 16.08, 1.26; R2, 28.58, 2.47; and after 3 mo: I, 32.33, 1.78; R1, 15.33, 0.72; R2, 20.08, 0.87; R1 significantly more improved after 3 mo than I; no significant differences on pain intensity among groups

ADLs, activities of daily living; EMG, electromyography; I, index treatment; R, reference treatment; ROM, range of motion; SD, standard deviation.

TABLE 12.7. *Details of trials on the effectiveness of exercise therapy for chronic low back pain*

Investigators (ref.)	Exercise regimen (no. of patients)	Reference treatment (no. of patients)	Results
Deyo et al. (21)	I1: stretching exercises and TENS (34) I2: stretching exercises and sham TENS (29)	R1: TENS (31) R2: sham TENS (31)	Mean improvement pain (VAS 0–100%) and activity (VAS 0–100%) after 4 and 12 wk: I1 and I2, 52%, 48%; R1 and R2, 37%, 41%; exercise significantly better
Hansen et al. (33)	I: intensive dynamic back muscle training (60)	R1: physical therapy: manual traction, hot packs, massage and flexibility, co-ordination and slowly progressive back and abdominal muscle exercises (59) R2: placebo control: semihot packs and light traction (61)	No significant differences in pain level (10-point scale) between groups posttreatment and after 1, 6, and 12 mo; overall treatment effect (10-point scale) of I and R1 significantly higher at all evaluations than R2; no significant changes over time.
Manniche et al. (66, 67)	I1: intensive back extensor (27) I2: mild isometric exercises/massage/hot compresses (32) I3: mild back extensor (31)	—	Median improvement in combined pain, disability, physical impairment index (0–100 points) after 3 and 9 mo: I1, 14.7, 15.0; I2, 2.0, 5.5; I3, 5.7, 7.0; I1 significantly better than I2 and I3
Elnaggar et al. (26)	I1: McKenzie extension (28) I2: Williams flexion (28)	—	Mean (SD) scores on McGill Pain Questionnaire (range, 0–78) pretreatment and posttreatment: I1, 15.9 (7.8) and 10.6 (8.6), vs. I2, 14.1 (9.8) and 8.9 (9.4); no significant difference
Lidström and Zachrisson (59)	I1: isometric strengthening and pelvic traction (20) I2: mobilizing/strengthening, hot packs and massage (21)	R: hot packs and rest (21)	No. of patients with noticeable improvement after 4 wk: I1, 17; I2, 9; R, 12; patients in I1 significantly better than I2 and R
Manniche et al. (65)	I1: intensive dynamic exercises, plus hyperextension (31) I2: intensive dynamic exercises (31)	—	Overall improvement posttreatment and after 3 and 12 mo not significantly different in I1 and I2; improvement on low back pain rating scale (0–100) posttreatment and after 3 and 12 mo in I1 of 10, 8, 3 vs. 7, 1, 0 in I2; significant at 3 mo
Lindström et al. (60, 61)	I: individual, submaximal, gradually increased exercise program: endurance and strength training, lifting, walking, jogging, swimming, fitness (51)	R: traditional care (52)	Proportion of patients returned to work within 6 wk or 12 wk after randomization: I, 59%, 80%; vs. R, 40%, 58%; significant; mean (SD) duration of sick leave from low back pain during second follow-up year: I, 12.1 (18.4) wk, vs. R, 19.6 (20.7) wk; significant; no differences in functional status (whole-body mobility) after 1 yr

Study	Index treatment (I)	Reference treatment (R)	Results
Johanssen et al. (42)	I1: dynamic back, neck, abdominal endurance exercises/stretching (20); I2: coordination/balance exercises (20)	—	Median pain score (scale, 0–8) pretreatment and after 3 and 6 mo: I1, 6, 3, 4, vs. I2, 6, 5, 4; not significant; median disability score (scale, 0–12); I1, 6, 2, 1, vs. I2, 5, 3, 2; not significant
Turner et al. (103)	I1: aerobic exercises (24); I2: aerobic exercises and operant-conditioning behavioral therapy (24)	R1: operant-conditioning behavioral therapy (25); R2: waiting-list control group (23)	Mean scores on McGill Pain Questionnaire and SIP pretreatment: I1, 19.42, 8.42; I2, 25.54, 8.50; R1, 20.96, 7.90; R2, 21.17, 6.24; and posttreatment: I1, 17.52, 5.49; I2, 12.41, 4.59; R1, 17.71, 4.72; R2, 20.95, 5.37; I2 significantly more improved than I1 and R2; no significant differences among I1, I2, and R1 after 6 and 12 mo
Kendall and Jenkins (46)	I1: isometric flexion (14); I2: mobilization (14); I3: extension (14)	—	No. of patients symptom free or improved after 1 and 3 mo: I1, 13, 11; I2, 11, 8; I3, 7, 6; I1 significantly better than I2 and I3
Risch et al. (89)	I: dynamic extension exercise program (31)	R: waiting-list control group (23)	Mean (SD) pain score pre- and posttreatment: I, 3.4 (1.6), 2.9 (1.7), vs. R, 3.7 (1.6), 4.1 (1.5); significant; mean (SD) physical disability score (SIP): I, 9.1 (9.3), 7.7 (9.4), vs. R, 15.2 (10.4), 19.3 (15.6); significant
Martin et al. (69)	I1: mobilizing abdominal and back muscles (12); I2: isometric abdominal and pelvic floor muscles (12)	R: detuned ultrasound and detuned short-wave diathermy (12)	Change in pain intensity (5-point scale) after 5 wk: I1, decrease; I2, increase; R, decrease; no significant difference in physiologic and clinical measures
Buswell (16)	I1: flexion program (25); I2: extension program (25)	—	Similar improvement of pain and function after treatment for I1 and I2; data not given
Sachs et al. (91)	I1: rehabilitation program: stretching/strengthening/cardiovascular conditioning exercises plus exercises on B-200 isostation (14)	R: rehabilitation program (16)	No significant difference in range of motion after 3-wk treatment period
Frost et al. (28)	I: fitness program and back school education (36)	R: back school education (35)	Mean (SD) scores on functional status (Oswestry) and pain (0–100 scale) pretreatment (I) 23.6 (9.7), 20.9 (12.3) vs (R) 23.6 (12.3), 25.6 (17.9) and posttreatment (I) 17.6 (10.9), 12.1 (9.9) vs (R) 21.7 (13.6), 22.1 (20.1). (I) significantly more improved than (R). After 6 months (I) significantly more improved functional status than (R).
White (107)	I1: mild static trunk and short-wave diathermy (76); I2: vigorous flexion and extension (72)	—	Proportion of patients showing improvement after treatment (maximum 7 wk) 38% (11) vs. 35% (12); not significant

I, index treatment; R, reference treatment; SD, standard deviation; SIP, Sickness Impact Profile; TENS, transcutaneous electrical nerve stimulation; VAS, visual analog scale.

TABLE 12.8. *Details of trials on the effectiveness of traction and orthoses for chronic low back pain*

Investigators (ref.)	Index treatment (no. of patients)	Reference treatment (no. of patients)	Results
Traction			
Beurskens et al. (11,12)	I: traction, 35–50% of body weight, 12 times, 5 wk, 20 min/session (77)	R: sham traction, maximum 20% of body weight, 12 times, 5 wks, 20 min/session (74)	Differences between groups (95% CI) after 5 weeks for global improvement: −7% (−23%; 9%), functional status (RDQ) −1.3 (−2.9; 0.3), pain last week (100 mm VAS) −3.0 (−11.8; 5.8), return to work (days of absence) −1.8 (−5.5; 1.9); no significant differences
Heijden et al. (36)	I: continuous motorized traction, 30–50% of body weight, 20 min, 3 times/wk, 4 wk (13)	R: continuous motorized traction, 0–25% of body weight, 20 min, 3 times/wk, 4 wk (12)	Median improvement of pain and functional status after 5 wk: I, 14, 2, vs. R, 16, 1; and after 9 wk: I, 14, 2, vs. R, 4, 2; no. of patients completely recovered or much improved after 5 and 9 wk in I, 7/13, 5/13, vs. R, 4/12, 3/12; no significant differences
Orthoses			
Million et al. (76)	I: corset with lumbar support for 8 wk (9)	R: corset without lumbar support for 8 wk (10)	Overall subjective improvement index: I, highly significant improvement; R, no change; overall objective improvement index: I and R improvement over the study period but no difference between groups

CI, confidence interval; I, index treatment; R, reference treatment; RDQ, Roland Disability Questionnaire.

B. Moderate evidence: provided by generally consistent findings in one high-quality RCT and one or more low-quality RCTs or by generally consistent findings in multiple low-quality RCTs.

C. Limited or contradictory evidence: one RCT (either high- or low-quality) or inconsistent findings in multiple RCTs.

D. No evidence: no RCTs.

An RCT was (arbitrarily) considered to be of high quality if the methodologic score was 50 points or more and of low quality if the methodologic score was less than 50 points.

RESULTS

Analgesics

Only one high-quality RCT (38) was identified (Tables 12.2 and 12.11), which showed a better overall improvement with diflunisal (NSAID) compared with paracetamol. There are no RCTs of analgesics versus placebo in chronic LBP. Although there is limited scientific evidence (level C) for chronic LBP, considerable evidence in other situations indicates that analgesics provide short-term symptomatic pain relief.

Nonsteroidal Antiinflammatory Drugs

Six RCTs (Tables 12.2 and 12.11) were identified, of which three were considered to be of high quality and three of low quality. The scores ranged from 27 to 62 points. One low-quality RCT compared two types of NSAIDs with a placebo in a crossover design and had a positive outcome (10). Of the two pragmatic RCTs comparing NSAIDs with other conservative types of treatment, the high-quality RCT reported a positive outcome with overall improvement compared with paracetamol (38,87). The results of the four RCTs comparing two different types of NSAIDs, two of high quality and two of low quality, did not show any differences (10,70,94,104). There is limited evidence (level C) that NSAIDs are more effective than paracetamol and placebo, and there is strong evidence (level A) that the various types of NSAIDs (piroxicam, indomethacin, ibuprofen, diclofenac, ketoprofen, naproxen, and diflunisal) are equally effective. NSAIDs can have serious adverse effects, particularly at high doses and in elderly patients. Ibuprofen has the lowest risk of gastrointestinal complications of the most commonly used NSAIDs, followed by diclofenac, mainly because of the low doses used in clinical practice.

Muscle Relaxants and Benzodiazepines

Only one high-quality RCT (4) was identified (Tables 12.2 and 12.11), and it reported a positive result of tetrazepam compared with a placebo on overall efficacy and pain intensity. There is limited evidence (level C) that muscle relaxants can provide short-term symptomatic relief. Muscle relaxants have potential side effects including drowsiness in up to 30% of patients.

Antidepressants

One high-quality and three low-quality RCTs were identified with scores ranging from 35 to 64 points. All four RCTs (Tables 12.2 and 12.11) compared an antidepressant

TABLE 12.9. *Details of trials on the effectiveness of behavioral/cognitive/relaxation therapy for chronic low back pain*

Investigators (ref.)	Index treatment (no. of patients)	Reference treatment (no. of patients)	Results
Turner and Clancy (101)	I1: aerobic exercises and operant conditioning (Fordyce); 2 hr/wk/8 wk (30) I2: cognitive-behavioral approach: systematic progressive muscle relaxation (Bernstein and Borkovec) and imagery; 2 hr/wk/8 wk (26)	R: waiting-list control group (25)	Mean (SD) scores on McGill Pain Questionnaire and SIP pretreatment, posttreatment, and after 6 and 12 mo: I1, 23.07 (12.37), 18.50 (12.43), 19.57 (15.31), 15.07 (11.62); vs. I2, 18.30 (10.43), 15.91 (11.63), 12.70 (12.75), 10.80 (6.38); not significant; I1 significantly better posttreatment than R on pain and physical and psychosocial functioning
Nicholas et al. (82)	I: cognitive-behavioral approach, including progressive muscle relaxation training (Bernstein and Borkovec) and physical therapy; one 2-hr and one 1.5-hr session/wk/5 wk (10)	R: physical therapy: information, exercises and handouts (one 2-hr and one 1.5-hr session/wk/5 wk) and attention (5 sessions) (10)	Mean (SD) scores of pain intensity (6-point nominal scale) and functional status (SIP) pretreatment, posttreatment, and after 6 mo: I, 3.13 (0.88), 3.07 (0.79), 2.89 (0.64) and 30.87 (12.17), 18.81 (10.97), 18.30 (11.18), vs. R, 2.84 (0.85), 2.72 (0.77), 2.75 (1.11) and 32.10 (13.45), 26.08 (16.40), 25.31 (14.34); not significant; I significantly better posttreatment than R on coping strategies, pain self-efficacy, and medication use; after 6 mo, I significantly better coping strategies
Nicholas et al. (81)	I1: behavioral treatment (operant-conditioning Fordyce) and physical therapy; one 2-hr and one 1.5-hr session/wk/5 wk (10) I2: behavioral treatment and physical therapy and progressive muscle relaxation training; one 2-hr and one 1.5-hr session/wk/5 wk (9) I3: cognitive treatment (coping strategies) and physical therapy; one 2-hr and one 1.5-hr session/wk/5 wk (10) I4: cognitive treatment and physical therapy and progressive muscle relaxation training; one 2-hr and one 1.5-hr session/wk/5 wk (8)	R1: physical therapy: information, exercises and handouts (one 2-hr and one 1.5-hr session/wk/5 wk) (11) R2: physical therapy (one 2-hr and one 1.5-hr session/wk/5 wk) and attention (5 sessions) (10)	Posttreatment I1, I2, I3, and I4 significantly more improved on pain intensity (6-point nominal scale), self-rated functional impairment (SIP), and pain beliefs than R1 and R2, but no significant differences after 6 and 12 mo; I1 and I2 significantly more improved posttreatment on self-rated SIP than I3 and I4; no other differences between index treatments after 6 and 2 mo on any of the outcome measures
Turner (100)	I1: progressive muscle relaxation training (Bernstein and Borkovec) (14 posttreatment; 18 follow-up) I2: cognitive-behavioral therapy: relaxation, coping, imagery (13 posttreatment; 16 follow-up)	R: waiting-list control group (9)	Mean (SD) score on self-rated functional impairment (SIP) and pain (VAS) pretreatment: I1, 14.6 (8.2), 57.9 (21.6); I2, 18.6 (7.9), 55.2 (24.8); R, 20.2 (11.1), 54.0 (32.0); and posttreatment: I1, 9.1 (8.3), 42.3 (20.2), I2, 10.2 (6.9), 36.5 (22.7); and R, 20.2 (8.2), 77.0 (21.6); I1 and I2 significantly better posttreatment than R; pain score for I1 after 1 mo significantly better than for I2; no other differences between I1 and I2 posttreatment, after 1 mo and 1.5 yr on pain, depression, and functional status

Study	Index treatment	Reference treatment	Results
Turner et al. (103)	I1: behavioral therapy: operant conditioning (Fordyce); 2 hr/wk/8 wk (25) I2: behavioral therapy, 2 hr/wk/8 wk, and aerobic exercise, 10–20 min, 5 times/wk/8 wk (24)	R1: aerobic exercise 10–20 min, 5 times/wk, 8 wk (24) R2: waiting-list control group (23)	Mean scores on McGill Pain Questionnaire, SIP, and depression pretreatment: I1, 20.96, 7.90, 10.40; I2, 25.54, 8.50, 12.38; R1, 19.42, 8.42, 11.95; and R2, 21.17, 6.24, 10.48; and posttreatment: I1, 17.71, 4.72, 8.08; I2, 12.41, 4.59, 7.31; R1, 17.52, 5.49, 7.38; and R2, 20.95, 5.37, 7.03; I2 significantly more improved than R1 and R2; no significant differences after 6 and 12 mo among I1, I2, and R1
Turner and Jensen (102)	I1: progressive muscle relaxation training (Bernstein and Borkovec) and imagery (24) I2: cognitive therapy (Beck) (23) I3: cognitive therapy and relaxation training (25)	R: waiting-list control group (30)	Mean (SD) pain score (VAS) pretreatment vs. posttreatment: I1, 51.29 (21.68), vs. 37.88 (20.07); I2, 56.91 (18.47) vs. 36.88 (20.45); I3, 60.68 (22.04) vs. 44.33 (28.45); and R, 50.07 (21.14) vs. 48.06 (20.97); I1, I2, and I3 significantly more improved than R; no significant differences among I1, I2, and I3 posttreatment and after 6 and 12 mo on pain, global measure of improvement, or functional status (SIP)
Stuckey et al. (96)	I: Relaxation training: progressive relaxation, breathing techniques, autogenic training, visual imagery; 8 sessions of 45 min (8)	R1: EMG biofeedback training; 8 sessions of 45 min (8) R2: placebo EMG: no feedback, no relaxation instructions; 8 sessions of 45 min (8)	Mean scores of pain intensity during function test (range, 0–100) at first and last treatment session: I, 36.8, 28.0, R1, 26.2, 31.6; R2, 42.4, 44.4; and ADLs (range, 1–7): I, 2.4, 2.9; R1, 2.6, 2.5; R2, 2.2, 2.4; I significantly more improved on pain intensity than R1 and R2, and significantly more improved on ADLs than R1
Newton-John et al. (80)	I: cognitive-behavioral therapy: education, goal setting, autogenic relaxation, cognitive pain control and restructuring techniques, homework tasks; groups of 4 subjects, 8 sessions of 1 hr, twice/wk (?)	R1: EMG biofeedback: multiple, short, criterion-oriented feedback trials, sitting position, plus psychoeducational session, diaphragmatic breathing exercises, 1 hr, twice/wk, 8 sessions (?) R2: waiting-list controls (?)	Mean (SD) pretreatment, posttreatment, and after 6 mo for pain: I, 15.72 (13.97), 10.38 (11.37), 8.68 (10.54); R1, 16.81 (11.66), 8.42 (6.05), 8.40 (7.31); R2, 16.37 (11.47), 17.56 (9.05); for disability: I, 27.25 (19.71), 18.00 (15.19), 16.38 (14.02); R1, 22.56 (9.93), 15.12 (8.38), 23.06 (23.28); R2, 25.17 (13.80), 26.33 (17.09); no significant differences between I and R1 for pain, disability, and several behavioral outcomes posttreatment and after 6 mo
McCauley et al. (71)	I: progressive muscle relaxation training (Bernstein and Borkovec) and differential relaxation; 50 min/wk/8 wk (8)	R: self-hypnosis (Barber) and hypnoanalgesic techniques; 50 min/wk/8 wk (9)	Mean scores on pain (VAS) pretreatment, posttreatment, and after 3 mo: I, 56.9, 39.1, 35.9, vs. R, 63.1, 43.6, 42.2; no significant differences between groups on pain or depression
Donaldson et al. (23)	I: progressive relaxation training (Lehrer and Woolfolk), 10 35-min sessions (12)	R1: single motor unit biofeedback training (Johnson, Mulder), 10 35-min sessions (12) R2: education on anatomy exercise, depression, stress, etc., 10 35-min sessions (12)	Mean scores on McGill Pain Questionnaire and pain intensity (VAS) pretreatment: I, 31.08, 2.51; R1, 28.75, 2.23; R2, 34.50, 3.48; posttreatment: I, 27.67, 1.90; R1, 16.08, 1.26; R2, 28.58, 2.47; and after 3 mo: I, 32.33, 1.78; R1, 15.33, 0.72; R2, 20.08, 0.87; R1 significantly more improved after 3 mo than I; no significant differences on pain intensity among groups

ADLs, activities of daily living; EMG, electromyography; I, index treatment; R, reference treatment; SD, standard deviation; SIP, Sickness Impact Profile; VAS, visual analog scale.

TABLE 12.10. Details of trials on the effectiveness of transcutaneous electrical nerve stimulation or acupuncture for chronic low back pain

Investigators (ref.)	TENS/acupuncture (no. of patients)	Reference treatment(s) (no. of patients)	Results
		TENS	
Deyo et al. (21)	I: TENS 3 times/d 45 min; high-frequency (80–100 pulses/sec, amplitude 30) 2 wk plus low-frequency (2–4 pulses/sec, amplitude 100) 2 wk or high-frequency 4 wk (65)	R: placebo TENS 4 wk (60)	Difference (95% CI) between I and R posttreatment: functional status (SIP) −0.5 (−2.2, 1.3), pain (100-mm VAS) −2.3 (−9.6, 4.9), Schober test (cm) 0.13 (−0.24, 0.50); no significant differences on any of the outcome measures
Moore and Shurman (79)	I: TENS 5 hr, 2 d, asymmetric biphasic square pulse, 100 sec, frequency 100 Hz, amplitude 0–60 mA (24)	R1: NMES, symmetric biphasic square pulse, 200 sec, frequency 70 Hz, amplitude 0–100 mA (24) R2: combination NMES/TENS, 5 hr with 3 times 10 min/treatment, 2 d (24) R3: Placebo TENS (24)	Mean (SD) of present pain intensity and pain relief (VAS) pretreatment and posttreatment: I, 2.58 (1.03), 46.23 (26.88) and 2.27 (1.13), 40.58 (27.55); R1, 2.67 (1.00), 48.83 (27.66) and 2.21 (0.99), 39.67 (30.94); R2, 2.75 (1.14), 48.46 (28.81) and 1.94 (1.06), 36.33 (31.29); R3, 2.79 (1.07), 50.56 (29.13), 2.42 (1.15), 44.81 (30.67); combined treatment most effective
Marchand et al. (68)	I: TENS high-frequency (125 μsec) pulses, low-intensity, 30 min, twice 10 wk (14)	R1: placebo TENS (12) R2: no treatment (16)	I significantly more effective in pain intensity than R1 after 1 wk, but not after 3 and 6 mo; pain unpleasantness ratings not different (data in graphs)
Lehmann et al. (57, 58)	I: TENS 250 pulses/sec, 60 Hz, subthreshold intensity, 3 wk (18)	R1: placebo TENS (18) R2: electroacupuncture 2 times/wk, 2–4 Hz, 3 wk (17)	R2 significantly more relief of peak pain posttreatment and after 6 mo and significantly more relief of average pain posttreatment and after 6 mo than I and R1; no differences between I and R1; (data in graphs)
		Acupuncture	
Coan et al. (18)	I: acupuncture/electroacupuncture (±10 treatments) (25)	R: waiting-list control group (25)	Reduction in pain score (11-point scale) and ADLs (4-point scale) after 10–15 wk: I, 51%, 19% vs. R, 2%, 0%; inadequate treatment in 11 of the 50 patients treated with acupuncture

286

Study	I (intervention)	R (reference)	Results
Mendelson et al. (74, 75)	I: acupuncture 30 min, twice/wk, 4 wk (36)	R: placebo acupuncture (41)	Reduction in pain score (100-mm VAS): I, 40%, vs. R, 26% after 4 wk; not significant; crossover: reduction in pain score for I now placebo, 40%, vs. R now acupuncture, 19%; significant; overall mean percentage decrease in pain score 26.1 for acupuncture and 21.8 for placebo; not significant
MacDonald et al. (64)	I: acupuncture/electroacupuncture 5–20 min, once/wk/7 wk (8)	R: placebo acupuncture (9)	Mean percentage reduction posttreatment in pain score and ADLs: I, 57.1, 52.0, vs. R, 22.7, 5.83; ADLs significant
Edelist et al. (25)	I: manual acupuncture plus electroacupuncture 3–10 Hz, 30 min, 3 treatments (15)	R: placebo acupuncture (15)	No. of patients improved posttreatment on pain and spinal mobility: I, 7, 7, vs. R, 6, 6; not significant
Molsberger et al. (78)	I: conventional conservative orthopedic treatment plus verum acupuncture, 30 min, 12 treatments, traditional acupuncture points, manual stimulation, Teh Chi (?)	R1: conventional conservative orthopedic treatment plus placebo acupuncture, 30 min, 12 treatments (?) R2: conventional conservative orthopedic treatment (?)	Patients with pain relief at least 50% posttreatment and after 3 mo: I, 64%, 75%; R1, 35%, 30%; R2, 44%, 17%; I significantly better than R1 and R2; percentage of patients with good or excellent overall improvement posttreatment and after 3 mo: I, 82%, 73%; R1, 70%, 55%; R2, 57%, 27%
Lehmann et al. (57, 58)	I: electroacupuncture 2 times/wk, 2–4 Hz, 3 wk (17)	R1: placebo TENS (18) R2: TENS 250 pulses/sec, 60-Hz, subthreshold intensity, 3 wk (18)	I significantly more relief of peak pain posttreatment and after 6 mo and significantly more relief of average pain posttreatment and after 6 mo than R2 and R1; no differences between R2 and R1; (data in graphs)
Gunn et al. (32)	I: rehabilitation program plus acupuncture 1–2 times/wk, 10 treatments maximum (29)	R: rehabilitation program (27)	No. of patients with good or total improvement at discharge and after 12 wk in I, 18, 17, vs. R, 4, 4; significant

ADLs, activities of daily living; I, index treatment; MNES, neuromuscular electrical stimulation; R, reference treatment; SD, standard deviation; SIP, Sickness Impact Profile; TENS, transcutaneous electrical nerve stimulation; VAS, visual analog scale.

TABLE 12.11. Randomized trials on the efficacy of various types of drugs in chronic low back pain in order to methodologic score

Scores for methodologic criteria

Investigators (ref.)	A 2	B 5	C 4	D 3	E 4	F 12	G 10	H 5	I 5	J 5	K 9	L 8	M 8	N 5	O 5	P 5	Q 5	Score 100	Conclusion[a]
Analgesics																			
Hickey (38)	2	1	4	2	4	—	10	5	5	—	5	8	8	3	—	5	—	62	Negative
Muscle relaxants																			
Arbus et al. (4)	1	—	—	3	2	—	10	—	5	5	5	6	6	3	—	5	5	51	Positive
Antidepressants																			
Goodkin et al. (30)	1	4	—	3	4	—	10	—	—	5	7	6	6	3	5	5	5	64	Negative
Alcoff et al. (2)	—	4	—	3	2	—	10	—	—	5	5	6	6	3	5	—	—	49	Positive
Jenkins et al. (41)	1	2	—	—	—	—	10	—	—	5	5	5	5	3	—	—	—	36	Negative
Pheasant et al. (86)	1	—	—	—	—	—	10	—	—	5	5	3	3	3	—	5	—	35	No conclusion
NSAIDs																			
Hickey (38)	2	1	4	2	4	—	10	5	5	—	5	8	8	3	—	5	—	62	Positive
Siegmeth and Sieberer (94)	—	—	—	2	4	—	10	5	5	—	—	8	8	3	—	5	—	50	No conclusion
Videman and Osterman (104)	1	3	—	2	4	—	10	5	—	—	5	6	6	3	—	5	—	50	Negative
Berry et al. (10)	2	—	—	2	4	—	10	5	5	5	5	4	4	3	—	—	—	49	Positive
Matsumo et al. (70)	1	—	—	—	4	6	8	5	5	—	5	3	1	3	—	5	—	46	Negative
Postacchini et al. (87)	2	—	—	—	2	—	8	5	—	—	—	5	—	5	—	—	—	27	No conclusion

Investigators (ref.)	A 2	B 5	C 4	D 3	E 4	F 17	G 10	H 5	I 5	J 5	K 5	L 10	M 10	N 5	O 5	P 5	Score 100	Conclusion[a]
Epidural steroid injections																		
Carette et al. (17)	2	5	4	3	4	8	10	5	5	5	5	10	10	—	5	5	81	Negative
Breivik et al. (13)	1	2	4	3	4	—	10	—	5	5	5	6	6	—	5	5	59	Positive
Bush and Hillier (15)	2	3	—	3	2	—	10	—	—	5	3	6	6	5	5	5	55	Positive
Cuckler et al. (20)	2	4	4	3	4	—	10	—	—	5	3	2	2	5	5	5	54	Negative
Serrao et al. (92)	2	4	—	4	4	—	10	—	—	—	3	6	6	3	5	5	51	Negative
Rocco et al. (90)	1	3	4	—	4	—	10	—	—	—	3	4	4	5	—	5	43	Negative
Ridley et al. (88)	2	4	2	2	2	—	10	—	—	5	3	4	4	5	—	—	41	Positive short-term only

NSAIDs, nonsteroidal antiinflammatory drugs.

[a] Conclusion of the author(s); positive indicates that analgesics were better than the reference treatment; negative indicates that analgesics were worse than or equally effective as the reference treatment.

with a placebo (2,30,41,86). The studies reported no statistically significant differences in pain and depression. There is moderate evidence that antidepressants are not effective (level B).

Epidural Steroid Injections

Five high-quality and two low-quality RCTs on epidural steroid injections were identified (Tables 12.3 and 12.11). The scores ranged from 41 to 81. Two high-quality and one low-quality trials compared the epidural steroid injection with a placebo injection (saline) (15,17,88). The high-quality trials reported conflicting results of pain relief from epidural steroid injection. In the other four trials, the epidural steroid injection was compared with an injection of bupivacaine (13), procaine (20), midazolam (92), or lidocaine and morphine (90). Three of these four trials were of high quality, and one was of low quality. Only one high-quality RCT reported a positive outcome. The study population in six trials was small, and the trials included patients with various indications such as chronic LBP, chronic LBP with sciatica, sciatica, lumbar radicular pain syndrome, and postlaminectomy pain syndrome. There is conflicting evidence that epidural steroid injections provide better short-term pain relief than placebo for patients with radicular symptoms (level C). There is moderate evidence (level B) that epidural steroid injections are not effective for chronic LBP without radicular symptoms. Because of inconsistent findings, it is not possible to judge whether epidural injections are more effective than injections of a local anesthetic alone (level C).

Exercise Therapy

Sixteen trials were identified on specific back exercises (Tables 12.7 and 12.12), three high-quality and 13 low-quality RCTs. The methodologic scores ranged from 24 to 61. The number of RCTs reporting positive and negative results was equal (n = 8), but the four high-quality RCTs all reported positive results. In nine trials, exercises were compared with various reference treatments such as traditional care, physical modalities, hot packs and rest, behavioral therapy, no exercise, a waiting-list control group, or a placebo treatment (21,28,33,59–61,69,89,91,103). Six of these nine trials, including three high-quality RCTs, reported a positive result, whereas three low-quality RCTs reported a negative result. The effectiveness of different types of exercises was examined in nine trials, of which six did not find any differences (16,26, 42,46,59,65–67,69,107). There is strong evidence that exercise therapy is effective (level A), and there is moderate evidence that the various exercises are equally effective (level B).

Back Schools

Eight RCTs, one of high quality (39,40,43) and seven of low quality (24,37,44, 45,47,56,87), were identified on the efficacy of some type of back school (Tables 12.5 and 12.12). The scores ranged from 19 to 55 points. Three trials, including the high-quality RCT, reported positive results for a back school, three reported negative results, and in two studies no clear conclusion was drawn (we considered one of these trials positive [37] and one as negative [44]). In four trials, a back school was compared with various types of reference treatments, including exercises, manipulation, NSAIDs, and physical therapy (24,37,47,87). Three of these low-quality trials reported positive

TABLE 12.12. *Randomized trials on the efficacy of various conservative treatments in chronic low back pain in order of methodologic score*

Investigators (ref.)	Scores for methodologic criteria																Total Score 100	Conclusion[a]
	A 2	B 5	C 4	D 3	E 4	F 17	G 10	H 5	I 5	J 5	K 5	L 10	M 10	N 5	O 5	P 5		
Manipulation																		
Koes et al. (51–54)	1	3	4	3	—	8	—	5	—	5	3	8	4	3	5	5	57	Positive
Ongley et al. (85)	2	4	2	—	4	—	5	5	—	—	5	4	4	5	5	5	50	Positive
Triano et al. (97)	1	1	4	3	—	8	5	5	—	5	2	4	—	3	—	5	43	Positive
Gibson et al. (29)	2	3	—	—	4	—	—	5	5	5	—	4	2	3	—	5	41	Negative
Herzog et al. (37)	—	1	—	—	—	—	1	5	5	5	—	6	2	3	—	5	37	No conclusion
Evans et al. (27)	—	—	2	—	2	—	0	5	5	—	—	6	2	3	—	5	35	Positive
Waagen et al. (105)	1	2	—	—	—	—	5	5	5	—	5	4	2	3	—	—	32	Positive
Arkuszewski (5)	—	1	2	—	4	—	5	5	—	—	—	4	—	5	5	5	31	Positive
Postacchini et al. (87)	1	3	—	—	2	—	—	5	—	—	—	6	—	5	—	—	27	Negative
Back schools																		
Hurri and Julkunen et al. (39,40,43)	2	3	—	—	4	8	5	5	—	—	—	8	—	5	5	5	55	Positive
Lankhorst et al. (56)	2	3	2	—	2	—	1	5	—	—	3	6	—	5	—	5	38	Negative
Keijsers et al. (45)	1	—	—	3	2	—	0	5	—	—	—	8	—	5	—	5	29	Negative
Donchin et al. (24)	—	3	—	—	—	—	5	5	—	—	—	4	—	5	5	—	27	Negative
Postacchini et al. (87)	1	3	—	—	2	—	5	5	—	—	—	6	—	5	—	5	27	Positive
Herzog et al. (37)	1	1	—	—	—	—	5	5	—	—	—	6	2	3	—	5	23	No conclusion
Klaber et al. (47)	1	3	—	—	2	—	5	5	—	—	—	4	—	3	5	—	23	Positive
Keijsers et al. (44)	1	1	—	—	—	—	5	5	—	—	—	4	—	3	—	—	19	No conclusion
Electromyographic Biofeedback																		
Asfour et al. (6)	1	3	—	—	4	—	10	5	—	—	—	4	—	3	5	5	40	Negative
Bush et al. (14)	1	4	—	—	4	—	10	—	—	5	3	4	—	3	5	—	39	Negative
Nouwen (84)	1	2	—	3	4	—	10	—	—	—	—	2	—	3	5	5	35	Negative
Newton-John et al. (80)	1	3	—	—	—	—	10	—	—	—	—	6	—	5	—	5	30	Negative
Stucky et al. (96)	1	—	—	—	—	—	—	5	—	5	3	4	4	3	—	5	30	Negative
Donaldson et al. (23)	1	—	—	—	—	—	5	5	—	—	—	4	—	3	—	5	23	Positive

290

Table (rotated on page). Columns read left-to-right after the study name; the final two columns are a total score and the overall conclusion. Treatment groups ("Exercise therapy", "Traction", "Orthoses") are shown as section sub-headers.

Study															Total	Conclusion
Exercise therapy																
Deyo et al. (21)	1	3	4	3	2	8	10	—	—	—	10	2	3	5	5	61	Positive
Hansen et al. (33)	1	4	2	3	—	8	10	—	5	3	4	4	5	—	5	59	Positive
Lindström et al. (60,61)	2	2	4	—	4	8	5	—	—	—	4	2	5	5	5	51	Positive
Manniche et al. (66,67)	2	1	4	3	2	—	10	—	—	—	10	2	5	5	5	54	Positive
Elnaggar et al. (26)	1	3	2	3	4	—	10	—	—	—	4	2	3	5	5	47	Negative
Lidström and Zachrisson (59)	1	2	—	3	4	—	10	—	—	—	6	2	3	5	5	46	Positive
Manniche et al. (65)	—	3	2	3	—	—	10	—	—	—	8	2	5	—	5	44	Negative
Johanssen et al. (42)	—	2	—	3	—	—	10	—	—	—	10	—	5	—	5	41	Negative
Turner et al. (103)	—	1	—	—	—	—	10	—	—	—	8	2	5	—	5	37	Negative
Kendall and Jenkins (46)	1	—	2	—	2	—	10	—	—	—	6	2	3	5	5	36	Positive
Risch et al. (89)	—	3	2	—	4	—	5	—	5	—	4	—	3	—	5	36	Positive
Martin et al. (69)	2	—	2	—	—	—	10	—	—	—	6	2	5	5	—	35	Negative
Buswell et al. (16)	—	1	—	—	—	—	10	—	—	—	4	—	3	5	—	30	Negative
Sachs et al. (91)	—	1	—	—	4	—	10	—	—	—	2	—	5	—	5	30	Negative
Frost et al. (28)	2	4	2	—	—	—	—	—	—	—	6	—	5	—	5	29	Positive
White (107)	1	—	—	—	—	8	—	5	—	—	2	—	3	5	5	24	Negative
Traction																
Beurskens et al. (11,12)	1	5	4	3	4	8	10	—	5	5	10	1	3	5	5	83	Negative
Heijden et al. (36)	1	2	—	—	2	—	10	—	5	5	6	0	5	5	5	56	Positive
Orthoses																
Million et al. (76)	2	2	5	—	—	—	10	5	—	3	8	—	3	—	—	38	Positive

continued

TABLE 12.12. Continued

Scores for methodologic criteria

Investigators (ref.)	A 2	B 5	C 4	D 3	E 4	F 17	G 10	H 5	I 5	J 5	K 5	L 10	M 10	N 5	O 5	P 5	Total Score 100	Conclusion[a]
Behavioral therapy																		
Turner and Clancy (101)	1	1	—	—	4	—	10	5	—	—	—	8	—	5	5	5	44	Positive
Nicholas et al. (82)	1	1	—	—	2	—	10	5	5	—	—	6	—	5	—	5	40	Positive
Nicholas et al. (81)	1	1	—	—	—	—	10	5	5	—	—	6	—	5	—	5	38	Positive
Turner (100)	—	2	—	—	—	—	10	5	—	—	—	10	—	5	—	5	37	Positive
Turner et al. (103)	1	1	—	—	—	—	10	5	—	—	—	8	2	5	—	5	37	Positive
Turner and Jensen (102)	1	1	—	—	—	—	10	5	—	—	—	8	2	5	—	5	37	Positive
Stuckey et al. (96)	1	—	—	—	—	—	10	5	—	—	3	4	—	3	—	5	31	Positive
Newton-John et al. (80)	1	3	—	—	—	—	10	—	—	—	—	6	—	5	—	5	30	Negative
McCauley et al. (71)	1	3	—	—	—	—	10	5	—	—	—	6	—	3	—	—	28	Negative
Donaldson et al. (23)	1	—	—	—	—	—	5	5	—	—	—	4	—	5	—	5	25	Negative
Transcutaneous electrical nerve stimulation																		
Deyo et al. (21)	1	3	4	3	2	8	10	5	5	5	5	10	1	3	5	5	79	Negative
Moore and Shurman (79)	1	5	—	—	2	—	10	5	5	5	3	6	0	3	—	5	56	Negative
Marchand et al. (68)	1	3	—	—	4	—	10	5	—	5	5	2	6	5	5	5	52	Positive short-term
Lehmann et al. (57,58)	1	—	—	—	—	—	10	5	—	5	3	4	2	3	—	5	35	Negative
Acupuncture																		
Coan et al. (18)	1	3	4	—	4	—	5	5	—	—	—	8	—	5	5	5	45	Positive
Mendelson et al. (74,75)	1	3	—	—	—	—	10	—	—	5	3	6	6	3	—	5	42	Negative
MacDonald et al. (64)	—	—	—	—	4	—	10	—	—	5	3	6	6	3	5	—	42	Positive
Edelist et al. (25)	—	—	—	—	4	—	10	5	—	5	3	2	6	3	5	5	39	Negative
Molsberger et al. (78)	—	—	4	—	—	8	5	5	—	5	3	4	2	—	—	—	38	Positive
Lehmann et al. (57,58)	1	—	—	—	—	—	10	5	—	5	3	4	4	3	—	—	35	Positive
Gunn et al. (32)	1	2	2	—	—	—	5	5	—	—	—	2	4	5	—	5	27	Positive

																	Conclusion[a]
Spa therapy																	
Constant et al. (19)	2	4	4	3	4	8	5	—	5	—	—	8	2	5	5	5	60	Positive
Guillemin et al. (31)	2	4	2	3	4	8	5	5	5	—	—	6	2	5	5	5	56	Positive
Nguyen et al. (83)	1	3	2	—	—	—	—	5	—	—	5	6	—	5	—	5	27	Positive
Multidisciplinary treatment																	
Harkapaa and Mellin et al. (34,35,72,73)	1	3	—	—	4	17	10	5	5	5	5	10	—	5	5	5	70	Positive
Alaranta et al. (1)	2	3	—	3	4	17	10	5	5	—	—	8	2	5	5	5	69	Positive
Mitchell and Carmen (77)	2	3	2	—	4	17	10	5	5	5	—	4	4	5	5	—	66	No conclusion
Lindström et al. (60,61)	2	2	4	—	4	8	5	5	—	—	—	4	2	5	5	5	51	Positive
Linton et al. (62)	1	1	—	3	4	—	5	5	—	—	—	6	—	5	5	5	45	Positive
Bendix et al. (7)	1	4	2	3	2	—	5	5	—	—	—	8	8	5	—	—	43	Positive
Bendix et al. (9)	2	3	2	3	2	—	5	5	—	—	—	6	6	5	—	—	39	Positive
Altmaier et al. (3)	1	2	—	—	2	—	5	5	—	—	—	6	—	5	—	5	36	Negative
Loisel et al. (63)	2	2	4	—	—	—	5	5	—	—	—	6	—	5	—	—	34	Positive
Strong (95)	—	2	—	—	—	—	5	5	—	—	—	4	—	5	5	5	31	Positive

[a] Conclusion of the author(s) of the study; positive conclusion indicates that the index treatment was better than the reference treatment; negative conclusion indicates that the index treatment was worse than or equally effective as reference treatment.

293

results (37,47,87), and one reported negative results (24). In four trials, a back school was compared with no treatment, a waiting-list control group, or a placebo treatment (detuned short-wave diathermy) (24,39,40,43–45,56). The high-quality RCT reported positive outcomes of an intensive modified Swedish back school program compared with no actual treatment in an occupational setting (39,40,43). There is limited evidence (level C) that an intensive back school program in an occupational setting in Scandinavia is more effective than no actual treatment. There is conflicting evidence (level C) on the effectiveness of back schools in nonoccupational settings and outside Scandinavia.

Behavioral Therapy

Ten low-quality RCTs were identified (Tables 12.9 and 12.12) on the effectiveness of behavioral therapy by itself for chronic LBP (23,71,80–82,96,100–103). The overall methodologic quality appeared to be low, ranging from 25 to 44 points. Seven of the ten trials reported positive results for behavioral therapy, and three trials reported negative results. The four trials by Turner et al. (100–103) reported positive results compared with a waiting-list control group for various kinds of behavioral therapies, such as progressive relaxation training, cognitive-behavioral therapy (relaxation, coping, imagery), and aerobic exercises plus operant conditioning. Newton-John et al. (80) found cognitive-behavioral therapy to be more effective than a waiting-list control group, but equally effective as EMG biofeedback. In six trials, behavioral therapy was compared with other conservative types of treatment, including traditional care, physical therapy, aerobic exercises, EMG biofeedback, self-hypnosis, and usual care (23,71,80,81,96,103). Three of these trials had positive results, and three had negative results. Five RCTs compared different types of behavioral therapies: operant conditioning, cognitive treatment (coping strategies), and progressive muscle relaxation (80,100–103). Three trials reported negative results and two reported positive results for this comparison. For a more extensive and detailed review of behavioral treatment and for the final grading of evidence, we refer the reader to Chapter 17.

Multidisciplinary Pain Treatment Programs

Ten RCTs evaluated the effectiveness of multidisciplinary treatment programs for chronic LBP, four high-quality RCTs (1,34,35,60,61,72,73,77) and six low-quality RCTs (3,7,9,62,63,95) (Tables 12.12 and 12.13). Eight RCTs, including three high-quality studies, reported positive results for the multidisciplinary treatment programs compared with traditional inpatient rehabilitation or usual care. The low-quality RCT reporting negative results did not find any differences between a standard rehabilitation program with a behavioral approach compared with the standard rehabilitation program (3). Seven of the trials, including the four high-quality trials, evaluated some type of functional restoration program. Six of these trials reported positive results on either pain or functional status or return to work. In one high-quality RCT, no clear overall conclusion was drawn because there was no difference in any of the clinical (physical or psychologic) outcomes, but the total costs of the multidisciplinary program were lower after 2-year follow-up. There is strong evidence (level A) that a multidisciplinary treatment program aimed at functional restoration is useful for patients with long-lasting, severe chronic LBP.

Manual Therapy

Two high-quality and seven low-quality RCTs (Tables 12.4 and 12.12) were identified, with scores ranging from 27 to 57 points. Six trials, including the two high-quality RCTs, reported positive results, two trials reported negative results, and in one trial no clear conclusion was drawn (we considered this trial negative). In five nonpragmatic trials, manual therapy was compared with a placebo therapy (29,51–54,85,87,97). The two high-quality RCTs reported a positive result for manual therapy compared with placebo (51–54,85). Eight trials (one high-quality RCT) were identified that compared manual therapy with other conservative types of treatment, such as normal care by a general practitioner, physical therapy (including short-wave diathermy, massage, exercises), back schools, and drug therapy (5,27,29,37,51–54,87,97,105). In five of these RCTs, including one high-quality RCT, the results were positive, and in three RCTs, the results were negative. A positive result of manual therapy was reported in studies that compared manual therapy with back education (97), massage and sham manipulation (105), and bed rest, analgesics and massage (5), usual care by the general practitioner (51–54), and analgesics (27). A negative outcome was reported in the high-quality trial comparing manual therapy with physical therapy (51–54). There is strong evidence that manual therapy provides more effective short-term pain relief than a placebo treatment (level A). There is moderate evidence (level B) that manual therapy is more effective than usual care by the general practitioner, bed rest, analgesics, and massage for short-term pain relief. There is limited and conflicting evidence of any long-term effects (level C).

Electromyographic Biofeedback

Six low-quality trials (Tables 12.6 and 12.12) were identified on the efficacy of EMG biofeedback (6,14,23,80,84,96). The methodologic scores of the trials ranged from 23 to 40 points. The sample sizes of all study groups were small, not exceeding 22 patients. Five RCTs reported negative results (6,14,80,84,96), and only one RCT reported a positive result (23). EMG biofeedback was compared with various reference treatments, such as placebo EMG (14,96), a waiting-list control group (14,84), cognitive-behavioral therapy, and relaxation training (23,96). There is moderate evidence that EMG biofeedback is not effective (level B).

Traction

Two high-quality RCTs (11,12,36) were identified (Tables 12.8 and 12.12). Both trials compared traction of 35% to 50% of the body weight with "placebo" traction of maximum 20% or 25% of the body weight. There were no significant differences in pain, overall improvement, functional status, or return to work. There is strong evidence (level A) that traction has no effect in treating chronic LBP.

Orthoses

Only one low-quality RCT (76) was identified (Tables 12.8 and 12.12), in which a lumbar corset with a synthetic support was compared with the same corset without support. The corset with support provided better subjective improvement, but there were no differences in spinal movements or straight leg raising. There is limited evidence (level C) that a lumbar corset with support may produce some subjective improvement.

TABLE 12.13. *Details of trials on the effectiveness of multidisciplinary treatment programs for chronic low back pain*

Investigators (ref.)	Treatment program (no. of patients)	Reference treatment(s) (no. of patients)	Results
Harkapaa and Mellin et al. (34,35,72,73)	I1: Inpatient group: 3-wk rehabilitation period in groups of 6–8 patients: modified Swedish back school (4 sessions), 15 sessions back exercises, 9 sessions relaxation exercises, supervised by physical therapist; heat or electrotherapy and massage, and session with physiologist and physician; refresher course 2 wk after 1.5 yr (156) I2: Outpatient group: 15 sessions during a 2-mo period, twice/wk in groups of 6–8 patients: modified Swedish back school (4 sessions), 15 sessions back exercises, 9 sessions relaxation exercises, supervised by physical therapist, and session with physiologist and physician; refresher course 8 sessions after 1.5 yr (150)	R: no systematic treatment; written and oral instructions on back exercises and ergonomics (153)	Changes in pain index and disability index after 3-mo follow-up: significantly greater reduction in I1 and I2 than in R (data in graphs and by ANOVA); at 2.5-yr follow-up, no clear differences; mean no. of days of sick leave from back pain pretreatment: I1, 5.2; I2, 6.0; R, 3.7; mean difference between pretreatment and 1.5-yr and 2.5-yr follow-up: I1, +0.3, +1.6; I2, −0.2, +2.2; R, +3.8, 4.8; not statistically significant
Alaranta et al. (1)	I: multidisciplinary treatment program (AKSELI): intensive physical and psychosocial training program, inpatient rehabilitation, 37 hr guided or self-controlled physical exercises, 5 hr of discussion groups/wk, no passive physical therapy; team of physician, psychologist, social worker, physical therapist, occupational therapist, work trainer; 3 wk (152)	R: current national (Finland) type of inpatient rehabilitation: passive physical therapy (massage, electrical therapies, traction, etc.), muscle training, pool exercises, back school education, 3 wk (141)	Decrease in Million Pain Index at baseline and after 3 and 12 mos: I, 43, 28, 29; R, 42, 34, 35; decrease significantly greater in I after 3 and 12 mo; mean number of yearly sick leave days decrease in I from 57.8 to 33.9 and in R from 58.5 to 36.9; not significant; decrease in number of yearly visits to physician: I, 74%; R, 67%; decrease in number of yearly outpatient physical therapy periods: I, 69%; R, 77%; no significant differences in psychologic outcomes; I significantly better in muscle strength and flexibility than R after 3 and 12 mo
Mitchell and Carmen (77)	I: functional restoration: active exercise program, physical exercise, mobility, strengthening, endurance, flexibility, ice, stretching, cognitive-behavioral therapy, education, relaxation, biofeedback, functional simulation, groups 10–12 patients, 8 wk, 40 treatment d, 7 hr/d, 5 d/wk (271)	R: referred back to primary care provider for usual care (271)	After 12 mo, 79% of group I and 78% of group R were back at work; average number of days of absence after 24 mos for back pain patients: I, 406; R, 450; not statistically significant; average savings of wage loss benefits for back pain $3,172 per patient over 24 mo; treatment costs were $2,507 higher in I; total costs per average injured worker were lower in group I than in group R $51,693
Lindström et al. (60, 61)	I: individual, submaximal, gradually increased exercise program (graded activity) with an operant-conditioning behavioral approach (Fordyce) (51)	R: traditional care (52)	Proportion of patients returned to work within 6 wk or 12 wk after randomization: I, 59%, 80%, vs. R, 40%, 58%; significant; mean (SD) duration of sick leave from low back pain during the second follow-up yr: I, 12.1 (18.4) wk, vs. R, 19.6 (20.7) wk; no differences in functional status after 1 yr

Study	Index (I) / Reference (R) treatment	Results
Linton et al. (62)	I: 5-wk period in a back clinic; 8 hr/d mostly in groups of 6 patients; exercise activities (walking, swimming, jogging, cycling) 4 hr/d; ergonomic education; individual physical therapy programs, behavioral therapy techniques (36) R: waiting-list control: no additional active treatment (30)	Pain intensity (VAS) significantly better in I than R after 6 wk and 6 mo (data in graphs and by ancova for repeated measures); other outcome measures (fatigue, anxiety, sleep quality, etc.): similar results
Bendix et al. (7,9)	I: intensive, multidisciplinary treatment program: aerobics, weight training, occupational therapy, relaxation, psychologic treatment (behavioral approach), stretching, theoretic class and recreation; 3 weeks, 39 hr/wk, dynamic groups of 7 patients (55) R: usual care: 61% physical therapy, 35% chiropractic manipulation, 15% hospitalized, 4% surgery (51)	Median back pain, leg pain (11-point scale), functional status (31-point scale), days of sick leave after 4 mo: I, 5.7, 3.5, 12.1, 10; R, 6.9, 5.4, 16.8, 122; I significantly better on back pain, functional status, and return to work; median back pain, leg pain (11-point scale), functional status (31-point scale), days of sick leave after 2 yr: I, 6, 4.5, 16, 15; R, 6.5, 4, 15, 123; I significantly less sick leave
Bendix et al. (7,8)	I: intensive, multidisciplinary treatment program: aerobics, weight training, occupational therapy, relaxation, psychologic treatment (behavioral approach), stretching, theoretic class and recreation; 3 wk, 39 hr/wk, dynamic groups of 7 patients (46) R1: active physical training, aerobics, weight training, traditional Swedish back school, 7–8 patients, 2 hr, twice/wk for 6 wk (43) R2: psychophysical program: psychologic pain management, active physical training, weight training, 7–8 patients, 2 hr, twice/wk for 6 wk (43)	Median back pain, leg pain (11-point scale), functional status (31-point scale), days of sick leave after 4 mo: I, 2.7, 0.4, 8.5, 25; R1, 4.4, 2.6, 13.5, 13; R2, 5.6, 3.1, 16.1, 122; group I significantly better than R1 and R2 regarding pain and functional status; I and R1 significantly better than R2 regarding return to work; median back pain, leg pain (11-point scale), functional status (31-point scale), days of sick leave after 2 yr: I, 3, 2, 10, 2.5; R1, 5, 4, 14, 11; R2, 6, 5, 17, 37; I significantly less pain, less sick leave, and better overall improvement after 2 yr
Altmaier et al. (3)	I: standard rehabilitation program and operant conditioning and relaxation training and biofeedback and cognitive-behavioral coping skills (24) R: standard inpatient rehabilitation program: physical therapy, aerobic exercises, education, vocational rehabilitation; 3 wk (21)	Mean scores on McGill Pain Questionnaire pretreatment, posttreatment, and after 6 mo: I, 24.24, 23.76 and 22.66, vs. R, 20.33, 18.05, and 18.19; no significant differences on any outcome measures
Loisel et al. (63)	I: intensive multidisciplinary treatment program of occupational medicine, ergonomic intervention, clinical and rehabilitation intervention, back school (25) R1: clinical intervention (31) R2: occupational intervention (22) R3: usual care (26)	Median no. of days lost from regular work: I, 60.0; R1, 131.0; R2, 67.0; R3, 120.5; I significantly better than R3; I significantly better functional status after 1 yr than R3; occupational interventions I and R2 had significantly better results for return to regular work
Strong (95)	I: inpatient pain management program plus 4 2-hr psychoeducational individual treatment sessions (video, information on pain and anatomy, importance of behaviors, cognitions and emotions, pain management strategies) (15) R: inpatient pain management program (anesthesia, psychiatry, occupational therapy, physical therapy) plus 8-hr nonspecific program (15)	Mean (SD) illness behavior pretreatment, posttreatment, and after 12 mo: I, 0.528, 0.311, 0.031; R, 0.231, 0.035, −0.038; mean (SD) depressed and negative cognitions: I, −0.33, −3.55, −0.033; R, 0.304, 0.663, 0.197; mean (SD) using acute pain strategies: I, 0.441, 0.278, 0.279; R, −0.316, −0.325, 0.484; I significantly better posttreatment reduction than R on depressed and negative cognitions

I, index treatment; R, reference treatment; SD, standard deviation; VAS, visual analog scale.

Transcutaneous Electrical Nerve Stimulation

Four trials studied the efficacy of transcutaneous electrical nerve stimulation (TENS) compared with placebo TENS for chronic LBP (Tables 12.10 and 12.12) (21,57,58,68,79). Three RCTs were of high quality, and one was of low quality, with methodologic scores ranging from 35 to 79 points. One high-quality RCT did not report any significant differences between TENS and placebo with regard to pain and functional status (21). Another high-quality RCT reported a positive short-term effect on pain intensity, but no long-term effect (68). The third high-quality study reported a significant difference between TENS and placebo TENS for pain relief, but not for pain intensity. Because of inconsistent findings (level C), it is not possible to judge the effectiveness of TENS in these patients.

Acupuncture

The seven trials we identified on the efficacy of acupuncture for chronic LBP (Tables 12.10 and 12.12) were all of low quality (18,25,32,57,58,64,74,75,78). The methodologic scores ranged from 27 to 45 points. Five of the trials reported positive results, and two trials reported negative results. Of the five trials using placebo acupuncture or a waiting-list control group as reference treatment, three reported a positive result and two a negative result (18,25,64,74,75,78). In the other two pragmatic trials, acupuncture was compared with TENS and placebo TENS (57,58), or a standard therapeutic regimen with acupuncture (dry needling) was compared with a standard therapeutic regimen alone (32). These two trials reported positive results. Because of inconsistent findings (level C) and poor quality of the studies, it is not possible to judge the effectiveness of acupuncture for chronic LBP.

Spa Therapy

Three trials were identified on the effectiveness of spa therapy, two high-quality (19,31) and one low-quality study (83) (Tables 12.12 and 12.14). All three trials reported 3 weeks of spa therapy to be significantly better for pain intensity and overall improvement or quality of life than usual or routine care in older patients with a mean age of around 60 years. There is strong evidence (level A) that spa therapy is an effective treatment for chronic LBP. However, the benefits were mainly short-term effects, and no data were reported either on return to work or on the cost-effectiveness of this seemingly expensive treatment. Furthermore, these spa therapies were intensive programs during a 3-week stay in a French or Hungarian spa resort. The interventions evaluated in these studies could be characterized as a passive multimodal program containing, for example, various types of mineralized water baths, underwater massage, and rest, and they are not similar to hydrotherapy. These findings seem only relevant to specific European areas with spa resorts (the Alps), and the generalizability therefore is low. Whether these results also apply to other countries is questionable.

CONCLUSION

In this systematic review, we assessed the effectiveness of the various interventions for the treatment of chronic LBP, by using a rating system for the strength of the scientific evidence. In general, there is no strong evidence for the effectiveness of most

TABLE 12.14. *Details of trials on the efficacy of spa therapy for chronic low back pain*

Investigators (ref.)	Spa therapy (no. of patients)	Reference treatment(s) (no. of patients)	Results
Constant et al. (19)	I: spa therapy: spa mineral water and specific techniques, including hot bath, pulsating showers, and local application of mud, 6 d/wk, 3 weeks, plus routine drug therapy (63)	R: routine drug therapy (63)	Mean change scores (SD) posttreatment and after 6 months: pain (VAS): I, −24.4 (28.6), −22.4 (28.0); R, −3.8 (20.5), 1.0 (22.6); functional status (RDQ): −3.5 (4.4), −5.1 (4.4); R, −0.1 (2.7), −0.9 (3.4); global measure (VAS): I, 27.5 (22.8), 28.7 (24.6); R, 5.4 (21.8), 1.6 (24.6); I significantly better regarding pain, global measure, and functional status after 3 wk and 6 mo
Guillemin et al. (31)	I: spa therapy: hydrotherapy, 15 min underwater, high-pressure showers, and series of 3-min showers with various pressures, low mineralization, 6 d/wk, 3 wk, no other interventions (52)	R: usual care, no massage or physical therapy (52)	Mean change scores (SE) posttreatment and after 9 mo: pain (VAS): I, −32.2 (2.9), −34.4 (2.9); R, −0.2 (2.7), 7.1 (2.3); functional status (Waddell score): I, −1.19 (0.24), 0.09 (0.32); R, −0.005 (0.15), 0.18 (0.3); I significantly better regarding pain, functional status, spinal mobility, and drug consumption after 3 wk; I significantly better regarding pain, spinal mobility, and drug consumption after 9 mo
Nguyen et al. (83)	I: spa therapy: journey, rest, balneotherapy, spring water, and medical attention, 21 d (91)	R: maintaining routine life and outpatient care, including physical therapies if necessary, 21 d (97)	Mean change scores (SD) for pain intensity (VAS), functional status, and quality of life after 24 wk: I, −12 (28), −1 (2), and −0.6 (0.9); R, 2 (22), −1 (2), and −0.2 (1.0); I significantly better on pain and quality of life

I, index treatment; R, reference treatment; RDQ, Roland Disability Questionnaire; SD, standard deviation; SE, standard error; VAS, visual analog scale.

of the interventions. Only one RCT on analgesics, muscle relaxants, traction, and orthoses, respectively, could be identified, and all RCTs on EMG biofeedback, behavioral therapy, and acupuncture were of low methodologic quality. Nevertheless, strong evidence was found for the effectiveness of manual therapy, exercise therapy, multidisciplinary pain treatment programs, and spa therapy, especially with regard to short-term effects. We only found moderate evidence for the effectiveness of behavioral therapy and limited evidence for back schools in an occupational setting. According to international guidelines, the major goal in the treatment of chronic LBP is return to work or usual activities, and additional therapeutic options for symptomatic pain relief may facilitate this process. The available evidence suggests that NSAIDs may be effective for this purpose, but not physical modalities such as TENS, EMG biofeedback, acupuncture, and orthoses. There is no evidence to support any form of long-term maintenance therapy.

RECOMMENDATIONS FOR TREATMENT

The following recommendations are based on the evidence summarized earlier, the United Kingdom Report of the Clinical Standards Advisory Group Committee on

Back Pain (108), and the Dutch General Practice Guideline on Low Back Pain (109).

Information

The most important objective is to prevent or reduce disability, both physically and mentally, and to improve the patient's quality of life and functioning. Dependence on medical treatment should be prevented and avoided. The emphasis should be on coping with the symptoms together with control of pain.

Drug Therapy

Long-term drug treatment should be avoided. If necessary, analgesics should be prescribed only to facilitate a gradual increase in activities, and they should be prescribed for a fixed period at fixed times, independent of the presence of pain.

Manual Therapy

The patient should be referred for manual therapy for pain relief. There is no evidence to support the recommendation of one specific type of manual therapy.

Exercise Therapy

The patient should be referred for exercise therapy to improve daily functioning. No evidence supports the recommendation of one specific type of exercise. The intensity of the exercises should be increased gradually at fixed times for a fixed period, independent of the presence of pain.

Multidisciplinary Treatment

Patients with severe, long-lasting LBP and disability, or high use of medical services for back pain, should be referred to a multidisciplinary treatment program aimed at functional restoration, behavioral management, or pain management.

REFERENCES

1. Alaranta H, Rytökoski U, Rissanen A, et al. Intensive physical and psychosocial training program for patients with chronic low back pain: a controlled clinical trial. *Spine* 1994;19:1339–1349.
2. Alcoff J, Jones E, Rust P, et al. Controlled trial of imipramine for chronic low back pain. *J Fam Pract* 1982;14:841–846.
3. Altmaier EM, Lehmann TR, Russell DW, et al. The effectiveness of psychological interventions for the rehabilitation of low back pain: a randomized controlled trial evaluation. *Pain* 1992;49:329–335.
4. Arbus L, Fajadet B, Aubert D, et al. Activity of tetrazepam (myolastan) in low back pain: a bouble-blind trial vs placebo. *Clin Trials J* 1990;27:258–267.
5. Arkuszewski Z. The efficacy of manual treatment in low back pain: a clinical trial. *Manual Med* 1986;2:68–71.
6. Asfour SS, Khalil TM, Waly SM, et al. Biofeedback in back muscle strengthening. *Spine* 1990;15:510–513.
7. Bendix AF, Bendix T, Labriola M, et al. Functional restoration for chronic low back pain: two-year follow-up of two randomized clinical trials. *Spine* 1998;23:717–725.
8. Bendix AF, Bendix T, Ostenfeld S, et al. Active treatment programs for patients with chronic low back pain: a prospective, randomized, observer-blinded study. *Eur Spine J* 1995;4:148–152.

9. Bendix AF, Bendix T, Vægter K, et al. Multidisciplinary intensive treatment for chronic low back pain: a randomized, prospective study. *Cleve Clin J Med* 1996;63:62–69.
10. Berry H, Bloom B, Hamilton EBD, et al. Naproxen sodium, diflinisal, and placebo in the treatment of chronic back pain. *Ann Rheum Dis* 1982;41:129–132.
11. Beurskens AJ, de Vet HCW, Köke AJ, et al. Efficacy of traction for non-specific low back pain: a randomised clinical trial. *Lancet* 1995;346:1596–1600.
12. Beurskens AJHM, van der Heijden GJMG, de Vet HCW, et al. The efficacy of traction for lumbar back pain: design of a randomized clinical trial. *J Manipulative Physiol Ther* 1995;18:141–147.
13. Breivik H, Hesla PE, Molnar I, et al. Treatment of chronic low back pain and sciatica: comparison of caudal epidural injections of bupivacaine and methylprednisolone with bupivacaine followed by saline. *Adv Pain Res Ther* 1976;1:927–932.
14. Bush C, Ditto B, Feuerstein M. A controlled evaluation of paraspinal EMG biofeedback in the treatment of chronic low back pain. *Health Psychol* 1985;4:307–321.
15. Bush K, Hillier S. A controlled study of caudal epidural injections of triamcinolone plus procaine for the management of intractable sciatica. *Spine* 1991;16:572–575.
16. Buswell J. Low back pain: a comparison of two treatment programmes. *N Z J Physiother* 1982;10:13–17.
17. Carette S, Leclaire R, Marcoux S, et al. Epidural corticosteroid injections for sciatica due to herniated nucleus pulposus. *N Engl J Med* 1997;336:1634–1640.
18. Coan RM, Wong G, Liang Ku S, et al. The acupuncture treatment of low back pain: a randomized controlled study. *Am J Chin Med* 1980;8:181–189.
19. Constant F, Collin JF, Guillemin F, et al. Effectiveness of spa therapy in chronic low back pain: a randomized clinical trial. *J Rheumatol* 1995;22:1315–1320.
20. Cuckler JM, Bernini PA, Wiesel SH, et al. The use of steroids in the treatment of lumbar radicular pain. *J Bone Joint Surg Am* 1985;67A:63–66.
21. Deyo RA, Walsh NE, Martin DC, et al. A controlled trial of transcutaneous electrical nerve stimulation (TENS) and exercise for chronic low back pain. *N Engl J Med* 1990;322:1627–1634.
22. Dickersin K, Scherer R, Lefebvre C. Identifying relevant studies for systematic reviews. *BMJ* 1994;309:1286–1291.
23. Donaldson S, Romney D, Donaldson M, et al. Randomized study of the application of single motor unit biofeedback training to chronic low back pain. *J Occup Rehabil* 1994;4:23–37.
24. Donchin M, Woolf O, Kaplan L, et al. Secondary prevention of low-back pain: a clinical trial. *Spine* 1990;15:1317–1320.
25. Edelist G, Gross AE, Langer F. Treatment of low back pain with acupuncture. *Can Anaesth Soc J* 1976;23:303–306.
26. Elnaggar IM, Nordin M, Sheikhzadeh A, et al. Effects of spinal flexion and extension exercises on low-back pain and spinal mobility in chronic mechanical low-back pain patients. *Spine* 1991;16:967–972.
27. Evans DP, Burke MS, Lloyd KN, et al. Lumbar spinal manipulation on trial. I. Clinical assessment. *Rheumatol Rehabil* 1978;17:46–53.
28. Frost H, Klaber Moffet JA, Moser JS, et al. Randomised controlled trial for evaluation of fitness programme for patients with chronic low back pain. *BMJ* 1995;310:151–154.
29. Gibson T, Grahame R, Harkness J, et al. Controlled comparison of short-wave diathermy treatment with osteopathic treatment in non-specific low-back pain. *Lancet* 1985:1258–1261.
30. Goodkin K, Gullion CM, Agras S. A randomized, double-blind, placebo-controlled trial of trazodone hydrochloride in chronic low back pain syndrome. *J Clin Psychopharmacol* 1990;10:269–278.
31. Guillemin F, Constant F, Collin JF, et al. Short and long-term effect of spa therapy in chronic low back pain. *Br J Rheumatol* 1994;33:148–151.
32. Gunn CC, Milbrandt WE, Little AS, et al. Dry needling of muscle motor points for chronic low-back pain: a randomized clinical trial with long-term follow-up. *Spine* 1980;5:279–291.
33. Hansen FR, Bendix T, Skov P, et al. Intensive, dynamic back-muscle exercises, conventional physiotherapy, or placebo-control treatment of low-back pain. *Spine* 1993;18:98–107.
34. Harkapaa K, Jarvikoski A, Mellin G, et al. A controlled study on the outcome of inpatient and outpatient treatment of low-back pain. I. *Scand J Rehabil Med* 1989;21:81–89.
35. Harkapaa K, Mellin G, Jarvikoski A, et al. A controlled study on the outcome of inpatient and outpatient treatment of low-back pain. III. *Scand J Rehabil Med* 1990;22:181–188.
36. Heijden GJMG van der, Beurskens AJHM, Dirx MJM, et al. Efficacy of lumbar traction: a randomised clinical trial. *Physiotherapy* 1995;81:29–35.
37. Herzog W, Conway PJW, Willcox BJ. Effects of different treatment modalities on gait symmetry and clinical measures for sacroiliac joint patients. *J Manipulative Physiol Ther* 1991;14:104–109.
38. Hickey RF. Chronic low back pain: a comparison of diflunisal with paracetamol. *N Z Med J* 1982; 95:312–314.
39. Hurri H. The Swedish back school in chronic low-back pain. I. Benefits. *Scand J Rehabil Med* 1989; 21:33–40.
40. Hurri H. The Swedish back school in chronic low-back pain. II. Factors predicting the outcome. *Scand J Rehabil Med* 1989;21:41–44.

41. Jenkins DG, Ebbutt AF, Evans CD. Trofanil in the treatment of low back pain. *J Int Med Res* 1976;4[Suppl 2]:28–40.
42. Johanssen F, Remvig L, Kryger P, et al. Exercises for chronic low back pain: a clinical trial. *J Orthop Sports Phys Ther* 1995;22:52–59.
43. Julkunen J, Hurri H, Kankainen J. Psychological factors in the treatment of chronic low back pain: follow-up study of a back school intervention. *Psychother Psychosom* 1988;50:173–181.
44. Keijsers JFEM, Groenman NH, Gerards FM, et al. A back school in the Netherlands: evaluating the results. *Patient Educ Counseling* 1989;14:31–44.
45. Keijsers JFME, Steenbakkers WHL, Meertens RM, et al. The efficacy of the back school: a randomized trial. *Arthritis Care Res* 1990;3:204–209.
46. Kendall PH, Jenkins JM. Exercises for backache: a double-blind controlled trial. *Physiotherapy* 1968;54:154–157.
47. Klaber Moffett JA, Chase SM, Portek I, et al. A controlled prospective study to evaluate the effectiveness of a back school in the relief of chronic low-back pain. *Spine* 1986;11;120–122.
48. Koes BW, Hoogen HMM van den. Efficacy of bed rest and orthoses for low back pain: a review of randomized clinical trials. *Eur J Phys Med Rehabil* 1994;4:86–93.
49. Koes BW, Assendelft WJJ, Heijden GJMG van der, et al. Spinal manipulation and mobilization for back and neck pain: a blinded review. *BMJ* 1991;303:1298–1303.
50. Koes BW, Bouter LM, Beckerman H, et al. Physiotherapy exercises and back pain: a blinded review. *BMJ* 1991;302:1572–1576.
51. Koes BW, Bouter LM, Knipschild PG, et al. A blinded randomized clinical trial of manual therapy and physiotherapy for chronic back and neck complaints: physical outcome measures. *J Manipulative Physiol Ther* 1992;15:16–23.
52. Koes BW, Bouter LM, Mameren H van, et al. Randomised clinical trial of manual therapy and physiotherapy for persistent back and neck complaints: results of one year follow-up. *BMJ* 1992;304:601–605.
53. Koes BW, Bouter LM, Mameren van H, et al. The effectiveness of manual therapy, physiotherapy and treatment by the general practitioner for non-specific back and neck complaints: a randomized clinical trial. *Spine* 1992;17:28–35.
54. Koes BW, Bouter LM, van Mameren H, et al. A randomized clinical trial of manual therapy and physiotherapy for persistent back and neck complaints: subgroup analysis and relationship between outcome measures. *J Manipulative Physiol Ther* 1993;16:211–219.
55. Koes BW, Tulder MW van, Windt DAWM van der, et al. The efficacy of back schools: a review of randomized clinical trials. *J Clin Epidemiol* 1994;47:851–862.
56. Lankhorst GJ, Stadt van der RJ, Vogelaar TW, et al. The effect of the Swedish back school in chronic idiopathic low-back pain. *Scand J Rehabil Med* 1983;15:141–145.
57. Lehmann TR, Russell DW, Spratt KF. The impact of patients with nonorganic physical findings on a controlled trial of transcutaneous electrical nerve stimulation and electroacupuncture. *Spine* 1983; 8:625–634.
58. Lehmann TR, Russell DW, Spratt KF, et al. Efficacy of electroacupuncture and TENS in the rehabilitation of chronic low back pain patients. *Pain* 1986;26:277–290.
59. Lidström A, Zachrisson M. Physical therapy on low back pain and sciatica: an attempt at evaluation. *Scand J Rehabil Med* 1970;2:37–42.
60. Lindström I, Ohlund C, Eek C, et al. The effect of graded activity on patients with subacute low back pain: a randomized prospective clinical study with an operant-conditioning behavioral approach. *Phys Ther* 1992;72:279–293.
61. Lindström I, Ohlund C, Eek C, et al. Mobility, strength, and fitness after a graded activity program for patients with subacute low back pain. *Spine* 1992;17:641–652.
62. Linton SJ, Bradley LA, Jensen I, et al. The secondary prevention of low-back pain: a controlled study with follow-up. *Pain* 1989;36:197–207.
63. Loisel P, Abenhaim L, Durand P, et al. A population-based, randomized clinical trial on back pain management. *Spine* 1997;22:2911–2918.
64. MacDonald AJR, MacRae KD, Master BR, et al. Superficial acupuncture in the relief of chronic low back pain. *Ann R Coll Surg Engl* 1983;65:44–46.
65. Manniche C, Asmussen K, Lauritsen B, et al. Intensive dynamic back exercises with or without hyperextension in chronic back pain after surgery for lumbar disc protrusion: a clinical trial. *Spine* 1993;18:560–567.
66. Manniche C, Hesselsoe G, Bentzen L, et al. Clinical trial of intensive muscle training for chronic low back pain. *Lancet* 1988;2:1473–1476.
67. Manniche C, Lundberg E, Christensen I, et al. Intensive dynamic back exercises for chronic low back pain: a clinical trial. *Pain* 1991;47:53–63.
68. Marchand S, Charest J, Li J, et al. Is TENS purely a placebo effect? A controlled study on chronic low back pain. *Pain* 1993;54:99–106.
69. Martin PR, Rose MJ, Nichols PJR, et al. Physiotherapy exercises for low back pain: process and clinical outcome. *Int Rehabil Med* 1980;8:34–38.

70. Matsumo S, Kaneda K, Nohara Y. Clinical evaluation of ketoprofen (Orudis) in lumbago: a double blind comparison with diclofenac sodium. *Br J Clin Pract* 1991;35:266.
71. McCauley JD, Thelen MH, Frank RG, et al. Hypnosis compared to relaxation in the outpatient management of chronic low back pain. *Arch Phys Med Rehabil* 1983;64:548–552.
72. Mellin G, Harkapaa K, Hurri H, et al. A controlled study on the outcome of inpatient and outpatient treatment of low-back pain. IV. *Scand J Rehabil Med* 1990;22:189–194.
73. Mellin G, Hurri H, Harkapaa K, et al. A controlled study on the outcome of inpatient and outpatient treatment of low-back pain. II. *Scand J Rehabil Med* 1989;21:91–95.
74. Mendelson G, Kidson MA, Loh ST, et al. Acupuncture analgesia for chronic low back pain. *Clin Exp Neurol* 1978;15:182–185.
75. Mendelson G, Selwood TS, Kranz H, et al. Acupuncture treatment of chronic back pain. *Am J Med* 1983;74:49–55.
76. Million R, Nilsen KH, Jayson MIV, et al. Evaluation of low-back pain and assessment of lumbar corsets with and without back supports. *Ann Rheum Dis* 1981;40:449–454.
77. Mitchell RI, Carmen GM. The functional restoration approach to the treatment of chronic pain in patients with soft tissue and back injuries. *Spine* 1994;19:633–642.
78. Molsberger A, Winkler J, Schneider S, et al. *Acupuncture and conventional orthopedic pain treatment in the management of chronic low back pain: a prospective randomised and controlled clinical trial.* Proceedings of the ISSLS. Toronto: ISSLS, 1998:87.
79. Moore SR, Shurman J. Combined neuromuscular electrical stimulation and transcutaneous electrical nerve stimulation for treatment of chronic back pain: a double-blind, repeated measures comparison. *Arch Phys Med Rehabil* 1997;78:55–60.
80. Newton-John TRO, Spence SH, Schotte D. Cognitive-behavioural therapy versus EMG biofeedback in the treatment of chronic low back pain. *Behav Res Ther* 1995;33:691–697.
81. Nicholas MK, Wilson PH, Goyen J. Operant-behavioural and cognitive behavioural treatment for chronic low back pain. *Behav Res Ther* 1991;29:225–238.
82. Nicholas MK, Wilson PH, Goyen J. Comparison of cognitive behavioral group treatment and an alternative non-psychological treatment for chronic low back pain. *Pain* 1992;48:339–347.
83. Nguyen M, Revel M, Dougados M. Prolonged effects of 3 weeks therapy in a spa resort on lumbar spine, knee and hip osteoarthritis: follow-up after 6 months, a randomized controlled trial. *Br J Rheumatol* 1997;36:77–81.
84. Nouwen A. EMG biofeedback used to reduce standing levels of paraspinal muscle tension in chronic low back pain. *Pain* 1983;17:353–360.
85. Ongley MJ, Klein RG, Dorman TA, et al. A new approach to the treatment of chronic low-back pain. *Lancet* 1987:143–146.
86. Pheasant H, Bursk A, Goldfarb J, et al. Amitriptylene and chronic low-back pain: a randomized double-blind crossover study. *Spine* 1983;8:552–557.
87. Postacchini F, Facchini M, Palieri P. Efficacy of various forms of conservative treatment in low back pain: a comparative study. *Neurol Orthop* 1988;6:28–35.
88. Ridley MG, Kingsley G, Gibson T, et al. Outpatient lumbar epidural corticosteroid injection in the management of sciatica. *Br J Rheumatol* 1988;27:295–299.
89. Risch SV, Norvell NK, Pollock ML, et al. Lumbar strengthening in chronic low back pain: physiologic and psychological benefits. *Spine* 1993;18:232–238.
90. Rocco AG, Frank E, Kaul AF, et al. Epidural steroids, epidural morfine and epidural steroids combined with morphine in the treatment of post laminectomy syndrome. *Pain* 1989;36;297–303.
91. Sachs BL, Ahmad SS, LaCroix M, et al. Objective assessment for exercise treatment on the B-200 isostation as part of work tolerance rehabilitation: a random prospective blind evaluation with comparison control population. *Spine* 1994;19:49–52.
92. Serrao JM, Marks RL, Morley SJ, et al. Intrathecal midazolam for the treatment of chronic mechanical low back pain: a controlled comparison with epidural steroid in a pilot study. *Pain* 1992:48;5–12.
93. Scheer SJ, Watanabe TK, Radack KL. Randomized controlled trials in industrial low back pain. III. Subacute/chronic pain interventions. *Arch Phys Med Rehabil* 1997;78:414–423.
94. Siegmeth W, Sieberer W. A comparison of the short-term effects of ibuprofen and diclofenac in spondylosis. *J Int Med Res* 1978;6:369–374.
95. Strong J. Incorporating cognitive-behavioral therapy with occupational therapy: a comparative study with patients with low back pain. *J Occup Rehabil* 1998;8:61–71.
96. Stuckey SJ, Jacobs A, Goldfarb J. EMG biofeedback training, relaxation training, and placebo for the relief of chronic back pain. *Percept Mot Skills* 1986;63:1023–1036.
97. Triano JJ, McGregor M, Hondras MA, et al. Manipulative therapy versus education programs in chronic low-back pain. *Spine* 1995;20:948–955.
98. Tulder MW van, Koes BW, Bouter LM. Conservative treatment of acute and chronic nonspecific low back pain: a systematic review of randomized controlled trials of the most common interventions. *Spine* 1997;22:2128–2156.
99. Tulder MW van, Assendelft WJJ, Koes BW, et al. Method guidelines for systematic reviews in the Cochrane Collaboration Back Review Group for Spinal Disorders. *Spine* 1997;22:2323–2330.

100. Turner JA. Comparison of group progressive-relaxation training and cognitive-behavioral group therapy for chronic low back pain. *J Consult Clin Psychol* 1982;50:757–765.
101. Turner JA, Clancy S. Comparison of operant behavioral and cognitive-behavioral group treatment for chronic low back pain. *J Consult Clin Psychol* 1988;56:261–266.
102. Turner JA, Jensen MP. Efficacy of cognitive therapy for chronic low back pain. *Pain* 1993;52:169–177.
103. Turner JA, Clancy S, McQuade KJ, et al. Effectiveness of behavioral therapy for chronic low back pain: a component analysis. *J Consult Clin Psychol* 1990;58:573–579.
104. Videman T, Osterman K. Double-blind parallel study of piroxicam versus indomethacin in the treatment of low back pain. *Ann Clin Res* 1984;16:156–160.
105. Waagen GN, Haldeman S, Cook G, et al. Short term trial of chiropractic adjustments for the relief of chronic low-back pain. *Manual Med* 1986;2:63–67.
106. Weide WE van der, Verbeek JHAM, van Tulder MW. Vocational outcome of intervention for low back pain. *Scand J Work Environ Health* 1997;23:165–178.
107. White AWM. Low back pain in men receiving workmen's compensation. *Can Med Assoc J* 1966;95:50–56.
108. Rosen M (chairman). Clinical Standards Advisory Group: Back Pain. London, HMSO, 1994.
109. Faas A, Chavannes AW, Koes BW, et al. The Dutch College of General Practitioners' Guidelines on Low Back Pain. *Huisarts Wet* 1996;39:18–31.

*Neck and Back Pain: The Scientific Evidence
of Causes, Diagnosis, and Treatment,* edited
by Alf Nachemson and Egon Jonsson.
Published by Lippincott Williams & Wilkins,
Philadelphia 2000.

13

Surgical Treatment of Lumbar Disc Prolapse and Degenerative Lumbar Disc Disease

Gordon Waddell*, J. N. Alastair Gibson†, and
Inga Grant‡

*Department of Orthopaedics, The Glasgow Nuffield Hospital, Glasgow, Scotland
†Clinical Research Unit, Princess Margaret Rose Orthopaedic Hospital,
Edinburgh, United Kingdom
‡Clinical Research Unit, Princess Margaret Rose Orthopaedic Hospital,
Edinburgh, United Kingdom

In all studies of back pain, 10% to 15% of patients account for 80% to 90% of the total health care consumption and costs for spinal disorders, and the 1% to 2% of patients who undergo surgery are the most expensive group. Although surgical investigations and interventions account for up to one-sixth of direct costs for spinal disorders in Sweden (see Chapter 20), much surgical treatment of lumbar spine surgery is still not substantiated by good scientific evidence. The rapid development of many new and expensive surgical procedures is of particular concern. Randomized controlled trials (RCTs) should provide the proper scientific basis for surgical practice and any proposed changes.

This chapter is based on a Cochrane Collaboration review and metaanalysis of surgical interventions in the lumbar spine (23), which attempts to answer two main questions:

1. What evidence is available on the clinical effectiveness of lumbar spine surgery?
2. What evidence is available on alternative forms and techniques of lumbar spine surgery?

Although there are alternate, technical ways of classifying surgery of the lumbar spine, from clinical, social, and historical perspectives, the clearest division is between the following groups:

1. Surgery for acute lumbar disc prolapse. This relatively well-defined group of patients presents with the primary complaint of sciatica, and surgery is basically some form of decompression of a nerve root.
2. Surgery for degenerative lumbar disc disease. This is a more heterogeneous group of patients and clinical presentations, including lumbar spondylosis, spinal stenosis, and spondylolisthesis. Surgery may take the form of either fusion for back pain caused by instability or decompression of the nerves for spinal stenosis, although decompression and fusion are often combined.

This classification produces a more natural division of the types of patients and the types of surgery and clinical outcomes achieved. In addition, the amount and quality of available evidence and the conclusions drawn are different for these two groups.

METHODS

Selection of Studies

The search strategy consisted of a computer-based search of scientific databases, a hand search of relevant surgical journals, and correspondence with experts to identify all RCTs relevant to the surgical treatment of lumbar disc prolapse and degenerative lumbar disc disease. RCTs in any language were considered. Data were extracted from the published papers and abstracts, and frequently reported outcomes were pooled for analysis using the Cochrane software. Professor C. Melot and Dr. M. Szpalski obtained and analyzed additional data on clinical outcomes of instrumented versus noninstrumented fusion by correspondence with some of the original authors.

Methodologic Quality of the Studies

Lumbar Disc Prolapse

Many of the trials had defects of design, which, in general, were worse in the trials of surgery than those of chemonucleolysis. Some of the trials had few patients. Methods and published details of randomization were often poor, and there was lack of concealment of randomization. Because of the nature of some of the surgical interventions, complete double blinding was not possible, but often little attempt was made at any blinding of outcome assessment. The most common surgical outcomes were crude ratings by surgeons or patients, and there were few proper clinical outcomes of pain relief, disability, or return to work. Some of the assessments were by the operating surgeon or by a resident or fellow beholden to the primary investigator. Although 23 of 26 trials had follow-up rates of at least 90%, there was often considerable early code break or crossover of patients, particularly in the trials of chemonucleolysis, and this situation was not always properly allowed for in the presentation of results. Only 4 of 26 trials presented 2-year follow-up results as recommended for surgical studies. These defects of trial design introduced some potential for bias. Further, most of the conclusions of this review are about relatively short-term outcomes over 6 to 12 months, and there is a lack of information on longer-term outcomes. Information on return to work and work capacity is also limited.

Degenerative Disc Disease

There were many serious weaknesses of trial design, including poor methods of randomization, lack of blinding, and lack of independent assessment of outcome. These defects, at times, gave considerable potential for bias. Most of the published results were technical surgical outcomes with some crude ratings of clinical outcome, but they had few patient-centered outcomes of pain, disability, or capacity for work.

Levels of Evidence

A. Strong evidence: provided by generally consistent findings in multiple high-quality RCTs.

B. Moderate evidence: provided by generally consistent findings in one high-quality RCT and one or more low-quality RCTs or generally consistent findings in multiple low-quality RCTs.
C. Limited evidence: one RCT (of either high or low quality) or inconsistent findings in multiple RCTs.
D. No evidence: no RCTs.

SURGERY FOR LUMBAR DISC PROLAPSE

The primary goal of surgical treatment of a *disc prolapse* is the relief of nerve root compression by removing the herniated nuclear material. Several alternative techniques are available. *Open discectomy,* performed with (microdiscectomy), or without (standard) use of an operating microscope, is the most common procedure, but less invasive surgical techniques, such as automated percutaneous discectomy and laser discectomy, are also used. Claims have been made from uncontrolled case series that all these alternative procedures can produce satisfactory results with smaller wounds and fewer serious complications, but these claims remain unproved. *Chemonucleolysis* is an alternative technique of chemically dissolving the nucleus of the disc with the enzyme chymopapain, but after more than 30 years of use, it is still the subject of controversy. Ideally, it would be important to define the optimal type of treatment for specific types of prolapse. For example, different surgical procedures may be appropriate if disc material is sequestrated rather than contained within the outer layers of the annulus fibrosus. It is particularly important that the safety, efficacy, and cost benefits of innovative procedures be compared with currently accepted forms of treatment.

Results

Twenty-six RCTs of all forms of surgical treatment for lumbar disc prolapse were identified (Table 13.1). Sixteen of the 26 trials were of some form of chemonucleolysis.

What Evidence Is There on the Clinical Effectiveness of Surgery for Lumbar Disc Prolapse?

Only one RCT compared surgical treatment of lumbar disc prolapse with any form of conservative treatment (61,62). This trial is widely quoted as a comparison of discectomy and conservative treatment and as showing a temporary benefit in clinical outcomes at 1 year, but no difference on longer-term follow-up at 4 and 10 years. That summary is inaccurate. It was actually a trial of a subgroup of patients with uncertain indications for surgery that compared primary discectomy with initial conservative treatment followed by discectomy if the patients failed to improve. The trial was not blinded, and there was considerable crossover, with 26% of the "conservative" group undergoing surgical treatment, although there was an intention-to-treat analysis. Both patient and observer ratings showed that discectomy was significantly better than "conservative therapy" after 1 year, but there were no significant differences in outcomes by the 4- and 10-year reviews. What it also showed is that if the clinical indications are uncertain, postponing surgical treatment to assess clinical progress further may delay recovery, but it does no long-term harm.

TABLE 13.1. *Characteristics of studies of the surgical management of lumbar disc prolapse*

Investigators (ref.)	Methods	Participants	Interventions	Outcomes	Notes
Benoist et al., 1993 (1)	Randomization method: independently generated list; Allocation concealment: B; Blinding: double; Lost to follow-up: 34/118 at 1 yr	118 pts, 80 m; 38 f, age 21–70 yr; Paris; Lumbar disc herniation + radicular pain; Unsuccessful conservative treatment (6 wk)	Exp: chymopapain (2,000 U); Ctl: chymopapain (4,000 U)	Surgeon rating; Patient rating; At 1 yr	
Bontoux et al., 1990 (3)	Randomization method: randomization table; Allocation concealment: A; Blinding: assessor; Lost to follow-up: 0/80 at 6 mo	80 pts	Exp: chymopapain (4,000 U); Ctl: triamcinolone hexacetonide (70 mg)	Independent observer rating; Second procedure required; At 6 mo	French translation
Bourgeois et al., 1988 (6)	Randomization method: drawing of lot; Allocation concealment: C; Blinding: double; Lost to follow-up: 0/60 at 6 mo	60 pts, 40 m, 20 f, age 26–62 yr	Exp: chymopapain (4,00 U); Ctl: triamcinolone hexacetonide (80 mg)	Independent observer rating; Second procedure required; At 6 mo	French translation
Bromley et al., 1984 (8)	Randomization method: tables; Allocation concealment: A; Blinding: double; Lost to follow-up: 0/30 at 17 mo	30 pts, 15 m, 15 f, age 21–63 yr; New Jersey; Failed conservative therapy (incl. 2 wk bed rest); Myelogram: confirming a single herniated disc	Exp: collagenase (600 U/mL); Ctl: normal saline	Patient rating; At 17 mo	
Chatterjee et al., 1995 (10)	Randomization method: not stated; Allocation concealment: B; Blinding: assessor; Lost to follow-up: 0/71 at 6 mo	71 pts; 39 m; 32 f, age 20–67; Liverpool; Contained disc herniation at a single level; Unsuccessful conservative treatment (min 6 wk)	Exp: automated percutaneous lumbar discectomy (APLD); Ctl: microdiscectomy	Repeat surgery (microdiscectomy) required after failed APLD; Independent observer rating; At 6 mo	Parallel study of direct/social economic costs reported in different publication (M/0005)
Crawshaw et al., 1984 (12)	Randomization method: not stated; Allocation concealment: B; Blinding: nil; Lost to follow-up: 2/52 at 1 yr	52 pts, sex not stated, age 15–60 yr; England; Root involvement at a single level; Failed conservative treatment (min 3 mo)	Exp: chemonucleolysis (4,000 U chymopapain); Ctl: surgery (choice left to surgeon)	Surgeon rating; Second procedure required; At 1 yr	
Dabezies et al., 1988 (13)	Randomization method: not stated; Allocation concealment: A; Blinding: double; Lost to follow-up: 9/173 at 6 mo	173 pts, 112 m, 61 f, age 18–70 yr; Multicenter: United States; Proven classic lumbar disc syndrome with unilateral single-level radiculopathy; Failed conservative treatment (min 2 wk strict bed rest)	Exp: chymopapain (8 mg in 2 mL); Ctl: cysteine-edetate-iothalamate	Surgeon rating; Second procedure required; At 6 mo	

Study	Methods	Participants	Interventions	Outcomes	Notes
Ejeskar et al., 1983 (15)	Randomization method: not stated; Allocation concealment: B; Blinding: assessor; Lost to follow-up: 0/29 at 1 yr	29 pts, 22 m, 7 f, age 19–73 yr; Sweden; Obvious signs + symptoms of a herniated disc; Severe symptoms for longer than 4 mo; Positive myelogram	Exp: chymopapain (4,000 IU); Ctl: surgery (laminotomy)	Patient rating; Second procedure required; At 1 yr	French translation (not full)
Feldman et al., 1986 (17)	Randomization method: drawing of lot; Allocation concealment: B; Blinding: double; Lost to follow-up: 0/39	39 pts	Exp: chymopapain (4,000 U); Ctl: distilled water	Independent observer assessment; Reoperation; At 1 yr	
Fraser, 1982, 1984, and 1995 (20–22)	Randomization method: not stated; Allocation concealment: A; Blinding: double; Lost to follow-up: 0/60 at 2 yr, 4/60 at 10 yr	60 pts, 39 m, 21 f, age 19–69 yr; Multiple centers: United States; Failed conservative treatment (unknown duration) within preceding 6 mo; Myelogram demonstrating posterolateral herniated disc at single level	Exp: chymopapain (8 mg in 2 mL); Ctl: saline (2 mL)	Surgeon rating; Patient rating; Second procedure required; At 2 and 10 yr	6-mo, 2-yr, and 10-yr follow-ups reported in separate publications
Hedtmann et al., 1992 (27)	Randomization: not stated; Allocation concealment: B; Blinding: nil; Lost to follow-up: 0/100	100 pts, 65 m, 35 f; Contained disc at one level; Failed conservative treatment (min 6 wk)	Exp: chymopapain (4,000 U); Ctl: collagenase (400 ABC)	Surgeon rating: 1 yr; Second treatment required: 3 yr	German translation (full); 5-yr results included in separate publication (Wittenberg et al., 1996 (63))
Henriksen et al., 1996 (28)	Randomization method: closed envelopes; Allocation concealment: A; Blinding: single	79 pts, age 30–48 yr; Denmark; Single-level nerve root compromise	Exp: microsurgical discectomy; Ctl: standard lumbar discectomy	Back pain score, leg pain score, time to discharge	
Javid et al., 1983 and 1992 (31,32)	Randomization method: permuted blocks; Allocation concealment: A; Blinding: double; Lost to follow-up: 2/108 at 6 mo	108 pts, 63 m, 45 f, age 36–41 yr; Multicenter: United States; Period of study: 1981–1982; Positive myelogram for single disc herniation; Failed conservative treatment (min 6 wk)	Exp: chymopapain (3,000 U); Ctl: sterile saline solution	Patient rating; Physician rating; Second procedure required; Code break; At 6 mo	
Jensen et al. 1996 (33)	Randomization method: not stated; Allocation concealment: B; Blinding: single & assessor	118 pts, 53 m, 46 f, age 19–75 yr	Exp: implantation of free fat graft following discectomy; Ctl: nil following discectomy	Patient assessment	
Lagarrigue and Chaynes, 1994 (35)	Randomization method: drawing of lot; Allocation concealment: B; Blinding: assessor; Lost to follow-up: 0/80 at 15 mo	80 pts	Exp: microdiscectomy; Ctl: discectomy	Surgeon rating; At 15 mo	French translation (not full)

continued

TABLE 13.1. Continued

Investigators (ref.)	Methods	Participants	Interventions	Outcomes	Notes
Lavignolle et al., 1987 (36)	Randomization method: not stated Allocation concealment: B Blinding: nil Lost to follow-up: 0/358 at 2 yr	358 pts	Exp: chemonucleolysis (4,000 U) Ctl: surgery	Surgeon rating Independent observer rating Second procedure required At 2 yr	French translation (not full)
MacKay et al., 1995 (37)	Randomization method: not stated Allocation concealment: B Blinding: assessor Lost to follow-up: 36/154	154 pts; 106 m, 48 f, age 14–79 yr Michigan Radiographically proven single-level herniation Unsuccessful nonoperative treatment (min 6 wk)	Exp: free-fat graft/Gelfoam Ctl: nil	Independent observer assessment MRI scar formation At 1 yr	
Mayer and Brock, 1993 (40)	Randomization method: not stated Allocation concealment: B Blinding: nil Lost to follow-up: 0/40 at 2 yr	40 pts, 26 m, 14 f, age 12–63 yr Berlin Previous unsuccessful conservative treatment (time period not stated) Only small, "noncontained" disc herniations included	Exp: percutaneous endoscopic discectomy Ctl: microdiscectomy	Patient rating Surgeon rating Repeat surgery At 2 yr	
Muralikutan et al., 1992 (44)	Randomization method: computer-generated randomization list Allocation concealment: B Blinding: nil Lost to follow-up: 6/92 at 1 yr	92 pts, 55 m, 37 f, age 19–60 yr Belfast Nerve root pain with/without back pain Failed conservative treatment (min 4 wk incl. 2 wk bed rest)	Exp: chemonucleolysis (4,000 U Chymopapain) Ctl: discectomy	Second procedure required At 1 yr	
Petrie and Ross, 1996 (46)	Randomization method: closed envelope Allocation concealment: A Blinding: single + assessor	213 pts, 134 m, 79 f, mean age 40 yr ctl and 38 yr exp	Exp: ADCON-L antiadhesion barrier gel Ctl: nil	Patient rating, magnetic resonance imaging scar score At 6 mo	
Revel et al., 1993 (48)	Randomization method: permuted blocks Allocation concealment: B Blinding: nil Lost to follow-up: 2/141 at 6 mo	141 pts, 94 m, 47 f, age 21–65 yr Multicenter: Paris Unsuccessful conservative treatment (min 30 d) Proven disc herniation at one vertebral level	Exp: automated percutaneous discectomy Ctl: chemonucleolysis	Patient rating Second procedure required At 6 mo	

Study	Methods	Participants	Interventions	Outcomes	Notes
Schwetschenau and Martins et al., 1976 and 1978 (39,52)	Randomization method: not stated Allocation concealment: A Blinding: double Lost to follow-up: 0/66 at 1 yr	66 pts, 44 m, 22 f, age 32–40 yr Washington, DC One or more clinical signs of herniated lumbar disc Positive myelogram Failed conservative treatment (incl. at least 3 wk bed rest)	Exp: chymopapain (20 mg) Ctl: sodium iothalamate (20 mg)	Surgeon rating Second procedure required (laminectomy) At 1 yr	Radiographic changes reported in separate publication (M/0006)
Tullberg et al., 1993 (56)	Randomization method: not stated Allocation concealment: B Blinding: nil Lost to follow-up: 0/60 at 1 yr	60 pts, 39 m, 21 f, age 17–64 yr Sweden Single lumbar disc herniation Failed conservative treatment (min 2 mo)	Exp: microdiscectomy Ctl: standard discectomy	Surgeon rating Leg pain score Back pain score Repeat surgery required At 1 yr	
Weber, 1983 (62)	Randomization method: envelopes Allocation concealment: A Blinding: nil Lost to follow-up: 5/126 at 1 yr	126 pts, 68 m, 58 f, age 25–55 yr Norway Fifth lumbar +/or first sacral root lesion Failed conservative treatment (min 2 wk)	Exp: surgical treatment Ctl: conservative treatment	Author rating At 1, 4, and 10 yr	
Wittenberg et al., 1996 (63)	Randomization method: not stated Allocation concealment: B Blinding: nil Lost to follow-up: 16/100 at 5 yr	Pts: 65 m, 35 f, age: mean 35.5 yr chymopapain, 38 yr collagenase Germany Sciatica with/without back pain for more than 6 wk	Exp: chymopapain (4,000 IU) Ctl: collagenase injection (400 ABC U)	Surgeon rating Return to work	
van Alphen et al., 1989 (60)	Quasirandomized: method: alternation Allocation concealment: B Blinding: nil Lost to follow-up: 1/151 at yr	151 pts, 99 m, 52 f, age 18–45 yr Netherlands Proven disc herniation (myelography) Failed conservative treatment (incl. 2 wk min bed rest)	Exp: chemonucleolysis Ctl: discectomy	Patient rating Surgeon rating Second procedure required At 1 yr	

Ctl, control group; Exp, study group; m, male; f, female; pts, patients.

Five RCTs compared the efficacy of chemonucleolysis using chymopapain versus placebo. These trials had the highest quality scores in this review, with generally adequate randomization, double blinding, and independent outcome assessment. In all the trials, chymopapain was injected by standard technique. The combined results from the five trials compared data from 448 patients with an average follow-up of 97%. The metaanalysis clearly showed that chymopapain was more effective than placebo whether outcomes were rated by the patients (odds ratio [OR], 4.14; 95% confidence interval [95% CI], 2.04, 8.42), by the surgeons conducting the study, or by an independent observer (OR, 2.51; 95% CI, 1.33, 4.76) (Fig. 13.1).

Another five RCTs compared the efficacy of chemonucleolysis using chymopapain and surgical discectomy. In each instance, a standard dose of chymopapain was injected by standard technique and was compared with standard discectomy. In all the trials, there were weaknesses of randomization, and the nature of these studies precluded blinding of the patients. The combined results from the five trials compared data from 682 patients with an average follow-up of 97%. Metaanalysis of three trials showed a significantly better result at 1 year with surgical discectomy when the outcome was rated by the surgeon (fixed OR, 1.96; 95% CI, 1.31, 2.92; random effects OR, 2.81; 95% CI, 0.96, 8.23) (Fig. 13.2), whereas two trials showed a nonsignificant better result at 1 year as rated by the patients (OR, 1.65; 95% CI, 0.81, 3.38). About 30% of patients with chemonucleolysis had further disc surgery within 2 years, and metaanalysis clearly showed that repeat surgery was more likely after chemonucleolysis (OR, 15.1; 95% CI, 5.6, 41.2). However, chemonucleolysis may be regarded as the final step in conservative treatment before open surgery, and surgery after failed chemonucleolysis is not strictly comparable to a second operation after failed discectomy. There is some suggestion that the results of discectomy after failed chemonucleolysis are poorer than the results of primary discectomy, but data are insufficient to allow metaanalysis, and, in any event, the patient subgroups so derived are unlikely to be comparable. Nevertheless, the main metaanalysis shows that the final outcome of patients treated by chemonucleolysis, including the effects of further surgery when chemonucleolysis failed, remains poorer than the outcome in patients treated by primary discectomy (Fig. 13.2).

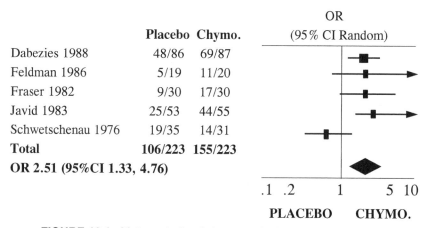

FIGURE 13.1. Metaanalysis of chemonucleolysis versus placebo.

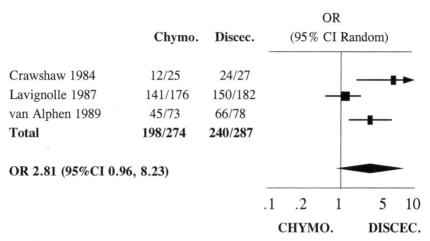

	Chymo.	Discec.	OR (95% CI Random)
Crawshaw 1984	12/25	24/27	
Lavignolle 1987	141/176	150/182	
van Alphen 1989	45/73	66/78	
Total	**198/274**	**240/287**	

OR 2.81 (95%CI 0.96, 8.23)

.1   .2   1   5   10

CHYMO.   DISCEC.

FIGURE 13.2. Metaanalysis of discectomy versus chemonucleolysis.

Conclusions

1. There is limited direct evidence from this review on the efficacy of surgical discectomy for lumbar disc prolapse (62), but there is strong indirect evidence from the RCTs of chemonucleolysis reviewed here that discectomy is more effective than chemonucleolysis, which, in turn, is more effective than placebo. Discectomy has survived the test of time after more than half a century in widespread use, and many clinical series have shown consistently that 70% to 95% of carefully selected patients have good or excellent outcomes, particularly for the relief of sciatica and for at least 6 to 24 months (30). We would conclude that despite the limited RCTs that directly compare surgical discectomy and conservative treatment, there is *moderate* evidence (*strength of evidence B*) on the efficacy of discectomy for carefully selected patients with sciatica resulting from lumbar disc prolapse that fails to resolve with conservative management. This procedure provides faster relief from the acute attack (*strength of evidence B*), although any positive or negative effects on the lifetime natural history of disc problems are unclear (*strength of evidence D*).

2. There is now good evidence on the efficacy of chemonucleolysis. There is *strong* evidence (*strength of evidence A*) from five generally high-quality trials that chemonucleolysis with chymopapain produces better clinical outcomes than placebo. One trial showed that these outcomes are maintained for 10 years (19–21,24). Despite some weaknesses of trial design, there is also *strong* evidence (*strength of evidence A*) from five trials that chemonucleolysis does not produce clinical outcomes as good as those in patients who undergo surgical discectomy. If chemonucleolysis is regarded as the final stage of conservative treatment, it will save about 70% of patients from requiring open surgery. However, the final results of a policy of chemonucleolysis followed by surgery if chemonucleolysis fails remain poorer than the results of primary discectomy. It is not possible to draw any conclusions about complication rates from these relatively small RCTs. That would require a completely different and much larger database, a finding that suggests that the complication rate of chemonucleolysis is lower than that of surgical discectomy (4,5) (*strength of evidence C*).

3. Although some of these trials reported on the proportion of patients who return to work, it is not possible to draw any firm conclusions about the efficacy or relative efficacy of any of these treatments for return to work (*strength of evidence C*). Scheer et al. (51) reached a similar conclusion from a systematic review of RCTs. Taylor (54) reviewed 19 uncontrolled case series and suggested that 82% of patients were able to return to their previous level of employment following primary back surgery compared with 59% after multiple back surgery.

What Evidence Is There on Alternative Forms and Techniques of Surgery for Lumbar Disc Prolapse?

Three trials, with data from 219 patients, compared microdiscectomy with standard discectomy. Only two trials gave data on clinical outcomes (28,35), and both showed no difference. Although they used different measures, metaanalysis was not possible. Use of the microscope lengthened the operative procedure, but it did not appear to make any significant difference to perioperative bleeding or other complications, length of inpatient stay, or the formation of scar tissue.

Three trials compared automated percutaneous discectomy with other surgical techniques, but these trials were not comparable, and they could not logically be combined for metaanalysis. Mayer and Brock (40) showed that clinical outcomes were comparable to those of standard discectomy, but these investigators considered that only 10% to 15% of patients needing surgical treatment may be suitable for automated percutaneous discectomy. Chatterjee et al. (10) reported only 29% satisfactory results for automated percutaneous discectomy compared with 80% for microdiscectomy. Revel et al. (48) also found automated percutaneous discectomy to be inferior to chemonucleolysis. This review did not identify any completed RCTs of laser discectomy.

Three trials including data on a total of 485 patients considered the effect of three different types of interposition membrane on the formation of intraspinal scarring following discectomy, as assessed by magnetic resonance imaging or enhanced computed tomography. One trial (46) claimed less scarring and better clinical outcomes after insertion of an antiadhesion barrier gel, but the published results were highly selected. The metaanalysis showed some reduction in moderate to severe scar formation, but that reduction did not reach statistical significance. There was no difference in clinical outcomes, whether assessed by patient or by surgeon. The only trial to report small numbers of reoperations found no difference (46).

No statistically significant differences in effect were demonstrated between low-dose and standard-dose chymopapain (1), between chymopapain and collagenase (26,27,63), or between chymopapain and steroid injection (3,6). Although one trial suggested that collagenase may be more effective than placebo, the study was small, and there was 40% code break by 8 weeks (8).

Conclusions

1. There is *strong* evidence (*strength of evidence A*) that microdiscectomy and standard discectomy give broadly comparable clinical outcomes. In principle, the microscope provides better illumination and teaching. These trials suggest that use of the microscope lengthens the operative procedure, but despite previous claims, they did not show any significant difference in perioperative bleeding, length of inpatient

stay, or the formation of scar tissue (*strength of evidence B*). However, it is not possible to draw any firm conclusions about complication rates from these trials (*strength of evidence C*)

2. There is *limited and contradictory* evidence (*strength of evidence C*) that automated percutaneous discectomy gives poorer clinical results than the alternative surgical techniques with which it has been compared.
3. There is *no* acceptable evidence (*strength of evidence D*) on laser discectomy.
4. It is possible that some form of interposition membrane may produce a slight reduction in the formation of severe scar tissue after discectomy, but any effect has not reached statistical significance and is probably weak (*strength of evidence B*). There is *moderate* evidence that it does not influence clinical outcomes (*strength of evidence B*) and *limited* evidence (*strength of evidence C*) that it does not influence the reoperation rate.
5. There is *limited and inconclusive* evidence (*strength of evidence C*) on the relative efficacy of different doses of chymopapain, chymopapain compared with collagenase, and collagenase compared with placebo, which does not permit any firm conclusions.

SURGERY FOR DEGENERATIVE LUMBAR DISC DISEASE

Degenerative lumbar disc disease is a common, age-related condition affecting most adults. Associated symptoms are variable and have a relatively low correlation with the severity of radiologic changes. Only a few patients come to surgery. Surgical treatment may consist of either fusion, with the basic aim of relieving discogenic and facet pain, or decompression of nerve root or cauda equina compression, with the basic aim of relieving neurogenic claudication. In general terms, severe disc degeneration, malalignment, and instability of the spine are treated by fusion, whereas associated spinal or root canal stenosis is treated by decompression. However, decompression and fusion are often combined. Decisions about surgery are usually based not only on the nature of the localized pathologic features and associated symptoms and disability, but also on the severity of pain and psychologic distress and on psychosocial issues. The choice of procedure may also be influenced by the surgeon's beliefs about the role of surgery in spinal disorders and the surgical instrumentation and skills available.

Results

Fourteen RCTs of all forms of surgical treatment for degenerative lumbar disc disease were identified (Table 13.2).

What Evidence Is There on the Clinical Effectiveness of Surgery for Degenerative Lumbar Disc Disease?

This review found no published RCTs comparing any form of surgery for degenerative lumbar disc disease with natural history, placebo, or any form of conservative treatment. No RCTs could be identified that dealt with the efficacy of fusion for degenerative disc disease. After more than 80 years of use, there is still considerable dispute whether lumbar fusion is an appropriate and effective method of treating back pain in patients with degenerative lumbar disc disease, in the absence of nerve root or cauda equina compression (53). There are heated debates and lack of clear evidence

TABLE 13.2. *Characteristics of studies of the surgical treatment of degenerative lumbar spondylosis*

Investigators (ref.)	Methods	Participants	Interventions	Outcomes	Notes
Bridwell et al., 1993 (7)	Randomization method: not stated Allocation concealment: C Blinding: nil Lost to follow-up: 1/44 at 2 yr	44 pts, 10 m, 34f, age 46–79 yr United States Spinal claudication symptoms Computed tomography scan/myelogram/magnetic resonance evaluation	Exp: no fusion Ctl: posterolateral fusion with/without instrumentation	Spondylolisthesis progression Reoperation At 2 yr	
Carragee, 1997 (9)	Randomization method: sealed envelopes containing random numbers Concealment: A Blinding: nil Lost to follow-up: 2 at 4.5 yr	Patients: 46 Grade I or II isthmic spondylolisthesis California	Exp: smokers with instrumented arthrodesis + decompressive laminectomy; nonsmokers with graft alone + decompressive laminectomy Ctl: same groups without decompressive laminectomy	Back pain Fusion Patient rating	
Emery et al., 1995 (16)	Randomization method: not stated Allocation concealment: B Blinding: nit Lost to follow-up: 5/84 at 22 mo	84 pts, age not stated United States Heterogeneous clinical conditions	Exp: fusion + luque plate/screw system Ctl: posterolateral fusion with autogenous graft	Fusion rate At 22 mo	
Fischgrund et al., 1997 (18)	Randomization method: closed envelope technique Allocation concealment: A Blinding: assessor Lost to follow-up: 8/76 at 2.4 yr	76 pts, 17 m, 59 f, age 52–86 yr United States Degenerative spondylolisthesis and spinal stenosis	Exp: fusion + Steffee plate/pedicle screws Ctl: fusion	Fusion Patient rating Progression of spondylolisthesis At 2 yr	
France et al., 1999 (19)	Randomization method: Not stated Allocation concealment: B Blinding: nit Lost to follow-up: 12/83 at 40 mo	83 pts, 51 m, 19 f, age 19–76 yr United States Heterogeneous spinal conditions	Exp: fusion + Steffee plate Ctl: posterolateral fusion	Patient rating Fusion rate	
Grob et al., 1995 (25)	Quasirandomized: method: date of admission to hospital Allocation concealment: C Blinding: nil Lost to follow-up: 0/30 at 28	45 pts, 21 m, 24 f, age 48–87 yr Switzerland History + clinical exam + CT scan Systemic disease excluded A midsagittal diameter of the spinal canal of less than 11 mm = stenotic	Exp: decompression with arthrodesis (both mono- + multisegmental) Ctl: decompression without arthrodesis	Patient rating Surgeon rating Reoperation required At 28 mo (mean)	Author contacted for data (pain figs + standard deviations)

Study	Methods	Participants	Interventions	Outcomes
Herkowitz and Kurz, 1991 (29)	Quasirandomized: alternately assigned to treatment; Allocation concealment: B; Blinding: nil; Lost to follow-up: 0/50 at 3 yr	50 pts, 36 f, 14 m; age 52–84 yr; Michigan; Spinal stenosis assoc. with degenerative lumbar spondylolisthesis	Exp: decompression alone; Ctl: decompression + fusion	Surgeon rating At 3 yr (mean)
McGuire and Amundson, 1993 (41)	Randomization method: not stated; Allocation concealment: B; Blinding: nil; Lost to follow-up: 1/27 at 2 yr	27 pts, 23 m, 4 f; age 24–42 yr; Symptomatic grade I to II spondylolisthesis refractory to conservative care; All treated with laminectomy + nerve root decompression	Exp: posterolateral fusion; Ctl: internal fixation + Steffee plate + screw system	Reoperation; Fusion rate At 2 yr
Mooney, 1990 (43)	Randomization method: not stated; Allocation concealment: B; Blinding: double; Lost to follow-up: 11/206 at 1 yr	195 pts; California; Pts undergoing initial attempts at interbody spinal fusion (anterior or posterior approach)	Exp: electromagnetic brace 8 hr/d; Ctl: placebo brace 8 hr/d	Surgeon rating At 1 yr
Postacchini et al., 1993 (47)	Randomization method: allocation by pathology and then assigned alternately number; Allocation concealment: C; Blinding: nil; Lost to follow up 3/70 at 3.7 yr	70 pts, 34 m, 36 f; 9 pts changed groups at surgery	Exp: multiple laminotomy; Ctl: laminectomy	Patient rating; Surgeon rating; Progression of spondylolisthesis; Operating time and blood loss
Rogozinski and Rogozinski, 1995 (49)	Randomization method: not stated; Allocation concealment: B; Blinding: nil; Lost to follow-up: nil at 2 yr	26 pts; Florida; Condition not specified	Exp: implanted bone stimulation wire; Ctl: no implant	Fusion
Thomsen et al., 1997 (55)	Randomization method: Not stated; Allocation concealment: B; Blinding: assessor; Lost to follow-up: 3/129—at 2 yr	130 pts, 60 m, 69 f; age 20–67 yr; Denmark; Severe low back pain of various causes	Exp: fusion + Cotrel-Dubousset pedicle screw/rod; Ctl: posterolateral fusion	Fusion; Secondary surgery; Patient rating
Zdeblick, 1993 (64)	Randomization method: random number generator; Allocation concealment: C; Blinding: nil; Lost to follow-up: 1/124	124 pts, age 20–80 yr; For lumbar or lumbosacral fusion for degenerative conditions of the spine; Wisconsin	Exp: fusion with autogenous bone graft; Ctl: fusion + semi-rigid/rigid fixation	Surgeon rating; Repeat surgery At 16 mo (mean)
Zdeblick et al., 1996 (65)	Randomization method: not stated; Concealment: B; Blinding: assessor; Lost to follow-up: Nil	Patients: 39; L5-S1 degenerative disc disease with normal proximal discs; Wisconsin	Exp: TSRII + PLIF; Exp: ALIF; Ctl: TSRII	Pain requiring medication; Incidence of second procedure; Fusion; Blood loss

ALIF, Anterior lumbar intervertebral fusion; Ctl, control group; Exp, study group; m, male; f, female; PLIF, Posterior lumbar intervertebral fusion; pts, patients; TSRH, Texas Scottish Rite Hospital.

on the nature and role of "instability," and the clinical indications for surgery are not well defined. The surgical techniques and the technical success rate of fusion vary widely, whereas reported satisfactory clinical outcomes range from 16% to 95% (57,58).

No RCTs could be identified that dealt with the efficacy of surgical decompression for degenerative disc disease or spinal stenosis. Attempted metaanalyses of largely retrospective case series by Turner et al. (59) suggested that 64% of patients treated surgically for spinal stenosis had good or excellent outcomes. Deyo et al. (14) and Ciol et al. (11) analyzed a large Medicare cohort and found that mortality increased from less than 0.8% in those aged less than 75 years to 2.3% in those aged more than 80 years. The complication rate was double in that older age group. Eleven percent of these patients had repeat back surgery within 6 years.

A previous metaanalysis of published reports of degenerative spondylolisthesis by Mardjetko et al. (38) suggested that decompression without fusion gave 69% satisfactory outcomes, but many reports described progressive slipping. Addition of fusion to the decompression appeared to give 90% satisfactory outcomes and 86% solid fusion. However, that metaanalysis was based mainly on case series that were retrospective.

Conclusions

1. There is no acceptable evidence (*strength of evidence D*) on the efficacy of any form of fusion for back pain or "instability."
2. There is no acceptable evidence (*strength of evidence D*) on the efficacy of any form of decompression for degenerative lumbar disc disease or spinal stenosis.
3. There is no evidence (*strength of evidence D*) on whether any form of surgery for degenerative lumbar disc disease is effective in returning patients to work.

What Evidence Is There on Alternative Techniques of Surgery for Degenerative Lumbar Disc Disease?

All the trials identified in this review of degenerative lumbar disc disease compared two or more surgical techniques. From a surgical perspective, the trials fell into two broad groups: the first considered techniques of fusion, whereas the second considered techniques of dealing with spinal stenosis and nerve compression. Each of two trials compared three techniques, and the trials are included in both groups. Analysis is complicated by the finding that the trials dealt with varied disorders, including degenerative disc disease, spinal stenosis, isthmic spondylolisthesis, and degenerative spondylolisthesis. Some of the trials did not distinguish among these conditions and only presented total results from mixed disorders.

Techniques of Fusion

There is considerable interest in and controversy about instrumented fusion. Posterior pedicle instrumentation was first used in Europe in the early 1960s (50). In the last few years, there has been an explosion of surgical and commercial interest in a wide variety of methods of instrumented fusion in both Europe and the United States. The foregoing metaanalysis of published case series of degenerative spondylolisthesis (38) suggested that fusion with pedicle screws produced a higher fusion rate

(93% versus 86%) than fusion without instrumentation, but that rate was not statistically significant, and the clinical outcomes were comparable (86% versus 90%).

The present review found nine RCTs that addressed the question whether instrumentation improved the outcome of posterolateral fusion, but only seven of these trials provided data that could be used. This gave a total of 649 patients with a mean 95% follow-up at 16 months to 4.5 years (median 2 years). However, this was a heterogeneous group of studies. Only one trial (65) dealt purely with patients with degenerative disc disease and back pain, although one other trial presented results separately for this subgroup of patients (64). One of the nine trials was in patients with degenerative lumbar spinal stenosis without instability (25), two in patients with isthmic spondylolisthesis (7,55), and another two in patients with degenerative spondylolisthesis (18,41). Three trials had patients with mixed diagnoses (16,19,64), and only one of these presented the results for each group separately (64). Many different instrumentation systems were used, and only three trials used the same system (Steffee plates). There was a wide variety of outcome measures, the most common measures being technical surgical outcomes of fusion rates, progression of spondylolisthesis, and reoperation rates. In the published papers, four trials gave some form of patient rating, but only three trials gave any detail on pain (9,18,19), and one reported on functional outcomes (55). Melot and Szpalski (personal communication) obtained further data on pain improvement in one trial by correspondence with the original authors (42).

Analysis of the data available from these trials showed the following:

1. Metaanalysis showed that instrumentation is more likely to lead to solid fusion (OR, 2.32; 95% CI, 0.95 to 5.68) (Fig. 13.3), although there are problems with assessing fusion in the presence of metalwork (2,34), an issue few of these trials considered.
2. Six RCTs provided clinical outcome data on instrumented versus noninstrumented fusion (analyzed by Prof. C. Melot). Preliminary metaanalysis of all six trials suggested that instrumented fusion may produce better clinical outcomes (OR, 1.36;

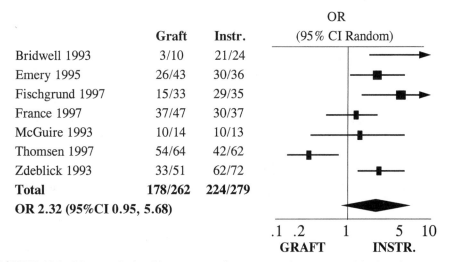

FIGURE 13.3. Metaanalysis of instrumented versus noninstrumented fusion: fusion rate.

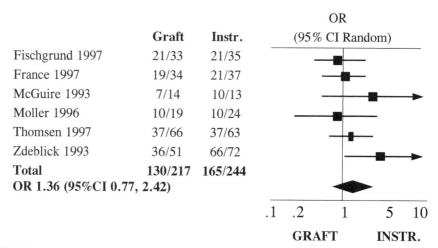

FIGURE 13.4. Metaanalysis of instrumented versus noninstrumented fusion: clinical outcomes. (Courtesy of Prof. C. Melot.)

95% CI, 0.77, 2.42) (Fig. 13.4), although this did not reach statistical significance. However, only one of the six trials (64) showed a significant difference in outcomes, and this was markedly different from the results of all the other trials. This was the only trial based entirely on crude outcome ratings by the operating surgeon, who claimed 92% excellent and good results from instrumented fusion. The other five trials all used various patient-centered measures of pain or functional status. Metaanalysis of the 338 patients in these five trials showed no difference in patient outcomes of pain and disability in instrumented versus noninstrumented fusion (OR, 1.05; 95% CI, 0.68, 1.62). Both of the two trials that provided actual patient ratings of pain (18,19) showed no significant difference in pain relief.

3. It was not possible to assess complication rates from RCTs, although other evidence suggests that complications may be more frequent or more serious with instrumented fusion (38). The RCTs showed no significant difference in the reoperation rate over 2 years.

4. Because of the heterogeneity of the trials, it was not possible to draw any conclusions about the results of instrumented fusion for any particular pathologic condition or about any particular instrumentation system.

Once again, however, we emphasize that this is a heterogeneous analysis of different patient groups, different instrumentation systems, and different outcomes; Any conclusions must be tentative.

Only one trial compared small numbers of patients with anterior and posterior interbody fusion (65), but it did not have sufficient power to demonstrate any significant difference in any outcome. Two trials assessed whether electrical stimulation could enhance fusion. Mooney (43) produced significantly improved fusion with pulsed electromagnetic stimulation in lumbar interbody fusion, but the improvement in clinical outcomes was not significant. Rogozinski and Rogozinski (49), in contrast, had inconclusive results with implanted direct current stimulation as an adjunct to instrumented posterolateral fusion.

Conclusions

1. There is *strong* evidence (*strength of evidence A*) that instrumented fusion produces a higher fusion rate (although that needs to be qualified by the difficulty of assessing fusion) but does not improve clinical outcomes (*strength of evidence A*), and other evidence (*strength of evidence D*) indicates that this type of fusion may be associated with higher complication rates.
2. There is *limited* evidence (*strength of evidence C*) that does not demonstrate any clear difference between anterior or posterior techniques of fusion.
3. There is *limited and inconclusive* evidence (*strength of evidence C*) that some forms of electrical stimulation may enhance fusion rates, but *moderate* evidence (*strength of evidence B*) that they do not influence clinical outcomes.

Techniques for Spinal Stenosis and Nerve Compression

This is a small and heterogeneous group of five studies. One RCT considered techniques of decompression for spinal stenosis by comparing laminectomy or multiple laminotomy (47), but that study had several confounding factors. Nine of the 35 patients scheduled for laminotomy actually had a laminectomy for technical reasons, and several patients in each group also had an intertransverse arthrodesis for degenerative spondylolisthesis. That trial did not demonstrate any difference in clinical outcomes or spondylolisthesis progression between the two treatment methods.

Three trials considered whether some form of posterolateral fusion, with or without instrumentation, was a useful adjunct to decompression alone (7,25,29) and provided data on a total of 139 patients with 99% follow-up at 2 to 3 years. Comparison of the three trials showed no difference in outcomes between fusion of any type or laminectomy (OR, 0.80; 95% CI, 0.31 to 2.10), as rated by the surgeon 18 to 24 months after the procedure. One of these trials (25) considered fusion with and without instrumentation in patients with degenerative spinal stenosis with no evidence of instability. It showed no difference in clinical outcomes or relief of pain, provided the posterior elements were preserved at operation. The other two trials considered the role of adjunct fusion in spinal stenosis associated with single-level or two-level degenerative spondylolisthesis. Herkowitz and Kurz (29) studied noninstrumented fusion alone. The results showed that fusion produced significantly less self-reported back pain and leg pain and significantly better surgeon ratings of outcome. Bridwell et al. (7) studied both instrumented and noninstrumented fusion and showed that patients who had a successful fusion had less spondylolisthesis progression and better patient ratings of improvement. These results were only significant in the group with an instrumented fusion, however, whereas successful noninstrumented fusion produced no such benefit.

Caragee (9) compared the results of fusion alone with fusion plus laminectomy and decompression for patients with an isthmic L5-S1 spondylolisthesis. The trial was confounded by the fact that nonsmokers had fusion by bone grafting alone, whereas smokers had their fusion supplemented by instrumentation. In neither group did the addition of decompression to the arthrodesis appear to improve the clinical outcomes.

Conclusions

The few and heterogeneous trials on spondylolisthesis, spinal stenosis, and nerve compression permit limited conclusions to be drawn.

1. There is *limited* evidence (*strength of evidence C*) that adjunct fusion to supplement decompression for degenerative spondylolisthesis produces less progressive slip and better clinical outcomes than decompression alone.
2. There is *limited* evidence (*strength of evidence C*) that fusion alone may be as effective as combined decompression and fusion for patients with grade I or II isthmic spondylolisthesis and no significant neurologic features.

UNCLASSIFIED

There is a single RCT of repeat surgery versus dorsal column stimulation for failed back surgery syndrome (45), but it is a preliminary report of a small number of patients, no detail is given of the patients or surgical procedures, and it does not provide sufficient data for analysis.

IMPLICATIONS AND FUTURE RESEARCH

Lumbar Disc Prolapse

There is only one RCT on the efficacy of surgical treatment for lumbar disc prolapse, although other types of RCT provide indirect evidence suggesting that surgical treatment does offer good clinical outcomes at least up to 1 year. Many RCTs of chemonucleolysis have been conducted and permit reasonably confident conclusions on the effectiveness of this treatment method. Numerous RCTs permit tentative conclusions on certain technical aspects of surgical discectomy. Further RCTs are required, however, with improved trial design and outcome assessment. In particular, there is a need for better evidence on the optimum selection and timing of surgical treatment in the overall management strategy, on the possible role of chemonucleolysis as a final stage of conservative management, and on the relative advantages and disadvantages of microdiscectomy versus standard discectomy. High-quality RCTs are required to determine the possible role of automated percutaneous discectomy or laser discectomy. There is a need for long-term studies that consider the effects of surgery on the lifetime natural history of disc problems.

Degenerative Disc Disease

There is no clear scientific evidence on the role or efficacy of any form of surgical decompression or fusion for degenerative disc disease compared with natural history, placebo, or conservative treatment. An urgent need exists for further RCTs of decompression for spinal stenosis and of fusion both as primary treatment and as an adjunct to decompression for specific disorders and clinical syndromes associated with lumbar spondylosis. There is a particular need to compare the clinical outcomes, morbidity and complications, costs, and cost-effectiveness of instrumented versus noninstrumented fusion. The quality of surgical RCTs still needs to be improved, and surgeons should seek expert methodologic advice when they plan trials.

Further Information

More detailed methodology and analysis are available in the Cochrane reviews (23).

ACKNOWLEDGMENTS

This chapter has been adapted and developed with permission from Gibson JNA, Grant IC, Waddell G. *Surgical treatment of lumbar disc prolapse and degenerative lumbar disc disease.* Oxford: Cochrane Library update software, issue 1, 1999; and Gibson JNA, Grant IC, Waddell G. The Cochrane review of surgery for lumbar disc prolapse and degenerative lumbar spondylosis. *Spine* 1999;24:1820–1832.

REFERENCES

1. Benoist M, Bonneville JF, Lassale B, et al. A randomized, double-blind study to compare low-dose with standard-dose chymopapain in the treatment of herniated lumbar intervertebral discs. *Spine* 1993;18:28–34.
2. Blumenthal SL, Gill K. Can lumbar spine radiographs accurately determine fusion in post-operative patients? Correlation of routine radiographs with a second surgical look at lumbar disc fusions. *Spine* 1993;18:1186–1189.
3. Bontoux D, Alcalay M, Debiais F, et al. Traitement des hernies discales lombaires par injection intradiscale de chymopapaine ou d'hexacetonide de triamcinolone: étude comparée de 80 cas [Treatment of lumbar disk hernia by intra-disk injection of chymopapain or triamcinolone hexacetonide: comparative study of 80 cases]. *Rev Rhum Mal Osteoartic* 1990;57:327–331.
4. Bouillet R. Complications of discal hernia therapy: comparative study regarding surgical therapy and nucleolysis by chymopapain. *Acta Orthop Belg* 1983;49[Suppl 1]:48–77.
5. Bouillet R. Complications de la nucleolyse discale par la chymopapaine. *Acta Orthop Belg* 1987;53:250–260.
6. Bourgeois P, Benoist M, Palazzo E, et al. Étude en double aveugle randomisée multicentrique de l'hexacetonide de triamcinolone versus chymopapaine dans le traitement de la lombosciatique discale: premiers résultats à six mois [Multicenter randomized double-blind study of triamcinolone hexacetonide versus chymopapain in the treatment of disk lumbosciatica: initial results at 6 months]. *Rev Rhum Mal Osteoartic* 1988;55:767–769.
7. Bridwell KH, Sedgewick TA, O'Brien MF, et al. The role of fusion and instrumentation in the treatment of degenerative spondylolisthesis with spinal stenosis. *J Spinal Disord* 1993;6:461–472.
8. Bromley JW, Varma AO, Santoro AJ, et al. Double-blind evaluation of collagenase injections for herniated lumbar discs. *Spine* 1984;9:486–488.
9. Caragee EJ. Single-level posterolateral arthrodesis, with or without posterior decompression, for the treatment of isthmic spondylolisthesis in adults: a prospective, randomised study. *J Bone Joint Surg Am* 1997;79:1175–1180.
10. Chatterjee S, Foy PM, Findlay GF. Report of a controlled clinical trial comparing automated percutaneous lumbar discectomy and microdiscectomy in the treatment of contained lumbar disc herniation. *Spine* 1995;20:734–738.
11. Ciol MA, Deyo RA, Howell E, et al. An assessment of surgery for spinal stenosis: time trends, geographic variations, complications and reoperations. *J Am Gerontol Soc* 1996;44:285–290.
12. Crawshaw C, Frazer AM, Merriam WF, et al. A comparison of surgery and chemonucleolysis in the treatment of sciatica: a prospective randomized trial. *Spine* 1984;9:195–198.
13. Dabezies EJ, Langford K, Morris J, et al. Safety and efficacy of chymopapain (Discase) in the treatment of sciatica due to a herniated nucleus pulposus: results of a randomized, double-blind study. *Spine* 1988;13:561–565.
14. Deyo RA, Ciol MA, Cherkin DC, et al. Lumbar spine fusion: a cohort study of complications, reoperations and resource use in the Medicare population. *Spine* 1993;18:1463–1470.
15. Ejeskar A, Nachemson A, Herberts P, et al. Surgery versus chemonucleolysis for herniated lumbar discs: a prospective study with random assignment. *Clin Orthop* 1983;174:236–242.
16. Emery SE, Stephens GC, Bolesta MJ, et al. Lumbar fusion with and without instrumentation: a prospective study. *Orthop Trans* 1995;19:362(abst).
17. Feldman J, Menkes CJ, Pallardy G, et al. Étude en double-aveugle du traitement de la lombosciatique discale par chimionucleolyse [Double-blind study of the treatment of disc lumbosciatica by chemonucleolysis]. *Rev Rhum Mal Osteoartic* 1986;53:147–152.

18. Fischgrund JS, Mackay M, Herkowitz HN, et al. Degenerative lumbar spondylolisthesis with spinal stenosis: a prosprective, randomized study comparing decompressive laminectomy and arthrodesis with and without spinal insturumentation. *Spine* 1997;22:2807–2812.
19. France JC, Yaszemski MJ, Lauerman WC, et al. A randomized prospective study of posterolateral lumbar fusion: outcomes with and without pedicle screw instrumentation. *Spine* 1997;24:553–560.
20. Fraser RD. Chymopapain for the treatment of intervertebral disc herniation: a preliminary report of a double-blind study. *Spine* 1982;7:608–612.
21. Fraser RD. Chymopapain for the treatment of intervertebral disc herniation: the final report of a double-blind study. *Spine* 1984;9:815–818.
22. Fraser RD, Sandhu A, Gogan WJ. Magnetic resonance imaging findings 10 years after treatment for lumbar disc herniation. *Spine* 1995;20:710–714.
23. Gibson JNA, Grant IC, Waddell G. *Surgical treatment of lumbar disc prolapse and degenerative lumbar disc disease.* Oxford: Cochrane Library update software, issue 1, 1999. (Also *Spine,* 1999;24:1820–1832.)
24. Gogan WJ, Fraser RD. Chymopapain: a 10-year, double-blind study. *Spine* 1992;17:388–394.
25. Grob D, Humke T, Dvorak J. Degenerative lumbar spinal stenosis: decompression with and without arthrodesis. *J Bone Joint Surg Am* 1995;77:1036–1041.
26. Hedtmann A, Steffen R, Kramer J. Prospective comparative study of intradiscal high-dose and low-dose collagenase versus chymopapain. *Spine* 1996;12:388–392.
27. Hedtmann A, Fett H, Steffen R, et al. Chemonukleolyse mit Chymopapain und Kollagenase: 3-Jahres-Ergebnisse einer prospektiv-randomisierten Studie [Chemonucleolysis using chymopapain and collagenase: 3-year results of a prospective randomized study]. *Z Orthop Ihre Grenzgeb* 1992;130:36–44.
28. Henrikson L, Schmidt V, Eskesen V, et al. A controlled study of microsurgical versus standard lumbar discectomy. *Br J Neurosurg* 1996;10:289–293.
29. Herkowitz HN, Kurz LT. Degenerative lumbar spondylolisthesis with spinal stenosis: a prospective study comparing decompression with decompression and intertransverse process arthrodesis. *J Bone Joint Surg Am* 1991;73:802–808.
30. Hoffman RM, Wheeler KJ, Deyo RA. Surgery for herniated lumbar discs: a literature synthesis. *J Gen Intern Med* 1993;8:487–496.
31. Javid MJ. A 1- to 4-year follow-up review of treatment of sciatica using chemonucleolysis or laminectomy. *J Neurosurg* 1992;76:184–190.
32. Javid MJ, Nordby EJ, Ford LT, et al. Safety and efficacy of chymopapain (chymodiactin) in herniated nucleus pulposus with sciatica. *JAMA* 1983;249:2489–2494.
33. Jensen T, Asmussen K, Berg-Hansen E, et al. First-time operation for lumbar disc herniation with or without free fat transplantation: prospective triple-blind randomized study with reference to clinical factors and enhanced CT scan 1 year after operation. *Spine* 1996;21:1072–1076.
34. Kant AP, Daum WJ, Dean SM, et al. Evaluation of lumbar spine fusion: plain radiographs versus direct surgical exploration and observation. *Spine* 1995;20:2313–2317.
35. Lagarrigue J, Chaynes P. Comparative study of disk surgery with or without microscopy: a prospective study of 80 cases [in French]. *Neurochirurgie* 1994;40:116–120.
36. Lavignolle B, Vital JM, Baulny D, et al. Études comparées de la chirurgie et de la chimionucleolyse dans le traitement de la sciatique par hernie discale [Comparative study of surgery and chemonucleolysis in the treatment of sciatica caused by a herniated disk]. *Acta Orthop Belg* 1987;53:244–249.
37. MacKay MA, Fischgrund JS, Herkowitz HN, et al. The effect of interposition membrane on the outcome of lumbar laminectomy and discectomy. *Spine* 1995;20:1793–1796.
38. Mardjetko SM, Connolly PJ, Shott S. Degenerative lumbar spondylosis: a meta-analysis of literature 1970–1993. *Spine* 1994;20S:2256S–2265S.
39. Martins AN, Ramirez A, Johnston J, et al. Double-blind evaluation of chemonucleolysis for herniated lumbar discs: late results. *J Neurosurg* 1978;49:816–827.
40. Mayer HM, Brock M. Percutaneous endoscopic discectomy: surgical technique and preliminary results compared to microsurgical discectomy. *J Neurosurg* 1993;78:216–225.
41. McGuire RA, Amundson GM. The use of primary internal fixation in spondylolisthesis. *Spine* 1993;18:1662–1672.
42. Moller H, Hedlund R. Fusion or conservative treatment in adult spondylolisthesis: a prospective randomized study. *Acta Orthop Scand* 1996;65[Suppl 260]:12(abst).
43. Mooney V. A randomized double-blind prospective study of the efficacy of pulsed electromagnetic fields for interbody lumbar fusions. *Spine* 1990;15:708–712.
44. Muralikuttan KP, Hamilton A, Kernohan WG, et al. A prospective randomized trial of chemonucleolysis and conventional disc surgery in single level lumbar disc herniation. *Spine* 1992;17:381–387.
45. North RB, Kidd DH, Piantadosi S. Spinal cord stimulation versus reoperation for failed back surgery syndrome: a prospective randomized study design. *Acta Neurochir* 1995;64:106–108.
46. Petrie JL, Ross JS. Use of ADCON-L to inhibit postoperative peridural fibrosis and related symptoms following lumbar disc surgery: a preliminary report. *Eur Spine J* 1996;5[Suppl 1]:S10–S17.
47. Postacchini F, Cinotti G, Perugia D, et al. The surgical treatment of central lumbar stenosis: multiple laminotomy compared with total laminectomy. *J Bone Joint Surg Br* 1993;75:386–392.

48. Revel M, Payan C, Vallee C, et al. Automated percutaneous lumbar discectomy versus chemonucleolysis in the treatment of sciatica. *Spine* 1993;18:1–7.
49. Rogozinski A, Rogozinski C. Efficacy of implanted bone growth stimulation in instrumented lumbosacral spinal fusion. *Orthop Trans* 1995;19:362.
50. Roy-Camille R, Saillant G, Mazel C. Internal fixation of the lumbar spine with pedicle screw plating. *Clin Orthop* 1986;203:7–17.
51. Scheer SJ, Radack KL, O'Brien DR. Randomised controlled trials in industrial low back pain relating to return to work. II. Discogenic low back pain. *Arch Phys Med Rehabil* 1996;77:1189–1197.
52. Schwetschenau PR, Ramirez A, Johnston J, et al. Double-blind evaluation of intradiscal chymopapain for herniated lumbar discs: early results. *J Neurosurg* 1976;45:622–627.
53. Szpalski M, Gunzburg R, Pope MR, eds. *Lumbar segmental instability*. Philadelphia: Lippincott Williams & Wilkins, 1999.
54. Taylor ME. Return to work following back surgery: a review. *Am J Ind Med* 1989;16:79–88.
55. Thomsen K, Christensen FB, Eiskjaer SP, et al. The effect of pedicle screw instrumentation on functional outcome and fusion rates in posterolateral lumbar spinal fusion: a prospective randomized clinical study. *Spine* 1997;22:2813–2822.
56. Tullberg T, Isacson J, Weidenhielm L. Does microscopic removal of lumbar disc herniation lead to better results than the standard procedure? Results of a one-year randomized study. *Spine* 1993;18:24–27.
57. Turner JA, Herron L, Deyo RA. Meta-analysis of the results of lumbar spine fusion. *Acta Orthop Scand* 1993;64[Suppl 251]:120–122.
58. Turner JA, Ersek M, Herron L, et al. Patient outcomes after lumbar spinal fusions. *JAMA* 1992;268:907–911.
59. Turner JA, Ersek M, Herron L, et al. Surgery for lumbar spinal stenosis: attempted meta-analysis of the literature. *Spine* 1992;17:1–8.
60. van Alphen HA, Braakman R, Bezemer PD, et al. Chemonucleolysis versus discectomy: a randomized multicenter trial. *J Neurosurg* 1989;70:869–875.
61. Weber H. *Lumbar disc herniation: a prospective study of prognostic factors including a controlled trial.* Thesis, University of Oslo, 1978.
62. Weber H. Lumbar disc herniation: controlled, prospective study with ten years of observation. *Spine* 1983;8:131–140.
63. Wittenberg RH, Oppenl SC, Steffen R. Intradiscal therapy with chymopapain or collagenase: five year results of a prospective randomized investigation. *Orthop Trans* 1996–1997;20:1064–1065.
64. Zdeblick TA. A prospective, randomized study of lumbar fusion: preliminary results. *Spine* 1993;18:983–991.
65. Zdeblick TA, Ulschmid S, Dick JC. The surgical treatment of L5-S1 degenerative disc disease: a prospective randomized study of laparoscopic fusion. *Orthop Trans* 1996–1997;20:1064–1065.

Neck and Back Pain: The Scientific Evidence
of Causes, Diagnosis, and Treatment, edited
by Alf Nachemson and Egon Jonsson.
Published by Lippincott Williams & Wilkins,
Philadelphia 2000.

14

Acute and Subacute Neck Pain: Nonsurgical Treatment

Karin Harms-Ringdahl* and Alf Nachemson†

*Departments of Physical Therapy and Rehabilitation Medicine, Karolinska Institute,
Stockholm, Sweden
†Department of Orthopaedics, Sahlgrenska University Hospital, Göteborg, Sweden

Numerous noninvasive treatments are used for acute and subacute neck pain. However, only a few of them have been evaluated in randomized controlled trials (RCT) or in clinically controlled studies, and these trials provide little evidence that one treatment method is more effective than another. This diversity probably results from a lack of understanding both of the pathophysiologic mechanisms of acute neck pain and of the reasons that the pain persists, in some cases, for 3 to 6 weeks. Acute and subacute neck disorders are conditions in which pain and pain-related decreased cervical range of motion are major problems. Thus, most studies use these outcome variables, and studies using outcome and/or screening variables reflecting disability and handicap (according to the 1980 World Health Organization definitions) are few. Although many different methods have been used to relieve pain, few have been documented in RCTs of patients aged 18 to 64 years who have with acute and subacute neck pain (lasting less than 12 weeks). Thus, many common treatment strategies in these patients encompass several pain-relieving methods on a trial-and-error base without an analysis of patients' characteristics, of the possible advantage of one method over another, and of the presence of relative contraindications to certain approaches. This practice makes it difficult to compare the various interventions used in different studies.

LITERATURE SEARCH

A literature search was carried out in the MEDLINE and CATS databases through December, 1997. The search was restricted to RCTs or review articles concerning the treatment of neck or cervical spinal pain or whiplash injuries and pain. Titles and abstracts were scrutinized, and studies concerning acute and subacute neck pain were included, as were some extensive review articles (1,10,11,13). Nonrandomized studies were excluded, as were articles not published in English. In addition, we excluded studies of patients with neck pain who also had an underlying known disease, such as rheumatoid arthritis, or infection. Studies including results for patients with undefined "neck *and/or* low back pain" and studies pooling results from patients with acute, subacute, and chronic neck pain were also excluded. Studies reporting results from patients with episodes of recurrent pain were included when the duration of the last episode of pain was less than 3 months. However, some studies were included in which it was clear that the patients' pain was considered by the authors to be mechanical in origin, provided the neck pain was acute or subacute or recurrent for the majority in the group, even if for a few patients the first episode had occurred more than 3 months earlier. To summarize, this chapter includes a discussion of conservative treatment of patients, aged 18 to 64 years, with acute or subacute neck pain. Patients were included independent of the proposed cause and symptoms of the neck pain as long as these patients were not considered candidates for operative treatment and/or the pain was not related to a systemic disease. Studies of patients in whom headache was the main focus were not included.

The studies were read applying the quality criteria, as described in Cochrane Collaboration Back Review Group (34) and shown in Table 1.4 in Chapter 1. The following grading system was used:

A. Strong evidence: support from metaanalysis or systematic review of good quality of two or more studies (RCTs).
B. Moderate evidence: provided by generally consistent findings in one high-quality RCT and one or more low-quality RCTs or by generally consistent findings in multiple low-quality RCTs.
C. Limited or contradictory evidence: only one RCT (of either high or low quality) or inconsistent findings in multiple RCTs.
D. Not studied or supported at all in scientific studies.

The term *positive outcome* was used when the experimental group showed significant improvement in outcome variables, compared with the control group. The term *indifferent results* was used when no difference was found, and *negative outcome* meant that the treatment group showed a significantly worse outcome than the control group. In the presentation, the treatment modalities found from the different RCTs are grouped in the following order:

• Spray and stretch (vapocoolant spray) (n = 1)
• Laser therapy (n = 1)
• Infrared light (n = 1)
• Electromagnetic therapy (n = 1)
• Transcutaneous electrical nerve stimulation (n = 1)
• Traction by equipment (n = 3)
• Cervical orthoses (n = 3)
• Exercise (stretching, strengthening, aerobic training, work hardening, aquatic, postural correction, neuromuscular control exercise, movement awareness) (n = 5)
• Manual therapy (including slow mobilization and fast manipulation techniques) (n = 5)
• Patient education (n = 2)
• Drug therapy (n = 1)

Because some studies compared two or three treatment modalities, the same study may be referred to twice. No RCTs included acupuncture treatment for acute or subacute neck pain.

Of the interventions listed here, it is only in the "exercise" group and in some forms of "patient education" that the patient is active and can be guided to self-care under supervision. The other therapies are passive with regard to patient participation, and most of those interventions need to be performed while a therapist is present. The economic consequences are discussed in Chapters 19 and 20.

Physical therapy is a topic within a profession and is not a treatment. The basic knowledge of physical therapists differs worldwide with regard to scientific matters and evidence-based treatment strategies. Many of the interventions mentioned earlier are included in those that, by cultural tradition, are provided by physical therapists (14). Thus, when "unspecified physical therapy" is used as a treatment modality in studies for the control group, any of the treatments listed earlier and combinations thereof may have been used, not only in different studies but also within the same study population. This situation has a grave impact on the power to detect significant differences among treatment modalities in several studies.

RESULTS

Review Articles

Gross et al. (10,11) and Aker et al. (1), in extensive, high-quality reviews, selected 25 RTCs for conservative management of mechanical neck disorders that met their inclusion criteria, which were similar to ours. However, they also included studies of patients with neck pain of more than 3 months' duration, not included in this chapter. According to Gross et al., additional 7 RCTs met their selection criteria, but they were multiple publications of the same patient groups. In general, the more detailed report was selected (1).

Among the 13 of the foregoing 25 RCTs discussed in the review by Gross et al. (11), 9 RCTs utilizing physical medicine or physical therapy modalities (except manual therapy) were included in this chapter (6,9,17,18,23–25,30,32). Eleven of these 13 RCTs were rated by Gross et al. (11) as moderately strong or better in terms of methodologic quality. In the metaanalysis by Aker et al. (1), 5 RCTs were combined, including patients with both acute and chronic neck pain. The conclusion was that there is too little research on effects of treatment modalities to "determine if therapies are of benefit, of no benefit or even harmful."

In their review of various forms of manual therapy, Gross et al. (10) included nine RCTs out of 25. One study overlapped with physical medicine modalities (23). Five of these RCTs had patients with acute or subacute neck pain and were included in the present study (4,5,21–23). Four of these RCTs were rated by Gross et al. (10) to have strong or moderately strong internal validity (4,5,22,23), and one was weak (21). In another high-quality review by Hurwitz et al. (13), the same studies, as well as one by Howe et al. (12), were included. In the study by Hurwitz et al. (13), only two of the studies included in the present chapter were considered to be of high quality (i.e., scored higher than 50 points out of possible 100 [5,16,34]), whereas three studies scored between 40 and 50 (4,12,23), and the remaining two studies (21,22) scored between 30 and 40. A metaanalysis of pooled effect size (10), not taking pain duration into account, indicated a moderate reduction in pain intensity (mean 16 points on a 100-point scale) after treatment when manual therapies were combined with other treatment modalities, as described later.

Treatment Modalities

Spray and Stretch (Vapocoolant Spray Followed by Passive Stretching)

In one controlled trial (30), no significant difference was noted between the active treatment technique and the placebo. Because the sample size was small, the results of this study must be interpreted with caution, and there is insufficient evidence about effectiveness of this treatment (level C).

Laser Therapy

One RCT used laser treatment for patients with subacute myofascial neck pain syndrome (32). Laser therapy did not reduce pain significantly. It is concluded that evidence about the effects of laser therapy is insufficient (level C).

Infrared Light

One RCT (17) studied the effect of infrared light compared with placebo (mock transcutaneous nerve stimulation) in a group of patients with cervical osteoarthrosis and neck pain with lasting more than 1 month. No significant treatment effect was reported. However, because of the small number of subjects included, the statistical power for the effect was low. The conclusion is that there is no evidence that infrared light has an effect on acute or subacute neck pain (level C).

Electromagnetic Therapy

In one small RCT (n = 40) (6), a pulsed electromagnetic therapy (PEMT) soft collar was used and was compared with a collar without PEMT. Patients in both groups were instructed to make neck movements each hour and were also prescribed antiinflammatory analgesics. The results indicated a significant short-term reduction of pain in the PEMT group after the first 2 and 4 weeks. After 12 weeks, when physical therapy treatments may have been included for both groups, there was no difference in pain but a small, clinical insignificant difference in range of motion and analgesic consumption. The theoretic basis for a possible effect by PEMT is not known. There is limited evidence that PEMT affects short-term analgesic intake and motion range in acute neck injuries. There is limited evidence that this treatment does not influence perceived pain intensity (level C). Because the effects of 2 weeks of soft collar wearing may be disadvantageous, studies are needed to compare soft collar and PEMT with no collar and advice to stay active.

Transcutaneous Electrical Nerve Stimulation

In one small RCT (23), transcutaneous electrical nerve stimulation was compared with a control treatment of collar, rest, education, and analgesics in patients with acute cervical pain. There was no significant difference in pain reduction between the groups (n = 10 in each group), but a difference was noted in the restoration of cervical mobility. Although the study was small, it indicated that transcutaneous electrical nerve stimulation may influence active pain-free range of motion in patients with acute cervical pain (level C).

Acupuncture

Two RCTs were found in which the effects of acupuncture were investigated: one versus placebo (25) and one versus traction combined with short-wave diathermy (19). However, both studies included patients with chronic pain (see Chapter 15). Thus, no studies have analyzed the effects of acupuncture in acute or subacute neck pain (level D).

Traction by Equipment

In one study (9), in which the statistical method was not reported, treatment using cervical traction was compared with postural advice and medication (analgesics and muscle relaxants), and the differences between groups were small. However, the population comprised patients with large differences in pain duration, and some of these patients had chronic pain. In another study in which a mixture of traction, exercise, and patient education was compared with collar and exercise, no significant treatment effect in pain or range of motion between the groups was reported. Time lost from work was significant and depended on the patients' social class.

Zylbergold and Piper (35) compared the efficacy of three commonly employed forms of traction in the treatment of cervical spine disorders with the efficacy of no traction. However, the patients were not homogeneous with regard to pain location and duration, and the short-term effects were absent after 6 weeks. Thus, there is limited evidence that cervical traction using equipment in addition to exercise is not effective (level C).

In a high-quality review (33) in which an older study (3) was also included, the investigators concluded that statistical power is often lacking because of small sample sizes, and no conclusions can be drawn about whether a specific traction modality is an effective therapy for neck pain.

Cervical Orthoses

In most studies that included patients with acute neck pain after a motor vehicle accident, *soft* collars were used for the first 14 days as a pain reliever in the standard treatment (8,20,22,24) or as the control treatment (6,23) (Table 14.1). Thus, the short-term use of collars was not included in the comparisons among interventions. However, in one RCT (8), patients with neck pain after a motor vehicle accident who were encouraged to wear a soft collar for the first 2 weeks were compared with those who were advised only to rest and to take analgesics. The results indicated that wearing a soft collar did not influence the duration or level of persistent pain in a positive way. A more active interventive approach enhancing activity and movements instead of prescribing rest and a collar seemed preferable (22). It is concluded that no studies indicated that soft collars had a positive effect on pain or a negative effect on mobility (level C).

In one study, published in 1998 (2) and thus not included in the search, the clinical outcome in two groups of patients with acute pain after whiplash injury was compared. One group received instructions to carry on as usual, whereas the other group of patients received a soft collar for 2 weeks and was certified as sick. Twenty-six weeks after inclusion in the study, there was a significantly better outcome for the "act-as-usual group" in terms of subjective symptoms, pain during daily activities, neck stiffness, memory and concentration, pain intensity, and headache. Thus, the results also indicated that when the use of soft collars was not combined with clear instructions to be physically active, these collars prolonged the episode of pain. Thus, limited evidence exists that orthoses lack effect on acute and subacute neck pain.

Exercise

Muscle training compared with stretching plus heat and massage (18) showed a significant difference in favor of the active exercise group after five treatments, at 3

TABLE 14.1. *Overview of studies, treatment modalities used for the treatment of acute or subacute neck pain, and their short-term and long-term effects*

Investigators (ref.)	Condition	Treatment	Effect parameters	Short-term outcome	Long-term outcome	Treatment compared
Brodin (4) (mixed pain duration)	Cervical pain, restricted cervical movements 36% <6 mo, the remainder longer	Manual mobilization (medication and neck school) (n = 23)	Pain intensity, cervical ROM	1 wk after conclusion of 3-wk treatment: positive for pain intensity and ROM	—	1. Medication (n = 23) 2. Medication, massage, electrical stimulation, traction, neck school (n = 17)
Cassidy et al. (5)	Mechanical neck pain of mixed duration	1. Manipulation (n = 52) 2. Mobilization (n = 48)	Pain intensity, ROM	5 min after treatment: positive both groups but 1 >2; however, 6% in both groups worse	—	—
Foley-Nolan et al. (6)	Acute whiplash injuries	Soft collar with PEMT 8 hr/d during 12 wk; antiinflammatory analgesics; advice to mobilize the neck 1/hr (n = 20)	Pain scores, movement scores, number of analgesics	2 and 4 wk: positive for pain and analgesics, no difference in movement scores	After 4 wk: patients not happy with progress referred to physical therapists 12 wk: indifferent for pain, positive but clinically small differences in movement scores and analgesics	Soft collar without PEMT; antiinflammatory analgesics; advice to mobilize the neck 1/hr (n = 20)
Friedrich et al. (7)	Neck muscle pain >6 wk	Neck exercises supervised during 8 sessions by a physical therapist (n = 47)	Quality of exercise performance, muscle status Pain relief	Positive	Lacking	Instructions from a brochure to exercise
Gennis et al. (8)	Acute neck pain after motor vehicle accident	Soft collar "as much as they could tolerate" for 2 wk; advice to rest and take analgesics	Degree of pain intensity, recovery, improvement, detorioration	—	6–10 wk after injury: no difference between groups	Advice to rest and take analgesics (n = 92)
Goldie and Landquist (9)	Cervical pain radiating into the arm, mixed pain duration (n = 73)	1. Isometric exercise 2. Intermittent traction	Neck mobility, overall improvement	Indifferent	24 wk after start: indifferent	Control
Howe et al. (12)	Neck, arm, or hand pain from cervical lesion with reduced ROM <4 wk (87%), previous attacks 81%	Rotational manipulations (1–3 treatments) and muscle relaxant medication (n = 21)	Pain intensity, ROM	Positive, immediate effect on pain and ROM, after 1 wk only on ROM	After 3 wk: indifferent on pain, positive for ROM	Muscle relaxant medication (Azapropazone) (n = 26)
Lewith (17)	Cervical osteoarthrosis: neck pain >1 mo	Infrared light (local heat)	Pain score, analgesics, sleep disturbance	Indifferent	—	Mock TNS
Levoska and Keinänen-Kiukaanniemi (18)	Recurrent neck and shoulder symptoms, including muscle tenderness of mixed duration (n = 47)	Physical therapy-guided muscle training	Neck muscle strength, isometric grip strength, shoulder endurance, tender points and pain thresholds, pain	After 5 treatments and after additional 4 wk, positive outcome	After 1 yr: positive outcome	1. Passive physiotherapeutic modalities (stretching, massage, and heat) 2. No treatment

Study	Condition	Treatment	Outcome measures	Result	Result (follow-up)	Control
McKinney et al. (21)	Acute <72 hr after whiplash	1. Active out patient physical therapy (n = 29) 2. Mobilization, advice (n = 30) 3. Two weeks rent + advice (n = 30)	Pain intensity, ROM	Positive: however, indifferent between 1 and 2	2 mo: positive; however, indifferent between 1 and 2	General advice about mobilization after a rest period of 10–14 d (n = 30); analgesics and neck collar given all three groups
Mealy et al. (22)	Acute whiplash injuries (emergency department)	Active treatment (n = 31) (ice first 24 hr thereafter Maitland mobilization and daily active exercises)	Pain intensity, ROM	After 4 wk: positive for pain intensity	After 8 wk: positive for pain intensity and ROM	Standard treatment (n = 30) (i.e., soft collar and advice to rest for 2 wk; thereafter gradual mobilization
Nordemar and Thörner (23)	Acute neck pain <3 d	TENS (n = 10)	Pain at rest and in motion, ROM	Positive ROM	—	Neck collar (n = 10)
Nordemar and Thörner (23)	Acute neck pain <3 d	Manual therapy (n = 10)	Pain at rest and in motion, ROM	Indifferent	—	Neck collar (n = 10)
Pennie and Agambar (24)	Acute neck pain after whiplash	Intermittent traction (10 min twice a wk), simple neck and shoulder exercises, traction (n = 61)	Pain intensity, mobility, time lost from work	Indifferent for mobility or pain intensity: time lost from work varied with social class (n = 128)	After 6–8 wk: patients who did not improve in the collar group referred to physical therapist	2-wk rest in neck collar, thereafter a program of active exercises (n = 74)
Provinciali et al. (26)	<2 mo after neck injury	Multimodal: postural training, manual techniques, and psychologic support (n = 30)	Pain intensity, ROM, self-rated treatment efficacy, return to work	30 d: indifferent for ROM, positive for pain intensity	6 mo: indifferent for ROM, positive for pain intensity, and return to work	Physical agents only, e.g., electrical and sonal modalities (n = 30)
Snow et al. (30)	Myofascial neck pain (n = 34 + 40)	Spray and stretch	—	Indifferent	—	Placebo, control
Takala et al. (31)	Frequent neck symptoms in an industry	Group gymnastics once/wk for 10 wk; crossover design (n = 22 + 13)	Pain intensity, localization, thresholds	Indifferent	Seasonal variation	Control not specified (n = 22 + 17)
Thorsén et al. (32)	Laboratory technicians with neck and shoulder tender points	Low lever laser therapy (n = 47)	Pain intensity, analgesics	Indifferent	—	Placebo
Zylbergold and Piper (35)	Cervical disorders, brachialgia included; mixed pain duration (n = 100)	Traction (static, intermittent, manual) twice/wk for 6 wk	Pain intensity (McGill Pain Questionnaire), ROM	Positive for 2 vs. 3, and vs. control for pain, forward flexion, right and left rotation	After 6 wk: Indifferent	Instructions, exercises, moist heat

PEMT, pulsed electromagnetic therapy; ROM, range of motion; TENS, transcutaneous electrical nerve stimulation; TNS, transcutaneous nerve stimulation.

months, and at the 1-year follow-up. Conversely, a randomized, crossover study with weekly group gymnastics for women who had recurrent neck pain in the workplace showed seasonal variation of neck pain, rather than an effect of intervention (31). Mealy et al. (22) compared active treatment comprising mobilization and exercises with a more passive intervention of soft collar and advice to rest in patients with an acute whiplash injury. A significant difference in range of motion and pain intensity was seen in favor of the active treatment.

Multimodal treatment (26) comprising postural training, manual techniques, and psychologic support was compared with the use of physical agents only, such as electrical and sonic modalities, in patients with subacute pain, who were included in the study within 2 months of a neck injury. Although there was no difference in range of motion, the multimodal-treatment group showed positive short-term and long-term effects of therapy, with a lower pain intensity level, higher self-rated treatment efficacy, and a faster return to work.

Thus, when one considers studies in which both mobilization and exercises were pooled and were compared with passive modalities, there is moderate evidence that active exercises are more efficacious than passive treatment modalities with massage, heat, and stretching (evidence level B). There may be a dosage problem because organized gymnastics given only once a week does not seem to influence pain intensity.

In a small study, comprising few patients (n = 17) with recent onset of neck complaint and simultaneous complaints of dizziness or vertigo (15), patients were randomized to physical therapy treatment or waiting-list control. The patients manifested significantly poorer postural control than did healthy subjects (n = 17). Physical therapy treatments including soft tissue treatment, stabilization exercises of the trunk and cervical spine, passive and active mobilization, relaxation techniques, home training programs, and minor ergonomic changes at work significantly reduced neck pain, intensity of dizziness, and postural performance. Although the study was too small to be conclusive, it showed the complexity of patient-perceived problems and their treatments.

Manual Therapy

In only one study (23) was manual therapy used alone, in a trial of manual mobilization versus cervical collar plus rest and patient education. There were no significant effects compared with the control treatment. However, because each group had only ten study subjects, the statistical power was low.

One RCT (21) of patients with acute neck sprains after traffic accidents showed no difference between a group receiving instructions and advice from a physical therapist about mobilizing exercises after a 2-week rest period and another group having physical therapy treatments including combinations of hot and cold applications, short-wave diathermy, hydrotherapy, traction and active and passive manual repetitive movements, instructions about posture, and home exercises. However, both groups were significantly improved compared with a group who only were given general advice about increasing mobilization after an initial rest period of 2 weeks.

Mealy et al. (22) showed that, in patients with acute whiplash injury, early treatment that combined manual therapy with active exercises had a positive outcome for pain intensity and, after 8 weeks, for cervical range of motion as well, compared with the standard treatment of advice to rest and the use of a soft collar for 2 weeks before gradually increasing movement.

A regimen of manual mobilization plus education and analgesics was compared with a regimen of massage plus electrotherapy, traction, and analgesics (4). Mobilization therapy decreased pain statistically better than massage therapy when mobilization was used in combination with other treatment modalities.

In one study (5), the immediate effects (defined as 5 minutes after treatment) of high-velocity manual manipulation versus low-velocity manual mobilization on pain and range of motion in the cervical spine were compared in a group of patients with a history of mechanical neck pain, lasting from 1 week to more than 6 months, that radiated to the trapezius muscle. Both techniques gave the same increase in range of motion and improved to the same intensity level (mean, 20.5/100).

Different specific subtypes of mobilization techniques were also used in the other studies mentioned earlier. For example, Mealey et al. (22) used Maitland mobilization techniques, Nordemar and Thörner (23) used static muscle work followed by passive rotations, and McKinney et al. (21) used Maitland and McKensey mobilization techniques.

At the 1-year follow-up in a later study published in 1998 (29), there was no difference in treatment outcome or recurrence rate for patients seeking primary health care for neck problems when these patients were randomized to treatment by a chiropractor or a physical therapist. However, the duration of neck pain seemed to influence the effects of the treatments provided by the two professional groups.

It is concluded that evidence about the effect of manual therapy (mobilization, manipulation, massage) when used alone and when compared with other treatments is insufficient (level C). However, when manual therapy is used in combinations with other, active treatment modalities, there is moderate evidence that some patient groups may benefit from mobilizing techniques as part of an activating program (evidence level B). Shekelle and Coulter (28) reported, in a consensus-type summary from a multidisciplinary expert panel, on the clinical characteristics of those patients with neck pain who are most likely to benefit from spinal manipulation.

Patient Education

In patients with acute pain related to whiplash injury (21), one group had physical therapeutic treatment comprising a combination of cold or heat application, hydrotherapy, traction, and active and passive repetitive movements using the principles of McKenzie and Maitland, in addition to instructions about postures and exercises to do at home. Another group received verbal and written reinforcing instructions on posture correction, use of analgesics and collars, use of heat sources, and muscle relaxation. This latter group was also encouraged to perform mobilizing exercises, which were also demonstrated and practiced. After 1 or 2 months, respectively, there was no difference in pain intensity and range of motion between the groups. However, both groups showed short-term and long-term benefits compared with a control group who only received analgesics, a cervical collar, and general advice to rest for the first 10 to 14 days (21).

The effect of brochure use versus physical therapist–guided teaching on neck muscular pain for more than 6 weeks was compared in 87 patients regarding performance of therapeutic exercise (7). The quality of exercise performance at follow-up correlated both with muscle status improvement and pain relief, as did muscle status improvement with pain relief. The pain relief was significant greater in the group of patients who received eight sessions of physical therapy–guided exercises, compared with those who received the instructions and a brochure at a single session.

It is concluded that there is moderate evidence that supervised instructions about home exercises and possibilities to stay active improve patient compliance compared with a brochure (level B). However, there is limited evidence that patient education as such can help to relieve acute or subacute pain (level C).

Drug Therapy

No RCTs published in English were found in which drug therapy was compared with placebo drugs in patients with acute or subacute neck pain. However, in a small study published in German (27) on the effects on patient-assessed pain, increased range of motion, and global activity, respectively, 20 patients seeking hospital treatment for acute neck pain were randomized to a group treated with tetrazepam or a group given placebo medication. Both groups were instructed to use paracetamol in addition if needed. After 3 and 7 days, there were significant differences between the groups in favor of those treated with tetrazepam.

It is concluded that there is insufficient evidence (level C) that pain relievers can relieve acute or subacute neck pain. There exists, however, an abundant literature on nonsteroidal antiinflammatory drugs for the treatment of acute low back pain, with strong evidence (level A) of pain relief (see Chapter 11).

SUMMARY AND CONCLUSIONS

There is support in the literature that staying active (i.e., to continue or return to usual activities as early as possible) reduces pain and decreases the consequences of acute neck pain (evidence level B). Painkillers and/or cervical collars should only be used for a limited period, to enable patients to perform physical activity. There is moderate evidence that mobilization techniques, when combined with other treatment modalities, helps to improve range of motion and to reduce pain faster than no treatment (level B). There is also moderate evidence that active exercises are more effective than passive treatments such as massage, heat, traction, and stretching (level B). Only one short-term study indicated that PEMT may reduce pain and may increase range of motion. Possible adverse effects of this therapy, which entails wearing a soft collar for 2 weeks, were not analyzed. There are no studies in which effects of acupuncture for acute or subacute neck pain are analyzed. Although some evidence indicates that patient-guided instructions enhance compliance, there is no evidence that patient education as such reduces pain (level C). RCTs are missing that analyze the influence of a therapist's reassuring attitude in combination with different treatment modalities (level D).

There is obviously a great need for more scientific studies in this area of increasing clinical and socioeconomic importance. The lack of strong or even moderate evidence for all the passive modalities currently used for acute or subacute neck pain should constitute an immediate challenge for the practitioners of these methods. In addition, those paying for these modalities should have wanted such studies to be performed.

REFERENCES

1. Aker PD, Gross AR, Goldsmith, CH et al. Conservative management of mechanical neck pain: systematic overview and metaanalysis. *BMJ* 1996;313:1291–1296.

2. Borchgrevink GE, Kaasa A, McDonagh D, et al. Acute treatment of whiplash neck sprain injuries. *Spine* 1998;23:2531.
3. British Association of Physical Medicine. Pain in the neck and arm: a multicentre trial of the effects of physiotherapy. *BMJ* 1966;1:253–258.
4. Brodin H. Cervical pain and mobilization. *Manual Med* 1985;2:1822.
5. Cassidy JD, Lopes AA, Yong-Hing K. The immediate effect of manipulation versus mobilization on pain and range of motion in the cervical spine: a randomized controlled trial. *J Manipulative Physiol Ther* 1992;15:570–575.
6. Foley-Nolan D, Moore K, Codd M, et al. Low energy high frequency pulsed electromagnetic therapy for acute whiplash injury. *Scand J Rehabil Med* 1992;24:51–59.
7. Friedrich M, Cermak T, Maderbacher P. The effect of brochure use versus therapist teaching on patients performing therapeutic exercise and changes in impairment status. *Phys Ther* 1996;76:1082–1088.
8. Gennis P, Miller L, Gallagher EJ, et al. The effect of soft cervical collars on persistent neck pain in patients with whiplash injury. *Acad Emerg Med* 1996;3:568–573.
9. Goldie I, Landquist A. Evaluation of the effects of different forms of physiotherapy in the cervical pain. *Scand J Rhabil Med* 1970;2–3:117–121.
10. Gross AR, Aker PD, Quartly C. Manual therapy in the treatment of neck pain. *Rheum Dis Clin North Am* 1996;22:579–598.
11. Gross AR, Aker PD, Goldsmith CH, et al. Conservative management of mechanical neck disorders: a systematic overview and meta-analysis. *Online J Curr Clin Trials* 1996;doc. no. 200–201.
12. Howe DH, Newcombe RG, Wade MT. Manipulation of the cervical spine: a pilot study. *J R Coll Gen Pract* 1982;33:574–579.
13. Hurwitz EL, Aker PD, Adam AH, et al. Manipulation and mobilization of the cervical spine: a systematic review of the literature. *Spine* 1996;21:1746–1760.
14. Jette DU, Jette AM. Physical therapy and health outcomes in patients with spinal impairments. *Phys Ther* 1996;76:930–945.
15. Karlberg M, Magnusson M, Malmstrom EM, et al. Postural and sympotomatic improvement after physiotherapy in patients with dizziness of suspected cervical origin. *Arch Phys Med Rehabil* 1996;77:874–882.
16. Koes BW, Bouter LM, van Mameren H, et al. Randomised clinical trial of manipulative therapy and physiotherapy for persistent back and neck complaints: results of one year follow-up. *BMJ* 1992:304:601–605.
17. Lewith GT. A randomised trial to evaluate the effect of infra-red stimulation of local trigger points, versus placebo, on the pain caused by cervical osteoarthrosis. *Acupunct Electrother Res* 1981;6:277–284.
18. Levoska S, Keinänen-Kiukaanniemi S. Active or passive physiotherapy for occupational cervicobrachial disorders? A comparison of two treatment methods with a 1-year follow-up. *Arch Phys Med Rehabil* 1993;74:425–430.
19. Loy TT. Treatment of cervical spondylosis: electroacupuncture versus physiotherapy. *Med J Aust* 1983;2:32–34.
20. McKinney LA. Early mobilisation and outcome in acute sprains of the neck. *BMJ* 1989;299:1006–1008.
21. McKinney LA, Dornam JO, Ryan M. The role of physiotherapy in the management of acute neck sprains following road traffic accidents. *Arch Emerg Med* 1989;6:27–33.
22. Mealy K, Brennan H, Fenelon GC. Early mobilisation of acute whiplash injuries. *BMJ* 1986;292:656–657.
23. Nordemar R, Thörner C. Treatment of acute cervical pain: a comparative study. *Pain* 1981;10:93–101.
24. Pennie BH, Agambar LJ. Whiplash injuries. A trial of early management. *J Bone Joint Surg Br* 1990;72:277–279.
25. Petrie JP, Hazleman BL. A controlled study of acupuncture in neck pain. *Br J Rheumatol* 1986;25:271–275.
26. Provinciali L, Baroni M, Illuminati L, et al. Multimodal treatment to prevent the late whiplash syndrome. *Scand J Rehabil Med* 1996;28:105–111.
27. Salzmann E, Wiedemann O, Lo L, et al. Tetrazepam in the treatment of acute cervical syndrome: randomized double-blind pilot study comparing tetrazam and placebo. *Fortschr Med* 1993;111:544–548.
28. Shekelle PG, Coulter I. Cervical spine manipulation: summary report of a systematic review of the literature and a multidisciplinary expert panel. *J Spinal Disord* 1997;10:223–228.
29. Skargren EI, Carlsson PG, Oberg BE. One-year follow-up comparison of the cost and effectiveness of chiropractic and physiotherapy as primary management for back pain: subgroup analysis, recurrence, and additional health care utilization. *Spine* 1998;23:1875–1883.
30. Snow CJ, Arves Wood R, Dowhopoluk V, et al. Randomized controlled clinical trial of spray and stretch for relief of back and neck myofascial pain. *Physiother Can* 1992;44:S8.
31. Takala EP, Viikari-Juntura E, Tynkkynen EM. Does group gymnastics at the workplace help in neck pain? A controlled study. *Scand J Rehabil Med* 1994;26:17–20.

32. Thorsén H, Gam AN, Svensson BH, et al. Low level laser therapy for myofascial pain in the neck and shoulder girdle: a double blind, cross over study. *Scand J Rheumatol* 1992;21:139–141.
33. van der Heijden, Beurskens AJ, Koes BW, et al. The efficacy of traction for back and neck pain: a systematic, blinded review of randomized clinical trial methods. *Phys Ther* 1995;75:93–104.
34. van Tulder MW, Koes BW, Bouter LM, et al. Method guidelines for systematic reviews in the Cochrane Collaboration Back Review Group for Spinal Disorders. *Spine* 1997;22:2323–2330.
35. Zylbergold RS, Piper MC. Cervical spine disorders: a comparison of three types of traction. *Spine* 1985;10:867–871.

Neck and Back Pain: The Scientific Evidence of Causes, Diagnosis, and Treatment, edited by Alf Nachemson and Egon Jonsson. Published by Lippincott Williams & Wilkins, Philadelphia 2000.

15

Nonsurgical Treatment of Chronic Neck Pain

Maurits W. van Tulder*, Mariëlle Goossens†, and Jan Hoving*

*Institute for Research in Extramural Medicine, Vrije Universiteit, van der Boechorststraat 7, Amsterdam, Netherlands
†Institute for Rehabilitation Research, Hoensbroek, Netherlands*

In this chapter, the effectiveness of the most common therapeutic interventions for chronic neck pain is evaluated. This chapter should answer the following questions:

Which interventions are the most effective in the treatment of chronic neck pain with and without radiation?
Are these interventions more effective than placebo, no treatment, or other conservative treatments (including other drugs)?
Are these interventions effective regarding relevant outcome measures, that is, overall improvement, functional status, return to work, pain intensity, or pain behavior?
Are these interventions effective in the short and/or long term?

The information provided in this chapter may be useful in the development of evidence-based guidelines for general practitioners, physical therapists, or other primary health care professionals.

METHODS

Selection of Studies

We used the results of an extensive literature search conducted by Gross et al. (13) for their review on neck pain. Their search included several computerized databases, manual searches of selected journals, reference checking, and information requests from authors to identify published and unpublished studies up to December 1993.

Additionally, we searched the MEDLINE and EMBASE databases from 1994 through July 1998 and used a highly sensitive search strategy for MEDLINE and for EMBASE developed by the Cochrane Center in the United Kingdom. Subsequently, the references given in relevant identified publications (randomized controlled trials [RCTs] and reviews) were further examined (2,12,15,29,34). We reviewed the titles and abstracts of the identified articles to determine the relevance of the articles for our systematic review. When there was any doubt, the article was retrieved and read. Abstracts were not selected.

A study was included if it met the following criteria:

1. It concerned a true RCT; trials with quasirandom procedures such as alternate allocation or allocation based on dates of birth were excluded.
2. The treatment regimen consisted of a conservative type of intervention.
3. The results, exclusively or separately, concerned patients with chronic neck pain.
4. The article was published in English.

Chronic neck pain was defined as neck persisting for 12 weeks or more. Studies were included if they reported on a mix of patients with subacute (6 to 12 weeks) and chronic neck pain. Studies were excluded if they reported on patients with acute (6 weeks or less) neck pain or on a mix of patients with acute and chronic neck pain.

Methodologic Quality of the Studies

All trials were scored according to the criteria listed in Table 15.1. The criteria are based on generally accepted principles of intervention research and refer to various aspects of study population, description of interventions, outcome measurements, and data presentation and analysis. A weight was attached to each criterion, resulting in a maximum score of 100 points for each study. The methodologic quality of the RCTs was assessed by two independent reviewers (Maurits van Tulder and Mariëlle Goossens). Disagreements between the two reviewers were resolved by consensus. The assessments resulted in a hierarchic list in which higher scores indicate studies of higher methodologic quality (Table 15.2).

TABLE 15.1. *Criteria for the methodologic assessment of randomized clinical trials of therapeutic interventions for chronic neck pain*

	Study population
A	Homogeneity
B	Comparability of relevant baseline characteristics
C	Randomization procedure adequate
D	Dropouts described for each study group separately
E	<20% loss to follow-up
	<10% loss to follow-up
F	>50 subjects in the smallest group
	>100 subjects in the smallest group
	Interventions
G	Interventions standardized and described
H	Placebo controlled
I	Pragmatic study/control group adequated[a]
J	Cointerventions avoided
K	Compliance measured and satisfactory in all study groups
	Effect
L	Patients blinded
M	Outcome measures relevant
N	Blinded outcome assessment
O	Follow-up period adequate
	Data presentation and analysis
P	Intention-to-treat analysis
Q	Frequencies of most important outcomes presented for each treatment group

[a] Criterion I was defined as pragmatic study for randomized controlled trials (RCTs) of therapeutic interventions for which a placebo treatment was feasible (i.e., drug therapies, manipulation); criterion I was defined as control group adequate for RCTs of therapeutic interventions for which a placebo treatment was less feasible (i.e., exercise therapy and behavioral therapy).

TABLE 15.2. *Randomized controlled trials on the effectiveness of various types of interventions in chronic neck pain in order of methodologic score*

							Scores for methodologic criteria											
Investigators (ref.)	A 2	B 5	C 4	D 3	E 4	F 12	G 10	H 5	I 5	J 5	K 5	L 5	M 10	N 10	O 5	P 5	Q 5	Score 100
Muscle relaxants																		
Thomas et al. (31)	0	5	0	3	4	0	10	5	0	5	5	5	2	2	0	5	5	56
Basmajian et al. (4)	0	0	0	0	4	0	10	5	0	0	0	5	8	8	0	5	0	45
Steroid injections																		
Barnsley et al. (3)	2	3	2	3	4	0	10	0	5	5	5	5	2	2	0	5	5	58
Castagnera et al. (6)	2	4	0	3	4	0	10	0	5	0	5	0	4	0	5	5	5	52
Stav et al. (30)	1	4	0	3	2	0	10	0	5	0	5	0	6	2	5	0	5	48
Manual therapy																		
Koes et al. (18–21)	1	3	2	3	2	0	10	5	5	0	0	5	4	4	0	0	5	53
Jordan et al. (17)	2	4	2	3	2	0	10	0	5	0	5	0	8	2	5	0	5	53
Sloop et al. (28)	1	2	2	3	4	0	0	0	0	0	5	5	8	8	0	5	0	43
Physical therapy																		
Persson et al. (24,25)	2	4	4	3	4	0	10	0	5	0	0	0	8	0	5	5	5	55
Koes et al. (18–21)	1	3	2	3	2	0	10	5	5	0	0	5	4	4	0	0	5	53
Levoska and Keinänen-Kiukaanniemi (23)	1	1	0	3	4	0	10	0	5	5	5	0	4	0	5	5	5	53
Jordan et al. (17)	2	3	2	3	2	0	10	0	5	0	5	0	8	2	5	0	5	52
Vesseljen et al. (35)	1	2	0	3	4	0	10	0	5	0	5	0	6	0	5	5	5	51
Behavioral therapy																		
Jensen et al. (16)	1	2	0	0	0	0	10	0	5	5	5	0	8	0	5	0	5	46
Acupuncture																		
Thomas et al. (31)	0	5	0	3	4	0	10	5	0	5	5	5	2	2	0	5	5	56
Petrie and Hazleman (26)	1	3	0	3	4	0	10	0	0	0	0	5	8	8	0	0	5	52
Coan et al. (8)	1	5	4	3	4	0	0	0	0	0	5	0	6	0	0	5	5	38
Traction																		
Goldie and Landquist (11)	2	3	2	3	4	0	10	0	5	5	0	0	4	0	0	5	5	48
Neck collar																		
Persson et al. (24,25)	2	4	4	3	4	0	10	0	5	0	0	0	8	0	5	5	5	55
Pillows																		
Lavin et al. (22)	1	5	0	0	2	0	10	0	5	5	0	0	6	0	0	0	0	34
Laser therapy																		
Thorsen et al. (32)	1	5	0	3	4	0	10	5	0	5	0	5	4	4	0	0	5	51
Ceccherelli et al. (7)	1	3	0	3	4	0	10	5	0	0	0	5	2	2	0	5	5	45
(Electro)magnetic therapy																		
Trock et al. (33)	2	2	4	0	2	0	10	5	0	0	5	5	8	8	0	5	5	59
Foley-Nolan et al. (10)	1	2	4	3	4	0	10	5	0	0	5	5	6	6	0	5	0	56
Hong et al. (14)	0	1	0	0	4	0	10	5	0	0	0	5	2	2	0	5	5	39
Proprioceptive exercises																		
Fitz-Ritzon (9)	1	2	2	3	4	0	10	0	5	0	0	5	2	2	0	5	5	47
Revel et al. (27)	1	3	0	0	0	0	5	0	0	5	0	0	6	0	0	0	5	25

Outcome of the Studies

We extracted the main results from each study according to the most important patient-centered outcome measures: pain intensity, overall improvement, functional status, and return to work. A study was considered positive when the therapeutic intervention was statistically significantly more effective than the reference treatment with regard to at least one of these outcome measures (results section of Table 15.3). A study was considered negative when the investigators reported no differences between the intervention under study and the reference treatment on these outcome

TABLE 15.3. *Characteristics of randomized controlled trials on the effectiveness of conservative treatment for chronic neck pain*

Investigators (ref.)	Disorder	Index treatment (I)	Reference treatment (R)	Results
			Muscle relaxants	
Thomas et al. (31)	Chronic cervical osteoarthritis	I1: diazepam: one dose of 5 mg (orally) (n = 44) I2: acupuncture: experienced acupuncturist, traditional meridian, manual stimulation, Teh Chi, 7 points, 40 min (n = 44)	R1: placebo diazepam (orally) (n = 44) R2: placebo-acupuncture: needles were inserted superficially and left without eliciting any further sensation, 40 min (n = 44)	Mean (SD) affective pain score (VAS 10 cm) before and after treatment: I1, 3.0 (0.8), 2.2 (1.0); I2, 3.5 (1.2), 2.3 (1.5); R1, 2.7 (1.0), 2.2 (1.0); R2, 3.1 (1.1), 2.4 (1.2). Mean (SD) sensory pain score (VAS 10 cm) before and after treatment: I1, 1.9 (0.7), 1.6 (0.7); I2, 2.5 (0.8), 1.8 (1.2); R1, 1.9 (0.8), 1.7 (1.0); R2, 2.0 (0.9), 1.6 (1.1). I2 significantly better than R1, but not than I1 or R2
Basmajian (4)	Chronic muscle spasm	I: cyclobenzaprine hydrochloride, 10 mg, 1 tbl 3 times daily, 2 wk, dosage increased to 5 tbl daily if necessary, dosage decreased if adverse reactions (n = 27)	R: placebo, 1 tbl 3 times daily, 2 wk (n = 28)	I significantly larger decrease in muscle spasm and pain after 2 wk; no data presented
			Steroid injections	
Barnsley et al. (3)	Whiplash	I: corticosteroid injection: intraarticular (1 mL injection with betamethasone 5.7 mg in the cervical zygapophyseal joints), 1 or 2 injections (n = 21)	R: local anaesthetic injection (1 mL injection with bupivacaine 0.5% in cervical zygapophyseal joints) (n = 20)	No difference in return of pain, I 3 d, R 3.5 d; pain relief, severity of pain, McGill Pain Questionnaire and psychologic symptoms checklist: no results presented
Castagnera et al. (6)	Chronic cervical radicular pain	I: injection with solution of steroid (0.5% lidocaine with 10 mg/mL triamcinoline acetonide) and morphine (2.5 mg morphine sulfate) (n = 10)	R: injection with steroid (0.5% lidocaine with 10 mg/mL triamcinoline acetonide); the dose of triamcinoline acetonide was volume-dependent (n = 14)	Number of patients with good, excellent, or complete pain relief after 1 day, 1, 3, 6, 8, 12 mo: I, 10, 8, 8, 8, 8; R, 13, 10, 11, 11, 11; no differences; no differences in medical treatment or return to work
Stav et al. (30)	Chronic degenerative disc disease and/or osteoarthritis	I: injection with methylprednisolone (80 mg–2 mL) and lidocaine (1%–5 mL) into cervical epidural space (C5-6 or C6-7), 1–3 injections, 2-wk interval (n = 25)	R: injection with (80 mg–2 mL) methylprednisolone and lidocaine (1%–5 mL) into posterior neck muscles, 1–3 injections, 2-wk interval (n = 17)	Percentage of patients with very good and good pain relief after 1 wk and 1 yr: I, 76%, 68%; R, 35%, 12%; significant; recovery of capacity for work after 1 wk and 1 yr: I, 69%, 61%; R, 13%, 16%; significant; daily dose of analgesics after 1 wk and 1 yr: I, 82%, 64%; R, 9%, 9%; significant; ROM also significantly more improved after 1 wk and 1 yr in I, 80%, 69%, than in R, 40%, 14%; no complications of epidural injections

			Manual therapy	
Koes et al. (18–21)	Chronic nonspecific neck complaints	I: manual therapy: manipulation and mobilization, maximum 3 mo (n = 13)	R1: physical therapy: exercises, massage, modalities, maximum 3 mo (n = 21) R2: continued treatment by GP, maximum 3 mo (n = 16) R3: detuned short-wave diathermy (10 min) and detuned ultrasound, (10 min), twice/wk, 6 wk (n = 14)	Mean score on severity of main complaint (10-point NRS; blinded outcome assessor) at baseline and after 3, 6, and 12 wk: I, 7.15, 4.50, 3.23, 2.09; R1, 7.29, 4.85, 3.43, 3.30; R2, 7.19, 5.77, 4.85, 3.31; R3, 7.21, 5.18, 3.75, 1.90; Mean (SD) score on physical functioning (10-point NRS; blinded outcome assessor) at baseline and after 3, 6, and 12 wk: I, 6.11, 3.34, 2.22, 1.20; R1, 5.61, 3.86, 2.95, 2.52; R2, 5.29, 4.20, 2.84, 2.86; R3, 5.71, 3.68, 2.12, 1.26
Jordan et al. (17)	Chronic nonspecific neck pain	I: manipulation by chiropractor: high-velocity, low-amplitude spinal manipulation of the apophyseal joints of the cervical spine, manual traction, instruction, education, 15–20 min, twice/wk, 6 wk (n = 40)	R1: intensive training: stretching, isometric strengthening, instruction, education, ergonomic advice, 60–75 min, twice/wk, 6 wk (n = 40) R2: physical therapy: individual treatment plan, active and passive, hot packs, massage, ultrasound, manual traction, exercise, ergonomic advice, education, 30 min, twice/wk, 6 wk (n = 39)	Median (90% CI) pain level at baseline, and after 6 wk (posttreatment) and 4 and 12 mo: I, 13 (10–15), 6 (4–7), 6 (5–8), 6 (6–8); R1, 12 (10–15), 6 (3–9), 4 (3–10), 6 (4–9); R2, 12 (10–15), 6 (3–8), 4 (3–10), 8 (6–11); median (90% CI) disability level at baseline, and after 6 wk and 4 and 12 mo: I, 8 (7–10), 4 (4–5), 6 (4–7), 5 (3–6); R1, 8 (7–10), 5 (4–7), 5 (3–7), 5 (4–7); R2, 9 (8–11), 4 (3–6), 5 (3–8), 6 (4–7); median (90% CI) patient's perceived effect posttreatment and after 4 and 12 mo: I, 2 (1–5), 3 (1–5), 3 (1–4); R1, 2 (1–4), 3 (1–4), 3 (1–4); R2, 2 (1–4), 3 (1–4), 3 (1–4); median (90% CI) doctor's global assessment posttreatment: I, 2 (1–4); R1, 2 (1–4); R2, 2 (1–4); no differences.
Sloop et al. (28)	Chronic cervical spondylosis or chronic nonspecific neck pain	I: manipulation after amnesic dose of 20 mg diazepam IV by rheumatologist experienced in manipulation techniques, 1 session (n = 21)	R: placebo: amnesic dose of 20 mg diazepam IV (n = 18)	Number of patients (%) improved after 3 wk: I, 12 (57%); R, 18 (28%); not significant; mean (SD) improvement in pain intensity (VAS) after 3 wk: I, 5 (32); R, 18 (31); not significant; no differences in ROM and ADLs
Persson et al. (24,25)	Cervical root compression	I: physical therapy: exercises, instructions, manual traction, mobilization, heat therapy, relaxation exercises, 15 sessions, 30–45 min, 3 mo (n = 27)	Physical therapy R1: cervical collar: patients chose the most comfortable, shoulder-resting, rigid collar during daytime, soft collar at night if wanted, 3 mo (n = 27) R2: surgery: anterior cervical decompression and fusion technique, posterior approach in one patient (n = 27)	Mean worst pain intensity last week (VAS) pretreatment, after 14–16 wk, after 12 mo: I, 70, 51, 53; R1, 68, 64, 52; R2, 72, 43, 42; mean present pain intensity last week (VAS) pretreatment, after 14–16 wk, after 12 mo: I, 50, 41, 39; R1, 49, 48, 35; R2, 47, 27, 30; after 14–16 wk, R2 significantly better than R1; after 14–16 wk I and R2 significantly better in overall SIP score than R1; no differences after 12 mo; after 14–16 wk, R2 significantly better postural performance than I and R1.

continued

TABLE 15.3. Continued

Investigators (ref.)	Disorder	Index treatment (I)	Reference treatment (R)	Results
Koes et al. (18–21)	Chronic nonspecific neck complaints	I: physical therapy: exercises, massage, modalities, maximum 3 mo (n = 21)	R1: manipulation/mobilization, max 3 mo (n = 13) R2: continued treatment by GP, maximum 3 mo (n = 16) R3: detuned short-wave diathermy (10 min) and detuned ultrasound (10 min), twice/wk, 6 wk (n = 14)	Mean score on severity of main complaint (10-point NRS; blinded outcome assessor) at baseline and after 3, 6, and 12 wk: I, 7.29, 4.85, 3.45, 3.30; R1, 7.15, 4.50, 3.23, 2.09; R2, 7.19, 5.77, 4.85, 3.31; R3, 7.21, 5.18, 3.75, 1.90; mean (SD) score on physical functioning (10-point NRS; blinded outcome assessor) at baseline and after 3, 6, and 12 wk: I, 5.61, 3.86, 2.95, 2.52; R1, 6.11, 3.34, 2.22, 1.20; R2, 5.29, 4.20, 2.84, 2.86; R3, 5.71, 3.68, 2.12, 1.26
Levoska and Keinänen-Kiukaaniemi (23)	Occupational cervicobrachial disorders	I: active physical therapy: stretching, dynamic muscle training and daily 10-min home exercise program, 60 min, 3 times/wk, total of 15 visits (n = 22)	R: passive physical therapy: surface heat 20 min, massage 20 min, light stretching, physical exercises for neck and shoulder 20 min, 3 times/wk, total of 15 visits (n = 22)	No. of patients with neck-shoulder pain baseline, posttreatment, after 3 and 12 mo: I, 18, 2, 16, 14; R, 21, 5, 19, 18; duration of symptom-free period, no differences; no differences between I and R on no. of painful points, and muscle tone; strength: maximal isometric forces and endurance forces, maximal isometric muscle strength, and endurance force of shoulder muscles improved significantly in I, maximal isometric extension force significantly increased in R
Jordan et al. (17)	Chronic nonspecific neck pain	I: physical therapy: individual treatment plan, active and passive, hot packs, massage, ultrasound, manual traction, exercise, ergonomic advice, education, 30 min, twice/wk, 6 wk (n = 39)	R1: intensive training: stretching, isometric strengthening, instruction, education, ergonomic advice, 60–75 min, twice/wk, 6 wk (n = 40) R2: manipulation by chiropractor: high-velocity, low-amplitude spinal manipulation of the cervical spine, manual traction, instruction, education, 15–20 min, twice/wk, 6 wk (n = 40)	Median (90% CI) pain level at baseline, and after 6 wk (posttreatment) and 4 and 12 mo: I, 12 (10–15), 6 (3–8), 4 (3–10), 8 (6–11); R1, 12 (10–15), 6 (3–9), 4 (3–10), 6 (4–9); R2, 13 (10–15), 6 (4–7), 6 (5–8), 6 (6–8); median (90% CI) disability level at baseline, and after 6 wk, and 4 and 12 mo: I, 9 (8–11), 4 (3–6), 5 (3–8), 6 (4–7); R1, 8 (7–10), 5 (4–7), 5 (3–7), 5 (4–7); R2, 8 (7–10), 4 (4–5), 6 (4–7), 5 (3–6); median (90% CI) patient's perceived effect posttreatment and after 4 and 12 mo: I, 2 (1–4), 3 (1–4), 3 (1–4); R1, 2 (1–4), 3 (1–4); R2, 2 (1–5), 3 (1–5), 3 (1–4); median (90% CI) doctor's global assessment posttreatment: I, 2 (1–4); R1, 2 (1–4); R2, 2 (1–4) no differences

Source	Condition	Intervention	Results
Vasseljen et al. (35)	Work-related neck and shoulder pain	I: individual physical therapy: in a clinic; massage (5–10 min), strength and flexibility exercises (20–30 min), stretching (3–4 min), weight training on apparatus (5–10 min), passive mobilization when indicated, education (ergonomics), and written instructions (home exercises), 1 h, 2 times/wk, total of 10 treatments (n = 12) R: group exercises: group sessions at the workplace, 4 arm exercises with 1.1-kg dumbbells (10 reps, 3 times), exercises for abdomen, back and breathing, stretching for neck and shoulder, education (ergonomics), and written instructions (home exercises), 30 min, 3 times/wk, 6 wk (n = 12)	Mean pain intensity (VAS) and perceived general tension (VAS) before and after treatment similar for I and R; mean (95% CI) pain intensity (VAS) after 6 mo: I, 2.4 (0.4–3.9); R, 2.9 (0.2–4.1); not significant; mean (95% CI) general tension (VAS) after 6 mo: I, 3.8 (1.8–6.7); R, 5.0 (1.8–5.6); not significant; number (%) of patients improved (much better or pain free) after treatment and after 6 mo: I, 9 (75%); R, 2 (17%), 3 (25%); no significant differences in muscle activity between I and R
Jensen et al. (16)	Chronic neck and shoulder pain	Behavioral therapy I: inpatient program including physical fitness, improving health behavior and develop plans to return to work and a psychologic intervention in groups: MMCBT given directly by psychologist to patients, 3 hr/wk for 5 wk, follow-up by telephone for 6 mo (n = 29) R: inpatient program including physical fitness, improving health behavior and develop plans to return to work and coaching of involved health care professionals by a psychologist: approach of MMCBT with psychologist functioning as a coach to other health professionals, 5 wk (n = 37)	Mean (SD) pain intensity (VAS) pretreatment, posttreatment, and after 6 mo: I, 51.6 (20.6), 42.4 (22.7), 48.5 (23.2); R, 52.2 (16.8), 45.0 (17.2), 45.2 (13.5); disability (Stanford Health Assessment Questionnaire): I, 24.1 (9.1), 27.0 (10.6), 25.6 (11.2); R, 27.1 (7.7), 30.1 (11.3), 26.2 (9.1); no significant differences; no differences in psychologic outcome measures, absenteeism, or cost-effectiveness
Thomas et al. (31)	Chronic cervical osteoarthritis	Acupuncture R1: placebo diazepam (orally) (n = 44) R2: placebo acupuncture: needles inserted superficially and left without eliciting any further sensation, 40 min (n = 44) I1: diazepam: 5 mg (orally) (n = 44) I2: acupuncture: experienced acupuncturist, traditional meridian, manual stimulation, Teh Chi, 7 points, 40 min (n = 44)	Mean (SD) affective pain score (VAS 10 cm) before and after treatment: I1, 3.0 (0.8), 2.2 (1.0); I2, 3.5 (1.2), 2.3 (1.5); R1, 2.7 (1.0), 2.2 (1.0); R2, 3.1 (1.1), 2.4 (1.2); mean (SD) sensory pain score (VAS 10 cm) before and after treatment: I1, 1.9 (0.7), 1.6 (0.7); I2, 2.5 (0.8), 1.8 (1.2); R1, 1.9 (0.8), 1.7 (1.0); R2, 2.0 (0.9), 1.6 (1.1). I2 significantly better than R1, but not than I1 or R2
Petrie and Hazleman (26)	Chronic neck pain with or without radiation	I: acupuncture: traditional meridian, 5 points, manual stimulation, Teh Chi, 20 min (at 5-min intervals), 2 times/wk, 4 wk (n = 13) R: sham transcutaneous nerve stimulation without current, consisting of a signal generator with an oscilloscope for patient to view with electrodes attached to base of the neck, 20 min, 2 times/wk, 4 wk (n = 12)	Mean pain intensity (VAS) baseline, posttreatment and after 1 mo: I, 47.08, 36.59, 31.77; R, 31.67, 32.88, 24.72; mean disability score (VAS) baseline, posttreatment, and after 1 mo: I, 32.80, 25.98, 24.74; R, 20.92, 25.85, 22.67; number of patients moderately or greatly better posttreatment: I, 6; R, 4; mean change in ROM posttreatment: I, +0.96; R −1.37; no significant difference among groups in any outcome measure

continued

345

TABLE 15.3. Continued

Investigators (ref.)	Disorder	Index treatment (I)	Reference treatment (R)	Results
Coan et al. (8)	Cervical spine syndromes	I: traditional meridian acupuncture, variable acupuncture point selection, electroacupuncture and moxibustion on some patients, 10 or more treatments, 3–4 times/wk (n = 15)	R: waiting list control group: no treatment (n = 15)	Mean pain score (11-point NRS) pretreatment and after 12 wk: I, 6.0, 3.6; R, 5.3, 5.4; I, 40%; R, 2% reduction; no. of patients improved after 12 wk: I, 12 (80%); R, 2 (13%); mean limitation of activity pretreatment and after 12 wk: I, 1.6, 1.1; R, 1.7, 1.5; no statistical testing
Goldie and Landquist (11)	Cervical pain with irradiation to upper extremity	I: isometric exercises: cervical movements (in sitting and standing) with manual resistance from physical therapist; after treatment 10 min rest in supine position; 20 min, 3 times/wk for 3 wk (total 10 treatments), (n = 24)	Traction R1: traction: Trutrac intermittent mechanical traction, supine position (8-sec rest, 8-sec traction), 20 min, force 30–40 pounds for men and 25–30 pounds for women; after treatment 10-min rest in supine position, 3 times/wk, 3 wk (n = 26) R2: control treatment: only instructions (n = 23)	Global assessment (no. of patients improved after 6 wk according to physician): I, 11/24; R1, 18/26; R2, 11/23; no differences; global assessment (no. of patients improved after 6 wk according to patient): I, 17/24; R1, 17/26; R2, 7/23; no differences in mobility
Persson et al. (24,25)	Cervical root compression	I: cervical collar: patients chose the most comfortable, shoulder-resting, rigid collar during daytime, soft collar at night if wanted, 3 mo (n = 27)	Neck collar R1: physical therapy: exercises, instructions, manual traction, mobilization, heat therapy, relaxation exercises, 15 sessions, 30–45 min, 3 mo (n = 27) R2: surgery: anterior cervical decompression and fusion technique, posterior approach in one patient (n = 27)	Mean worst pain intensity last wk (VAS) pretreatment, after 14–16 wk and after 12 mo: I, 68, 64, 52; R1, 70, 51, 53; R2, 72, 43, 42; mean present pain intensity last wk (VAS) pretreatment, after 14–16 wk, after 12 mo: I, 49, 48, 35; R1, 50, 41, 39; R2, 47, 27, 30; after 14–16 wk R2 significantly better than I; after 14–16 wk R1 and R2 significantly better in overall SIP score than I; no differences after 12 mo; after 14–16 wk R2 significantly better postural performance than I and R1
Lavin et al. (22)	Benign neck pain (arthritis, trauma)	I: water-based pillow: first wk regular pillow followed by 2 wk of water-based pillow continued by 2 wk of the roll pillow (n = 22)	Pillows R1: roll pillow: first wk regular pillow followed by 2 wk of the water-based pillow continued by 2 wk of the roll pillow (n = 19) R2: standard pillow: this was the patient's current pillow; used only the first week of the 5-wk intervention (n = 41)	I: significantly better than R1 and R2 concerning morning pain relief; I and R2 had longer sleep duration than R1; SIP overall score: I, 43.0; R1, 57.2; R2, 58.0; number of patients satisfied (7-point NRS): I, 22; R1, 7; R2, 4; significant

Laser therapy

Study	Condition	Intervention (I) / Reference (R)	Results
Thorsen et al. (32)	Myofascial neck pain and shoulder girdle	R: placebo laser treatment: laser identical in sound, heat, and vibration; after initial treatment, patients crossed over to receive laser treatment (n = 22) I: laser treatment: 0.9 J per tender point, maximum 9 J per treatment, each tender point (maximum 10) treated for 1 min, 6 sessions, 2 wk; after initial treatment, patients crossed over to receive placebo (n = 25)	No differences after 3 wk in intensity of pain-rest (VAS) or pain-function; data in graphs; number (%) of patients reporting beneficial effect from treatment: I, 8 (17%); R, 20 (43%); R significantly better
Cecherelli et al. (7)	Cervical myofascial pain	R: placebo laser therapy: same as I but without emission, 3 times/wk for 3 wk for a total of 12 sessions (n = 14) I: laser therapy: diode laser, irradiation of 1 J of energy of the four most painful tender areas found with palpation and irradiation of 5 bilateral acupuncture points each irradiated with 0.1 J; total energy during treatment 5, 3 times/wk for 3 wk for a total of 12 sessions (n = 13)	Mean (SD) no. of words on McGill Pain Questionnaire pretreatment and posttreatment (3 wk): I, 12.76 (2.35), 6.53 (4.05); R, 11.42 (3.43), 11.64 (3.83); mean (SD) total pain score pre- and posttreatment: I, 29.84 (9.58), 13.53 (11.43); R, 27.71 (11.20), 25.71 (10.41); I significantly better than R

(Electro)magnetic therapy

Study	Condition	Intervention (I) / Reference (R)	Results
Trock et al. (33)	Osteoarthritis of the cervical spine (radiographs)	R: placebo, 30 min, 3–5 times/wk, 18 treatments, (n = 39) I: electromagnetic therapy: pulsed electromagnetic fields; patients lay on mattress in specially made polycarbonate half-shell device, extremely low frequency, <2 A with 120 V, stepwise application of energy 5 Hz, 10–15 gauss, 10 min; 10 Hz, 15–25 gauss, 10 min; 12 Hz, 15–25 gauss, 10 min, 3–5 times/wk, 18 treatments (n = 42)	Mean (SD) differences in pain posttreatment and after 1 mo compared to pretreatment: I, 27.9 (27.3), 25.9 (30.2); R, 16.3 (24.3), 14.7 (29.4); mean (SD) differences in ADL: I, 3.8 (6.7), 3.8 (7.4); R, 3.1 (5.8), 2.1 (5.6); mean (SD) patient's global improvement posttreatment and after 1 mo: I, 42.7 (35.6), 41.2 (35.9); R, 46.2 (31.7), 40.0 (32.3); pain posttreatment significantly different; baseline values of pain, pain on motion, and tenderness significantly higher in I than R
Foley-Nolan et al. (10)	Persistent neck pain (spondylosis, whiplash)	R: placebo electromagnetic therapy: for 3 wk followed by active treatment (real electromagnetic therapy); a placebo facsimile unit was used (n = 10) I: electromagnetic therapy: pulsed electromagnetic therapy; low-power pulsed short-wave approximately 27 MHz/ mean power 1.5 mW/cm², incorporated in a soft neck collar, using a collar 8 hr/d for 3 wk, followed by another 3 wk (n = 10)	Median pain score (10 cm VAS) pretreatment and after 3 wk: I, 7.0, 4.0; R, 6.75, 5.5; I significantly better; global improvement (much better, completely well) after 3 wk: I, 3; R, 1; median score range of movement pretreatment and after 3 wk: I, 3.6, 4.1; R, 3.3, 3.5; I significantly better
Hong et al. (14)	Chronic neck and shoulder pain	R: placebo, nonmagnetic necklace, 24 hr, 3 wk (n = 25) I: magnetic neck lace; samarium cobalt elements with brass chains plated with gold or rhodium, surface density 1,300 gauss, 24 hr/d, 3 wk (n = 27)	Mean (SD) pain intensity (5-point scale) pre- and posttreatment: I, 3.1 (0.5), 2.7 (0.7); R, 2.8 (0.6), 2.6 (0.6); mean (SD) pain frequency (5-point scale) pre- and posttreatment: I, 2.9 (0.6), 2.5 (0.7); R, 2.8 (0.6), 2.5 (0.6); no significant differences

continued

TABLE 15.3. Continued

Investigators (ref.)	Disorder	Index treatment (I)	Reference treatment (R)	Results
Fitz-Ritson (9)	Chronic motor vehicle accident patients with pain/soreness/stiffness of cervical musculature	I: chiropractic treatment plus "phasic" neck exercises, 5 days a week, 8 wk (n = 15)	Proprioceptive exercises R: chiropractic treatment plus rehabilitation exercises (ROM, stretching, isometric-toning, isokinetic strengthening), 5 d/wk, 8 wk (n = 25)	Improvement on Neck Pain Disability Index posttreatment: I, 48.3%; R, 7.4%; baseline differences between groups
Revel et al. (27)	Chronic nonspecific neck pain	I: rehabilitation: NSAIDs and analgesics, exercises concerned with eye-neck co-ordination using a standardized protocol consisting of 15 individual sessions (passive and active proprioception exercises) 30–40 min, 2 times/wk, 8 wk (n = 30)	R: symptomatic treatment with NSAIDs and analgesics (n = 30)	Mean (SD) decrease in pain intensity after 10 wk: I, 21.8 (25.2); R, 4.3 (19.6); significant; percentage of patients with good or very good functional improvement: I, 60%; R, 27%; significant; mean (SD) improvement in ROM-flexion/extension and ROM-rotation: I, 0.5 (1.7), 1.3 (2.6); R, 0.2 (1.4), 1.2 (4.3); significant for rotation; no differences in medication intake (daily amount of NSAIDs and analgesics)

ADLs, activities of daily living; CI, confidence interval; GP, general practitioner; MMCBT, multimodal cognitive behavioral therapy; NRS, Numerical rating scale; NSAIDs, nonsteroidal antiinflammatory drugs; ROM, range of motion; SD, standard deviation; SIP, Sickness Impact Profile; VAS, visual analogue scale.

measures or when the reference treatment was reported to be more effective with regard to at least one of these outcome measures. When the therapeutic intervention under study was reported to be statistically significantly more effective on one of the outcome measures but less effective on another, or when these outcome measures were not assessed in a study, no conclusion was drawn.

Levels of Evidence

Our conclusions on the effectiveness of the therapeutic interventions were based on the strength of the scientific evidence (1). The rating system consisted of four levels of scientific evidence, based on the quality and the outcome of the studies:

A. Strong evidence: provided by generally consistent findings in multiple high-quality RCTs.
B. Moderate evidence: provided by generally consistent findings in one high-quality RCT and one or more low-quality RCTs or by generally consistent findings in multiple low-quality RCTs.
C. Limited or contradictory evidence: only one RCT (either high- or low-quality) or inconsistent findings in multiple RCTs.
D. No evidence: no RCTs.

An RCT was (arbitrarily) considered to be of high quality when the methodologic score was 50 points or more and of low quality when the methodologic score was less than 50 points.

RESULTS

Study Selection

In the reviews by Gross et al. (13) and by Persson et al. (25), RCTs were identified on conservative treatment for neck pain. Thirteen of these RCTs were excluded for this review because they reported on patients with acute neck pain, on a mix of patients with lumbar and cervical back pain, or on secondary prevention of neck pain. Ten RCTs considered to represent conservative treatment for chronic neck pain and were selected from the review by Gross et al. (13). Additionally, 353 MEDLINE references and 173 EMBASE references from January 1994 to July 1998 were checked. Eleven additional RCTs were identified. One of these RCTs (5) was excluded because it concerned an experimental methodologic study. Overall, 20 RCTs on conservative treatment for chronic neck pain were included in this review.

Effectiveness of Interventions

Muscle Relaxants

One high-quality study (31) and one low-quality study (4) were identified that evaluated muscle relaxants for chronic neck pain. The high-quality study did not find a difference between diazepam and placebo (31). The low-quality study reported that cyclobenzaprine hydrochloride was significantly better after 2 weeks of treatment compared with placebo with regard to both measured and perceived muscle spasm and pain (4). Because of inconsistent findings, it is not possible to judge the effectiveness of muscle relaxants in chronic neck pain (evidence level C). Muscle relaxants have potential side effects, including drowsiness in up to 30% of patients (1).

Steroid Injections

Two high-quality studies and one low-quality study were identified (3,6,30). One of the high-quality RCTs reported no differences between intraarticular steroid injections in the cervical zygapophyseal joint and injection of a local anesthetic with regard to pain relief (3). The other high-quality RCT reported no additional benefit of epidural steroid injection with morphine compared with epidural steroid injection without morphine with regard to pain relief or return to work (6). The low-quality RCT reported that epidural steroid injections were associated with significantly better pain relief, return to work, and improved range of motion compared with an intramuscular steroid injection, even after 1 year (30). There is limited evidence (level C) that steroid injections are not an effective treatment for chronic neck pain.

Manual Therapy

Two high-quality studies (17–21) and one low-quality study (28) were identified. One high-quality RCT compared manipulation or mobilization (provided by specifically trained physical therapists) with nonmanipulative physical therapy, usual care by a general practitioner, and a "placebo" (18–21). The other high-quality study compared manual therapy with physical therapy and intensive training (17). The low-quality study compared a single manipulation after an amnestic dose of diazepam with a "placebo" consisting of diazepam only (28). There were no statistically significant differences among the groups in all three studies. Therefore, strong evidence (level A) indicates that manual therapy is not more effective than physical therapy, and moderate evidence (level B) indicates that manual therapy is not an effective treatment for chronic nonspecific neck pain.

Physical Therapy

Five high-quality studies were identified that evaluated physical therapy for chronic nonspecific neck pain (17–21), occupational neck and shoulder pain (23,35), and cervical nerve root compression (24,25). In Table 15.3, the content of physical therapy evaluated in the studies is described. In all studies, physical therapy consisted of individual treatment including some type of exercises in addition to massage and/or instructions and/or heat therapy and/or manual traction. The number of treatment sessions varied from 10 to 15, and the duration of the treatment period ranged from 5 weeks to 3 months. There were no differences among physical therapy and group exercises (17,35) or manual therapy (17–21), continued care by the general practitioner, and "placebo" (detuned short-wave diathermy and detuned ultrasound) (18–21). Again, manipulative and nonmanipulative physical therapy showed better short-term results in terms of overall improvement and physical functioning than the other two groups, but this difference was not statistically significant. Moreover, no differences were noted between active and passive physical therapy (23). There is strong evidence (level A) that unspecified physical therapy is no different from alternative treatments with which it has been compared for chronic nonspecific neck pain, such as group exercises, manual therapy, or usual care by a general practitioner. There is limited evidence (level C) that physical therapy is no more effective than "placebo" physical therapy and that there is no difference between active and passive physical therapy. Physical therapy was equally effective as surgery in the short term but better than a cervical collar, and in the long term (after 12 months), physical therapy, cervical collars, and surgery were equally effective for patients with chronic cervical nerve root compression (24,25).

Behavioral Therapy

One low-quality RCT (16) reported no differences between multimodal cognitive-behavioral treatment with the behavioral component directly administered and multimodal cognitive-behavioral therapy with the psychologist functioning as a "coach," with regard to pain intensity, disability, psychologic outcomes, absenteeism from work, and cost-effectiveness. Therefore, there is limited evidence (level C) that these types of therapy equally effective. However, scientific evidence is not sufficient to permit any judgment on the efficacy or effectiveness of behavioral therapy for patients with chronic neck pain.

Acupuncture

Three RCTs were identified on the effectiveness of acupuncture for chronic neck pain (8,26,31). Two RCTs were considered to be of high methodologic quality (26,31), and one was of low methodologic quality (8). The two high-quality studies reported no differences between traditional meridian acupuncture and sham transcutaneous electrical nerve stimulation, placebo acupuncture, or diazepam. There is strong evidence (level A) that acupuncture is not effective for treating chronic neck pain.

Traction

The one low-quality study that was identified on traction for chronic neck pain reported no differences among traction, isometric exercises, and a control group receiving instructions only (11). Therefore, there is limited evidence (level C) that traction is not an effective treatment for chronic neck pain.

Cervical Collar

Only one high-quality study was identified, and it reported a smaller short-term effect of cervical collars compared with surgery or physical therapy (24,25). There were no differences after 12 months. Therefore, limited evidence (level C) suggests that cervical collars are not effective in the treatment of patients with chronic cervical nerve root compression.

Pillows

One low-quality RCT (22) reported a water-based pillow to be significantly better than a standard pillow or a roll pillow regarding morning pain relief, general health status, and satisfaction. Because only one low-quality trial was identified, there is limited evidence (level C) that a water-based pillow is an effective treatment for chronic neck pain. However, a conflict of interest existed in this study.

Laser Therapy

Two RCTs were identified that compared laser therapy with placebo laser (7,32). The high-quality study reported no differences in pain intensity, but a significantly larger percentage of patients in the placebo group reported a beneficial effect from treatment (32). The low-quality study reported laser to be significantly better than placebo (7). Because of inconsistent findings, it is not possible to make any judgment on the effectiveness of laser therapy for chronic neck pain (level C).

Electromagnetic Therapy

Three RCTs were identified (10,14,32). Two high-quality studies (10,33) reported pulsed electromagnetic therapy to be significantly better than placebo, although in one study baseline values were significantly different (32). There is strong evidence (level A) that electromagnetic therapy provides effective short-term pain relief. The low-quality RCT did not find any differences between a magnetic necklace and placebo, a finding indicating that limited evidence suggests that a magnetic necklace is not effective (level C).

Proprioceptive Exercises

Two low-quality studies were identified that evaluated proprioceptive exercises for chronic neck pain (9,27). One study reported better short-term improvement on disability with chiropractic treatment plus proprioceptive exercises compared with chiropractic treatment plus rehabilitation exercises (9). The other study showed proprioceptive exercises with medication to be better than medication alone regarding decrease in pain intensity and improvement in physical functioning (27). There is limited evidence that proprioceptive exercises provide good short-term outcomes (level C) in these patients.

CONCLUSION

Because of methodologic problems, we believe that it is not opportune to make any recommendations in favor of any type of treatment for chronic neck pain at this time. Only a small number of studies could be identified, and the studies were heterogeneous with regard to methodologic quality, study populations, interventions, reference treatments, and outcome measures. Patients included in the studies were diagnosed as having whiplash, radicular pain, muscle spasm, osteoarthritis, spondylosis, root compression, myofascial pain, or undefined nonspecific pain. The effectiveness of treatments may vary among these diagnostic categories of neck pain, but scientific data are insufficient to perform subgroup analyses. Another problem encountered was the small sample sizes of the RCTs. These trials may lack power to detect clinically relevant differences among treatments simply because the sample sizes were not large enough. Furthermore, the content of the interventions at issue, as well as the type and content of the control interventions varied widely. Partly for these reasons, we conclude that there is no clear evidence that any form of treatment studied is particularly effective for patients with chronic neck pain. There is definitely a need for more high-quality studies with larger sample sizes to evaluate the cost-effectiveness of commonly used treatments for chronic neck pain. More studies on chronic neck pain are needed, especially because neck pain has become more and more common in industrialized countries and is becoming an important medical and socioeconomic problem.

REFERENCES

1. Agency for Health Care Policy and Research. *Acute low back problems in adults: assessment and treatment.* Clinical practice guideline no. 14. Rockville, MD: Agency for Health Care Policy and Research, 1994.
2. Aker PD, Gross AR, Goldsmith CH, et al. Conservative management of mechanical neck pain: systematic overview and meta-analysis. *BMJ* 1996;313:1291–1296.
3. Barnsley L, Lord SM, Wallis BJ, et al. Lack of effect of intraarticular corticosteroids for chronic pain in the cervical zygapophyseal joints. *N Engl J Med* 1994;330:1047–1050.
4. Basmajian JV. Cyclobenzaprine hydrochloride effect on skeletal muscle spasm in the lumbar region and neck: two double-blind controlled clinical and laboratory studies. *Arch Phys Med Rehabil* 1978;59:58–63.
5. Byrn C, Olsson I, Falkheden L, et al. Subcutaneous sterile water injections for chronic neck and shoulder pain following whiplash injuries. *Lancet* 1993;341:449–452.
6. Castagnera L, Maurette P, Pointillart V, et al. Long-term results of cervical epidural steroid injection with and without morphine in chronic cervical radicular pain. *Pain* 1994;58:239–243.
7. Ceccherelli F, Altafini L, Lo Castro G, et al. Diode laser in cervical myofascial pain: a double-blind study versus placebo. *Clin J Pain* 1989;5:301–304.
8. Coan RM, Wong G, Coan PL. The acupuncture treatment of neck pain: a randomized controlled trial. *Am J Chin Med* 1982;9:326–332.
9. Fitz-Ritson D. Phasic exercises for cervical rehabilitation after "whiplash" trauma. *J Manipulative Physiol Ther* 1995;18:21–24.
10. Foley-Nolan D, Barry C, Coughlan RJ, et al. Pulsed high frequency (27 MHz) electromagnetic therapy for persistent neck pain: a double-blind, placebo-controlled study of 20 patients. *Orthopedics* 1990;13:445–450.
11. Goldie I, Landquist A. Evaluation of the effects of different forms of physiotherapy in cervical pain. *Scand J Rehabil Med* 1970;2–3:117–121.
12. Gross AR, Aker PD, Quartly C. Manual therapy in the treatment of neck pain. *Rheum Dis Clin North Am* 1996;22:579–598.
13. Gross AR, Aker PD, Goldsmith CH, et al. Conservative management of mechanical neck disorders: a systematic overview and meta-analysis. *Online J Curr Clin Trials* 1996;5:doc. 200 + 201.
14. Hong C-Z, Lin JC, Bender LF, et al. Magnetic necklace: its therapeutic effectiveness on neck and shoulder pain. *Arch Phys Med Rehabil* 1982;63:462–466.
15. Hurwitz EL, Aker PD, Adams AH, et al. Manipulation and mobilization of the cervical spine: a systematic review of the literature. *Spine* 1996;21:1746–1760.
16. Jensen I, Nygren A, Gamberale F, et al. The role of the psychologist in multidisciplinary treatments for chronic neck and shoulder pain: a controlled cost-effectiveness study. *Scand J Rehabil Med* 1995;27:19–26.
17. Jordan A, Bendix T, Nielsen H, et al. Intensive training, physiotherapy, or manipulation for patients with chronic neck pain: a prospective, single-blinded, randomized clinical trial. *Spine* 1998;23:311–319.
18. Koes BW, Bouter LM, Knipschild PG, et al. The effectiveness of manual therapy, physiotherapy and continued treatment by the general practitioner for chronic nonspecific back and neck complaints: design of a randomized clinical trial. *J Manipulative Physiol Ther* 1991;14:498–502.
19. Koes BW, Bouter LM, van Mameren H, et al. The effectiveness of manual therapy, physiotherapy, and treatment by the general practitioner for nonspecific back and neck complaints. *Spine* 1992;17:28–35.
20. Koes BW, Bouter LM, van Mameren H, et al. A blinded randomized clinical trial of manual therapy and physiotherapy for chronic back and neck complaints: physical outcome measures. *J Manipulative Physiol Ther* 1992;1:16–23.
21. Koes BW, Bouter LM, van Mameren H, et al. A randomized clinical trial of manual therapy and physiotherapy for persistent back and neck complaints: subgroup analysis and relationship between outcome measures. *J Manipulative Physiol Ther* 1993;16:211–219.
22. Lavin RA, Pappagallo M, Kuhlemeier KV. Cervical pain: a comparison of three pillows. *Arch Phys Med Rehabil* 1997;78:193–198.
23. Levoska S, Keinänen-Kiukaanniemi S. Active or passive physiotherapy for occupational cervicobrachial disorders? A comparison of two treatment methods with a 1-year follow-up. *Arch Phys Med Rehabil* 1993;74:425–430.
24. Persson L, Carlsson C-A, Carlsson JY. Long-lasting cervical radicular pain managed with surgery, physiotherapy, or a cervical collar: a prospective, randomized study. *Spine* 1997;22:751–758.
25. Persson L, Karlberg M, Magnusson M. Effects of different treatments on postural performance in

patients with cervical root compression: a randomized prospective study assessing the importance of the neck in postural control. *J Vestib Res* 1996;6:439–453.

26. Petrie JP, Hazleman BL. A controlled study of acupuncture in neck pain. *Br J Rheumatol* 1986;25:271–275.

27. Revel M, Minguet M, Gergoy P, et al. Changes in cervicocephalic kinesthesia after a proprioceptive rehabilitation program in patients with neck pain: a randomized controlled study. *Arch Phys Med Rehabil* 1994;75:895–899.

28. Sloop PR, Smith DS, Goldenberg E, et al. Manipulation for chronic neck pain: a double-blind controlled study. *Spine* 1982;7:832–835.

29. Spitzer WO, Skovron ML, Salmi LR, et al. Scientific monograph of the Quebec task force on whiplash-associated disorders: redifining "whiplash" and its management. *Spine* 1995;20[Suppl 8]:1S–73S.

30. Stav A, Ovadia L, Sternberg A, et al. Cervical epidural steroid injection for cervicobrachialgia. *Acta Anaesthesiol Scand* 1993;37:562–566.

31. Thomas M, Eriksson SV, Lundeberg T. A comparative study of diazepam and acupuncture in patients with osteoarthritis pain: a placebo controlled study. *Am J Chin Med* 1991;19:95–100.

32. Thorsen H, Gam AN, Svensson BH, et al. Low level laser therapy for myofascial pain in the neck and shoulder girdle: a double-blind, cross-over study. *Scand J Rheumatol* 1992;21:139–142.

33. Trock DH, Bollet AJ, Markoll R. The effect of pulsed electromagnetic fields in the treatment of osteoarthritis of the knee and cervical spine: report of randomized, double blind, placebo controlled trials. *J Rheumatol* 1994;21:1903–1911.

34. van der Heijden GJMG, Beurskens AJHM, Koes BW, et al. The efficacy of traction for back and neck pain: a systematic, blinded review of randomized clinical trial methods. *Phys Ther* 1995;75:93–104.

35. Vasseljen O, Johansen BM, Westgaard RH. The effect of pain reduction on perceived tension and EMG-recorded trapezius muscle activity in workers with shoulder and neck pain. *Scand J Rehabil Med* 1995;27:243–252.

*Neck and Back Pain: The Scientific Evidence
of Causes, Diagnosis, and Treatment,* edited
by Alf Nachemson and Egon Jonsson.
Published by Lippincott Williams & Wilkins,
Philadelphia 2000.

16

Surgical Treatment of Neck Pain

Carl-Axel Carlsson* and Alf Nachemson†

*Department of Neurosurgery, University Hospital, Lund, Frölunda, Sweden
†Department of Orthopaedics, Sahlgrenska University Hospital, Göteborg, Sweden

Pain in the neck may arise from several causes, such as nerve root compression and soft tissue injuries. This chapter concentrates on chronic cervical pain symptoms of more than 3 months' duration that are caused by cervical spondylosis, cervical disc herniation, and whiplash injuries.

Relevant studies were obtained through a MEDLINE search of the literature from 1987 to 1998, a search that was supplemented by earlier articles mentioned in the primary search and considered important. Review articles in the current orthopedic and neurosurgical literature were also collected for evaluation.

The aim of this chapter was to answer, if possible, the following questions. Which is the most effective surgical treatment in the three selected diagnoses with respect to relief or reduction of chronic pain: What evidence of effectiveness is available?

CERVICAL SPONDYLOSIS AND CERVICAL DISC HERNIATION

These two conditions are discussed together. Both can affect the nerve root and can cause radiculopathy, the main symptom of which is pain.

The most common causes of compression are *spondylosis* with hypertrophic facet and uncovertebral joints and a bulging or herniated disc. *Disc herniations* have been divided into "soft" and "hard" types. The literature includes hard disc herniation in the diagnosis of cervical spondylosis (2,4,22).

The mechanisms whereby spondylosis and disc herniation cause pain are still unclear. Direct, constant pressure on the nerve root does not cause persistent pain. Small movements and increased sensitivity of the root caused by "algogenic" substances and/or an intraradicular edema have been suggested as possible pain-producing mechanisms (see Chapter 7). Changes causing compression can also be seen on magnetic resonance imaging (MRI) scans in asymptomatic patients (2).

The average annual incidence of cervical radiculopathy is less than 0.1 per 1,000 (14,15,24). Spondylolytic changes are more common causes of cervical radiculopathy than are pure disc herniations.

The most frequently affected level is C5-6, followed by C6-7 and C-C5. The main symptom is pain, radiating from the neck to the shoulder and arm, usually on one side. The location of the pain is determined by the level of the compressed nerve root.

Many uncontrolled case series, with varying follow-up times, of patients with cervical radiculopathy who were treated using different surgical approaches have been presented (3,5,6,7,9–12,19,23,25,29,35). Some of these authors were pioneers in the field of cervical spinal surgery. The reports usually followed a common pattern. They were written by one surgeon alone or together with colleagues, who presented the results of their own series of operated patients. These open studies reported clinical outcomes as excellent and good, fair and poor, with good results almost invariably around 70% to 80%. These studies have a historical interest, but they have no true scientific value in the present era of evidence-based medicine.

For nonvalidated reasons, cervical radiculopathy caused by nerve root compression has been considered a definite indication for surgery. This belief in surgical treatment may stem from the "successful" results in the reports exemplified in the previous paragraph and possibly from a fear of neurologic deterioration if conservative therapies are used instead.

Many early uncontrolled studies dealt with surgical techniques alone (5,11,19). The question whether to fuse has been the subject of controversy ever since Hulth, in the late 1950s, introduced the "disc fenestration" technique (11,12).

One prospective and controlled study (32) supported the view that satisfactory results could be achieved by performing an anterior single-level cervical disc resection alone, a relatively simple operation compared with fusion, with or without additional plating. After a 4-year follow-up, even the bony union rate, difficult to judge (38), seemed to be the same in the three groups of patients, with no significant differences in clinical outcome; the rate of excellent or good results was around 75% in all groups.

Another adequately controlled study (34) compared stabilization with acrylate with discectomy alone. The results did not favor the use of "bone cement" for fusion.

One prospective randomized trial, which was small but with a satisfactorily high percentage of follow-up, compared one-level and two-level fusion with autologous bone grafting with and without plates (37). Only when two levels were fused did plating offer significant benefit. None of the 17 patients operated on for symptoms after whiplash injury had an excellent outcome. As in many studies, these authors used the criteria developed by Odom et al. (25) for determining success.

We could only find one single controlled randomized study comparing conservative therapy (physical therapy or cervical collar) with a one-level fusion procedure using bank bone for cervical radiculopathy (26–28). The patient's diagnosis was always verified by MRI. The root compressions resulted either from spondylosis or from a combination of spondylosis and a bulging disc. The results revealed that all three groups of patients (27 in each group) improved, but the improvement rate differed. The surgically treated patients improved faster than the conservatively treated patients, but at the 1-year follow-up, there was no difference between the groups. This finding was valid for pain (intensity and distribution), tender points, sensory loss, muscle strength, well-being, and mood (26–28). Many patients in the surgical group had undergone reoperation. The authors concluded that surgery and conservative treatments were equally effective after 1 year, but surgery could be used in patients with unbearable and intractable pain, to provide faster pain relief.

This controlled study was supported by a few open comparative studies. Saal et al. (30) followed 26 patients with radiculopathy caused by MRI-verified disc herniation. The follow-up time was more than 1 year. Twenty of the 26 patients were successfully treated by physical therapy and pharmacologic pain control. Ellenberg et al. (8) concluded in a review article that when patients with proven cervical radiculopathy were treated with nonoperative methods, successful outcome occurred in 80% to 90%. Busch et al. (4) prospectively followed 13 patients with neurologic and MRI signs of large disc herniations treated by epidural corticosteroid injections; 12 months later, regression was seen by repeat MRI scans and independent observeration in 12 patients. In a review of cervical spondylosis, McCormack and Weinstein (22) pointed out that surgical results were initially modestly good but declined with long-term follow-up. These authors concluded that this finding raised the question whether, and how much, surgical treatment affects the natural course of the disease.

A prospective multicenter study Sampath et al. (31) with an independent clinical review by members of the Cervical Spine Research Society failed to demonstrate significant differences between those patients who were surgically treated and those who received medical treatment. The surgical group was followed-up for a mean of 11 months (8–13 months) by telephone interviews. Only 63% of the patients were available for follow-up. They seemed to improve more than the medically treated patients, but a significant number (26%) reported persistent excruciating or horrible pain on follow-up. The conclusion of this uncontrolled study was that a randomized study should be performed. We have already mentioned the only such randomized trial.

Conclusions

One randomized controlled trial comparing surgical and conservative treatments of one-level cervical radiculopathy resulting from spondylosis with or without an additional bulging disc did not prove the efficacy of surgery for this condition. In addition, three available controlled studies on techniques have not solved the problem of which method is more effective: disc fenestration discectomy, fusion, or fusion with plating.

WHIPLASH INJURY

Whiplash injury is a common and troublesome disorder. Approximately 10% to 20% of these patients develop chronic neck symptoms after car collisions (20,21,36).

The clinical entities associated with the injury are called *whiplash-associated disorders*. These conditions were reviewed by a multiprofessional group, the Quebec Task Force on Whiplash Injuries, which performed a systematic analysis of whiplash injury and whiplash-associated disorders (33).

One contribution of the group was the classification of whiplash-associated disorders, as follows:

Grade 0: no complaints about the neck; no physical signs.
Grade I: neck complaint of pain, stiffness, or tenderness; no physical signs.
Grade II: neck complaint and musculoskeletal signs.
Grade III: neck complaint and neurologic signs.
Grade IV: neck complaint and fracture or dislocation.

Grade 0 was excluded by the Quebec Task Force, as was grade IV, because fractures and dislocations did not fall within the framework of their task or of this review. Our report focuses on grades I, II, and III, and the specific aim is to try to answer the following question: Which is the most effective surgical method to treat whiplash-induced neck pain syndromes?

Neck pain is the most common complaint, followed by headache. Radiculopathy seems rare (20,33). Few reports are available on the results of surgical treatment of patients with persisting symptoms after whiplash injury (1,13,37).

Except for the small number of patients included in the Zoëga studies (37,38), the results of surgical procedures in patients with chronic neck pain after whiplash injury have not been subjected to controlled studies (33). Even in the uncontrolled studies, however, the results have been generally unsatisfying. Jonsson et al. (13), in a case series, demonstrated acceptable results after early surgical intervention in patients with radicular symptoms and MRI evidence of bulging or herniated discs; these findings were supported by the large follow-up study from Arhus, Denmark (9,10).

Thus, perhaps the time interval between injury and treatment is of some importance. This concept is only an assumption, however, and is not yet supported by controlled studies.

In spite of extensive diagnostic measures, it is difficult to identify the origin of pain (33). Many structures may cause the pain associated with whiplash injury. Based on their repeat double-blind studies and using an intricate injection technique of the nerves to the zygapophyseal joints, Lord et al. (16–18) demonstrated, in a randomized study of patients who respond properly to these injections, that an electrocoagulation neurectomy can relieve pain in patients who had 6 months or more of pain after a whiplash injury. The results of neurectomy, however, were not long lasting; pain recurred after 6 to 12 months in most patients. These authors, however, claimed that the intervention could be repeated with similar, good results.

Conclusions

We have not been able to find any controlled randomized studies concerning the effect of surgery on neck pain in patients with whiplash injuries. One small study (37), comparing plating with no plating and fusion, did not obtain satisfactory results in this group of patients. Because of the lack of controlled studies at present, no surgical method is available that can be recommended to reduce neck pain after whiplash (level of evidence D).

OVERALL CONCLUSIONS

There is little evidence in support of surgical treatment versus conservative treatment for patients with neck pain and/or cervical radiculopathy, supposedly caused by spondylosis, so-called "hard" or "soft" disc herniation, or whiplash injury. A multitude of surgical methods has been proposed, including fixation by various types of metallic devices. It is not possible at present to support any particular method of fusion. Given the increasing numbers of patients with neck syndromes, various types of treatment including surgery must have a higher priority for clinically well-controlled studies.

REFERENCES

1. Algers G, Pettersson K, Hildingsson C, et al. Surgery for chronic symptoms after whiplash injury. *Acta Orthop Scand* 1993;64:654–656.
2. Boden SD, McCowin PR, Davis DO, et al. Abnormal magnetic resonance scans of the cervical spine in asymptomatic subjects. *J Bone Joint Surg Am* 1990;72:1178–1184.

3. Bohlman H, Emery SE, Goodfellow DB, et al. Robinson anterior cervical discectomy and arthrodesis for cervical radiculopathy. *J Bone Joint Surg Am* 1993;75:1298–1307.
4. Busch K, Chaudhuri R, Hillier S, et al. The pathomorphologic changes that accompany the resolution of cervical radiculopathy: a prospective study with repeat magnetic resonance imaging. *Spine* 1997;22:183–187.
5. Cloward RB. The anterior approach for removal of ruptured cervical discs. *J Neurosurg* 1958;15:602–611.
6. Connolly ES, Seymour BJ, Adams JE. Clinical evaluation of anterior cervical fusion for degeneration cervical disc disease. *J Neurosurg* 1965;23:431–437.
7. DePalma AF, Rothman RH, Lewinneck RE, et al. Anterior interbody fusion for severe cervical disc degeneration. *Surg Gynecol Obstet* 1972;134:755–758.
8. Ellenberg MB, Hornet JC, Treanor WJ. Cervical radiculopathy. *Arch Phys Med Rehabil* 1994;75:342–352.
9. Eriksen EF, Buhl M, Fode K, et al. Treatment of cervical disc disease using Cloward's technique: the prognostic value of clinical preoperative data in 1,106 patients. *Acta Neurochir (Wien)* 1984;70:181–197.
10. Espersen JO, Buhl M, Eriksen EF, et al. Treatment of cervical disc disease using Cloward's technique. I. General results, effect of different operative methods and complications in 1,106 patients. *Acta Neurochir (Wien)* 1984;70:97–114.
11. Hirsch C. Cervical disc rupture: diagnosis and therapy. *Acta Orthop Scand* 1961;30:172–186.
12. Hirsch C, Wickbom I, Lidstrom A, et al. Cervical disc resection: a follow-up of myelographic and surgical procedure. *J Bone Joint Surg Am* 1964;46:1811–1821.
13. Jonsson H Jr, Cesarini K, Sahlstedt B, et al. Findings and outcome in whiplash-type neck distorsions. *Spine* 1994;19:2733–2743.
14. Kelsey JL, Githens PB, Walter SD, et al. An epidemiologic study of acute prolapsed cervical interverte-bral disc. *J Bone Joint Surg Am* 1984;66:907–914.
15. Kondo K, Molgaard CA, Kurland LT, et al. Protruded intervertebral cervical disc. *Minn Med* 1981;64:751.
16. Lord SM, Barnsley L, Bogduk N. The utility of comparative local anesthetic blocks versus placebo-controlled blocks for the diagnosis of cervical zygapophysial joint pain. *Clin J Pain* 1995;11:208–213.
17. Lord SM, Barnsley L, Wallis BJ, et al. Chronic cervical zygapophysial joint pain after whiplash: a placebo-controlled prevalence study. *Spine* 1996;21:1737–1744.
18. Lord SM, Barnsley L, Wallis BJ, et al. Percutaneous radio-frequency neurotomy for chronic cervical zygapophyseal-joint pain. *N Engl J Med* 1996;335:1721–1726.
19. Lundsford LO, Bissonette DJ, Jannetta PJ, et al. Anterior surgery for cervical disc disease. *J Neurosurg* 1980;53:1–15.
20. Macnab I. The "whiplash syndrome." *Orthop Clin North Am* 1971;2:389–403.
21. Marshall LL. The "whiplash" injury. *Med J Aust* 1976;2:26–27.
22. McCormack RM, Weinstein PR. Cervical spondylosis: an update. *West J Med* 1996;165:43–51.
23. Murphy MG, Gado M. Anterior cervical discectomy without interbody bone grafts. *Clin Neurosurg* 1972;37:71–74.
24. Mäkelä M, Heliövaara M, Sievers K, et al. Prevalence, determinants and consequences of chronic neck pain in Finland. *Am J Epidemiol* 1991;194:1356–1367.
25. Odom GL, Finney W, Woodhall B, et al. Cervical disc lesions. *JAMA* 1958;166:23–28.
26. Persson LC, Carlsson C-A, Carlsson J. Long-lasting cervical radicular pain treated with surgery, physio-therapy or a cervical collar: a prospective randomised study. *Spine* 1997;22:751–758.
27. Persson L, Karlberg M, Magnusson M. Effects of different treatments on postural performance in patients with cervical root compression: a randomised prospective study assessing the importance of the neck in postural control. *J Vestib Res* 1996;6:439–453.
28. Persson LC, Moritz U, Brandt L, et al. Cervical radiculopathy: pain, muscle weakness, and sensory loss in patients with cervical radiculopathy treated with surgery, physiotherapy or cervical collar. A prospective, controlled study. *Eur Spine J* 1997;6:256–266.
29. Robinson RA, Walker AE, Felic DC, et al. The results of anterior interbody fusion of the cervical spine. *J Bone Joint Surg* 1962;44:1569–1587.
30. Saal JS, Saal JA, Yurth EF. Nonoperative management of herniated cervical disc with radiculopathy. *Spine* 1996;21:1877–1883.
31. Sampath P, Bendebba M, Davis JD, et al. Outcome in patients with cervical radiculopathy. *Spine* 1999;24:591–597.
32. Savolainen S, Rinne J, Hernesniemi J. A prospective randomized study of anterior single-level cervical disc operations with long-term follow-up: surgical fusion is unnecessary. *Neurosurgery* 1998;43:51–55.
33. Spitzer WO, Skovron ML, Salmi LR, et al. Scientific monograph of the Quebeck Task Force on Whiplash-Associated Disorders: redefining "whiplash" and its management. *Spine* 1995;20:8S:1S–73S.
34. van den Bent MJ, Oosting J, Wouda EJ, et al. Anterior cervical discectomy with or without fusion with acrylate: a randomized trial. *Spine* 1996;21:834–839.

35. White AA, Southwick WO, Deponte RJ. Relief of pain by anterior cervical spine fusion for spondylosis: a report of sixty-four patients. *J Bone Joint Surg* 1973;55:525–534.
36. Wickström J, LaRocca H. Head and neck injuries from acceleration-deceleration forces. In: Rage D, Wilke L, eds. *Spinal disorders.* Philadelphia: Lea & Febiger, 1977:349–356.
37. Zoëga B. *Cervical discectomy and fusion with or without plate fixation: a randomized clinical and radiographic study on outcome and cost-utility.* Thesis, Göteborg University, Sweden, 1998.
38. Zoëga B, Karrholm J, Lind B. One-level cervical spine fusion: a randomised study, with or without plate fixation, using radiostereometry in 27 patients. *Acta Orthop Scand* 1998;69:363–368.

*Neck and Back Pain: The Scientific Evidence
of Causes, Diagnosis, and Treatment,* edited
by Alf Nachemson and Egon Jonsson.
Published by Lippincott Williams & Wilkins,
Philadelphia 2000.

17

Utility of Cognitive-Behavioral Psychological Treatments

Steven J. Linton

*Program for Behavioral Medicine, Department of Occupational and Environmental
Medicine, Örebro Medical Center, Örebro, Sweden*

Because neck and back pain are currently viewed from a multidimensional perspective, there has been considerable interest in psychologic treatment methods. Indeed, the development of a chronic pain problem from an acute injury has often highlighted psychologic processes. As a result, psychologic treatments would appear to be logical as a method of meeting the behavioral, cognitive, and emotional dimensions of the problem. Many programs aimed at treating neck and back pain employ some form of psychologic treatment. A question remains as to the utility of these techniques.

AIM

The aim of this chapter is to review systematically the evidence concerning psychologic treatments for neck and back pain. The following questions are posed:

1. Is there evidence that psychologic approaches such as cognitive-behavioral therapy (CBT) are helpful in the treatment of neck and back pain?
2. What is the evidence when psychologic approaches are employed as part of a multidimensional team?
3. Do studies specifically isolating the effects of psychologic treatments provide evidence to justify the use of these treatments?
4. What is the evidence for using psychologic approaches at the various stages (acute to chronic) of pain?

EFFECT OF PSYCHOLOGIC TREATMENT

Because psychologic factors are related to pain and the development of persistent pain problems, many treatment approaches have embraced psychologic therapies. Indeed, the current multidimensional view of pain encompasses psychologic as well as other forms of therapy. *CBT* for pain has been developed to be an integral part of the multidimensional treatment program (10,13). It was conceptualized as a way of enhancing treatment by addressing pertinent cognitive (e.g., negative emotions and thoughts) and behavioral (e.g., altered activity and medication taking) aspects.

In addition, the cognitive-behavioral approach offers an educational concept, whereby learning encompasses the entire rehabilitation process. As a result, all staff members are encouraged to use the techniques, and specific methods such as for physical and occupational therapy have been developed. In a true multidimensional CBT program then, it is difficult to separate the effects of psychology from the other parts of the treatment. Moreover, the content of these programs is by no means standardized, and the CBT methods vary enormously, as does the amount of time spent on the psychologic aspects. Consequently, many reviews have looked at multidimensional programs as a whole in which CBT has been employed. This approach provides information pertaining to one of our questions, namely, "What is the evidence about efficacy when psychologic approaches are employed as part of a multidimensional team?" However, it is also of interest to determine more exactly the contribution CBT may make. Thus, reviews that have looked only at studies that isolate these effects experimentally are also included, keeping in mind the difficulties of attempting to separate the effects of psychologic aspects from other parts of the treatment.

CBT techniques have been incorporated into a number of different settings for the treatment of neck and back pain problems. Several studies have attempted to judge the effects of CBT techniques such as in prospective, randomized investigations. Although other psychotherapeutic approaches are sometimes employed, they were not included in the review articles or tables in this chapter because no randomized controlled trials (RCTs) were located. Indeed, several authors have bemoaned the lack of controlled studies investigating the effects of psychodynamic and other psychotherapies (14).

Several difficulties are encountered in reviewing the effects of psychologic treatment. These include specifying the treatment, controlling for the amount of treatment, determining the specifics of the therapist, assessing the combination with other treatments, providing large samples resulting from the work involved, comparing the samples, evaluating the quality of the design, and determining the measurement methods, as well as understanding the setting and orientation of the program. In essence, each investigation has a unique combination of techniques, delivery, patients, and setting that influences the execution of the study and its results.

Cognitive-behavioral pain management has developed from at least two traditions. First, a learning or operant approach was founded in the 1970s that was based on a quota (graded activity) system of physical activity training, a program for reducing medication consumption (often referred to as the "pain cocktail" because the medication was given in a glass of syrup), and the use of social reinforcement to encourage "well" behaviors and to discourage "pain" behaviors. The second tradition involved relaxation training either in the form of biofeedback or relaxation based on breathing, muscle contraction and relaxation, and guided imagery (some forms are called "progressive" relaxation.) Stress inoculation training, which is based on relaxation, was sometimes employed in pain treatment settings.

A focus on the cognitive and emotional aspects of pain resulted in the addition of a "coping" approach. The ideas were to examine and to alter negative thoughts and beliefs that could hinder recovery. Instead, positive coping strategies were taught that were designed to enhance recovery.

Psychologically oriented pain management programs subsequently added other interesting techniques that have been standard in psychologic treatment such as goal setting and problem solving. Many of these techniques are added to address some important aspect of the consequences of pain of life, and they may involve such diverse areas as stress, family, or workplace issues.

Consequently, the main forms of CBT may include relaxation training, coping strategies, operant activity training, operant medication reduction, biofeedback, compliance enhancement, problem solving, social skills training, stress reduction, assertiveness training, and return-to-work skills. Moreover, a true behavioral approach involves a thorough analysis on which the content of treatment is based. Theoretically, each patient should therefore receive unique treatment. Many studies have attempted to provide a standardized treatment protocol to allow scientific investigation. Nevertheless, the content of these approaches varies tremendously, and this variation should be kept in mind when one evaluates the results.

Many reviews and original studies sometimes included patients who did not specifically have a back pain problem. Because CBT is often provided in a multidimensional setting and because it is not disease specific, studies of chronic pain and musculoskeletal pain were sometimes included. Among others, Turk (39) argued that there may be more in common within the category of chronic pain irrespective of diagnosis than there are differences among diagnostic subgroups. Critical and systematic reviews of RCTs were given priority.

REVIEW METHODOLOGY

Literature Search

To identify as many relevant review and research articles as possible, three data bases were searched. These were MEDLINE (1985 to September, 1998), PsychInfo (1967 to September 1998), and ArbLine. The MEDLINE search strategy was to include articles about psychologic aspects and treatment of neck pain, back pain, or musculoskeletal pain. Because many of the psychologic factors are not believed to be disease specific, evidence regarding "mixed" populations were included when a substantial number of participants reported neck or back pain problems. Therefore, the following words were employed in the search: behavior or psychotherapy, adaptation, psychologic, probability, risk factors, predictors, prognosis, self-care, exercise therapy, back school, and health education. The search was restricted to include RCTs, review articles, comparative studies, follow-up studies, prospective studies, evaluation studies, and clinical trials because all these may include evaluations of CBT methods. This search resulted in 550 citations in MEDLINE. The PsychInfo strategy was similar, including back and neck pain and prevention, predictor, or risk factors, as well as treatment. This search produced 152 citations. A similar ArbLine search gave 14 citations.

Finally, articles and reviews were perused to identify additional relevant citations that were not included in these database searches. In all, more than 900 articles were identified.

Review Procedure

This review is organized such that review articles in the literature are examined first, and then key articles are evaluated. Critical and systematic reviews were given precedence in the overview, whereas RCTs were selected as key studies.

Original studies were included when the population consisted mainly of patients with back or neck pain, when a clear CBT was employed, when the effect of the CBT could be isolated, and when an RCT design was employed. The criteria for inclusion ensured a minimum methodologic standard, although the level may have been more generous than some reviews that employ quality ratings. Although the contribution of studies using other methodologies was recognized, such methods may be subject to a multitude of biases.

A table of quality studies was constructed to provide an overview of the best current recommendations specific to neck and back pain. Each reference was located and examined. The summary data were retrieved from the study by the author and were cross-checked with the abstract and conclusion provided in the report. Information about the population, interventions, control groups, and outcome were summarized.

Key outcome domains were as follows: (a) psychologic variables (e.g., depression, anxiety, fear, distress); (b) pain (e.g., intensity ratings, duration, descriptors); (c) function (e.g., activities of daily living, work); (d) medication consumption (e.g., number or dosage of painkillers consumed); and (e) health care utilization. If the CBT produced a statistically significant greater improvement on at least two domains, then it was classified as a "positive" outcome. If a control condition produced a significantly better result than the CBT intervention on at least one domain and the other domains showed no difference, then it was classified as a "negative" outcome. Finally, when no significant difference among the groups was found in any domain, it was classified as a "neutral" outcome.

Conclusions were based on the findings of the review articles in addition to the results from the tables. Each conclusion was evaluated with regard to the level of evidence supporting it. A grading system was used in which level A evidence entails support from a systematic review of good quality or two or more good-quality studies, whereas level B represents support from one or more RCTs or a good observational study. Level C means that data are insufficient or inconclusive, and level D means that no acceptable studies are available. This differs somewhat from the evidence levels in Table 1.4 (Chapter 1.)

Limitations

Although every effort has been made to include all relevant articles and to appraise them in a fair and scientific way, there are nevertheless limitations to this review. First, the search may not have identified all articles, and some important articles may not have been identified. A second problem concerns the criteria for inclusion in the evaluation. Methodologic criteria have been suggested (34,46). However, although there is considerable agreement concerning the basic criteria, the exact weight of each aspect may be debated. Quality ratings were therefore not applied. Although this may have led to the inclusion of studies of questionable merit, the criteria employed do establish a basic and relatively high standard while avoiding the problem of eliminating valuable RCT studies because of low ratings. Third, summarizing studies in tables inevitably results in the loss of information that may color interpretation. Finally, studies summarized in tables tend to be evaluated simplistically, such as "positive" or "negative," although reality is considerably more complex. Therefore, the tendency is to draw conclusions in a "box score" fashion that may not do justice to the differences among studies. Taken together, these factors represent limitations that need to be considered when one reads the evaluation.

SUMMARY OF PREVIOUS REVIEWS

Many reviews of the literature exist, although many of these are not systematic reviews. In this section, reviews employing systematic techniques are examined.

Flor et al., 1992

Flor et al. (9) identified 65 studies, although many of these were not RCTs, that evaluated the outcome of interdisciplinary treatment. Treatment techniques varied but included psychologic interventions in combination with medical treatments and physical or occupational therapy. The average duration of treatment was 7 weeks. Studies were graded in terms of quality based on, for example, the type of control groups, sampling, and dependent variables employed.

Overall, the review found that patients who were provided a multidimensional treatment had superior results as compared with various control groups. At follow-up (average of 95 weeks), an effect size of 0.81 was noted between treatment and the controls that indicated a 38% improvement. Within-group effect sizes were larger for the multidisciplinary group (1.31 at follow-up), a finding suggesting a 55% improvement. The results implied ". . . that the groups treated in a multidisciplinary pain clinic demonstrate at least twice the change reported by control groups" (9).

Moreover, when treatment was compared with single-modal treatments, the multidisciplinary results were also superior. Interestingly, the size of improvement did not depend on the quality of the study or the type of control group.

A detailed look at the behavioral outcome variables showed substantial improvements. The effect size for return to work was 0.67, a finding showing that treated patients had more than twice the rate of returning to work (68%) than did treated or single-modal treated controls (36%). Health care utilization followed a similar pattern. At long-term follow-up, 75% of patients receiving multidimensional treatment functioned better than those who were untreated or treated by conventional, unimodal approaches.

Flor et al. (9) concluded that the results supported the efficacy of multidisciplinary pain treatment. However, these investigators suggested caution, given the quality of the studies and difficulties in conducting a metaanalysis of them.

Cutler et al., 1994

Cutler et al. (5) employed metaanalysis to determine the effect of "nonsurgical pain center treatment" for chronic pain. In addition, they looked only at return to work as the outcome variable. They identified 37 studies evaluating nonsurgical treatments that also provided empiric data on return to work after treatment. Many of these studies reflected the "functional restoration" approach to rehabilitation in which psychologic techniques were part of a multidisciplinary team. However, several of the studies included in the review were not truly RCTs.

The articles were subjected to a metaanalysis, and it was found that treated patients returned to work significantly more often than did controls. Treatment was found approximately to double the chance of return to work. The authors concluded that evidence indicated that treatment did increase return-to-work rates.

Turner, 1996

This article reviewed CBT-oriented interventions designed to manage patients at the primary care level (41). Databases were searched to locate RCTs for CBT for chronic pain. The search of the literature identified 14 RCTs employing CBT treatments. Metaanalyses were performed on specific posttreatment effect variables. However, because the various studies employed different outcome variables, the number of studies for each outcome variable was small, the largest being four studies. Turner found that relative to waiting-list controls at posttest, CBT interventions were statistically superior on measures of pain report, self-reported pain behavior, and functional disability, but not for depression or observed pain behavior. Comparisons with other active treatments were hampered by the small number of studies, and metaanalyses did not produce significant effect sizes.

With regard to CBT in primary care settings, two studies were found dealing with acute pain (both showing some effect), and one concerning patients with chronic pain that showed a considerable effect. Turner concluded that CBT interventions could be useful in primary care settings, but that additional research was needed to evaluate their efficacy for specific outcome variables.

Van Tulder et al., 1997

This systematic review was concerned with conservative treatment of acute and chronic nonspecific back pain and therefore included a variety of treatments (45). One section dealt with "behavior therapy." Studies were selected from a systematic search of several data bases and included only RCTs with acute or chronic LBP. Furthermore, each study was rated for methodologic quality. One difficulty was classifying studies because some may have included more than one type of treatment or may have used exercise according to a learning paradigm.

Only one study was found for behavior therapy for acute pain, and the authors gave it a low methodologic rating. For chronic pain, five studies evaluating biofeedback were included in the review, and these were said to provide little support because four were negative. Eleven studies of behavior therapy were included of which eight reported significant, positive results. Because the authors viewed these RCTs as being of "low quality," they concluded that "there is limited evidence that behavior therapy is an effective treatment modality for chronic LBP with good short-term results. . . ." (45).

Flor, 1997

This metaanalytic review asked the pertinent question whether adding CBT techniques to pain management enhanced the effects (67). Eighty studies were identified, although once again many of the studies were not RCTs, with a total population of more than 3,000 patients with chronic back pain or mixed pain symptoms and in whom psychologic interventions were employed. Average improvement was then calculated for patients who received "additional" psychologic treatment as compared with patients who received medical treatment only. A mean additional improvement of 47% was seen at 3 months after treatment. This statistic remained largely unchanged at $1/2$ year, at which a 48% average improvement was noted. This finding shows, according to Flor, that patients undergoing interdisciplinary treatment with a psychologic component felt, on average, 48% better than patients who received purely medical treatment.

The improvements were categorized, and Table 17.1 shows the improvement that may be attributed to the addition of psychologic treatment for outcomes in the behavioral domain. The average improvement was 54%. Other improvements by outcome domain were as follows: pain, 37%; impairment, 23%; mood, 20%; and psychophysiology, 54%.

TABLE 17.1. *Additional behavioral improvements from psychologic treatment compared with medical treatment*

Improvement	Percentage (%)
Ability to work	43
Medication consumption	63
Health costs	35
Physical activity	53
Pain behavior	62

Adapted from Flor H. *A way out of the vicious circle: learning to manage chronic pain through self-control.* Berlin: Humboldt University, 1997, with permission.

An analysis was also made of the various psychologic techniques. Flor (6) found that operant (behavioral, learning) techniques produced an average improvement of 53%, whereas biofeedback had 46%, as compared with all other psychologic methods at 36%. It is concluded that clear improvement in these domains has been shown, with an average improvement across outcome domains and psychologic treatments of 50%.

Finally, no correlation was found between organic injury and the effects of adding psychologic techniques. In other words, CBT techniques were also effective when the problem was clearly linked to somatic problems.

Compas et al., 1998

This review focused on clearly identifying psychologic treatments and then evaluating the evidence for their effectiveness in RCTs (4). These authors identified five types of psychologic treatment: operant behavioral treatment, CBT, biofeedback, hypnosis, and psychodynamic therapy. However, no evidence was available for hypnosis and psychodynamic therapies that was directly relevant to neck and back pain. The authors, moreover, established a criterion for determining the success of the outcome. This involved an effect that significantly reduced pain, as well as improved psychologic and physical functioning.

For chronic pain, mainly chronic low back pain, studies were identified that fulfilled the definitions for the therapy and used an RCT design. These investigators found that operant behavioral treatment was efficacious because all three RCTs showed improvements as compared with controls. Likewise, CBT was found to be effective because all four studies demonstrated superior results as compared with a waiting-list control. It was concluded that biofeedback was effective because three studies showed results superior to those with pseudotherapy or a standard medical therapy. However, these authors did note that two early studies did not show positive results. Interestingly, this review also found that CBT was effective for rheumatic diseases (operant behavioral and biofeedback were not tested).

These investigators concluded that these cognitive and behaviorally oriented psychologic treatments were often effective in reducing pain and improving the psychologic and physical functioning of people with persistent pain. "Taken together, the findings are impressive, particularly because most of the participants in these studies have had long histories of pain and multiple failures to respond to conventional medical treatments" (4).

Morley et al., 1999

These authors conducted a systematic review of RCTs of psychologic treatments for chronic pain (27). They excluded headache, but they included other categories than neck and back pain. However, this was the only metaanalysis specifically oriented toward the effects of CBT. Moreover, these investigators went to considerable lengths to classify the studies correctly with regard to the content of the treatment, as well as including a broad range of outcome variables. Eight domains of outcome were considered. Effect sizes were calculated in which treatment was compared with a waiting-list control group, as well as when compared with active alternative treatments.

These authors identified 27 trials in 33 published articles; 25 RCTs contained data suitable for calculating effect sizes. The outcome domains were as follows:

1. Pain experience.
2. Mood/affect.
3. Cognitive coping and appraisal.
4. Behavioral activity.
5. Biology/fitness.
6. Social role functioning.
7. Use of health care.
8. Miscellaneous.

The treatments were classified as follows:

1. Biofeedback and relaxation.
2. Behavioral therapy.
3. CBT.
4. Coping skills training.
5. Cognitive therapy.

The results revealed consistent evidence that these cognitive and behavioral techniques were effective when compared with a waiting-list control group. For example, significant z scores were found for all the domains. When the comparison was made with the active treatment comparison groups, significant z scores were found for three of the domains (pain, coping, and abnormal behavior), and the effect sizes for the other domains were positive but not statistically significant. These investigators concluded that the effect sizes were modest, but nevertheless similar to other areas in which, for example, psychologic treatments were included or chronic problems were treated.

SUMMARY AND EVALUATION OF KEY STUDIES

Table 17.2 summarizes the RCTs in which some form of CBT was compared with a control group or active treatment in an English-language publication. Only studies that in some way isolated the specific effects of CBT were included; thus, studies of multidimensional programs employing CBT as one part of treatment were included only when the specific effect of CBT could be determined. In addition, only studies using patients with neck and back pain or mixed chronic pain including a substantial proportion of patients with neck or back pain were included. In all, 29 trials were isolated and summarized.

The content, duration, and administration of the CBT programs varied tremendously across studies. They ranged from electromyographic biofeedback, applied relaxation, and stress management to activity training and medication reduction. Duration was from a few hours to weeks. Moreover, the settings were different, ranging from participants in study groups to outpatients, day patients, and hospitalized patients. Some programs utilized medical rehabilitation or pain services, whereas other treatments were administered at spas or in nonmedical settings.

Waiting-list control groups and "treatment as usual" groups were the most common types of comparison groups. The studies all had follow-ups and broad-based assessments of several variables. Outcome evaluation stressed psychologically relevant factors such as function and activity levels, pain perception, mood, anxiety, and coping.

Table 17.2 is organized so four domains were evaluated at posttest. These domains were chosen to reflect the aims of psychologic treatment and to cover important areas underscored in previous reviews. The domains are psychologic function, pain, physical function, and medication use. At follow-up, work status or sick leave was included as a domain. Each domain was rated such that a plus sign indicated a significant improvement in favor of the CBT on a key variable in the domain and no significant differences in favor of the control condition. A minus sign indicated that the control group had a significantly better result, whereas a zero indicated no significant difference among the groups. When no data were collected in the domain, the domain was deemed "not applicable."

Despite the difficulties and possible limitations noted earlier, an overall classification of each study is also provided. To ascertain the effects as compared with the type of control group employed, results compared with a waiting-list control group or an active control were specified separately. A positive rating was given if at least *two* of the four key domains showed a significant advantage for the CBT and there were no significant differences in any other domains. A negative rating means that the control condition was superior or that a waiting-list control group was equal to the CBT treatment, whereas a neutral rating indicates less than two significant differences among the groups.

As Table 17.2 indicates, CBT was found to fulfill the definition of being superior to the waiting-list control group in 14 of the 16 trials employing such a design (18–20,23,24,26,28,31,32,35,40,42,44,48). The remaining 2 studies had significant improvements in favor of the CBT treatment in 1 of the 4 domains (36,43). These 16 studies represented a range of populations and CBT programs, but they consistently produced superior results particularly with regard to the psychologic, pain, function, and medication use domains.

When CBT was compared with active treatments, 12 of the 14 studies found CBT to be superior on at least 2 variables (1,3,8,12,22,24,29,30,33,37,38,47), whereas Fordyce et al. (11) reported a significant difference in favor of the psychologically oriented treatment. One study found no significant differences between standard rehabilitation as compared with standard rehabilitation plus a CBT program (2).

The RCTs consequently provided considerable evidence to support the efficacy of CBT for neck and back pain. The investigations consistently reported significantly larger improvements for CBT as compared with a waiting-list control group or active treatment, and these differences were maintained at follow-up. Most of the studies (26 of 29) employed patients with chronic pain, although patients with subacute and acute pain were also treated (11,22,47). Long-term follow-up examinations ranging from 3 to 24 months were conducted in 28 of the 29 studies. Improvements were reported to be maintained in 27 of the 28 studies reporting positive results at the

TABLE 17.2. *Randomized controlled trials in which cognitive-behavioral therapy for neck or back pain was isolated (at least two positive significant differences are needed for a + conclusion)*

Investigators (ref.)	No. of patients	Pain	Control	Psychologic treatment	Posttreatment status[a]	Follow-up	Conclusion WLC	Active
Alaranta et al., 1994 (1)	293 f = 55%	Chronic low back	1. Standard rehabilitation	2. Home training + exercise + CBT modeled after functional restoration programs (relaxation, stress management, coping)	Psych: + Pain: NA Function: + Meds: NA	12 mo Psych: + Pain: + Function: + Meds: NA Work: 0	NA	+
Altmaier et al., 1992 (2)	45 f = 27%	Low back	1. Standard rehabilitation	2. Standard + CBT (relaxation, coping, exercise reinforcement)	Psych: NA Pain: 0 Function: 0 Meds: NA	6 mo Psych: NA Pain: 0 Function: 0 Meds: NA Work: 0	NA	0
Basler et al., 1997 (3)	76 f = 76%	Chronic low back, average duration, 11 yr	1. Usual pain center treatment, e.g., TENS, medication, physical therapy	2. Usual pain center treatment (1) + CBT (education, relaxation, modifying thoughts and feeling, enhancing pleasant activities)	Psych: + Pain: + Function: + Meds: NA	6 mo Control not available Improvements maintained	NA	+
Flor and Birbaumer, 1993 (8)	78 f = 60%	Chronic back, tempromandibular joint	1. Conservative	2. CBT (pain and stress management) 3. EMG biofeedback	Psych: + (3>1) Pain: + (3>2,1) Function: NA Meds: NA	24 mo, EMG superior Psych: + Pain: NA Function: + Meds: NA Work: NA Health care: +	NA	+
Fordyce et al., 1986 (11)	107 f = 39%	Acute low back (1–10 d)	1. Usual management	2. Behavioral management (operant exercise quotas, medication program)	Psych: NA Pain: 0 Function: 0 Meds: NA	12 mo Psych: NA Pain: NA Function: + Meds: NA Work: 0	NA	0

continued

Study	Population	Condition	Intervention groups	Outcomes	Follow-up		
Friedrich et al., 1998 (12)	93 f = 49%	Chronic low back (mean duration 48 mo)	1. Standard exercise 2. Standard exercise + compliance (instructions, reinforcement, contract, reminders, monitoring)	Psych: 0 Pain: 0 Function: + Meds: NA work: +	12-mo compliance 2>1 Psych: 0 Pain: 0 Function: + Meds: NA Work: +	NA	+
Keller et al., 1997 (18)	63 f = 71%	Chronic	1. WLC 2. CBT (exercise goals, coping, relaxation education)	Psych: + Pain: + Function: + Meds: NA	6-mo follow-up WLC: NA Improvements maintained	+	NA
Kerns et al., 1986 (19)	28 f = 18%	Chronic	1. WLC 2. Behavioral (social reinforcement, rehearsal, monitoring, relaxation) 3. CBT (reconceptualization, coping, relaxation, role playing)	Psych: + (3>2, 1) Pain: + (3>2, 1) Function: + (3>2, 1) Meds: NA Health care: + (2,3>1)	3/6 mo WLC: NA Differences between types of treatment marginal	+	NA
Kole-Snijders et al., 1999 (20)	148 f = 64%	Chronic low back, average 9.8 yr	1. WLC 2. Usual treatment (graded activity); note this is WLC after waiting period 3. Operant (graded activity, spouse training) + cognitive and relaxation (reconceptualization, applied relaxation) 4. Operant (as 2) + group discussion (discussed pain as attrition control for group 3)	Psych: + (4,3>1) Pain: + (3>4,1) Function: + (4,3>1) Meds: NA	12 mo Effects maintained, no significant differences among the three CBT groups (2,3,4)	+	NA
Lindström et al., 1992 (22)	103 f = 31%	Subacute low back	1. Traditional care 2. Graded activity + workplace visit + back school	None	24-mo follow-up Psych: NA Pain: NA Function: + Meds: NA Work: +	NA	+

TABLE 17.2. Continued

Investigators (ref.)	No. of patients	Pain	Control	Psychologic treatment	Posttreatment status[a]	Follow-up	Conclusion WLC	Conclusion Active
Linton and Götestam, 1984 (23)	20 f = 55%	Chronic back	1. WLC	2. Applied relaxation 3. 2 + operant (applied relax + medication reduction, exercise quotas, social reinforcement)	Psych: + (3,2>1) Pain: + (2>1) Function: + (3,2>1) Meds: + (3,2>1)	9 mo WLC: NA Gains maintained by 3 and 2	+	NA
Linton et al., 1985 (24), and Melin and Linton, 1988 (25)	28 f = 54%	Chronic back	1. WLC	2. Usual treatment 3. 2 + applied relaxation and operant activity	Psych: 0 Pain: + (3>2,1) Function: + (3>1) Meds: + (3>1)	20 mo Psych: 0 Pain: + (3>2,1) Function: + (3>2,1) Meds: 0 Work: 0	+	+
Moore and Chaney, 1985 (26)	43 f = 2%	Chronic, 29 low back	1. WLC	2. CBT (relaxation operant conditioning principles) 3. CBT couples (same as 2, but provided to couple)	Psych: + (3,2>1) Pain: + (3,2>1) Function: + (3,2>1) Meds: NA	7 mo WLC: NA Maintained	+	NA
Newton-John et al., 1995 (28)	44 f = 61%	Chronic low back	1. WLC	2. CBT (goal setting, activity scheduling, relaxation, diversion, relabeling) 3. EMG biofeedback	Psych: + (3,2>1) Pain: + (3,2>1) Function: + (3,2>1) Meds: NA	6 mo WLC: Na Maintained	+	NA
Nicholas et al., 1992 (30)	20 f = 45%	Chronic low back	1. Attention control + back education + exercise	2. 1 + CBT (activity goals, depression therapy, coping, cognitions)	Psych: + Pain: 0 Function: + Meds: NA	6 mo Psych: + Pain: 0 Function: + Meds: NA Work: NA	NA	+

Study	Sample	Population	Treatment conditions	Outcomes	Follow-up		
Nicholas et al., 1991 (29)	58 f = 52%	Chronic low back	1. Physical therapy 2. 1 + Attention 3. 1 + cognitive (negative cognitions, relaxation, pain management) 4. 1 + behavioral (activity goals, depression, relax)	Psych: + (3,4>2,1) Pain: + (3,4>2,1) Function: + (3,4>2,1) Meds: + (3,4>2,1)	12 mo Psych: + (3,4>2,1) Pain: + (3,4>2,1) Function: + (3,4>2,1) Meds: 0 Work: NA	NA	+
Peters and Large, 1990 (31)	68 f = 62%	Chronic, 29 back	1. No-treatment control 2. CBT inpatient 3. CBT outpatient (education, relaxation, coping, exercise, counseling, medications, social reinforcement)	Psych: + (2,3>1) Pain: + (2,3>1) Function: + (2,3>1) Meds: NA	12 mo Psych: 0 Pain: + (2,3>1) Function: 0 Meds: NA Work: NA	+	NA
Puder, 1988 (32)	69 f = 71%	Chronic, 70% musculoskeletal	1. WLC 2. CBT (stress inoculation)	Psych: + Pain: 0 Function: + Meds: + Health care: +	6 mo WLC: NA Maintained	+	NA
Rose et al., 1997 (33)	84 f = ?	Chronic back (8.1 yr)	1. Group CBT (education, cognitions, graded activity, relaxation) 2. Individual CBT (same as 1)	Psych: + Pain: + Function: + Meds: NA	6 mo Psych: + Pain: + Function: + Meds: NA Work: NA	NA	+
Spence, 1989 (35)	45 f = 98%	Chronic neck, upper limbs	1. WLC 2. Individual CBT (relaxation, goal setting, cognitive restructuring, coping assertion) 3. Group CBT	Psych: + (3,2>1) Pain: 0 Function: + (3,2>1) Meds: 0	24 mo WLC: NA Maintained, 2 = 3	+	NA
Spence et al., 1995 (36)	48 f = 84%	Chronic neck, upper limb	1. WLC 2. Applied relaxation 3. EMG biofeedback 4. 2 + 3	Psych: + (4,3,2>1) Pain: 0 Function: 0 Meds: NA	6 mo WLC: NA Some relapse, still significant gains on depression, beliefs, and anxiety	0	NA

continued

TABLE 17.2. Continued

Investigators (ref.)	No. of patients	Pain	Control	Psychologic treatment	Posttreatment status[a]	Follow-up	Conclusion WLC	Conclusion Active
Strong, 1998 (37)	30 f = ?	Chronic low back (7 yr)	1. Placebo (nonspecific health info.) + usual rehabilitation	2. CBT psychoeducation stressing cognitive, emotional, and behavioral change + usual rehabilitation	(Used three factors in analyses) Psych: + Pain: + Function: + Meds: NA	3 mo Only 18 patients available	NA	+
Stuckey et al., 1986 (38)	24 f = 54%	Chronic low back for at least 6 mo	1. Placebo (same setting as 2, but no feedback)	2. EMG biofeedback (upper trapezius) 3. Relaxation (progressive)	Psych: + (3>2,1) Pain: + (3>2,1) Function: + (3>2) Meds: NA relatively small differences.	None	NA	+
Turner and Jensen, 1993 (43)	102 f = 54%	Chronic low back with mild disability	1. WLC	2. cognitive (stress management, coping, negative emotions) 3. relaxation (progressive) 4. 2 + 3	Psych: 0 Pain: + (4,3,2>1) Function: 0 Meds: NA	12 mo WLC: NA All three treatment groups improved before follow-up	0	NA
Turner and Clancy, 1988 (42)	81 f = 37%	Chronic low back with mild disability	1. WLC	2. Operant (social reinforcement, communication, exercise goals) 3. CBT (relaxation, negative emotions, cognitions, coping)	Psych: + (2>1) Pain: + (2>1) Function: + (2>1) Meds: NA	12 mo WLC: NA 2 = 3 both improved	+	NA
Turner et al., 1990 (44)	96 f = 48%	Chronic low back with mild disability	1. WLC	2. Aerobic exercise 3. Behavioral therapy only (social reinforcement, communication, goal setting) 4. Behavioral therapy + 2	Psych: + (4>1) Pain: + (4>1) Function: + (4>1) Meds: NA	12 mo WLC: NA Remain improved, no difference between treatment groups	+	NA

Study	N, sex	Pain	Intervention	Results	Follow-up		
Turner, 1982 (40)	36 f = 85%	Chronic low back	1. Attention control 2. Relaxation (progressive) 3. CBT (relaxation, stress inoculation)	Psych: + (3,2>1) Pain: + (3,2>1) Function: + (3,2>1) Meds: NA	24 mo WLC: NA Gains maintained relax = CBT	+	NA
Von Korff et al., 1998 (47)	255 f = 62%	Back (6–8 wk after primary care)	1. Usual care + self-care book 2. Self-management (problem solving, activity management, educational videos)	Psych: + Pain: 0 Function: + Meds: NA	12 mo attitude toward self-care 2>1 Psych: + Pain: 0 Function: + Meds: NA Work: NA	NA	+
Williams et al., 1996 (48)	121 f = 53%	Chronic 74% neck or back	1. WLC 2. CBT inpatient (exercise quotas, goal setting, pacing, education, problem solving, drug reduction, family) 3. CBT outpatient	Psych: + (2>3>1) Pain: + (2>3>1) Function: + (2>3>1) Meds: + (2>3>1)	12 mo WLC: NA Maintained, in-patients better than outpatients	+	NA

F, female; CBT, cognitive-behavioral therapy; EMG, electromyography; TENS, transcutaneous electrical nerve stimulation; WLC, waiting list control.

[a]Key variables are defined as follows: Psych., psychological variable such as depression, anxiety or tension, emotions, and coping; Pain, such as intensity or an index; Function, e.g., activity level or disability; Meds, medication usage such as amount of analgesics consumed; Work, representing time lost from work such as sick days or return-to-work status; and health care utilization. Designations are as follows:

+ positive: if the psychologic treatment intervention is more effective (statistically significant difference) than the control intervention on at least two domains variable), and there are no statistically significant differences on the other domains.

− negative: if the psychologic treatment intervention is less effective (statistically significant difference) than a control intervention on at least one domain, and there are no statistically significant differences on the other key variables or if the psychologic treatment is not more effective than no intervention at all.

0 neutral: if there is no statistically significant difference between the psychologic treatment intervention and control intervention on any of the domains.

NA: not applicable; if the variable was not recorded or the design did not allow for a comparison to be made.

posttest. Altmaier et al. (2) reported no difference. However, in 15 of the trials, the control group was no longer available for comparison. This was a particular problem for studies using waiting-list control groups because 13 of the 16 studies did not have the control group available for comparison at the follow-up. Although this situation is understandable when a waiting-list control means withholding treatment, it does create problems for drawing conclusions about the long-term effects of the treatment.

Example Studies

To present a more in-depth description of how studies in this field are designed and what results are produced, three studies are described here. First, Jensen et al. (17) conducted an outpatient study of the effects of a CBT package program administered to Swedish workers with spinal pain who had been home from work for less than 6 months. A matched controlled design was employed in which 70 participants were matched with regard to age, employment status, employment type, diagnosis, and duration of sick leave. The 35 participants in the CBT group received 5 modules ranging from education (interdisciplinary view of pain), CBT skills (a tailored program with 8 sessions involving problem solving, goal setting acquisition skill, and applied relaxation), physical therapy (emphasized physical activity and self-care), occupational support (a meeting with representatives of the workplace and insurance representatives), and a short course for the patient's supervisor. All modules were integrated and designed from a CBT perspective. The comparison group received treatment as usual. Outcome was assessed before and after treatment as well as at a 6-month follow-up. The results indicated that the CBT group made significantly larger improvements with regard to disability, pain, and depression. Interestingly, the greatest benefits, by far, were observed for women. An 18-month follow-up (16) showed that the differences were maintained. However, there was no significant difference between the groups for sick leave because both groups showed a decreasing trend.

An excellent study that compared the results of an inpatient and an outpatient CBT program with a waiting-list control group was reported (48). One hundred twenty-one patients with mixed pain, but predominantly spinal pain, of an average of more than 90 months' duration were randomized to a 4-week inpatient course or 8 half-days of outpatient CBT or to a waiting-list control group. The staff, teaching materials, and setting were the same for both groups. The program included exercise and training, goal setting, pacing, education, problem solving, changing maladaptive coping behaviors and thoughts, drug reduction, relaxation, sleep management, relapse prevention, and family involvement. Results were assessed with a broad battery of measures before treatment and at 1, 6, and 12 months after discharge. The results showed that although there was virtually no change in the control group, inpatients and outpatients made significant improvements in physical performance and psychologic function, and they reduced medication use. However, the inpatients made greater gains, maintained them better, and used less health care at the 1-year follow-up than did the outpatients.

Keller and associates (18) studied the effects of a CBT-oriented multidimensional program on patients with chronic low back pain in an outpatient setting. Sixty-five patients were randomly allocated to a treatment or a waiting-list control group. The treatment was provided in groups and consisted of 18 meetings lasting 2 hours each in addition to 18 individualized training sessions of 30 minutes. The components of treatment were education, relaxation training, pleasant activity scheduling and distraction, and physical exercise and posture training. Outcome was assessed with a broad range of variables including functional capacity, disability, muscular strength, pain and posture self-efficacy, attitudes, depression, well-being, behavioral habits, and posture at pretreatment and posttreatment evaluation, as well as at a 6-month follow-up. At posttest, the treatment group showed significant improvements on all variables except depression and muscular strength. The improvements for the group receiving CBT treatment were maintained at follow-up, although the waiting-list control was no longer available for statistical comparison.

Finally, an evaluation based in Bergen, Norway, (15) assessed a multimodal CBT program for outpatients who were certified for illness because of musculoskeletal pain. Four hundred sixty-nine patients on sick leave were randomly assigned to the CBT intervention that comprised a 4-week program of physical treatment, cognitive-behavioral modification, education, and workplace-based interventions or to a control group treated by their general practitioner. At a 1-year follow-up, the patients who received multimodal CBT had significantly better improvements on ergonomic behavior, work potential, quality of life, and physical and mental health. However, the return-to-work rate was about equivalent to that of the control group. Although this study does not meet our inclusion criteria, it does illustrate an interesting application of CBT in a multidimensional program.

Summary

The results of the RCTs demonstrate a consistent effect in which CBT is superior to waiting-list control groups or other forms of active treatments. Notwithstanding the generally favorable results, there are several critical points to be considered when evaluating the CBT studies. First, few studies identified the necessary content of CBT or the effects of specific techniques; that is, many designs compared a package, and these packages generally varied considerably from study to study. Therefore, there was a lack of information about the components needed to achieve an adequate CBT program. Second, although the results included variables relevant to the treatment, they often employed different assessment methods. This makes it difficult to compare across studies, as well as to determine the exact impact from a broader perspective. Finally, although the studies showed statistically and clinically significant results, most studies employed a limited number of participants and were conducted in unique settings that may have reduced their generalizability to other patients and settings.

EVIDENCE-BASED CONCLUSIONS

Based on the studies identified in Table 17.2 as well as the systematic reviews, the following conclusions concerning the effects of CBT on primarily chronic neck and back pain may be drawn at this time:

1. Multidimensional programs that include CBT programs are statistically and clinically superior to control groups on key outcome variables: level A evidence.

2. CBT programs produce moderate to large improvements on the key outcome variables as compared with waiting-list controls: level A evidence.

3. Compared with active treatment, CBT has a small to moderate effect on key outcome variables: level B evidence.

4. The CBT programs appear to have their largest effects on psychologic function, pain, physical function, and medication intake. Few studies examined the variable of return-to-work because this was not relevant for many of the patients: level C evidence.

5. There is weak evidence indicating equivalence between components and techniques in CBT treatment; that is, there is little indication at present that one form of CBT is better than another: level C evidence.

6. There is some evidence to show that the significant posttreatment improvements are maintained at long-term follow-up, but only limited evidence to show that CBT remains significantly superior to control conditions because control groups are often not available at follow-up: level C evidence.

Thus, there is considerable evidence that CBT may be useful especially for patients with chronic neck or back pain. Most of the studies dealt with the treatment of patients with long histories of a back pain problem. Consequently, a return-to-work was not a primary goal for the patients in most of these studies. The evidence to date suggests that CBT programs may help to improve quality of life. Moreover, the original concept of behavioral treatment seems to have been incorporated into many guidelines because graded (operant) activity training and the medication reduction program are central aspects of pain treatment today, and relaxation and cognitive techniques are common as well. Although the idea of applying CBT at an earlier point is interesting and some preliminary studies have shown promise, there is a dire lack of properly controlled studies from which to draw accurate conclusions about the specific effects of CBT on acute or subacute neck or back pain.

The conclusions in this chapter may be compared with those in Chapter 12 on conservative treatment of chronic low back pain. In Chapter 12, only patients with chronic low back pain are included. Moreover, multidisciplinary programs that usually employ CBT methods of some sort are evaluated separately, whereas only studies using behavioral techniques are included. This differs from the present chapter, which includes reviews of multidisciplinary programs, while Table 17.2 is based on studies that isolated a broader array of treatment, that is, CBT techniques. Another difference is that Chapter 12 systematically evaluates the quality of the studies, whereas to ensure quality, this chapter has included only RCTs. As a result, this chapter has 29 studies in Table 17.2, whereas Chapter 12 includes 10 studies on behavior therapy. Nevertheless, the conclusions are t similar because Chapter 12 notes strong evidence for the utility of multidisciplinary programs and moderate evidence for behavioral treatments as compared with a waiting-list control.

Several methodologic points deserve mention. The difficulties in conducting a proper RCT in this area make the review procedure cumbersome. For example, CBT has been conceptualized as part of a multidimensional treatment, and therefore isolating the effect of psychologic treatments presents a considerable challenge. Most often, CBT, by itself, has been compared with a waiting-list control group. Although a check of the 29 studies showed that waiting-list control groups tended to remain the same or to improve slightly during this period and thus constituted a feasible control, these groups unfortunately did not control for nonspecific effects, and the groups were often terminated on ethical grounds at posttest, thus precluding statistical comparisons at long-term follow-up.

Moreover, there is a lack of description specifying the content of the treatment, the amount provided, the therapists involved, and the way in which the psychologic component may have been combined with other approaches. These details are important in sorting out the effects of the treatment, particularly when comparing studies. Further, investigators usually use convenience samples from their own clinics, and these samples may be limited in size by availability and by the expense of the treatment. Certainly, samples from one clinic may not be comparable with those of another.

Nevertheless, the evidence in the review articles and in Table 17.2 showed a consistent effect relative to a waiting-list control group or a group receiving active treatment. The size of the effect, when CBT was isolated, was moderate, although the effect sizes in the reviews on multidimensional treatment were larger. Some indication that the effects were maintained at long-term follow-up was the rule.

RESEARCH NEEDS

1. Properly designed, long-term follow-up comparisons, such as comparisons with other cost-effective alternative treatments.
2. Studies of the process of "change," that is, what techniques enable patients to feel better.
3. Development and evaluation of CBT methods to enhance the treatment of problems early on as well as to prevent recurrence.
4. The identification of prognostic factors for CBT.
5. Matching CBT techniques to the patient to produce tailored treatment. This is relevant to questions of which techniques to choose for which person, as well as the question of which techniques are most effective within CBT.

REFERENCES

1. Alaranta H, Rytökoski U, Rissanen A, et al. Intensive physical and psychosocial training program for patients with chronic low back pain: a controlled clinical trial. *Spine* 1994;19:1339–1349.
2. Altmaier EM, Lehmann TR, Russell DW, et al. The effectiveness of psychological interventions for the rehabilitation of low back pain: a randomized controlled trial evaluation. *Pain* 1992;49:329–335.
3. Basler HD, Jäkle C, Kröner-Herwig B. Incorporation of cognitive-behavioral treatment into the medical care of chronic low back patients: a controlled randomized study in German pain treatment centers. *Patient Educ Counseling* 1997;31:113–124.
4. Compas BE, Haaga DAF, Keefe FJ, et al. A sampling of empirically supported psychological treatments from health psychology: smoking, chronic pain, cancer, and bulimia nervosa. *J Consult Clin Psychol* 1998;66:89–112.
5. Cutler RB, Fishbain DA, Rosomoff HL, et al. Does nonsurgical pain center treatment of chronic pain return patients to work? A review and meta-analysis of the literature. *Spine* 1994;19:643–652.
6. Flor H. *A way out of the vicious circle: learning to manage chronic pain through self-control.* Berlin: Humboldt University, 1997.
7. Flor H. Der Stellenwert verhaltenstherapeutischer Ansaetze bei der Behandlung chronischer Schmerzen [The value of behavior therapy in the treatment of chronic pain]. *Der Kassenarzt* 1999;39:40–46.
8. Flor H, Birbaumer N. Comparison of the efficacy of electromyographic biofeedback, congnitive-behavioral therapy, and conservative interventions in the treatment of chronic musculoskeletal pain. *J Consult Clin Psychol* 1993;61:653–658.
9. Flor H, Fydrich T, Turk DC. Efficacy of multidisciplinary pain treatment centers: a meta-analytic review. *Pain* 1992;49:221–230.
10. Fordyce WE. *Behavioral methods for chronic pain and illness.* St. Louis: CV Mosby, 1976.
11. Fordyce WE, Brockway JA, Bergman JA, et al. Acute back pain: a control-group comparison of behavioral vs traditional management methods. *J Behav Med* 1986;9:127–140.
12. Friedrich M, Gittler G, Halberstadt Y, et al. Combined exercise and motivation program: effect on the compliance and level of disability of patients with chronic back pain. *Arch Phys Med Rehabil* 1998;79:475–487.
13. Gatchel RJ, Turk DC, eds. *Psychological approaches to pain management: a practitioner's handbook.* New York: Guilford Press, 1996.
14. Grzesiak RC, Ury GM, Dworkin RH. Psychodynamic psychotherapy with chronic pain patients. In: Gatchel RJ, Turk DC, eds. *Psychological approaches to pain management: a practitioner's handbook,* vol 1. New York: Guilford Press, 1996.

15. Haldorsen EMH, Kronholm K, Skouen JS, et al. Multimodal cognitive behavioral treatment of patients sicklisted for musculoskeletal pain: a randomized controlled study. *Scand J Rheumatol* 1998;27: 16–25.
16. Jensen IB, Bodin L. Multimodal cognitive-behavioural treatment for workers with chronic spinal pain: a matched cohort study with an 18-month follow-up. *Pain* 1998;76:35–44.
17. Jensen IB, Nygren Å, Lundin A. Cognitive-behavioral treatment for workers with chronic spinal pain: a matched and controlled cohort study in Sweden. *Occup Environ Med* 1994;51:145–151.
18. Keller S, Ehrhardt-Schmelzer S, Herda C, et al. Multidisciplinary rehabilitation for chronic back pain in an outpatient setting: a controlled randomized trial. *Eur J Pain* 1997;1:279–292.
19. Kerns RD, Turk DC, Holzman AD, et al. Comparison of cognitive behavioral and behavioral approaches to the outpatient treatment of chronic pain. *Clin J Pain* 1986;1:195–203.
20. Kole-Snijders AMJ, Vlaeyen JWS, Goossens MEJB, et al. Chronic low back pain: what does cognitive coping skills training add to operant behavioral treatment? Results of a randomized clinical trial. *Journal of Consulting and Clinical Psychology.* 1999;67:931–944.
21. Lindström I, Öhlund C, Nachemson A. Validity of patient reporting and predictive value of industrial physical work demands. *Spine* 1994;19:888–893.
22. Lindström I, Öhlund C, Eek C, et al. The effect of graded activity on patients with subacute low back pain: a randomized prospective clinical study with an operant-conditioning behavioral approach. *Phys Ther* 1992;72:279–293.
23. Linton SJ, Götestam KG. A controlled study of the effects of applied relaxation and applied relaxation plus operant procedures on the regulation of chronic pain. *Br J Clin Psychol* 1984;23:291–299.
24. Linton SJ, Melin L, Stjernlöf K. The effects of applied relaxation and operant activity training on chronic pain. *Behav Psychother* 1985;13:87–100.
25. Melin L, Linton SJ. A follow-up study of a comprehensive behavioural treatment programme for chronic pain patients. *Behav Psychother* 1988;16:313–322.
26. Moore JE, Chaney EF. Outpatient group treatment of chronic pain: effects of spouse involvement. *J Consult Clin Psychol* 1985;53:326–334.
27. Morley S, Eccleston C, Williams A. Systematic review and meta-analysis of randomised controlled trials of cognitive behaviour therapy and behaviour therapy for chronic pain in adults, excluding headache. *Pain* 1999;80:1–13.
28. Newton-John TR, Spence SH, Schotte D. Cognitive-behavioural therapy versus EMG biofeedback in the treatment of chronic low back pain. *Behav Res Ther* 1995;33:691–697.
29. Nicholas MK, Wilson PH, Goyen J. Operant-behavioural and cognitive-behavioural treatment for chronic low back pain. *Behav Res Ther* 1991;29:225–238.
30. Nicholas MK, Wilson PH, Goyen J. Comparison of cognitive-behavioral group treatment and an alternative non-psychological treatment for chronic low back pain. *Pain* 1992;48:339–347.
31. Peters JL, Large RG. A randomised control trial evaluating in- and outpatient pain management programmes. *Pain* 1990;41:283–293.
32. Puder RS. Age analysis of cognitive-behavioral group therapy for chronic pain outpatients. *Psychol Aging* 1988;3:204–207.
33. Rose MJ, Reilly JP, Pennie B, et al. Chronic low back pain rehabilitation programs: a study of the optimum duration of treatment and a comparison of group vs. individual therapy. *Spine* 1997;22:2246–2253.
34. Sackett DL, Richardson WS, Rosenberg W, et al. *Evidence-based medicine: how to practice and teach EBM.* New York: Churchill Livingstone, 1997.
35. Spence SH. Cognitive-behavioral therapy in the management of chronic, occupational pain of the upper limbs. *Behav Res Ther* 1989;27:435–446.
36. Spence SH, Sharpe L, Newton-John T, et al. Effect of EMG biofeedback compared to applied relaxation training with chronic, upper extremity cumulative trauma disorders. *Pain* 1995;63:199–206.
37. Strong J. Incorporating cognitive-behavioral therapy with occupational therapy: a comparative study with patients with low back pain. *J Occup Rehabil* 1998;8:61–71.
38. Stuckey SJ, Jacobs A, Goldfarb J. EMG biofeedback training, relaxation training, and placebo for the relief of chronic back pain. *Percept Mot Skills* 1986;63:1023–1036.
39. Turk DC. Biopsychosocial perspective on chronic pain. In: Gatchel RJ, Turk DC, eds. *Psychological approaches to pain management: a practitioner's handbook,* vol 1. New York: Guilford Press, 1996.
40. Turner JA. Comparison of group progressive-relaxation training and cognitive-behavioral group therapy for chronic low back pain. *J Consult Clin Psychol* 1982;50:757–765.
41. Turner JA. Educational and behavioral interventions for back pain in primary care. *Spine* 1996;21:2851–2859.
42. Turner JA, Clancy S. Comparison of operant behavioral and cognitive-behavioral group treatment for chronic low back pain. *J Consult Clin Psychol* 1988;56:261–266.
43. Turner JA, Jensen MP. Efficacy of cognitive therapy for chronic low back pain. *Pain* 1993;52:169–177.
44. Turner JA, Clancy S, McQuade KJ, et al. Effectiveness of behavioral therapy for chronic low back pain: a component analysis. *J Consult Clin Psychol* 1990;58:573–579.

45. van Tulder MW, Koes BW, Bouter LM. Conservative treatment of acute and chronic nonspecific low back pain. *Spine* 1997;22:2128–2156.
46. van Tulder MW, Assendelft WJJ, Koes BW, et al. Methodologic guidelines for systematic reviews in the Cochrane Collaboration Back Review Group for spinal disorders. *Spine* 1997;22:2323–2330.
47. von Korff M, Moore JE, Lorig K, et al. A randomized trial of a lay-led self-management group intervention for back pain patients in primary care. *Spine* 1998;23:2608–2615.
48. Williams ACDC, Richardson PH, Nicholas MK, et al. Inpatient vs outpatient pain management: results of a randomised controlled trial. *Pain* 1996;66:13–22.

*Neck and Back Pain: The Scientific Evidence
of Causes, Diagnosis, and Treatment*, edited
by Alf Nachemson and Egon Jonsson.
Published by Lippincott Williams & Wilkins,
Philadelphia 2000.

18

Treatment of Neck and Low Back Pain in Primary Care

Margareta Söderström* and Lars Englund†

*Department of Family Medicine, Göteborg University, Göteborg, Sweden
†Department of Public Health and Caring Sciences, Family Medicine Section, Uppsala
University, Uppsala Science Park, Uppsala, Sweden

Evidence-based guidelines for treating patients with neck and low back pain have been developed from previously published systematic reviews of the scientific literature. The guidelines give high priority to primary care as an appropriate source of treatment for these patients (18,22,31,39).

Furthermore, studies suggest that primary care may be the only treatment source required for most patients with back problems. The research emphasizes the importance of a thorough medical history (anamnesis) and a physical examination adequate to identify the few patients who should be referred to other specialties for diagnosis and treatment of cancer, severe infection, specific rheumatic disease, and other severe conditions that may cause back pain. For other patients with back pain, the most important role of the primary care physician is to intervene as little as possible and to avoid subjecting patients to ineffective examinations or treatments that may lead to the development of chronic problems.

The guidelines for general practitioners (GPs) developed by the Royal College of General Practitioners in England (40) state that: "A simple but fundamental change, away from the traditional recommendation of bed rest toward a positive recommendation to remain active would improve clinical outcomes and reduce the personal and social impact of back pain." This advice is particularly important when psychosocial factors are involved because such factors may encourage and accelerate a transition from temporary to chronic back pain (24). One way to avoid this is to inform patients (after history taking and physical examination) that their pain is not the result of back damage and that it is not harmful to resume normal daily activities (49). Nevertheless, many important questions remain unanswered, and much more research is needed on how best to address and treat patients who visit primary care clinics for back problems.

The findings presented in previous chapters are also relevant in primary care of patients with neck and low back pain. Strict application of evidence-based medicine may be difficult in practice for the GP in primary care. Physicians often see patients who have vague symptoms, which in some cases may be typical of low back problems, but these problems may also be combined with symptoms of other disorders. Many randomized controlled studies that assess the effects of different treatment methods do not include patients with vague or complex combinations of symptoms and diseases.

Studying such situations requires other types of complementary studies, including those using qualitative methods (43).

This chapter differs from the other treatment chapters in this book. Although the chapter is based on a review of the scientific literature, it was neither meaningful nor possible to classify and grade the studies systematically on the strength of the evidence because few studies assessed the problem from a broader perspective, and they dealt only indirectly with the outcomes of various treatment strategies. Rather, we selected studies that covered broader aspects that we judged to be particularly relevant to primary care.

LITERATURE SEARCH

The keyword "family practice" yielded a voluminous number of studies in the various databases. Few of these (150 references) addressed the treatment of patients with back problems. However, not all were found to be relevant to this chapter. Considering the outcomes of treatment methods discussed in the previous chapters, we found selected studies that addressed other important aspects of back pain from a primary care perspective.

PATIENT-DOCTOR RELATIONSHIP

Knowledge about the meaning of the patient-doctor relationship is important to clinical decisions and the quality of care (26,34). General practice in medicine is characterized by a focus on the patient-doctor relationship. Biomedical, personal, and more holistic perspectives characterize the diagnosis.

The importance of the patient-doctor relationship in different contexts has received increasing interest (1). The Swedish Council on Technology Assessment in Health Care, for example, published a scientific review on the topic (35). Earlier, the prevailing attitude had been that a good patient-doctor relationship was no more than a superficial polish, whereas biologic factors and medical interventions actually determined the outcome of treatment. This perspective is now shifting toward a more holistic biomedical and psychosocial view toward complicated and complex problems such as back pain. Hence, the consultation itself should be viewed as a valuable treatment resource, and when it takes place in a positive atmosphere with mutual respect, it promotes the patient's recovery.

Patients' attitudes about their symptoms and diseases are influenced by a range of factors such as previous experience, expectations, psychosocial resources, and the perceptions of other people. Patients have perceptions concerning the nature of disease, its causes, its severity, and how it can be cured. In addition, gender—both of the patient as well as the doctor—may influence the outcome of a consultation (23,30). Although the patient's understanding of a disease differs from the physician's, it is no less important. Numerous studies (many of which are presented in earlier chapters) have shown that patients' attitudes are important factors in the progression of disease and in medical treatment decisions (29).

A descriptive study from Ontario, Canada analyzed factors that influenced treatment results in approximately 200 patients from 13 different general practice clinics. The patients had symptoms that they had not earlier experienced, involving gastrointestinal distress, back and/or neck pain, chest pain, headache, fatigue, or blood in the feces (2). The patients were followed-up after 1 month, and if they continued to demonstrate symptoms, a second follow-up was scheduled 2 months later. Two independent observers conducted telephone interviews with the patients and reviewed the records to determine the quality of the consultation based on the patients' history, medical examination, and medications. Thereafter, factors that may have played a role in alleviating the symptoms were analyzed. The factor that was most strongly associated with the alleviation of symptoms after 1 month was that the physician and the patient had the same perception concerning the nature of the problem. After 3 months of follow-up, the physician's level of awareness about relevant psychosocial problems was the factor most strongly related to the alleviation of symptoms. No association was demonstrated between symptom alleviation and medical history, physical examination, use of laboratory tests, and prescription of drugs.

In a descriptive study from Mexico City, an anthropologist studied factors responsible for symptom alleviation (17). The study included 267 patients with problems such as back pain, headache, fatigue, and gastrointestinal disorders. These patients were interviewed before visiting an outpatient clinic in internal medicine. Each physician gave a diagnosis immediately after the consultation. After approximately 1 month, the patients were visited in their homes, and changes in their symptoms were documented using interviews and questionnaires. The survey showed that 17% had no remaining symptoms, 25% reported no change, and varying degrees of symptom relief were reported in the remaining patients. These three groups (completely recovered, partially recovered, and unchanged) were related to a series of variables such as specific symptoms, number of diagnoses per patient, number of laboratory tests taken, prescribed drugs, and number of days with symptoms before the physician visit. The following five variables were most strongly correlated with the degree of recovery: (a) whether the physician had explained the cause of the symptoms to the patient, (b) whether the physician had given the patient a diagnosis, (c) whether the physician and the patient held the same perception about the problem, (d) whether the patient was active and asked questions during the visit, and (e) how long the patient had experienced symptoms. The authors distinguished two different types of patients. One type included patients with chronic or long-term symptoms, for whom the patient-doctor relationship played a secondary role in recovery. The second type included patients who had symptoms for a shorter period, and the patient-doctor relationship played an important role in the recovery of these patients.

A study from Seattle analyzed how satisfaction with care was influenced by the attitudes of GPs toward patients with back pain (7). The results showed that the GPs' attitudes did not correlate with any of the measures used to assess patient satisfaction with care. Patients of doctors who were more secure in their role as physicians were, however, significantly more satisfied with the information they received than patients visiting physicians who seemed less secure in their role as physicians.

A study by von Korff et al. analyzed the effects of three different physician styles, based on the degree of "intervention" (52). The study included 44 GPs who treated approximately 1,000 patients presenting with back pain. The physicians were classified into three groups based on their rates of prescribing painkillers and recommending bed rest. In the follow-up study after 1 month, the patients of physicians who prescribed fewer painkillers and recommended less bed rest reported fewer limitations in activity than the other patients. In the 1-year follow-up, these patients were also more satisfied than others with the information they received on how they should deal with their back pain. Furthermore, their care required fewer resources. However, the long-term outcomes, measured as satisfaction with care, pain, and functional status, were similar in all three groups.

A study from England, based on in-depth interviews, analyzed patients' perspectives on low back pain and their perceptions about treatment delivered by GPs (44) (Table 18.1). A cohort consisting of 52 adult patients with low back pain who visited 12 GPs was invited to participate in the study. The prerequisites included the following: no signs of nerve root involvement, no indications of inflammatory disease, and no previous back surgery. The cohort was considered representative of patients with low back pain who visited primary care services in various parts of Great Britain. The results of the study showed that most patients visit their family doctor only when pain is intense. They hesitated to seek care because they were afraid to waste the doctor's time or they were skeptical about the doctor's ability to help. Some patients were also concerned about their possibilities for employment if they sought medical care. The few patients who consulted a GP usually wanted their disease confirmed, or they viewed the consultation as an opportunity to discuss alternative treatment strategies. Equally as many in the cohort were satisfied as were dissatisfied with the physician's treatment. Those who were satisfied placed greatest value on the physician's communication skills and the thoroughness of the diagnosis. In particular, they valued the physician's approach in addressing the disease history, the thoroughness of the examination, and how well the physician explained the results of diagnostic tests. The patients reported that they were not looking for a magic cure for low back pain because they did not believe such a cure existed. However, they wanted the physician to listen to them and to offer appropriate treatment advice.

A study of primary care in Sweden (30) described a cognitive treatment method in the consultation process. The study randomized 92 patients, all young immigrants, to a treatment group or a control group. The patients had been on sick leave for more than 6 weeks for pain, including low back pain. The treatment consisted of three long, structured dialogues with an emphasis on the patient's focus on pain. Physical and structured dialogues, psychologic examinations, and self-assessment of working capacity and fear of pain were performed before and after the program. The progression of the disorder during the sick leave period was discussed, and follow-up took place at 3 and 6 months. After completion of the program, significant differences benefiting the treatment group were identified; for example, fewer patients were afraid of pain, fewer were diagnosed with depression, more assessed their working capacity higher, and more had returned to work at 8-month follow-up. The study also showed that primary care physicians normally use a range of treatment methods, including cognitive therapy.

In summary, these studies suggest that physician involvement, empathy, and ability to listen but to intervene as little as possible are of major importance. During the consultation, a shared perception on the nature of low back pain by the patient and the physician can improve the course, at least in patients with short-term pain in the low back.

PATIENT AND PHYSICIAN EDUCATION

Patient Education

One of the few randomized controlled studies in primary care addressed the effects of education on patients with low back pain (13). In this study, one group of patients received a brochure on the problem of low back pain, and a second group received a presentation of the contents in the brochure during a 15-minute consultation by a nurse. The follow-up time was lengthy, but the result was modest. The only positive

TABLE 18.1. *Patients' and physicians' perception of low back pain*

Investigators (ref.)	Design	Population	Patients' perception	Physicians' perception	Comments
Lonnberg 1997 (27,28)	Descriptive, questionnaire I. Health care provider sample II. Population sample	I. n = 1,018 a. GPs: 436 men, 103 women b. Physical therapists: 57 men, 221 women c. Chiropractors: 109 men, 61 women d. Reumatologists: 13 men, 5 women II. n = 3,204, >16 yr e. With back problem: 595 men, 700 women f. Without back problem: 95 men, 959 women	When comparing the reasons given to seek health care to GPs, the authors concluded that patients' foremost interests were to know whether the pain could be caused by some underlying serious disease and to be treated Patients mostly considered the problem caused by "overuse" or "muscular tension" Patients were relatively more interested in having an explanation of their symptoms	GPs considered the backache to be caused by too little exercise or too much sitting in routine work GPs were more occupied with giving good treatment	
Skelton et al., 1996 (44)	In-depth interview in 1993 to elicit the view of low back pain and its management in general practice Categorized into seven themes: 1. Impact on low back pain on quality of life 2. Expectation on prognosis 3. Commitment to secondary prevention 4. Readiness to consult GPs 5. Satisfaction with explanation of their pain 6. Satisfaction with GPs management 7. Willingness to consult complementary therapists	52 selected patients with low back pain; mean age, 41 yr (range 18–66 yr), 26 men, 26 women from 12 general practices Themes: 1. 39 patients had reduced quality of life 2. 10 were optimistic, 11 pessimist, 31 worried about the prognosis 3. 29 were active, 4 thought about it, 16 did not work with prevention 4. 15 thought it appropriate; 29 visited during unusually severe episodes 5. 20 received an explanation 6. 22 were satisfied	Patients have complex views on a common problem, and there is a rich heterogeneity in patients' perceptions; it appears that patients do not want a "magical cure" for low back pain when one does not exist, but rather would like their GPs to listen to them and to offer a comprehensive approach to management		

GP, general practitioner; yr, year

outcome was that knowledge about low back pain increased, and more patients in the nurse's group tried to perform the recommended exercises.

Many authors have advocated the use of educational materials for patients with back problems. Earlier, such material was based largely on biomedical perceptions of back pain that were neither evidence-based nor in agreement with more recent guidelines. A study on patient information in primary care, based on contemporary research on the combined importance of biomedical and psychosocial factors in back pain, showed that patients' knowledge about their back problems, in fact, increased (6).

Physician Education

Cherkin et al. developed a program for teaching physicians about low back pain (11,12). The program was tested on 29 medical providers in primary care. The physicians' perception and attitudes were assessed before and after the program. The percentage of physicians who felt more knowledgeable about the subject increased significantly. After the program, the physicians indicated that they knew how to treat low back pain best and thought that the patients probably were more satisfied with the treatment. In addition, the physicians could more often assure their patients that the back pain was not the result of a serious disease. Nevertheless, the educational program had little impact on the frequently negative attitude of physicians toward patients with back pain as well as their frustration with patients who expected them to cure the problem. The study also included patients of physicians who received the education. The researchers wanted to know how the education was perceived by their patients. The results were assessed by telephone interviews with 148 patients who had visited physicians before the education program and 157 patients who had visited them afterward. Despite the markedly positive attitude toward the program among the physicians, it did not lead to any significant improvements for the patients, including those patients whom the physicians expected to benefit the most from the education.

VIEWS ON TREATMENT OF LOW BACK PAIN IN PRIMARY CARE

Deyo and Phillips are two researchers who considered the care of patients with low back pain to be a major challenge to primary care (16). They claimed that there is a major difference in how this challenge is perceived by orthopedic surgeons, who focus on the low back itself, and by GPs, who focus on the symptoms of low back pain. The authors summarized their observations from many studies as follows: "The primary care physician has to consider not only the biology of the low back but also the symptom of back pain *and* the patient—the whole body, history, family, psychosocial situation including working conditions, and the patient's rational and irrational fears. This is a major task, and indeed it is not enough to examine the low back only."

This view received support from Croft et al., who conducted a prospective study of the population registered at two family practice clinics (15). The authors used a questionnaire that measured psychologic distress and correlated their observations with the patient's follow-up visits for low back pain in primary care. The researchers found that symptoms of psychologic distress among persons without back pain can, to some extent, predict back problems. It was calculated that the proportion of new episodes of low back pain that may be attributable to such psychologic factors in the general population is 16%.

In primary health care in England, various therapies of low back pain were tested, including psychiatric consultations assessed in a randomized controlled study (25). In Finland, couple therapy was tested in patients with chronic low back pain, also in a randomized controlled study (41). None of these methods, however, were shown to have any effect on common outcome measures. However, couple therapy was shown to have good effects on variables such as psychologic anxiety and communication within the marriage (42).

Von Korff et al. questioned the value of the "acute" versus "chronic" classification of low back pain in primary care (53). They suggested that it is more meaningful to focus on pain-related functional capacity and the number of days with pain than to be confined to the date when pain commenced. Their study found that two-thirds of the consecutive patients with low back pain in primary care recovered, whereas one-third developed a more chronic course. In comparison with earlier studies based on occasional episodes of low back pain, these investigators found the prognosis of "acute" low back pain worse and that of "chronic" low back pain better.

In a critical review, von Korff and Saunders attempted to determine the functional impact of short-term and long-term back pain on patients who sought treatment in primary care (51). These investigators suggested that back pain in primary care patients demonstrated a typical relapse pattern, with variation and change, rather than an acute and self-defined course. Hence, most patients experienced relapses. Presenting the results of treatment for the first pain episode only could result in a more favorable profile of the long-term outcome than was justified. In the follow-up, the outcome substantially improved during the first 4 weeks. One month after patients had sought medical help, 66% to 75% experienced only mild back pain. After 1 month, approximately 33% of the patients reported continued and at least moderately severe pain, whereas 20% to 25% reported substantial limitations in activity. At follow-up after 1 year or longer, approximately 33% reported periodic recurrent or consistent pain of at least moderate intensity, whereas approximately 15% reported severe pain, and 20% reported substantial limitations in activity.

In a commentary to the foregoing review, the suggestion was made that the weak correlation between pain and self-reported functional limitation motivates one to view these as two separate concepts (38). The finding that "objective" measures of functional limitations, such as work absenteeism and sick leave, have little to do with the biomedical aspects of the disorder should also be noted.

Different Caregivers

A study of 208 caregivers and their 1,500 patients compared the treatment for acute low back pain provided by physicians in primary care with care provided by chiropractors and orthopedic surgeons (9). After 6 months, the authors measured the time it took for patients in the three groups to achieve functional recovery, to return to work, and to recover fully. The patients recovered equally well independently of the type of care provider consulted. The costs for health care were highest among orthopedic surgeons and chiropractors and lowest among primary care physicians.

In another study of patients with various musculoskeletal symptoms, the results of treatment provided by different types of care providers were analyzed (45). The authors reported that "low back pain was treated by different types of care providers without major differences in outcomes." Should, perhaps, this be viewed as a good reason to select the caregiver who achieves the same outcome at the lowest cost?

In a study by Cherkin et al., the differences in diagnostic examinations among physicians in various specialties were investigated (14). A questionnaire with hypothetic descriptions of patients with acute and chronic low back pain and sciatica was sent to a stratified national random sample of 2,604 physicians representing 8 different specialties. The response rate was 43%. Neurologists and neurosurgeons referred to x-ray examinations at twice the rate of other specialists, psychiatrists and neurologists referred to electromyograms three times as often as others, and rheumatologists ordered laboratory tests for both acute and chronic low back pain at twice the rate of others. In the authors' judgment, the use of diagnostic tests was both excessive and premature when compared with existing guidelines. The lack of consensus among the specialties suggests a need for additional guidelines and greater compliance with existing guidelines.

In commenting on the article by Cherkin et al. (14), Carey (8) suggested: "Physicians need an arsenal of simple, inexpensive treatments which they can confidently recommend to their patients. The excessive use of ineffective treatment methods suggests that the medical experts do not yet recognize any effective methods. The challenge to our researchers and educators who are interested in back pain is to develop better treatment alternatives for patients and recommend these methods to providers in an acceptable way."

In comparison with the English study by Skelton et al. (44) referred to earlier, a study from the United States presented a completely different image of how family physicians treat back pain (10). The purpose of this study was to compare treatment by GPs with treatment by chiropractors. Of 320,000 registered patients, 718 had visited a GP during a 2-week period. One-half of these patients were selected to participate in the study. All patients who had visited a chiropractor during the same period (181 patients) were recruited for the study. The questionnaire design was based on focus groups among patients consulting GPs or chiropractors. The response rates were 80% and 94%, respectively. Because the patients themselves could select their care providers, the results should be interpreted with caution. Age and sex distribution were similar in both groups, but more patients in the GP-treated group characterized their health as "poor." Patients in the chiropractor-treated group experienced more and longer episodes of pain.

General satisfaction with care of the back pain was much higher in the chiropractor group than in the GP group in spite of the satisfaction with the caregiver for other reasons in both groups. Chiropractic patients were also more satisfied with the information they received and the interest shown in them by the care provider. They also expressed a greater level of confidence with the care provider. The GPs' patients found it much more difficult to agree with the physician concerning the causes underlying the pain. These patients were also less inclined to return to the physician for care.

Treatment Based on Guidelines

The impact of a medical back care program in a health maintenance organization in the United States was assessed by Branthaver et al. (5). These investigators compared two medical centers in California, one that used a back care program and one that did not. The GPs at the center with the program referred 42% fewer patients for consultation with specialists, sent 59% fewer to physical therapy, and ordered 33% fewer x-ray examinations. Despite these findings, there were no differences in the clinical course of these patients, and the doctors were more satisfied with the care they had given. Other differences between the two centers may have presented confounders that could have explained the observed differences, thus placing some limitations on the study.

An article from the Quebec Task Force group described a prospective cohort study of back pain (39). After 7 weeks of treatment, 58% of the patients had not been referred to a specialist. Hence, the authors of the study considered applying guidelines as a means to increase referral rates. These investigators stated that those responsible for financing care must be given clear information from clinical guidelines on whether it is appropriate to engage a specialist for consultation. Discussing the results, Waddell (48) suggested that the appropriate referral rate is unknown, and even if one could identify it, the referral rate alone does not provide adequate information about appropriate practice. He suggested that it is not only necessary to refer the right number of patients, but also, and more important, to refer the right patients. Only 1% to 2% of patients actually need to be referred to a specialist, and such a referral would be meaningless for approximately 95% of primary care patients with low back pain. Waddell also emphasized that the effectiveness of clinical practice guidelines remains unproven when it comes to treating low back pain. He also stated: "Creating an evidence base and designing guidelines is one thing, but implementing them and changing clinical practice is another."

This theme was also addressed in an article by Freeborn et al. (18). Their study involved primary care physicians, including practitioners in both internal medicine (n = 67) and family medicine (n = 28) in a controlled intervention study of clinical practice guidelines for low back pain. The guidelines had been introduced to reduce variations in treatment of patients with low back pain and to reduce the utilization of radiology examinations of the low back. From 4 months after the start of the study, the experimental group, which used the guidelines, received feedback every second month on their utilization of x-ray examinations. Neither the guidelines alone nor the guidelines combined with feedback correlated with any significant reduction in radiology utilization rates or with the variability of the caregiver compared with the treatment suggested in the guidelines. The conclusion here is that guidelines must be adapted both to the practice design and to patient expectations and behavior.

A retrospective, descriptive study including 524 primary care patients with chronic low back pain showed, conversely, that treatment of low back pain lacks a solid evidence base (50). For that reason, clinical guidelines are needed.

CHANGING PERSPECTIVES

Sweden

It was not easy to find high-quality studies of treatment of primary care patients with low back pain in Sweden. In a Swedish study on the effects of manual therapy and steroid injections for patients with low back pain, a control group received routine "good" back treatment in primary care (4). A treatment model was developed for the control group in collaboration with the GPs who participated in the study. They decided that "active, optimal, and standardized conventional treatment" should consist of the following: "drugs, ergonomic advice and recommendations, both verbal and printed, back school, sick leave, active back training, corsets, bandages, bandaging, short-wave treatment, ultrasound, transcutaneous nerve stimulation, electrostimulation, heat treatment (Steam pac), cold (Cold pac, ice), posture instructions, posture training, and, in some cases, exercise and massage in a pool" (4). Most of these interventions were later shown to be ineffective and cannot be considered optimal treatment. Nevertheless, even though that model is based on inactivity, this treatment strategy has been described as an active model of treatment. Other studies of Swedish patients with back pain have confirmed the common use of the foregoing modalities among GPs (3,47).

Another Swedish study from 1992 (33) involved hypothetic cases of low back pain. The cases were presented to 200 GPs at primary care clinics in mid-Sweden. Responses were obtained from 159 of the physicians, who were asked to order diagnostic tests from a list of commonly used alternatives. The physicians were also asked to prescribe drugs and sick leave as though the patient had paid a first visit to the practice.

The interventions proposed by the GPs were as follows: full-time sick leave was granted by 97% of the participating physicians, return visits were ordered by 96%, at least one drug was prescribed by 90%, and physical therapy was ordered by 77%. Erythrocyte sedimentation rates, which at that time were presumably the most common screening test in primary care for suspected serious disease, were ordered by 56% of the physicians. Other interventions ordered included the following: dipstick urine analysis (48%), rehabilitation (33%), x-ray examination of the low back (36%), rectal examination (29%), prescription of two different drugs (17%), breast examination (6%), computed tomography of the low back (6%), urine microscopy (6%), three drugs (3%), and gynecologic examination (2%). Only 6% of the GPs would have referred patients to an orthopedic clinic for investigation on the first visit, even if the case description suggested lumbar herniated disk, a condition for which surgical treatment may be appropriate.

To some extent, the results reflect what providers considered "routine treatment" when the study was conducted in 1992. The disadvantage of questionnaires with hypothetic cases is that participating doctors tend to give overambitious answers. In real day-to-day practice, less direct measures are probably the norm.

Denmark

The study described earlier from Denmark (27,28) also showed that 40% of the Danish population had experienced back pain during the previous year, and 24% of these persons, or nearly 10% of the population, had visited a GP for their back problems. The study was based on questions to a sample of GPs who were representative of rural areas, mixed rural and suburban areas, and densely populated areas. In part, the study attempted to identify how patients with low back pain were routinely treated in primary care. The physicians were asked to describe their routines, and corresponding information was also obtained from physical therapists and chiropractors. The study investigated how people in general viewed professional care of back pain, and therefore questions were sent to a representative sample of inhabitants in the respective areas.

Only 55% of the professional caregivers responded to the questionnaire. Because dropout was poorly described, the question of possible bias cannot be answered. Dropout rates in the questionnaire to the general public were not reported.

The diagnoses reported by Danish GPs revealed how these physicians viewed their patients. Of 12 diagnostic alternatives, "myosis regio dorsi" was the most common diagnosis, followed by lumbago. Sciatica was in the sixth place. Regarding factors of importance in selecting a treatment method, the physicians were asked to choose among several alternatives. "The decision to establish a clinical diagnosis" was viewed by 67% of the GPs as the most important factor in the choice of treatment method. "The information given by the patients" was reported by 61% of the physicians, "knowledge about the patient's family or social situation" by 27% of the physicians, and "the patient's age" by 19%. Only 9% of the physicians indicated that "findings from x-ray examination" were of importance, as compared with 37% of the physical therapists and 54% of the chiropractors who viewed x-ray examination as important. Thirty-three percent of the GPs agreed with the statement that "most patients who seek care for back problems do not require special examination or treatment."

When the authors compared the patients' reasons for seeking help from a GP, they found that the patients mainly wanted to know whether their pain was caused by a serious underlying disorder. "Desire to be treated" was in second place as a motive for seeking care. The second article, written by the same authors and based on the same data, addressed how the differences between caregivers and the population are perceived (28). More women than men, and more young people, reported that they desired professional care. Although physicians perceived that back problems were caused by too little exercise or too much sedentary work, most patients believed that exertion and muscle tension caused their pain. In contrast to patients' preference for consultations, physicians were more oriented toward providing appropriate treatment. The patients were more interested in having their symptoms explained.

SCOPE OF PROBLEM IN PRIMARY CARE IN SELECTED COUNTRIES

Sweden

After infectious diseases, musculoskeletal diseases represent the second most common reason for primary care visits in most Western countries (21,46). Nevertheless, since the early 1990s, the number of physician visits resulting from musculoskeletal disorders has declined in Sweden. The decline in physician visits does not necessarily reflect a real reduction in the incidence or prevalence of musculoskeletal disorders. Other factors may be the cause.

A population-based questionnaire directed toward persons aged 20 through 64 years and living in Dalarna, Sweden, showed that 25% of the respondents reported at least one episode of low back pain during the past 3 months (19). Only 15% of those interviewed had visited a caregiver because of low back pain. Of these patients, 27% reported that they had visited a physician in primary care, 4% had visited an orthopedist, and 12% had visited a chiropractor or naprapath. Most had visited a physical therapist. Per 100,000 population, on average a single visit was made to a primary care physician for back pain, whereas nearly 10 visits were made to a physical therapist (20). A study conducted in 1987 in southern Sweden showed that each GP received, on average, two patients with low back pain per week (21).

Denmark, Finland, and Canada

The Danish study found that, on average, GPs were visited by five patients with back problems per week (28) (Table 18.2). Hence, the number of patients who visit primary care physicians does not appear to be particularly great.

More than one-fourth of all adults with musculoskeletal symptoms in Denmark and Finland visit primary care centers or GPs. GPs, physical therapists, and chiropractors have different treatment routines, and the patients who visit these three provider categories reflect different sociodemographic and disease profiles. Although providers

TABLE 18.2. *Health care providers chosen and the treatment given patients with low back pain*

Investigators (ref.)	Design	Population	Result 1: description	Result 2: treatment	Comments
Lonnberg, 1997 (28)	Descriptive questionnaire I. Health care providers II. Population sample	I. n = 1,018 a. GPs: 436 men, 103 women b. Physical therapists: 57 men, 221 women c. Chiropractors: 109 men, 61 women d. Reumatologists: 13 men, 5 women II. n = 3,204, >16 yr e. With back problem: 595 men, 700 women f. Without back problem: 950 men, 959 women	I. Number of patients in 14 days (who made a first consultation): a. 10 (5) b. 21 (7) c. 183 (17) d. m.d. II. 482 (37%) visited a health care provider; men and women made the same choices: 306 (24%) to GPs, 125 (10%) to physical therapists, 147 (11%) to chiropractors, 56 (4%) to rheumatologists	I. treatments given to patients by health care providers a. Analgesics (73%), blockades (34%), manipulations (25%), physical training (70%), bed rest (27%) b. Dynamic training (98%), massage (93%), hot packs (75%), ultrasound (73%), physical training (98%), bed rest (9%) c. Manipulations (100%), massage (68%), triggerpoint treatment (67%), physical training (92%), bed rest (22%)	Mean time for consultation with GPs for back pain was 14 min GPs' patients were more troubled or burdened by their backache and were younger, fewer were employed, and more had concomitant diseases
McKinnon et al., 1997 (32)	Retrospective study of medical records for 12 mo plus a postal questionnaire to a sample of these patients in the intake area of three primary health care centers	n = 900	Annual prevalence of low back pain was 48%; 24% had contacted their GPs; 4% were referred to hospital specialists	Actions taken by GPs: 12%, illness certification 27%, analgesic prescriptions 16% physical therapy 10%, radiography	Low consultation rate, time off, and day-to-day disability indicate that most episodes are self-limiting; most believed that low back pain was self-limiting and would not consult health care professionals for future episodes; answering rate, 59%

GPs, general practitioners; m.d., missing data.

often report poor physical condition as the underlying cause for back problems, patients indicate that overexertion of the low back causes the problem.

Primary care in Finland is more like that in Sweden than in Denmark. The average number of patients per GP and the number of consultations per day are comparable to Swedish figures.

A study of primary care in Finland recorded all cases of a musculoskeletal nature, excluding violence-related trauma (36). During a 2-week registration period at 6 primary care centers, 6,526 individuals had visited these centers, and 21% of these patients had musculoskeletal symptoms. The study was conducted in a rural area, and the percentage of farmers was proportionally higher than in the country as a whole. Among women, neck pain (22%) was the most common reason for a physician visit related to musculoskeletal symptoms, followed by low back pain (16%). Among men, low back pain was the most common reason for the visit (21%), followed by neck pain (18%). These authors later confirmed that neck pain and shoulder pain in particular seem to be part of a complex of multisite musculoskeletal symptoms involving frequent primary care visits (37).

Great Britain

In a systematic review of studies on bed rest and studies in which patients were advised to remain active for acute low back pain, Waddell et al. found that a common approach in Great Britain involved analgesics and activity limitations, including bed rest (49). The report questioned the effectiveness of this treatment and referred to studies confirming that normal activity results in faster recovery. Waddell et al. stated that "some patients may need to rest in bed for several days, but this should be viewed as a consequence of their pain and not as a treatment"(49). Advice to remain active and to live normally appeared to result in quicker return to work, reduced chronic disability, and fewer recurring problems. Most studies cited in the review were representative of primary care, and the observations should be of major interest to family doctors and GPs in other countries.

A study based on a sample (n = 900) of the population in a catchment area for three primary care centers in Great Britain questioned whether the subjects had low back pain during the previous year (32) (Table 18.2). Ninety-five percent of the patients in the study had a medical record at the primary care centers. The annual prevalence of low back pain was 48%. Twenty-four percent had contact with their family doctor for low back pain, and 4% had been referred to hospital specialists. The consultation rate was approximately the same among those who contacted primary care centers for low back pain and those who had chronic diseases, and it was higher than the average consultation rate in the population. Treatment is shown in Table 18.2. Given the epidemiologic design of the study, it was clear that a limited percentage of patients with low back pain sought medical help. Few of them visited primary care centers or needed to be placed on sick leave. The low consultation rates for low back pain in relation to the high prevalence of symptoms is believed to exist in primary care in many countries.

SUMMARY

- Primary care is the appropriate treatment level for most patients with back pain.
- It is important to determine whether potentially serious disease is the cause of pain.

- The consultation process and the patient-doctor relationship are of major importance because they give the caregiver and the patient an opportunity to discuss their perceptions on the causes of back pain.
- An important message to the patient is to remain active, and to continue to live normally.
- Bed rest should be avoided and should not be prescribed as treatment.
- Being aware of potential psychosocial risk factors may help to prevent acute back pain from becoming chronic.
- Gender aspects should be taken into consideration to increase the understanding of the back pain problem.
- Only a small percentage of persons with low back pain seek care through primary care physicians, and even fewer seek care at the secondary level at hospitals and specialty clinics.
- The most common interventions for low back pain in primary care in Sweden are certification of sick leave, prescription of analgesic drugs, instructions for physical exercise, and scheduling of return visits.
- As a rule, GPs suggest that low back pain is caused by underuse of the back, whereas patients as a rule believe that back pain is due to overexertion.
- The type of caregiver does not appear to play a major role in the outcome.
- There are major variations among physicians in their choices of treatment for back pain and in the type of care provided by different specialists. This variation is more closely related to the specialty than to patient characteristics.
- Psychiatric treatment in primary care has not shown to be effective for treatment of patients with back pain.
- The prognoses for acute low back pain may be worse than previously believed because acute low back pain may often reflect an episode of recurring disease.
- Guidelines are recommended for treating back pain in general practice, but the effect of such guidelines has not been proven.
- Patient education has not been shown to be effective in treating back pain. Likewise, physician education has not been shown to benefit the patient, although it benefits the physician.

REFERENCES

1. Balint M. *The doctor, his patient and the illness.* London: Pitman, 1964.
2. Bass M, Buck C, Turner L, et al. The physician's action and the outcome of illness in family practice. *J Fam Pract* 1986;23:43–47.
3. Bergendorf S, Hansson E, Hansson T, et al. *Projektbeskrivnin och undersökningsgrupp: Rygg och Nacke 1.* Stockholm: Riksförsäkringsverket, 1998:1–119.
4. Blomberg S, Hallin G, Grann K, et al. Manual therapy with steroid injections: a new approach to treatment of low back pain. A controlled multicenter trial with an evaluation by orthopedic surgeons. *Spine* 1994;19:569–577.
5. Branthaver B, Stein GF, Mehran A. Impact of a medical back care program on utilization of services and primary care physician satisfaction in a large, multispecialty group practice health maintenance organization. *Spine* 1995;20:1165–1169.
6. Burton AK, Waddell G, Burtt R, et al. Patient educational material in the management of low back pain in primary care. *Bull Hosp Jt Dis* 1996;55:138–141.
7. Bush T, Cherkin D, Barlow W. The impact of physician attitudes on patient satisfaction with care for low back pain. *Arch Fam Med* 1993;2:301–305.
8. Carey TS. Comments to Cherkin et al. *Arthritis Rheum* 1994;37:22–23.
9. Carey TS, Garrett J, Jackman A, et al. The outcomes and costs of care for acute low back pain among patients seen by primary care practitioners, chiropractors, and orthopedic surgeons: the North Carolina Back Pain Project. *N Engl J Med* 1995;333:913–917.

10. Cherkin DC, MacCornack FA. Patient evaluations of low back pain care from family physicians and chiropractors. *West J Med* 1989;150:351–355.
11. Cherkin D, Deyo RA, Berg AO. Evaluation of a physician education intervention to improve primary care for low-back pain. II. Impact on patients. *Spine* 1991;16:1173–1178.
12. Cherkin D, Deyo RA, Berg AO, et al. Evaluation of a physician education intervention to improve primary care for low-back pain. I. Impact on physicians. *Spine* 1991;16:1168–1172.
13. Cherkin D, Deyo RA, Street JH, et al. Pitfalls of patient education: limited success of a program for back pain in primary care. *Spine* 1996;21:345–355.
14. Cherkin DC, Deyo RA, Wheeler K, et al. Physician variation in diagnostic testing for low back pain: who you see is what you get. *Arthritis Rheum* 1994;37:15–22.
15. Croft PR, Papageorgiou AC, Ferry S, et al. Psychologic distress and low back pain: evidence from a prospective study in the general population. *Spine* 1995;20:2731–2737.
16. Deyo RA, Phillips WR. Low back pain: a primary care challenge. *Spine* 1996;21:2826–2832.
17. Finkler K, Correa M. Factors influencing patient perceived recovery in Mexico. *Soc Sci Med* 1996;42:100–207.
18. Freeborn DK, Shye D, Mullooly JP, et al. Primary care physicians' use of lumbar spine imaging tests: effects of guidelines and practice pattern feedback. *J Gen Intern Med* 1997;12:619–625.
19. Fritzell P. *Ont i ländryggen: en rapport från DalaRyggs enkätundersökning november 1995–augusti 1996 i Dalarna, Falun, 1998.*
20. Granvik M. *1996 års befolkningsenkät. Resultatredovisning: Personer med värk i ländch korsryggen. Landstinghetskansliets epidemiologiska utredningsarbete 99:1997, Falun, 1997.*
21. Håkansson A. Basdata: till vad nytta? Redovisning av ett treårsmaterial från vårdcentralen Teleborg. *Allmänmedicin* 1987;8:154–157.
22. Jacobson L, Edwards A, Granier S, et al. Evidence-based medicine and general practice. *Br J Gen Pract* 1997;47:449–452.
23. Johansson E, Hamberg K, Lindgren G, et al. "How could I even think of a job?" Ambiguities in working life in a group of female patients with undefined musculoskeletal pain. *Scand J Prim Health Care* 1997;15:169–174.
24. Kendall NAS, Linton SJ, Main CJ. *Guide to assessing psychosocial yellow flags in acute low back pain: risk factors for long-terms disability and work loss.* Wellington, NZ: Accident Rehabilitation & Compensation Insurance Corporation of New Zealand and the National Health Committee, 1997.
25. Koopmans GT, Meeuwesen L, Huyse FJ, et al. Effects of psychiatric consultation on medical consumption in medical outpatients with low back pain. *Gen Hosp Psychiatry* 1996;18:145–154.
26. Larsen J-H, Risör O, Putnam S. P-R-A-C-T-I-C-A-L: a step-by-step model for conducting the consultation in general practice. *Fam Pract* 1997;14:295–301.
27. Lonnberg F. [The management of back problems among the population. II. Therapists' and patients' perception of the disease.] *Ugeskr Laeger* 1997;159:2215–2221.
28. Lonnberg F. [The management of back problems among the population. I. Contact patterns and therapeutic routines.] *Ugeskr Laeger* 1997;159:2207–2214.
29. Lunde IM. *Patienters egenvurdering: et medicinsk perspektivskift.* Thesis, University of Copenhagen, Denmark, 1992.
30. Löfvander M, Engström A, Theander H, et al. Rehabilitation of young immigrants in primary care: a comparison between two treatment models, *Scand J Prim Health Care* 1997;15:123–128.
31. Materson RS. The AHCPR practice guidelines for low back pain. *Bull Rheum Dis* 1996;45:6–8.
32. McKinnon ME, Vickers MR, Ruddock VM, et al. Community studies of the health service implications of low back pain. *Spine* 1997;22:2161–2166.
33. Peterson S, Eriksson M, Tibblin G. Practice variation in Swedish primary care. *Scand J Prim Health Care* 1997;15:68–75.
34. Putnam S, Lipkin M. The patient-centered interview: research support. In: Lipkin MP, Lazare A, eds. *The medical interview.* New York: Springer-Verlag, 1995.
35. Ottosson J-O, ed. *Patient-läkarrelationen: Läkekonst på vetenskaplig grund. Natur och Kultur.* Stockholm: Swedish Council on Technology Assessment in Health Care, 1999:1–374.
36. Rekola KE, Keinanen-Kiukaanniemi S, Takala J. Use of primary health services in sparsely populated country districts by patients with musculoskeletal symptoms: consultations with a physician. *J Epidemiol Community Health* 1993;47:153–157.
37. Rekola KE, Levoska S, Takala J, et al. Patients with neck and shoulder complaints and multiside musculoskeletal symptoms: a prospective study. *J Rheumatol* 1997;24:2424–2428.
38. Roland M. Point of view. *Spine* 1996;21:2838.
39. Rossignol M, Abenhaim L, Bonvalot Y, et al. Should the gap be filled between guidelines and actual practice for management of low back pain in primary care? The Quebec experience. *Spine* 1996;21:2893–2898.
40. Royal College of General Practitioners. *Clinical guidelines for the management of acute low back pain.* London: Royal College of General Practitioners, 1996.
41. Saarijärvi S. A controlled study of couple therapy in chronic low back pain patients: effects on marital satisfaction, psychological distress and health attitudes. *J Psychosom Res* 1991;35:265–272.

42. Saarijärvi S, Rytökoski U, Alanen E. A controlled study of couple therapy in chronic low back pain patients: no improvement of disability. *J Psychosom Res* 1991;35:671–677.
43. Sackett D, Wennberg J. Choosing the best research design for each question: it's time to stop squabbling over the "best" methods. *BMJ* 1997;315:1636.
44. Skelton AM, Murphy EA, Murphy RJ, et al. Patients' views of low back pain and its management in general practice. *Br J Gen Pract* 1996;46:153–156.
45. Solomon DH, Bates DW, Panush RS, et al. Costs, outcomes, and patient satisfaction by provider type for patients with rheumatic and musculoskeletal conditions: a critical review of the literature and proposed methodologic standards. *Ann Intern Med* 1997;127:52–60.
46. Svenninger K. *Statistik från verksamheten på vårdcentralen i Dalby 1988 hämtat ur journalsystem Dalby.* Dalby, Lunds Universitet Dalby/Lund, 1988.
47. Swedish National Board of Health and Welfare. *Yearbook of Health and Medical Care, 1995.* Stockholm: Socialstyrelsen, 1995.
48. Waddell G. Point of view. *Spine* 1996;21:2898.
49. Waddell G, Feder G, Lewis M. Systematic reviews of bed rest and advice to stay active for acute low back pain. *Br J Gen Pract* 1997;47:647–652.
50. van Tulder MW, Koes BW, Bouter LM, et al. Management of chronic nonspecific low back pain in primary care: a descriptive study. *Spine* 1997;22:76–82.
51. von Korff M, Saunders K. The course of back pain in primary care. *Spine* 1996;21:2833–2839.
52. von Korff M, Barlow W, Cherkin D, et al. Effects of practice style in managing back pain. *Ann Intern Med* 1994;121:187–195.
53. von Korff M, Deyo RA, Cherkin D, et al. Back pain in primary care: outcomes at 1 year. *Spine* 1993;18:855–862.

*Neck and Back Pain: The Scientific Evidence
of Causes, Diagnosis, and Treatment,* edited
by Alf Nachemson and Egon Jonsson.
Published by Lippincott Williams & Wilkins,
Philadelphia 2000.

19

Cost-Effectiveness of Treatment for Neck and Low Back Pain

Mariëlle Goossens* and Silvia Evers†

*Institute for Rehabilitation Research, Hoensbroek, The Netherlands
†Department of Health Organisation, Policy and Economics, University of Maastricht,
Maastricht, The Netherlands

Because the incidence and costs of back pain are great and the socioeconomic implications of disability are growing rapidly, it is becoming important to examine how much of the burden and costs can be avoided by effective therapies and at what cost. This question can be answered by means of economic evaluation studies. Economic evaluation studies, of which cost-effectiveness analyses are a specific example, compare both the costs and the outcomes of alternative health care interventions. This information can be used to support decision making about the allocation of scarce resources and to obtain the maximum gain in health. Many studies in the field of low back pain incorporate some cost issues in their analyses. However, previous research showed that sound economic evaluation in this area has received little attention, in contrast to some other chronic medical problems (41).

A systematic review of economic evaluation studies of back pain management has been published (10). In this chapter, the review has been updated by including all sound economic evaluation studies that were published between 1995 and December 1997. We also extended the literature search with different search strategies. The purpose of this chapter is threefold. First, we provide insight into the status and the quality of economic evaluation studies in the field of back pain. Second, we will compare the cost-effectiveness of different comparable treatments. Third, we try to draw conclusions about the most cost-effective therapy for acute and chronic back pain.

METHOD

Selection of Studies

In the published review (10), several strategies were combined to find literature in the field of the economic evaluation of back pain. Studies published between 1984 and 1995 were identified with a MEDLINE search, by using the keywords costs, cost analysis, cost-effectiveness analysis, back pain, spine, and economic evaluation. Additional articles were found by citation tracking and through an economic evaluation bibliography (11). Articles were included in the review if the field of study was back pain, the study used an economic evaluation, and the article was published in English.

For the update of the literature search, we searched the databases through December 1997. We also used the structured abstracts of economic evaluation of interventions for back pain from the references of the United Kingdom National Health Service economic evaluation database and the Health Economic Evaluation Database of the Office of Health Economics and the International Federation of Pharmaceutical Manufacturers Association (30,32).

Methodologic Quality of the Studies

A methodologic checklist (9) was used to select only those articles describing an economic evaluation study in the field of back pain treatment. Using the checklist, the studies were screened for general, epidemiologic, and economic aspects. Table 19.1 lists the main criteria used. The economic part of the checklist was based on the general principles of performing and evaluating the quality of economic evaluation studies (8). In the health care evaluation research, several evaluation designs are distinguished. Two features characterize economic analysis, regardless of the activities to which it is applied. A full economic evaluation study must make a comparison between two or more alternatives, and both the costs (inputs) and the consequences (outputs) have to be examined. Depending on the nature of the consequences resulting from the alternatives examined, there are four types of full economic evaluation: cost-minimization analysis, cost-effectiveness analysis, cost-benefit analysis, and cost-utility analysis. Apart from the foregoing full economic evaluation designs, we also included three other types of partial evaluations: outcome description, cost description, and cost analysis. The term *partial* means that they do not fulfill both conditions for economic evaluation, and the label *partial evaluation* indicates that they will not allow one to answer efficacy questions (8). However, the reason for including them in the review is that they may represent important intermediate stages in understanding the costs and consequences of health services and programs. When making conclusions, we take this distinction into account. Cost of illness studies are not considered to be economic evaluation studies and therefore are not included in this review.

When we talk about economic evaluation studies, we refer to both full economic evaluation and the three types of partial evaluation. The methods of partial evaluation and full economic evaluation are explained further in the review of studies in this chapter.

The quality of the studies was assessed by the two authors. Disagreement was resolved by consensus.

TABLE 19.1. *Main items of the checklist*

General	Economic
Country	Economic evaluation design used
Perspective of analysis	Costs identification (direct, direct nonmedical, in-
Nature of the study	direct costs)
Disease category	Costs measurement (sources direct, direct non-
Epidemiologic	medical, indirect costs)
Epidemiologic design used	Costs valuation (valuation direct, indirect costs)
Design characteristics (prestratification/match-	Identification consequences
ing, randomization, population size, number	Measurement consequences
of groups)	Valuation consequences
Adequate measurement of effect (blinding)	Discounting, differential timing
Results	Sensitivity analysis

TABLE 19.2. Conclusions on the cost-effectiveness of various types of interventions in back pain

Investigators (ref.)	Intervention	Reference treatment	Diagnosis	Results	Authors' conclusion	Statistics calculated
Injury prevention and back schools						
Brown et al. (3)	Back school	No-treatment control	Back injury/municipal employees (work-related)	Significantly fewer injuries; significant difference on lost work time, lost time cost, and medical costs for back school participants, difference between groups but not statistically, significant	Negative	No
Versloot et al. (48)	Back school	No-treatment control	Back pain	Decrease in absenteeism of 5 d, but no significance, difference between groups	Positive	No
Hochanadel and Conrad (12)	On-site industrial physical therapy program	Situation before	Musculoskeletal injury (50% low back pain)	Significant reduction in the absence rate; for the life of the program, net savings (program costs – savings)	Positive	Assumptions for the life of the program
Coleman and Hansen (5)	Educational program	No-treatment control	Work-related back injury (bus company employees)	Decrease in length of absenteeism by 5 d/yr per employee. Significant decrease in cost per back injury claim during second year of the program; total cost savings in 3 year; program costs – costs of back injuries (decreased).	Positive	No significant cost difference? Vague
Postincidence management and secondary prevention						
Aarås (1)	Ergonomic interventions (at the workplace)	No comparison	Musculoskeletal illness	Reduction in sick leave	Positive	No
Linton and Bradley (17)	Secondary prevention program	Situation before	Subacute low back pain (female nurses)	Significant decrease in pain and use of medication, increase in activity level, substantial reduction in absenteeism and employer costs	Positive	Assumptions, probably
Linton et al. (19)	Early active intervention	Treatment as usual	Acute musculoskeletal pain	Significantly less sick listing and eight times lower risk of developing chronic pain; fewer chronic cases would result in lower costs	Positive	Assumptions, probably
Mitchell et al. (27)	Back belts	No-treatment control	Low back injuries (warehouse workers)	Back belts are minimally effective in preventing injury and costs of injury are higher for workers wear a belt	Negative	Yes?
Mitchell and Carmen (29)	Functional restoration program	Treatment as usual	Soft tissue and back injuries (injured workers, 71% male)	Difference (not significant) in absence from work, compensation costs, and total costs	Positive but not significant	Yes
Ryan et al. (35)	Educational and early rehabilitation	No-treatment control	Early back pain	Program easy to institute and inexpensive succeeding in preventing back pain chronicity	Positive	
Ryden et al. (36)	Health promotion program; I: Back care program II: Light-duty program	Situation before	Back injuries (hospital employees)	Decrease in back injuries, and decrease in costs of back injuries (savings in medical bills, workers' compensation cost, and lost time)	Positive	?

continued

401

TABLE 19.2. Continued

Investigators (ref.)	Intervention	Reference treatment	Diagnosis	Results	Authors' conclusion	Statistics calculated
Simmons et al. (38)	Multidisciplinary therapy	Situation before	Chronic low back pain (with and without radiculopathy)	Reduction in medical costs	Positive	Yes
Sinclair et al. (39)	(Clinical) early active intervention	Usual care	Acute back injury	No advantages from the program compared with usual care on all outcome measures	Equally effective	Yes (partly)
Stieg et al. (43)	Interdisciplinary pain treatment	Situation before	Chronic pain	Reduction in health care costs	Positive	No
Medical treatment						
Manipulation and physical therapy						
Meade et al. (26)	Chiropractic treatment	Conventional hospital outpatient management	Low back pain of mechanical origin	Clinical improvement in pain intensity and disability, resulting in savings in social security payments	Positive	No (assumptions)
Nyiendo (31)	Chiropractic treatment	Other medical care	Low back pain	Increase (not significantly, different) in return to work	Negative	No
Skargren et al. (40)	Chiropractic treatment	Physical therapy	Low back and neck pain	Same effectiveness and costs for chiropractic and physical therapy	Negative	Yes
Tuchin and Bonello (45)	Chiropractic treatment	Conventional medical management	Back pain, spinal injuries	Possibly cost-effective	Possibly positive	Pilot study
Exercise therapy						
Malviaara et al. (23)	Ordinary activity	Bed rest vs. exercises	Acute low back pain	Light exercise resulted in slower recovery after 3 wk; avoiding bed rest leads to rapid recovery; difference but not significant in costs between groups	Positive	No
Mitchell and Carmen (28)	Intensive exercises	Treatment as usual	Back injuries, acute soft tissue	Treatment program resulted in earlier recovery, enabling a greater percentage to return to work sooner; increase in health care costs offset by savings in wave loss cost	Positive	No
Timm (44)	Active treatment	Passive treatment	Chronic low back pain	Active approaches of low-tech and high-tech exercise significantly improved objective functional measures; low-tech provides the longest interval of pain relief and may therefore be cost-effective	Positive	Assumptions
Surgery						
Bell et al. (2)	Spinal cord stimulation	Long-term maintenance	Failed back surgery syndrome	Improvements in clinical efficacy would result in less demand of medical care	Positive (long-term)	Assumptions
Devulder et al. (6)	Spinal cord stimulation		Failed back surgery syndrome	In 13 yr, resulted in pain relief and return to work; although is expensive, possibly cost-effective in the long term	Positive (long-term)	Assumptions

402

Reference	Intervention	Comparator	Condition	Findings	Result	Quality
Malter et al. (24)	Lumbar discectomy	No surgical treatment	Herniated intervertebral disc	For carefully selected patients unresponsive to conservative treatment, provides substantial benefit in quality of life; total costs greater for surgical treatment	Positive	No
Manucher and Javid (25)	Chemonucleolysis	Laminectomy	Herniated lumbar disc	Rates of return to work and patient improvement greater but not significantly different; no difference in results of clinical examination; resulted in cost savings	Positive	No (possible)
Ramirez and Javid(33)	Chemonucleolysis	Laminectomy	Herniated nucleus pulposus, low back pain, and neck pain	5-d difference in length of hospitalization resulting in cost savings for chemonucleolysis (less reoperation)	Positive	No (assumptions)
Ray (34)	Lumbar threaded fusion cage	Anterior composite interbody grafting with posterior pedicle screw fixation (360-degree fusion)	Back pain	Improvement in overall surgical and hospitalization costs, surgical time, and blood losses provided by threaded fusion cage technique (assumable similar clinical outcomes)	Positive	No
Stevenson et al. (42)	APLD	Microdiscectomy	Contained lumbar disc herniation	Worse outcomes on a four-point scale for the APLD, costs per successful outcome for microdescectomy 60% of the average cost per APLD successful outcome	Negative (for APLD)	No (weak analysis)
Tunturi et al. (46)	Posterior fusion of the lumbar spine	—	Patients subjected to fusion of lumbosacral spine	Profitable at a cost-benefit ratio of 1:29 cost-compared work output	Positive	No
Other therapies and procedures						
Liang and Komaroff (16)	Lumbar roentenograms	No treatment	Acute low back pain	To avert 1 d of physical suffering, the population would have to be subjected to the additional risk of 3,188 mrad of radiation and an additional cost of $2,072; benefit is too small to justify the costs and risk	Negative	Partly
Lissovoy et al. (20)	Intrathecal morphine therapy	Medical management	Failed back surgery syndrome	In a simulation model, the average patient achieved 43.8 mo of pain relief; may save money relative to conventional therapy	Positive	Model
MacLean (22)	Family physician's care	Hospital care	Medical back pain	Family physicians treat inpatients with back pain probably more cheaply than do other physicians without any comprise of effectiveness	Positive	No
Shekkele et al. (37)	General practitioner's care	Chiropractor, internist, orthopedist	Back pain	Lowest cost for care provided by general practitioners in comparison with care provided by chiropractors, internists and orthopedists	— (Comparison)	—

APLD, automated percutaneous lumbar discectomy.

TABLE 19.3. *Main characteristics of the studies*

Investigators (ref.)	Intervention and reference treatment	Diagnosis	Study design	Economic design	No. experimental	No. control	Costs[a]	Valuation costs	Main outcome measures	Discounting	Sensitivity analyses
Injury prevention and back schools											
Brown et al., 1992 (3)	Back school vs. no-treatment control	Back injury, municipal employees	Cohort	CEA	70	75	(1,2,4)	Charges HCA[d]	Sick days, lost time cost, medical expenses, number of back injuries	No	No
Coleman and Hansen, 1994 (5)	Educational program vs. no-treatment control	Back injury, bus company, employees	Cohort	CD	30	—	1,2,4	Unclear	—	No	No
Hochanadel and Conrad, 1993 (12)	Physical therapy and back school vs. situation before	Musculoskeletal illness (50% LBP)	Cohort	CD	5,301	—	1,4	Estimates	—	No	No
Versloot et al., 1992 (48)	Back school vs. no-treatment control	Back pain	RCT	CEA	200	300	1,4	Unclear	Sick days	No	No
Postincidence management and secondary prevention											
Aarås, 1994 (1)	Ergonomic interventions	Musculoskeletal illness	Cohort	CO[b]	420	—	1,4	Estimates	Reduction in recruitment costs, training costs, instructors' salary costs, sick leave	Yes	No
Linton and Bradley, 1992 (17)	Secondary prevention program vs. situation before	Subacute LBP, female nurses	Cohort	CEA[b]	36	—	1,4	Estimates	Pain intensity, fatigue, anxiety, sleep, activities of daily living, depression, helplessness, medication, absenteeism for illness	No	No
Linton, et al., 1993 (19)	Early active intervention vs. treatment as usual	Acute musculoskeletal pain	RCT	CEA	134	106	1	Estimates	Treatment satisfaction, pain, discomfort, pain-free days, sleep quality, stress, depression, well-being, pain control, sickness absenteeism	No	No
Mitchell et al., 1994 (27)	Back belts vs. no-treatment control	Low back injury, warehouse workers	Cohort	CEA	1,000	1,000	1,2,4	Unclear	Back injuries, lost time due to injuries, limited activity days	No	No
Mitchell and Carmen, 1994 (29)	Functional restoration vs. treatments as usual	Back injury (injured workers, 71% male)	RCT	CA	271	271	1,2,4	Unclear	Return to full-time work, number of patients granted income support	No	No

Study	Intervention	Design	Analysis	N	N	Perspective	Cost basis	Outcomes		
Ryan et al., 1995 (35)	Early rehabilitation and education vs. no-treatment control	Cohort	CA	Unclear	Unclear	1,2,4,	Charges	—	No	No
Ryden et al., 1988 (36)	Two health promotion programs; one educational, two light-duty programs vs. situation before	Cohort	CEA[b]	Unclear	—	1,2,4	Charges	Hospital costs, workers' compensation costs, and lost time	No	No
Sinclair et al., 1997 (39)	Early active intervention vs. usual care	Cohort	CEA	355	530	1,2,4	Unclear	Time to return to work, health care costs, health-related quality of life, functional capacity, pain	No	No
Simmons et al., 1988 (38)	Multidisciplinary therapy vs. situation before	Cohort	CO	60	—	1,2	Charges	Medical expenses	No	No
Stieg et al., 1986 (43)	Interdisciplinary pain management vs. situation before	Cohort	CO[b]	53	—	1,2,4	Unclear	Decreased health care costs to the insurers	No	No
Manipulation and physical therapy										
Meade et al., 1990 (26)	Chiropractic vs. conventional hospital outpatient treatment	RCT	CEA	384	357	1,4	Average costs	Oswestry pain disability index straight leg raising, and lumbar flexion	No	No
Nyiendo 1991 (31)	Chiropractic vs. medical treatment	Cohort	CD	94	107	1,2,4	Unclear	Medical expenses and decreased sick days	No	No
Skargren et al., 1997 (40)	Physical therapy vs. chiropractic therapy	RCT	CEA	219 chiropractic therapy	192 physical therapy	1,2,4	Charges	Pain intensity, use of painkillers, sick leave, Oswestry LBP disability index, general (global) health	No	No
Tuchin and Bonello, 1995 (45)	Chiropractic therapy vs. conventional medical management	Pilot study randomized	(20 CEA selected)	20	20	1,2	Not clear	Days lost from work	No	No
Exercise therapy										
Malmivara et al., 1995 (23)	Bed rest vs. exercises vs. ordinary activities	RCT	CEA	67 + 52	67	1,2,3,4	Charges, actual patient costs	Days of sick leave, intensity and duration of pain, Oswestry back disability index, quality of life, ability to work, lumbar flexion	Yes	No

continued

TABLE 19.3. Continued

Investigators (ref.)	Intervention and reference treatment	Diagnosis	Study design	Economic design	No. experimental	No. control	Costs[a]	Valuation costs	Main outcome measures	Discounting	Sensitivity analyses
Mitchell and Carmen, 1990 (28)	Intensive exercises and educational sessions vs. treatment as usual	Back injury	Cohort	CEA[b]	703	2,172	1,2,4	Unclear	Compensation costs for wage loss and health care	No	No
Timm, 1994 (44)	Active vs. passive treatment	Chronic LBP	RCT	CEA	4 × 50	50	1,2	Average costs	Pain status, episode of chronic LBP, length of pain relief, Oswestry pain disability index	No	No
Surgery											
Bell et al., 1997 (2)	Spinal cord stimulation	Failed back surgery syndrome	Cohort	CD	? Difference literature samples taken		1,2	Estimates and charges	Medical costs of spinal cord stimulation, medical resource use	Yes	Yes
Devulder et al., 1997 (6)	Spinal cord stimulation vs. long-term maintenance	Failed back surgery syndrome	Cohort (13 yr)	CO	69	1,2	(4)	Unclear	Use of stimulator, return to work, pain relief	No	No
Malter et al., 1996 (24)	Lumbar discectomy	Herniated intervertebral disc	Based on RCTs	CEA/CUA	Different literature samples		1	Cost estimates, tariffs	Quality of life, quality-adjusted life years	Yes	No
Manucher and Javid, 1995 (25)	Chemonucleolysis vs. laminectomy	Herniated lumbar disc	Cohort	CEA	100	100	1,2	Charges	Patient evaluation, clinical examination rate of return to work, change in job	No	No
Ramirez and Javid, 1985 (33)	Chemonucleolysis vs. laminectomy	Herniated nucleus pulposus, LBP, neck pain	Cohort	CEA[b]	40	40	1,2	Charges	Length of hospitalization, unsatisfactory results, repeat operations	No	No
Ray, 1997 (34)	Lumbar interbody fusions vs. anterior composite interbody composite	Back pain	Cohort	CMA	25	25	1,2	Charges	Blood loss, surgical time translated into costs	Yes	No
Stevenson et al., 1995 (42)	APLD vs. microdiscectomy	Contained lumbar disc herniation	RCT	CEA	31 (APLD)	40	1,3	Actual data	Treatment success on four-point scale	No	No

406

Author, year	Intervention	Condition	Study design	Analysis			Cost identified	Cost basis	Outcome		
Tunturi et al., 1979 (46)	Posterior fusion	??	Cohort	CO	118		1,3,4	Charges	Work output	Yes	No
Other therapies											
Liang and Komaroff, 1982 (16)	Roentgenograms in primary care vs. no roentgenograms	Acute LBP	Cohort	CEA	Unclear	Unclear	1	Charges	Day of suffering from undiagnosed and untreated disease, radiation exposure, (in milliards), dollar charges for lumbar roentgenograms	No	Yes
Lissovoy et al., 1997 (20)	Intrathecal morphine therapy vs. medical management	Failed back surgery syndrome	Model	CEA	Model	Model	1,2	Charges	Pain relief	Yes	Yes
MacLean, 1993 (22)	Hospital care given by family physicians or other physicians	Back pain	Cohort	CEA	68	560	1,2	Charges	MedisGroups major morbidity, in-hospital mortality, length of stay	No	Yes
Shekelle et al., 1995 (37)	Comparison of provider types of care	Back pain	Cohort	CA	686[c]		1,2	Charges	—	Yes	No

[a] Cost identified:
1. Program costs (direct)
2. Costs of other health care utilization (direct)
3. Out of pocket expenses of patients and their families (direct)
4. Costs of productivity losses due to absence from work (indirect)

[b] Some of the consequences in this study are valued in monetary terms.

[c] Six hundred eighty-six persons were divided in five subgroups depending on back pain care.

[d] Human capital approach

CA, cost analysis; CBA, cost-benefit analysis; CD, cost description; CEA, cost-effectiveness analysis; CMA, cost-minimalization analysis; CO, cost-outcome description; CUA, cost-utility analysis; HCA, human capital approach; LBP, low back pain; RCT, randomized controlled trial; APLD, automated percutaneous lumbar discectomy.

Levels of Evidence

Our conclusion on the cost-effectiveness of the interventions is based on several evidence levels. Because of the different character of this chapter, it is important to mention that these evidence levels are different from those in the other chapters. The following rating criteria are important for classification into the evidence levels. These criteria can also be found in Tables 19.2 and 19.3.

a. A study is classified as a complete economic evaluation study (cost-minimization analysis, cost-effectiveness analysis, cost-benefit analysis, and cost-utility analysis).
b. Effectiveness data must be supported by effect measures that are identified, quantified, and supported by statistical evidence.
c. Costing data have to be supported by cost components that are identified, quantified, and supported by statistical evidence.
d. A study is classified as a partial evaluation study.

Studies were (when possible) classified into the following evidence levels:

A. Sufficient evidence on cost-effectiveness: multiple studies with criteria a, b, and c.
B. Moderate evidence on cost-effectiveness: multiple studies with criterion a; one study with criteria a, b, and c.
C. Limited evidence on cost-effectiveness: multiple studies with criteria b, c, and d.
D. No evidence on cost-effectiveness: studies fulfilling only criterion d.

RESULTS

Study Selection

After excluding editorials, letters, non–English-language articles, and reviews, we included 30 articles referring to economic evaluation of back pain treatments (1,2,3,5, 6,12,17,19,20,23–28,30,33–40,42–46,48,50). In the review, we included three more studies that did not refer to the economic evaluation of a treatment but referred to either the evaluation of different types of care (22,37) or the evaluation of diagnosis (16). Many other studies were excluded because they did not appear to be economic evaluation studies. Some studies only mentioned the term "costs" or "cost-effectiveness" in their abstract or the conclusion, without further report. Most of the studies included in the review were performed in North America, two studies were performed in Australia, and 10 were conducted in Europe (Finland, Germany, the Netherlands, Norway, and Belgium).

Tables 19.2 and 19.3 give an overview of the studies reviewed for this chapter. Table 19.2 summarizes the most important findings in the economic evaluation, whereas Table 19.3 contains information about the intervention and the conclusions.

Nature of Economic Appraisal

The most frequently used economic evaluation design in our review (20 studies) was the cost-effectiveness analysis. The values used for consequences in these studies were in natural units, for example, pain intensity, pain duration, health care consumption, absenteeism, and continuation of activities. In three of the cost-effectiveness analyses, some of the consequences were translated into monetary terms (17,33,36). We did not classify them as cost-benefit analyses because this type of analysis measures all costs and benefits in pecuniary units and computes a net monetary gain or loss. The study by Ray (34) was classified as a cost-minimization analysis, because the effectiveness of threaded fusion cages and 360-degree fusions was assumed to be the same. Although Malter et al. (24) classified their study as a cost-effectiveness analysis, it can also be categorized as a cost-utility analysis because benefits were finally expressed in quality-adjusted life-years.

Three of the studies (28,36,37) analyzed only costs, without an economic assessment of outcomes. These studies were classified as cost-analyses. Another four partial evaluation studies (2,5,12,50) also restricted their analysis to costs but were classified as cost descriptions because they did not compare the costs of alternatives. Finally, five studies could be classified as cost-outcome descriptions because they evaluated the costs and outcomes of only one intervention (1,6,36,43,46).

Alternatives Compared

Another important standard in economic evaluation research is the comparison of at least two alternatives. The alternatives with which the various treatments were compared were not always explicitly mentioned in the articles. Of the 33 studies, 25 used a comparison of two or more alternative interventions or a "no-intervention control." Six studies compared the intervention with the situation at baseline. Two studies did not use a comparison at all.

The studies reviewed evaluated a wide range of different types of treatments. To provide an overview of the studies, we listed the treatments, according to Cats-Baril and Frymoyer (4), into three categories for which cost-effectiveness studies are important: injury prevention (e.g., back schools, workplace design, screening programs); postincidence management programs (return-to-work programs designed to bring the injured worker back to productive status as soon as possible and to avoid the downward spiral of unemployment); and back injury and pain remedies, which involve medical treatment.

Injury Prevention and Back Schools

Two of the studies evaluated the cost-effectiveness of a back school program (3,48). Both studies compared the treatment with a no-treatment control group. This approach is the most reasonable alternative in prevention programs because omitting the program will not harm the patient by worsening his or her current state of health. In a 6-year controlled study, Versloot et al. (48) evaluated a back school program aimed to decrease the length of absenteeism. Although no significant difference in length of absenteeism was found between participant and nonparticipant groups, Versloot et al. (48) assumed the back school program to be cost-effective in industry. Brown et al. (3) evaluated the cost-effectiveness of a back school rehabilitation program for municipal employees. The program resulted in significantly fewer injuries compared with the control group, but no significant decrease in lost work time, lost time cost, medical costs, and number of injuries in participants who had completed the back school course. In accordance with the conclusions from other evaluations of back schools (31), these two studies showed no significant differences between the back school participants and the control group (also see Chapter 6). Looking at the complete cost-effectiveness, there is limited evidence to conclude that back schools programs do not result in different cost-effectiveness compared with a no-treatment control group (Level C).

In a study by Hochanadel and Conrad (12), an on-site industrial physical therapy program was compared with the situation before implementation of the program, and these investigators found a reduction in absenteeism. The study by Coleman and Hansen (5) compared an educational program with a no-treatment control group. The program resulted in a decrease of total costs of back injuries in terms of lost time and medical expenses. Because both studies were only partial evaluation studies, the evidence at present is not enough to assume that these programs may be cost-effective (Level D).

Postincidence Management and Secondary Prevention Programs

As emphasized earlier, the indirect costs of lost work time are substantial for patients with back pain. Six of the studies dealt with management and secondary prevention programs (17,19,28,29,36,39) for persons with back injuries.

In a retrospective study of 53 patients with chronic pain, Stieg et al. (43) compared the expenditures for drugs, medical treatment, and disability payments before and after interdisciplinary chronic pain treatment. The program resulted in fewer disability payments.

In the study by Ryden et al. (36), the continuation of the status quo was the alternative to two health promotion programs in a hospital setting: a back education program tailored to individual job requirements and a light duty program for employees who were unable to return to their usual tasks that allowed a replacement worker to be found for the original position. The programs resulted in a decrease in the costs of back injuries, made up of savings to the hospital in medical bills, workers' compensation costs, and lost time.

Another type of secondary prevention program involves changes in the workplace. Aarås (1) showed that changes in workload because of an ergonomic intervention in the workplace produced substantial savings. Mitchell et al. (27) showed that the use of back belts in the workplace was minimally effective in preventing injury. Costs of injury were substantially higher than when patients were injured otherwise.

In an 18-month follow-up study by Linton and Bradley (17), a secondary prevention program for subacute back pain served as its own control. Results showed that subjects had significantly less pain, used fewer medications, and were more active at 18-month follow-up than at baseline. Assuming that, without the program, the rising trend in the number of sick days claimed by these participants would have continued, employers would save at least twice the cost of the program.

Mitchell and Carmen (28) undertook a study to determine whether an intensive and active exercise program for 703 patients was a more effective treatment for acute back and other soft tissue injuries than the current variety of treatments received by a matched comparison group of 2,172, who were treated in the community at large. There was an initial increase in health care costs resulting from the intensity of the treatment, but these costs were more than offset by cost savings in the number of days absent from work and in compensation benefits.

In addition, in the study by Linton et al. (19), sick leave was a major outcome measure. Two studies (18,19) (patients with and without a prior history of being listed as sick with acute musculoskeletal pain problems) were evaluated that compared the effects of an early active intervention with a treatment as a usual control group. The intervention group demonstrated significantly less time lost from work because of illness and fewer chronic cases in patients without a previous history of sickness-related absenteeism.

Mitchell and Carmen (29) compared a group provided with functional restoration with a control group receiving a therapy that varied with the preference of the treating practitioner. Duration of absence from work, compensation costs, disability costs, and total costs were less for those treated than for the control subjects, but these differences were not statistically significant.

Sinclair et al. (39) compared a clinical early active intervention program for acute back injury with a group receiving treatment as usual. After 1 year, there was no advantage from the program compared with the usual care on functional capacity, health-related quality of life, pain, time to return to work, and health care costs.

Although the content of these programs differs enormously, the overall conclusion is that limited evidence (Level C) indicates that secondary prevention programs and postincidence management programs, generally for acute back pain in a work setting, may be cost-effective, especially by reducing the number of lost work days and overall time loss. The conclusions in a review of Turk (47) concerning the cost-benefit analysis of multidisciplinary pain centers were more positive. Turk summarized that multidisciplinary pain centers improve overall functioning, reduce health care costs and return to work for chronic low back pain patients. However, Turk's calculations were based on assumptions and an extrapolation from treatment outcomes reported in several (noneconomic evaluation) studies that were selected on a systematic basis. Furthermore, only studies with conclusions in favor of the multidisciplinary pain centers were included, a factor that resulted in overall conclusions that were far too optimistic. Nevertheless, his conclusion points in the same limited (C) positive direction as the conclusion in the present review.

Back Injury and Pain Remedies: Clinical Treatment

This category was subdivided into manipulation and physical therapy, exercise therapy, surgery, other therapies. The treatments were usually compared with another treatment, or the usual treatment, rather than with a no-treatment control group.

Manipulation and Physical Therapy

Four studies, of which three were cost-effectiveness studies, compared chiropractic treatment with another type of therapy. Meade et al. (26) compared chiropractic therapy with conventional hospital outpatient management. There was an obvious clinical improvement in pain intensity and disability attributable to chiropractic treatment. These improvements may result in a reduction of days of absenteeism.

Moreover, Nyiendo (31) made a comparison between claimants with disabling work-related low back pain injuries in Oregon receiving chiropractic therapy and those receiving medical treatments. He found a difference between those receiving chiropractic and medical care in terms of lost working days or compensation amounts, but the difference was not significant.

Tuchin and Bonello (45) compared chiropractic treatment with standard medical management for back pain and spinal injuries, management that included bed rest, physical therapy and analgesics or antiinflammatory drugs. The authors concluded that chiropractic treatment may be associated with fewer days lost from work because of illness and may therefore be called cost-effective. However, this study was designed to serve as a pilot for a full-scale study in which the possibility of cost-effectiveness would be proven again. Because of the narrow perspective of the study, only days of work were evaluated. Patients' health outcomes were not considered.

Finally, Skargren et al. (40) undertook a cost-effectiveness analysis of a randomized clinical trial in 223 patients with (acute and chronic) back and neck problems who received either chiropractic treatment or physical therapy. The authors concluded that chiropractic treatment and physical therapy were equally cost-effective after therapy and after 6 months.

In conclusion, rather limited evidence indicates that chiropractic treatment may be cost-effective compared with conventional treatment and equally effective as physical therapy. The evidence was only limited because the conclusions concerning the costs were mainly based on assumptions (evidence level C).

Exercise Therapy

Three cost-effectiveness studies compared active treatment with several types of passive treatment (23,28,44). A study by Malmivaara et al. (23) compared three different types of treatments of acute low back pain: bed rest, exercises, and ordinary activity. It appeared that continuing ordinary activities led to less of a need for home help and less absenteeism than the two other alternatives (see also Chapter 11).

Timm (44) reported on the cost-effectiveness of passive treatment (physical agents, joint manipulation) and active treatment (low-tech and high-tech exercise) for chronic low back pain. The four treatment groups were compared with a control group of persons who did not receive treatment. The study found that only active treatment produced significant improvements of objective functional measurements of chronic low back pain. The low-tech exercise treatment provided the longest interval of pain relief and turned out to be the most cost-effective.

Mitchell and Carmen (28) compared an intensive active exercise program for acute back injury with a passive program. The active group turned out to be superior to the control group in earlier return to work.

Comparisons of active treatment with several types of passive treatment found that active treatment reduced absenteeism and increased mobility in patients with acute and chronic low back pain. Therefore, there is moderate evidence to believe that active treatment may result in cost-effectiveness (evidence level B).

Surgery

The economic consequences of spinal cord stimulation (SCS) for patients with failed back surgery syndrome (FBSS) were evaluated in two studies (2,6). The study by Bell et al. (2) described the economic implications of SCS by comparing the medical resource utilization of SCS with the traditional alternative of palliative care for patients with FBSS that consists of a mix of surgical procedures and other interventions labeled "chronic maintenance." The short term study resulted in many assumptions for the annual medical resource use by patients with FBSS who underwent nonsurgical chronic care. Devulder et al. (6) evaluated the costs of SCS, which was used in the treatment of 69 patients with FBSS during a period of 13 years. SCS resulted in lower costs for materials and hospital stay. Patients with SCS also reported pain relief, and several returned to work. The authors concluded that SCS may be a cost-effective method if others therapies fail. Because both studies based cost-effectiveness on assumptions, we concluded that, in the short term, there is limited evidence on the cost-effectiveness of SCS for patients with FBSS (evidence level C).

There is also moderate evidence that chemonucleolysis is cost-effective compared with laminectomy for the treatment of herniated lumbar disc. In the study by Ramirez and Javid (33), chemonucleolysis resulted in savings when the cost of repeat operations was taken into consideration. Most of the savings reflected the 5-day difference in length of hospitalization with the two treatments. Manucher and Javid (25) compared the cost-effectiveness of chymopapain chemonucleolysis with that of laminectomy. Based on the results, the authors assumed that the outcomes of both treatments were the same. The average savings were calculated to be $5,365 when chymopapain chemonucleolysis was performed instead of laminectomy. To use chymopapain chemonucleolysis rather than laminectomy would reduce short-term and long-term health costs. However, because the results of the study were based on nonrandom sample groups (and the clinical examination was partially carried out by the authors themselves), the results were applicable only to this particular study.

Two studies evaluated the cost-effectiveness of lumbar discectomy (45,42). Stevenson et al. (42) compared automated percutaneous lumbar discectomy (n = 31) with microdiscectomy (n = 40) in the treatment of contained lumbar disc herniation. From the results, these authors concluded that within the restrictions imposed by the data set, automated percutaneous lumbar discectomy was less cost-effective and less effective clinically than microdescectomy. However, many assumptions were made for the cost calculation, so it is difficult to make strong conclusions. The second study, by Malter et al. (24), described a cost-effectiveness analyses of lumbar discectomy for patients with herniated lumbar discs unresponsive to conservative management. In this study, part of the cost data and all the effectiveness data were based on previously published data. Part of the cost data was newly gathered from a commercially available datafile. The study from which the effectiveness data were taken compared surgical with nonsurgical therapy. Further, Malter et al. (24) combined the effectiveness data from the trial of Weber (49) with quality-of-life values from another study (in which patients with a current back pain episode were asked to rank their own quality of life). Finally, these values were used to calculate the number of quality-adjusted life-years gained with surgical versus medical treatment. The data source for the costs was a commercially available database including 2,175 patients insured by commercial insurers and self-insured businesses. The authors concluded that surgical discectomy was a cost-effective treatment. However, in this study, many assumptions were made to calculate the cost-effectiveness, and this approach raised questions concerning the conclusion. Because there was no comparison and only limited evidence concerning cost-effectiveness, we can conclude by saying that there is no evidence that lumbar discectomy is cost-effective compared with no surgical treatment or microdiscectomy (evidence level D).

The study by Ray (34) compared the surgical and hospitalization costs, operating times, and blood loss attributable to lumbar interbody fusions at one and two lumbar levels by the use of two device systems: the Ray threaded fusion cage and an anteroposterior interbody technique with pedicle screw and rod stabilization (360-degree fusions). The therapy was given to 50 patients with progressive disabling low back pain to arise from only one or two painful degenerated lumbar disc spaces. Ray concluded that the threaded fusion cage procedure was significantly more cost-effective than the well-established method of anterior composite interbody grafting with posterior pedicle screw fixation, even though the complication rates and clinical success rates were similar. Because the results of this study could not be compared with other findings, and there was no statistically significant evidence on the costs, there is no evidence to believe that use of the threaded fusion cage is a cost-effective procedure.

Finally, the study of Tunturi et al. (46) compared the costs (calculated from treatment, visits to outpatient department, and traveling) with the economic benefits (return to work) of posterior fusion of the lumbosacral spine. The calculations were based upon 118 operated patients followed-up for an average of 4.8 years. The authors concluded that the fusions were profitable at a cost-benefit ratio of 1:2.9. Because neither of these two studies (34,46) compared their own methods with an alternative, there is no evidence that fusions are cost-effective (Level D).

Other Therapies

Four studies could not be categorized into one of the previous headings. Two studies comparing different providers of back pain care concluded that care given by general practitioners was significantly less costly, compared with care provided by chiropractors, internists, orthopedists (37), or other caregivers in the hospital (22). Shekelle et al. (37) compared the costs of care given by chiropractors, general practitioners, internists, and orthopedists. It was concluded that the costs of care given by general practitioner was significantly the lowest, whereas care given by orthopedists was significantly the most expensive. MacLean (22), comparing the cost of family physicians' care with those of hospital care, also concluded that the costs of care by family physicians were lower. There is thus limited evidence (level C) that general practitioners are less costly compared to other specialists.

The next study was not comparable with the others in this review. This study from Liang and Komaroff (16) compared the benefits, risks, and costs of obtaining diagnostic roentgenograms in patients with acute low back pain and in patients not receiving diagnostic roentgenograms. The authors concluded that the risks and costs of performing lumbar roentgenograms at the initial visit in patients with acute low back pain did not seem to be justified by the relatively small benefit noted (level D).

Finally, the study of Lissovoy et al. (20) compared intrathecal morphine therapy with medical treatment in a simulated cohort of patients with FBSS. In this model, the average patient achieved 43.8 months of pain relief with intrathecal morphine therapy. This approach may result in cost savings relative to conventional therapy (Level D).

Methods Used in Determining Costs and Consequences

The next sections describe the evaluation methods used in the partial and full economic evaluation studies. A summary of the most important findings can be found in Table 19.3.

Costs Identified

Although the perspective of the study determined the costs and consequences that we examined, only 4 studies mentioned the perspective explicitly (2,20,24,34). All studies included the cost of the intervention itself, and 24 studies included the costs of other health care services (2,3,5,6,20,23,25,27–29,31,33–40,43–45,51). Costs borne by the patients and their families were included only in the studies by Malmivaara et al. (23), Stevenson et al. (42), and, partly, Tunturi et al. (46). Indirect costs were measured by patients' absenteeism in 21 studies (1,3,5,6,12,17,19,23,26–29,31,36,38–40,43,46,48,51).

Data Sources

After the selection of costs relevant to the study, one has to determine how these costs can be measured. To measure medical consumption, some studies used the databases of health care suppliers (3,6,23,25,34,36,40,42), insurance companies (1,12,23), workers' compensation boards (39), or questions to the patient (1,12,23,27,38,42). Once, a combination of two or more data sources was used to validate medical consumption measures independently (38). Information on absenteeism was obtained from (national) insurance companies (17,19,31,35,43), from the databases of employers (1,48,51), and from the patient (6). It was unclear how some studies obtained their cost data (16,28,29,44,46).

Cost Valuation

After identifying which costs are to be included in an economic evaluation and how they are measured, costs have to be valued. This means putting currency labels on the volumes found. Only the study by Stevenson (42) calculated the actual economic costs related to the intervention. Thirteen studies used charges (2,3,16,20,22,23,31,33-35,37,38,46), cost estimates (1,12,17,19), or average costs (26,44). The remaining studies were vague about how they obtained costs on fees.

In general, the human capital approach is the most frequently used method of valuing indirect costs. In this approach, lost production that results from temporary absence from work, disability, or premature death is valued using the average earnings (13,15). However, in our sample only Brown et al. (3) used the human capital approach to value indirect costs. The study by Skargren et al. (40) estimated the indirect costs from the mean income in different sex and age groups, including social costs. The other studies that took indirect costs into account were not clear about how they valued them.

Consequences Determined

An economic evaluation study should examine not only the costs of the alternatives but also the consequences (or the "output"). The studies included in the review used a large variety of outcome measures. To facilitate the comparison among the outcomes, we categorized the outcomes into therapeutic measures, quality-of-life measures, and return to work (8).

Clinical Outcomes

In principle, patient-centered outcomes can be measured objectively. The term *patient-centered outcomes* refers only to an individual's ability to function and not to the significance, preference, or value attached to this ability by the individual or by others (25). In several studies, these therapeutic outcomes were measured in terms of pain intensity, duration of pain, and number of back injuries (3,6,20,23,26,39,40,44).

Because back pain is frequently not an objectively demonstrable disorder, therapeutic outcomes can best be combined with other outcomes such as quality-of-life measures, because the issue of quality of life addresses different aspects of the disease (26).

Eight studies used quality-of-life measures of outcome (17,19,23,24,26,39,40,44). Seven of these studies used domain-specific questionnaires focusing on those aspects directly related to having pain and to pain-related complaints. Because economic evaluation studies are often directed toward overall comparisons among several interventions, generic and utility measures are considered important outcome measures. Only the studies by Malter et al. (24) and Sinclair et al. (39) used generic measures. The study by Malter et al. (24) also used time tradeoff scores to determine quality-adjusted life-years.

Changes in Resource Use or Benefits

Changes in resource use and benefits turned out to be the most important outcome measure in back pain studies. Some of the studies even restricted the outcome assessment to these intermediate effects of the intervention (1,22,23,28,29,31,36,38,43,45–47,51). In the studies selected for this review, outcomes dealing with absenteeism and return to work seemed important. This was not a surprise because most studies dealt with back pain—related injury and acute back pain. In many studies, the outcomes were measured in volumes and were translated into monetary units. For instance, days of absenteeism may be translated into compensation costs for wage loss, or length of hospitalization may be translated in terms of hospital costs. Therefore, such changes in resource use and benefits were considered in our review along with the methods of measuring costs, which are discussed in the previous section.

Discounting and Sensitivity Analysis

Another important factor in economic evaluation is that different studies may deal with costs and consequences that have different time dimensions. In some programs, the benefits and costs may occur immediately, whereas in others, the benefits of the intervention may continue or may only be realized in the future even though the costs are incurred immediately. In the latter case, one has to discount the figures, to convert future costs and benefits into equivalent present values. Only a few studies discounted their data (1,2,20,23,24,34,37,46,51), although other studies collected data over several years (3,6,17,26,31,33,36,38,43,48).

In the last step of performing an economic evaluation, one has to adjust for the assumptions made during the study. A sensitivity analysis should be performed, using different assumptions or estimates to examine the changes in results of the analysis. If the changes in results from the different assumptions are minor, the results may be held with greater confidence. If the sensitivity analysis produces significant changes in the results, then greater caution is necessary when interpreting the data, and more effort is required to reduce the uncertainty or to improve the accuracy of the critical variables. A sensitivity analysis was performed in only four studies (2,16,20,22).

Some Methodologic Aspects of the Studies

A sound epidemiologic design is important for an economic evaluation. The design of the study is one of the main determinants of the quality of the results of economic evaluation studies. The quality of results is especially important for clinical and public policy makers, who use them to make decisions concerning alternative treatments. Economic evaluation studies can be conducted preferably using prospective data (randomized clinical trials) or, more commonly, using retrospective data (21). Of the full economic evaluation studies in our review that used comparison groups, only 11 randomized the patients into these groups (3,19,23,26,29,31,40,42,44,45,48). Eight studies did not use an alternative therapy as a comparison at all (1,5,12,35,36,38,43,51). Several studies gave either ethical or practical reasons for not using a comparison group (18,43,46,51). Drummond (7) argued that if no comparison group is used, effectiveness information based on previous good-quality studies should be provided. Four of the 8 studies (12,17,36,38) reported the conclusions of other studies of the same treatment, but they did not generally say anything about the quality or validity of these earlier treatment results.

It was remarkable that at least 12 studies did not report on statistically significant evidence on the costs outcomes and the target variable for the economic evaluation (16,22,24,25,28,31,33,34,42,43,46,48). However, these studies did generally provide reasons that their findings could nevertheless be called significant. For example, MacLean (22) reported that the findings were not statistically significant but were financially significant, but this investigator did not explain what was meant by "financially significant."

CONCLUSIONS AND RECOMMENDATIONS

Despite the rising health care costs of low back pain and the increased interest in economic evaluations, the economic aspects of low back pain interventions have received little attention. A systematic search from 1984 through 1997 of several databases found only 30 studies in English that actually contained such an evaluation. Of these studies, 21 were classified as full economic evaluation studies.

The interventions for back pain have been divided into injury prevention programs, postincidence management programs, and clinical treatment. From this review, it was impossible to draw definite conclusions on the cost-effectiveness of each category. The small number of comparable treatments, the large differences in and low quality of the costing methodology, and the large differences among the back pain populations made comparisons among the estimates in the studies reviewed difficult. This was also the reason that we only concluded on moderate and limited evidence for the evaluated studies and did not find strong evidence of cost-effectiveness for either of the treatment modalities. Since we used less strict evidence gradings than in other chapters of this book, the moderate and limited evidence (B, C) should also be read with care. For work-related back injury or back pain, limited evidence (C) of equal cost-effectiveness was found for back schools and injury prevention programs compared with no treatment, limited evidence (C) was found for different forms of secondary prevention programs, and for multidisciplinary pain management programs. There was limited evidence (C) that chiropractic treatment was equally cost-effective compared with physical therapy and was cost-effective compared with conventional treatment. Furthermore, there was moderate evidence (B) for cost-effectiveness of exercise therapy (compared with passive treatment), and chemonucleolysis. Mainly because of low costing methodology, there was only limited evidence (C) on cost-effectiveness for lumbar discectomy and no evidence (D) for lumbar fusions.

Most of the studies in the review dealt with acute back pain and back pain—related injuries. The cost-effectiveness of the different therapies was therefore mostly expressed in reduced absenteeism. Interventions for patients with chronic low back pain were rarely subjected to economic evaluation.

In this chapter, a major purpose of reviewing economic evaluation was to use the results of the studies further for decision making and planning. However, to assess the results for this purpose, the methods employed in the different studies had to be valid and clearly documented. For some studies reviewed in this chapter, the main purpose was not the economic evaluation of the treatment, but the assessment of the effect of the treatment instead. As a result, the methodology of performing an economic evaluation was placed in the background. Differences found in cost-effectiveness possibly reflected the characteristics of the interventions or programs evaluated, rather than differences in costing.

The review showed a significant need to improve the application and clearness of economic evaluation in the area of back pain. Therefore, the conclusions in this chapter should be read while keeping in mind the mentioned shortcomings of these studies. Decisions about the most cost-effective therapies for back pain are not possible at this moment.

REFERENCES

1. Aarås A. The impact of ergonomic intervention on individual health and corporate prosperity in a telecommunications environment. *Ergonomics* 1994;37:1679–1696.
2. Bell GK, Kidd D, North RB. Cost-effectiveness analysis of spinal cord stimulation in treatment of failed back surgery syndrome. *J Pain Symptom Manage* 1997;13:286–295.
3. Brown KC, Sirles AT, Hilyer JC, et al. Cost-effectiveness of a back school intervention for municipal employees. *Spine* 1992;17:1224–1228.
4. Cats-Baril WL, Frymoyer JW. *The economics of spinal disorders. In: The adult spine: principles and practice.* New York: Raven Press, 1991.
5. Coleman S, Hansen S. Reducing work-related back injuries. *Nursing Manage* 1994;25:58–61.
6. Devulder J, De Laat M, Van Bastelaere M, et al. Spinal cord stimulation: a valuable treatment for chronic failed back surgery patients. *J Pain Symptom Manage* 1997;13:296–301.
7. Drummond MF. *Principles of economic appraisals in health care.* New York: Oxford University Press, 1980.
8. Drummond MF, O'Brien B, Stoddart GL, et al. *Methods for the economic evaluation of health care programmes,* 2nd ed. Oxford: Oxford University Press, 1997.
9. Evers SMAA, Wijk van AS. *Toolkit for reviewing literature.* Working paper, Department of Health Economics, University of Limburg, Maastricht, Netherlands, 1994:94–3.
10. Goossens MEJB, Evers SMAA. Economic evaluation of back pain interventions. *J Occup Rehabil* 1997;7:15–32.
11. Health Economics. Economic evaluation bibliography. *Health Econ* 1992;December[Suppl]:1.
12. Hochanadel CD, Conrad DE. Evolution of an on-site industrial physical therapy program. *J Occup Med* 1993;35:1011–1016.
13. Hodgson T, Meiners M. Cost-of-illness methodology: a guide to current practices and procedures. *Health Soc* 1982;60:429–462.
14. Keijsers JFEM. *The efficacy of back schools: empirical evidence and its impact on health care practice.* Dissertation, University of Maastricht, Maastricht, Netherlands, 1991.
15. Koopmanschap MA, Ineveld van BM. Towards a new approach for estimating indirect costs of disease. *Soc Sci Med* 1992;34:1005–1010.
16. Liang M, Komaroff AL. Roentgenograms in primary care patients with acute low back pain: a cost-effectiveness analysis. *Arch Intern Med* 1982;142:1108–1112.
17. Linton SJ, Bradley LA. An 18-month follow-up of a secondary prevention program for back pain: help and hindrance factors related to outcome maintenance. *Clin J Pain* 1992;8:227–236.
18. Linton SJ, Bradley LA, Jensen I, et al. The secondary prevention of low back pain: a controlled study with follow-up. *Pain* 1989;36:197–207.
19. Linton SJ, Hellsing AL, Andersson D. A controlled study of the effects of an early intervention on acute musculoskeletal pain problems. *Pain* 1993;54:353–359.
20. Lissovoy de G, Brown RE, Halpern M, et al. Cost-effectiveness of long-term intrathecal morphine therapy for pain associated with failed back surgery syndrome. *Clin Ther* 1997;19:96–85.
21. Luce B, Elixhauser A. Estimating costs in the economic evaluation of medical technologies. *Int J Technol Assess Health Care* 1990;6:57–75.
22. MacLean DS. Family practice and the health care system: outcome and cost of family physicians' care. Pilot study of three diagnosis-related groups in elderly inpatients. *J Am Board Fam Pract* 1993;6:588–593.
23. Malmivaara A, Häkkinen U, Aro T, et al. The treatment of acute low back pain: bed rest, exercises, or ordinary activity? *N Engl J Med* 1995;332:351–355.
24. Malter AD, Larson EB, Urban N, et al. Cost-effectiveness of lumbar discectomy for the treatment of herniated intervertebral disc. *Spine* 1996;21:1048–1055.

25. Manucher J, Javid MJ. Chemonucleolysis versus laminectomy: a cohort comparison of effectiveness and charges. *Spine* 1995;20:2016–2022.
26. Meade TW, Dyer S, Browne W, et al. Low back pain of mechanical origin: randomised comparison of chiropractic and hospital outpatient treatment. *BMJ* 1990;300:1431–1437.
27. Mitchell LV, Lawler FH, Bowen D, et al. Effectiveness and cost-effectiveness of employer-issued back belts in areas of high risk for back injury. *J Occup Med* 1994;36:90–94.
28. Mitchell RI, Carmen GM. Results of a multicenter trial using an intensive active exercise program for the treatment of acute soft tissue and back injuries. *Spine* 1990;15:514–521.
29. Mitchell RI, Carmen GM. The functional restoration approach to the treatment of chronic pain in patients with soft-tissue and back injuries. *Spine* 1994;19:633–642.
30. National Health Service Centre for Reviews and Dissemination. *NHS economic evaluation database.* York, UK: University of York, 1998.
31. Nyiendo J. Disabling low back Oregon workers' compensation claims. III. Diagnostic and treatment procedures and associated costs. *J Manipulative Physiol Ther* 1991;14:287–297.
32. *OHE-IFPMA database limited.* London: Health Economic Evaluation Database (HEED), 1998.
33. Ramirez LF, Javid MJ. Cost effectiveness of chemonucleolysis versus lamicectomy in the treatment of herniated nucleus pulposus. *Spine* 1985;10:363–367.
34. Ray CD. Threaded fusion cages for lumbar interbody fusions: an economic comparison with 360 fusions. *Spine* 1997;22:681–685.
35. Ryan WE, Krishna MK, Swanson CE. A prospective study evaluating early rehabilitation in preventing back pain chronicity in mine workers. *Spine* 1995;20:489–491.
36. Ryden LA, Molgaard CA, Bobbitt SL. Benefits of a back care and light duty health promotion program in a hospital setting. *J Community Health* 1988;13:222–230.
37. Shekelle PG, Markovich M, Louie R. Comparing the costs between provider types of episodes of back pain care. *Spine* 1995;20:221–227.
38. Simmons JW, Avant WS Jr, Demski J, et al. Determining successful pain clinic treatment through validation of cost effectiveness. *Spine* 1988;13:342–344.
39. Sinclair SJ, Hogg-Johnson S, Mondloch MV, et al. The effectiveness of an early active intervention program for workers with soft-tissue injuries: the early claimant cohort study. *Spine* 1997;22:2919–2911.
40. Skargren EI, Oberg BE, Carlsson PG, et al. Cost-effectiveness of chiropractic and physiotherapy treatment for low back pain and neck pain: six-month follow-up. *Spine* 1997;22:2167–2177.
41. Spilker B. *Quality of life assessment in clinical trials.* New York: Raven Press, 1990.
42. Stevenson RC, McCabe CJ, Findlay AM. An economic evaluation of a clinical trial to compare automated percutaneous lumbar discectomy with micodiscectomy in the treatment of contained lumbar disc herniation. *Spine* 1995;20:739–742.
43. Stieg RL, Williams RC, Timmermans-Williams G, et al. Cost benefits of interdisciplinary chronic pain treatment. *Clin J Pain* 1986;1:189–193.
44. Timm KE. A randomized-control study of active and passive treatments for chronic low back pain following L5 laminectomy. *J Orthop Sports Phys Ther* 1994;20:276–286.
45. Tuchin PJ, Bonello R. Preliminary findings of analysis of chiropractic utilization and cos in the workers compensation system of New South Wales, Australia. *J Manipulative Physiol Ther* 1995;18:503–511.
46. Tunturi T, Niemela P, Laurinkari J, et al. Cost-benefit analysis of posterior fusion of the lumbosacral spine. *Acta Orthop Scand* 1979;50:427–432.
47. Turk DC. Efficacy of multidisciplinary pain centers in the treatment of chronic pain. In: *Pain treatment centers at a crossroads: a practical and conceptual reappraisal. Progress in pain research and management.* Seattle: IASP Press, 1996:257–273.
48. Versloot JM, Rozeman A, Son van AM, et al. The cost-effectiveness of a back school program in industry: a longitudinal controlled field study. *Spine* 1992;17:22–27.
49. Weber H. Lumbar disc herniation: a controlled, prospective study with ten years of observation. *Spine* 1983;8:131–140.
50. Webster BS, Snook SH. The cost of compensable low back pain. *J Occup Med* 1990;32:13–15.
51. Wiesel SW, Boden SD, Feffer HL. A quality-based protocol for management of musculoskeletal injuries. *Clin Orthop* 1994;301:164–176.

Neck and Back Pain: The Scientific Evidence
of Causes, Diagnosis, and Treatment, edited
by Alf Nachemson and Egon Jonsson.
Published by Lippincott Williams & Wilkins,
Philadelphia 2000.

20

Cost of Back Pain in Some OECD Countries

Anders I. Norlund* and Gordon Waddell†

Swedish Council on Technology Assessment in Health Care, Stockholm, Sweden
†Department of Orthopaedics, The Glasgow Nuffield Hospital,
Glasgow, Scotland

Illness can be interpreted in different ways, depending on perspective: that of the patient (feeling sick), that of the physician (diagnosed illness), or that of the employer (absence from work). These perspectives overlap but are not synonymous. When cost of illness is calculated, a societal perspective is normally used.

Methods of calculation of cost of illness imply that health can be regarded as a type of capital asset (14). This asset can be depreciated in value by (among other things) illness and death and thus can cause losses or costs to society. The economic estimate of the burden of a disease on society is intended to give information of the value that can be gained from reduction of the incidence and prevalence of the specific disease (4). The economic estimates of costs of illness are normally calculated from two basic methods: the willingness to pay method and the human capital method. The burden on society caused by suffering from pain, the decline in well-being, and other social consequences should also be considered, but consensus is lacking regarding the methods for transforming these losses to costs.

Because of differences in several aspects–organization of health care, organization of the labor market, incentives procured by sickness benefit systems and control mechanisms, and levels of costs of living–these comparisons between calculations of costs of illness are seldom done. However, in this chapter we attempt to compare studies with similar methodologic approaches.

METHODS

A literature search on cost of illness from back pain yielded many references and gave the impression that comparisons could be made among many studies. However, use of critical analysis for inclusion of studies (5,7) reduced the number of possible comparisons. From the original list of references of 25 studies, only 14 could be used for further analysis in a meaningful way. However, some studies claimed to have a societal perspective, although the perspective was more limited, and prices or charges were used instead of costs.

One study from Germany (9) had a more limited perspective, basically that of health care, but calculations were made from costs. Another group of studies had a more limited perspective, such as occupational back pain, in which compensation was used as an indicator of costs. The limitation, however, is that costs of back pain generated from injury claims are difficult to use for comparisons with studies based on a societal perspective. Finally, there remained only three studies that seemed reasonable to use for comparison: an update of the Swedish Council on Technology Assessment (SBU)in Health Care report on back pain (11) and the reports by van Tulder et al. (12) and by Coyle and Richardson (2).

RESULTS

Costs of back pain in Sweden were calculated for 1987 (11) and were updated for this report through 1995. Briefly, the societal cost of back pain in Sweden remained relatively high in the 1990s (Table 20.1). The total estimated cost in 1995 of 29.4 billion SEK corresponded to approximately 1.7% of the Swedish gross national product (GNP). Compared with the situation in 1987, using the same price level, there was a minor (7%) decrease in total societal cost in Sweden from back pain; that is, the cost curve leveled and was slowly decreasing. Short-term sickness absence resulting from back pain was reduced by 30% as measured in number of days compared with 1987 (although days with compensation were less dramatically reduced). The number of early retirements decreased somewhat but remained high.

As regards the total structure of costs, there was a slight difference between direct and indirect costs in the study of the United Kingdom (2), on the one hand, and in those of Sweden (the present report) and the Netherlands (12), on the other hand (Table 20.2). The reason for this difference was the more conservative valuation of early retirements in the study by Coyle and Richardson (2). If, for instance, the report from the United Kingdom had used the same average cost per day for early retirements as for sickness absence, then the proportions of direct versus indirect costs would have been 5.5% and 94.5%; that is, the indirect costs would have been even more dominant than in the Dutch or Swedish reports. Compared with this finding, the reports from the United States often described another structure of costs; according to Webster and Snook (13), 32% of costs were direct, and 68% were indirect. If, however, claims are transformed according to average wage plus social security costs (claims represented only 63% of average salary [10]), the structure of costs would be 17% direct costs and 83% indirect costs, thus resembling the results of the European reports.

Looking at the direct costs only, there seemed to be some major differences among the three reports. According to the study by van Tulder et al. (12), there appeared to be an approach to treatment of back pain in health care in the Netherlands that differed from approaches in the other countries in this comparison. Outpatient physi-

TABLE 20.1 *Summary of direct health care costs for patients with back problems in Sweden in 1995 compared with 1987*

Type of care	Cost in million SEK, 1995	Cost in million SEK in 1987, transformed to 1995 price levels
Inpatient care	415	419
Outpatient care:	1,869	1,082
Physician visits: 797		
Physical therapy: 952		
Rehabilitation services: 120		
Pharmaceuticals	152	167
Total cost	2,436	1,794

TABLE 20.2. *Percentage distribution of costs in cost of illness studies*

	Investigators (ref.)		
	Coyle and Richardson (2)	SBU (11)	van Tulder (12)
Direct costs	11.5	8	7.4
Indirect costs	88.5	92	92.6
Total	100	100	100
Direct costs specified:			
Physician visits	36	33	8
Physical therapy	31	39	38
Pharmacy	10	6	—
Radiology	7	(11)[a]	—
Inpatient days	16	17	54
Other		5	
Total	100	100	100

[a] Calculated but not included, to avoid double counting, because included in the average cost of outpatient visits and inpatient care.

cian visits corresponded to only 8% of direct costs compared with 33% to 36% in the two other studies (Table 20.2). However, as regards physical therapy, there was a closer resemblance among the compared countries, that is, 39% of the total direct costs for Sweden compared with 38% for the Netherlands and 31% for the United Kingdom. The proportion of cost of pharmaceuticals out of total direct costs was about 10% in the United Kingdom. Compared with that proportion, the 6% calculated for Sweden, excluding costs of over-the-counter drugs, seemed reasonable.

There was a striking difference in inpatient care for the Netherlands–more than half, 54%, of the direct costs compared with 16% to 17% for the United Kingdom and for Sweden. This specific situation in the Netherlands was also described in the utilization per 1,000 inhabitants age 15 to 64 years (Table 20.3), that is, 47 days per 1,000 inhabitants compared with 21 and 24 days for the United Kingdom and for Sweden, respectively. Another striking result was the high frequency of physician visits in the United Kingdom, 371 per 1,000 inhabitants 16 to 64 years old.

Finally, there was an important difference in the utilization of the sickness benefit systems. Sweden had a high rate of sickness absence days resulting from back pain. With 3,522 absence days per 1,000 inhabitants 16 to 64 years old, this rate was almost three times higher in Sweden than in the United Kingdom or in the Netherlands. Furthermore, there was almost the double rate of utilization of days of inpatient care (per 1,000 inhabitants aged 16 to 64 years) in the Netherlands, compared with the United Kingdom, despite the same frequency of sickness absence days. This finding

TABLE 20.3. *Utilization per 1,000 inhabitants 15 to 64 years old (ref. nos. in parentheses.)*

	United Kingdom (2)	Sweden (11)	Netherlands (12)
Health care			
Physician visits	371	141	110[a]
Inpatient days	21	24	47
Sickness benefits			
Sickness days	1,379	3,522	1,239

[a] Not mentioned in the article but calculated from total cost ($2 + $2.8 + $22 million US) divided by the indicated cost per visit ($23.1 US).

TABLE 20.4. *Comparison of the societal cost of back pain in different countries[a]*

Country	Cost in millions (currency)		Cost in million original currency		Cost per inhabitant corrected exchange rate (US dollars −91)		
	Direct	Indirect	Direct	Indirect	Direct	Indirect	Total
United Kingdom							
UK (£)	678	5,200	385	2,948	7	113	120
Netherlands							
NL ($)	368	4,600	368	4,600	24	299	323
Sweden (SEK)	2,436	26,950	213	2,262	24	266	290

[a] According to Organization for Economic Cooperation and Development (OECD) retrospective statistics, 1996, table exchange rates.

seemed to indicate differences of traditions of organizing health care for people suffering from back pain.

A final comparison of the societal cost of back pain was made among the Swedish study and those conducted in the Netherlands in 1991 (12) and the United Kingdom in 1991 to 1992 (2). Cost estimations in each study were converted to United States dollars for the same base year, 1991, by using official currency statistics, and were divided per inhabitant according to demographic statistics from the Organization for Economic Cooperation and Development (OECD) (8).

Thus, the calculated cost per inhabitant of illness caused by back pain seemed to fall within approximately the same range for the studies in the Netherlands and in Sweden (Table 20.4). However, in the United Kingdom, costs were only about one-third, mainly because another way was used to calculate losses of production. Using the same method as implemented in the Dutch and the Swedish studies, that is, average wage plus costs for social security, the cost per inhabitant for the United Kingdom could be calculated to be about 80% of that in the Netherlands and 90% of that in Sweden. The low calculated cost per physician visit in the United Kingdom also added to the low total direct cost of back pain per inhabitant.

DISCUSSION

Several international studies indicated that the prevalence of back pain, especially 1-year or lifetime experience, was similar in most countries in the OECD. Yet, the utilization of resources for back pain differed among these countries, as described in the foregoing analysis.

Thus, as regards the number of physician visits, Yelin and Callahan (15) reported an average of 2.2 visits, which could be compared with 1.1 visits in the Netherlands (12), 1.4 visits in Sweden (an update of reference 11), and 3.71 visits in Great Britain (2). The average length of inpatient care in the United States was reported to be 9.2 days in the 1980s (6), and 7.0 days in the early 1990s (15), as compared with 10.5 days in the Netherlands (12).

The rate of surgery for back pain per 1 million inhabitants also differed among countries of the OECD and was by far higher in the United States than in most European countries (3). Differences in organizing and financing health care, as well as differences in social security systems, may have caused these differences of utilization of resources despite similarities in the prevalence of back pain.

However, estimates of the total burden to society from back pain indicated similarities among several countries of the OECD. Thus, the estimate of cost of back pain corresponded to 1.7% of GNP according to the Swedish report (an update of reference 11), which was also the estimate for the Netherlands (12). As a comparison, Yelin and Callahan (15) reported 2.5% for the United States, but this percentage also included patients with arthritis and fractures. In a review of reports on back pain, Cats-Baril and Frymoyer (1) reported estimates of cost of back pain in the range of 0.5% to 2.0% of the GNP.

CONCLUSIONS

There are but few studies from OECD countries with a comparable societal perspective on cost of illness from back pain. A tentative comparison among three European reports on back pain indicated high utilization of outpatient physician visits in the United Kingdom, high utilization of inpatient care in the Netherlands, and high utilization of sickness benefit absence in Sweden. However, the structure of cost was similar: about 10% direct cost and 90% indirect cost.

Estimates in several reports on back pain indicated that the total cost of back pain corresponded to 1% to 2% of the GNP. Although it was difficult to compare studies from Europe with those from the United States, there seemed to be some similarities in the cost of back pain as a share of the GNP and some similarities also exist regarding the use of health care services between European countries and the United States.

REFERENCES

1. Cats-Baril WL, Frymoyer JW. The economics of spinal disorders. In: *The adult spine: principles and practice.* New York: Raven Press, 1991.
2. Coyle D, Richardson G. The cost of back pain. In: *Clinical Standards Advisory Group report on back pain.* London: Her Majesty's Stationery Office, 1994:65–71.
3. Deyo RA, Cherkin D, Conrad D, et al. Cost, controversy, crisis: low back pain and the health of the public. *Annu Rev Public Health* 1991;12:141–156.
4. Drummond MF. *Principles of economic appraisal in health care.* Oxford: Oxford University Press, 1980.
5. Drummond MF, O'Brien B, Stoddard G, et al. *Methods for the evaluation of health care programmes,* 2nd ed. Oxford: Oxford University Press, 1997.
6. Frymoyer JW, Durett CL. The economics of spinal disorders. In: *The adult spine: principles and practice,* 2nd ed. Philadelphia: Lippincott–Raven, 1997.
7. Goossens MEJB, Evers SMAA. Economic evaluation of back pain interventions. *J Occup Rehabil* 1997;7:15–32.
8. OECD statistics directorate. *Historical statistics 1960–1994,* 1996 ed. Paris: Organization for Economic Cooperation and Development, 1996.
9. Pharmametrics. *Was kostet uns der Ruecken? Analyse der Krankheitskosten bei Rueckenschmertzen* [*cost of illness study*]. Freiburg: Sanofi/Winthrop, 1997.
10. Snook SH, Webster BS. The cost of disability. *Clin Orthop* 1987;221:77–84.
11. Swedish Council on Technology Assessment in Health Care (SBU). *Ont i ryggen* [*report on back pain*]. Stockholm: SBU, 1991.
12. van Tulder MW, Koes BW, Bouter LM. A cost of illness study of back pain in the Netherlands. *Pain* 1995;62:233–240.
13. Webster BS, Snook SH. The cost of compensable low back pain. *J Occup Med* 1990;32:13–15.
14. Williams A. The nature, meaning and measurement of health and illness: an economic viewpoint. *Soc Sci Med* 1985;20:1023–1027.
15. Yelin E, Callahan LF, for the National Arthritis Data Work Group. The economic cost and social and psychological impact of musculoskeletal conditions. *Arthritis Rheum* 1995;38:1351–1362.

Neck and Back Pain: The Scientific Evidence of Causes, Diagnosis, and Treatment, edited by Alf Nachemson and Egon Jonsson. Published by Lippincott Williams & Wilkins, Philadelphia 2000.

21

Review of Social Security Systems

Gordon Waddell* and Anders I. Norlund†

*Department of Orthopaedics, The Glasgow Nuffield Hospital, Glasgow, Scotland
†Swedish Council on Technology Assessment in Health Care, Stockholm, Sweden

AIMS

The aims of this chapter are:

1. To compare social security arrangements in various European Union (EU) countries against a background of demographics, economic situation, health, and health care.
2. To consider how social security arrangements may influence neck and back pain and disability.

When possible, the United States and Japan were included for comparison. Throughout this review, there is no definite evidence of any significant variation in the pathologic features or physical basis of neck and back pain over time or in different European countries (see Chapter 2).

All EU countries have state-sponsored "pay-as-you-go" social security systems (29). Welfare has three broad aims:

1. To provide insurance against the traditional risks such as unemployment, sickness, disability, and old age.
2. To alleviate poverty.
3. This often involves some degree of redistribution of wealth.

Particularly relevant to neck and back pain, social security provides various forms of benefits for those who are unable to work because of injury or illness. In general, sickness benefits aim to provide replacement income for those who are temporarily unable to work because of sickness. This is basically a short-term program, in expectation of recovery and return to work. Long-term or permanent incapacity is covered by invalidity benefits, which may alternatively be regarded as a form of disability pension for those who have not reached pension age. Most countries also make special arrangements for sickness resulting from work-related injury or disease.

Olsson et al. (36) and Folkesson et al. (18) offered a Swedish overview of social security in European countries in the early 1990s. They pointed out that the family is fundamental to all social security. In earlier times and in less developed countries today, support for sickness and disability was entirely from the family and its social networks. Even today and in the most highly developed welfare states, much basic support for sickness and disability still comes from the family. In addition, however, social security is now provided by the public sector, the market, and/or the family. Social security in Scandinavian countries is largely provided by the public sector: health care and social benefits are financed through taxes, to a large extent organized through the public sector, and are distributed on equitable grounds. However, the trend is toward some marketlike solutions. In the Netherlands, market-oriented solutions have been stronger, such as private social security funds and private health care. However, as the main funding agency, the government has taken an increasing regulatory role. In the United Kingdom, public-oriented systems of health care and parts of the social services are publicly financed, but there are also parts of the welfare system that depend on the family and voluntary organizations, and there is some trend toward more marketlike solutions. Finally, in countries such as France, Italy, and Germany, the long tradition of Catholic social teaching has encouraged family-oriented care and social support. However, the trend in these countries is toward increased public regulation, as in Germany, where there has been a reaction against large increases of the cost of health care resulting from the growth of a previously almost unregulated market. Thus, the tendency is for the social security systems in the various European countries to become more similar, a finding that is not surprising in view of common EU membership and the goal of gradual harmonizing of the social security systems. In the United States, in contrast, much social security and most health care is provided in the private sector, and the main role of the public sector is to provide a safety net for those who cannot afford private insurance.

REVIEW METHODS

None of this material is in the standard medical or scientific literature or is included in electronic databases, and standard search techniques identified little information. This material is almost all in the "gray literature" and was identified by citation tracking and correspondence. We particularly acknowledge the assistance of the Swedish National Social Security Board (RFV), Arbeiden Sociale Zekerheid, toegepaste research en informatie (AS/tri), the International Social Security Association (ISSA), and the United Kingdom Department of Social Security (DSS) library and database for assistance in finding and obtaining much of this material. This was supplemented by hand searching of European Community and ISSA publications starting from 1970, the *International Social Security Review* and the *Social Security Bulletin.* Although every effort was made to identify and review all relevant published material, the lack of proper databases or indexing means that it is not possible to fulfill the criteria of a systematic review.

Sources of Data

There is a wealth of material in various reports from European and national government departments, agencies, and research foundations. Official European reports—Mutual Information System on Social Protection in the Member States of the European Union (MISSOC) 1995 (29), 1996 (30), 1997 (31); annual *Eurostat Labour Force Surveys* to 1996 (14), *Eurostat Yearbook 1996* (15), *Eurostat Yearbook 1997* (16), *OECD Historical Statistics* published in 1997 (33)–provided the most comprehensive source of economic, demographic, and basic statistics. Official EU publications–MISSOC 1995 (29), 1996 (30), 1997 (31), annual *Eurostat Labour Force Surveys* to 1997 (14), *Eurostat Yearbook 1996* (15), *Eurostat Yearbook 1997* (16), ISSA reports from 1993 (24), Bloch (6,7), and ISSA reports from 1996 (25)—provided the most comparable and unbiased descriptions and statistics on the health care and social security systems in the widest range of European countries. Reports from Sweden (18,36), the United Kingdom (8,27), the Netherlands (11,42,43,50), and Denmark (40,41) each compared overlapping sets of European countries. These reports were often from a particular national perspective, but they also provided insight and the most accurate data on their own country. Gordon (19) and Simanis (48) looked at the European situation in the early to mid-1980s from the perspective of the United States. Otero-Sierra et al. (38) gave a more limited comparison of France and Spain.

MISSOC (31) provided the most comprehensive description of the social security arrangements in all European countries as of July 1, 1996. The AS/tri report from the Netherlands, which was commissioned by the Swedish Council on Technology Assessment in Health Care (SBU) (43), provided a succinct summary of the current arrangements, together with data on sickness and work incapacity rates and trends from 1980 to 1995. Earlier AS/tri reports (11,42) gave more detailed methodology.

Limitations of Data

These data have some basic problems:

1. Many authors quoted selected statistics that were sometimes out-of-date, or they used two isolated statistics over a short time to demonstrate trends, a practice that may give a false picture. Too often, they assumed links, ignored confounding influences, and assumed cause and effect.
2. There is a great deal of variation in the same statistics from different sources or even from the same EU source at different times, and this variation casts doubt on the accuracy of many of the statistics.
3. There is sometimes national or political bias in selecting, presenting, and interpreting the statistics.

RESULTS

Historical Background

Throughout history and still today, society has provided two distinct but linked forms of social support for the injured, sick, and disabled: compensation and social security (1).

Compensation

Ancient compensation codes such as the Code of Hammurabi (circa 1750 B.C.) and the Law of Moses (circa 800 B.C.) predate written history. The original concept of retribution in "an eye for an eye; a tooth for a tooth; a hand for a hand; a foot for a foot" was later replaced by scales of financial compensation, and this became embodied in common law and still remains the basis of civil litigation.

One of the key elements of the Industrial Revolution was the building of the railroads. The world's first railway line opened in England in 1825, and the carriage bore the legend "a public service free of danger," but rapid and uncontrolled growth of the railways led to casualties on a scale unprecedented except in war. Public anxiety led to legislation, in England as well as in other countries. When the Berlin-Potsdam railway opened in 1838, the railway companies were made legally responsible for any accidents. In England, the Fatal Accidents Act of 1846 first gave the right of compensation to the family of a person killed in an accident. From that time, there was progressive expansion in the scope and cover of the legal framework for the compensation of workers.

The new laws led to a spate of legal and medical activity. Some of the injuries were severe and fully justified compensation, but there was soon a problem of claims made for more minor injuries. Some of these claimants had subjective symptoms without much objective evidence of injury, and "sprains and strains" of the back were soon leading examples. The limitations of medical examination made the problem worse (55). As legislation extended the scope of compensation, so the scale of the problem grew. By 1915, "pain in the back as a result of injury is the most frequent affection for which compensation is demanded from the casualty company." After World War II, in most countries there was a progressive increase in the number of claims for work-related injury, largely because of expansion of the definition of injury. Low back pain was a prime example, supported by medical concepts of ruptured discs.

Social Security

Welfare was originally only concerned with tackling outright destitution. During the Middle Ages, social support for the destitute took the form of charity, initially led by the church and religious bodies. In England, the "Poor Laws" were passed in 1598 and 1601 during the feudal Elizabethan regime and remained in force well into the 18th century. This was the first recognition that the state had a responsibility to prevent destitution, to raise taxes to do so, and to ensure that there was an administrative framework to deliver help. The poor laws initially placed the onus on the landed classes to provide "poor houses" for the crippled, and during the 19th century that responsibility progressively passed to local government, but the poor laws remained in force in Britain until the passage of the Social Security Act in 1911. However, the poor laws provided only basic support, had severe social stigma, and were based on a distinction between the "worthy poor" and those who were undeserving. The deserving received grudging charity; those who were judged to be "unworthy" even if disabled could be warned out of town or subjected to corporal punishment. In North America, the same poor law approach was adopted. Despite the poor laws, however, private charity often played a more important role.

Present forms of social support for sickness and invalidity date from the social, industrial, and medical revolutions of the 19th century. As national wealth and income rose, there was gradual acceptance of society's responsibility to provide care for the sick and disabled, and the goal of welfare changed from dealing with absolute destitution to alleviating poverty. There had been war pensions for disabled soldiers since Greek times. Now, society also began to care for "the wounded soldiers of industry." The limitations of civil litigation led to schemes for compensation without going to the courts.

Bismarck in Germany introduced the first national system of social insurance against the risks of occupational injury, illness and invalidity, and old age, and this system was an integral part of his *Socialpolitik*. This social policy was partly a political response to the emerging working class and the fledgling labor movement. It was also key to the development of a nation state, by addressing the social situation of workers as a collective, to bring the industrial proletariat and employers together in social peace, with the state as a third party. The practical elements were modern actuarial private insurance (setting premiums to cover compensation for specified risks) and the thriving 19th century friendly societies (voluntary associations whose members paid dues in return for benefits to cover sickness, old age, burial, etc.). About the same time, German medicine led the world with a biomedical model of disease. The combination produced what Hadler (20) described as the *Prussian paradigm.*

Biomedical Basis According to Hadler (20)

Clinical and Administrative Decision	Criteria
Determine cause	Injury? Due to employment?
Determine whether permanent state reached	Can anything more be done to treat or rehabilitate?
Determine permanent (partial) disability	Based on objective evidence of pathology (impairment). (This now applies more in the United States than in the European Union.)

The social perspective was also a moral, Prussian approach, based on the Western work ethic. Who is more "worthy" than the man who wants to work to support his family, who is working, and in the course of his work is injured, so he becomes permanently disabled and unable to support his family?

Prussian Paradigm According to Hadler (20)

Level of worthiness	Insurance fund	Indemnification
Work incapacity from work injury	Workmen's Accident Insurance	Wage replacement until fit to return to work, medical care and rehabilitation, permanent partial awards
Work incapacity from illness in a worker	Public Pension Insurance	Wage replacement for a finite period while under medical treatment and unfit for previous work, medical care and rehabilitation, some level of monetary transfer if disability persists
Sickness in a non-worker	Public Aid	Sustenance, medical care

The combination of the Western work ethic and the concept of the worthy poor led to workers compensation. Bismarck introduced the first social legislation in Germany in 1884, with accident insurance and sickness benefits for the employed, followed by the Disability and Old Age Insurance Act in 1891, and a comprehensive National Insurance Act in 1911. The Prussian model spread soon through Europe and served as a model for most of the industrialized countries (e.g., the first Workman's Compensation Act in Britain in 1897). However, the United States was slow to follow the European example in workmen's compensation. The first legislation was in New York State in 1910, but it was not until 1949 that all States had workers' compensation legislation, and the United States still does not have a universal system of health care and sickness benefits. In Australia, workers' compensation legislation was enacted in almost all states by 1910. Japan did not have any such system until it was introduced by the occupying United States after World War II.

From Bismarck's initiative in 1884, no other single event had such a profound international impact on social security as the Beveridge Report on *Social insurance and allied services* in the United Kingdom in 1942 (36). Beveridge attacked the inadequacies of the existing system and aimed to create an all-encompassing social safety net. Beveridge did not wish the United Kingdom to revert to prewar class inequalities, and there were political elements of social obligation, solidarity, and redistribution of wealth. Beveridge was close to the economist Keynes, and social insurance was considered to have a macroeconomic function as an "automatic stabilizer." In 1944, Beveridge published *Full employment in a free society* and obviously believed in an intimate relationship between social insurance and employment and between work and welfare.

After Beveridge, concepts shifted from the German notion of social *insurance* to the broader United States New Deal concept of social *security* as part of the growth of citizenship. Marshall (28) expressed the view that citizens in a modern Western democracy had civil, political, and social rights including statutory social services. The emphasis shifted from the industrial worker to the citizen *per se*. Human and social rights are now enshrined in United Nations declarations and in many national constitutions. Titmuss (53), in an essay entitled *The social division of welfare,* pointed out that statutory provisions for social well-being could include the following:

- Social security.
- Fiscal policies, tax credits, or tax deductions, as well as cash benefits.
- Occupational benefits, from fringe benefits at enterprise level to provisions through nationwide contracts negotiated by employers' organizations and trade unions.
- Various types of voluntary assistance and charitable and mutual aid.

Social security must be considered in such a complete socioeconomic context. In Europe, concepts of the *welfare state* have increasingly embraced notions of universal support and solidarity as a fundamental social right (the institutional model). In contrast, in the United States and Japan, it has been assumed that most people can arrange their own social security through their employment and personal contract, and notions of *welfare* provided by the state have always remained a safety net associated with poverty and destitution and the distinction between the deserving and the undeserving poor (the residual model). The difference between Europe and the United States should not be overstated: there is the same debate about the role and impact of social security in Europe, and the recipients of social security benefits in the United States equally regard it a right upheld by the courts. As the economic situation has changed and as social security costs have risen during the last decade, most social security systems have also considered and experimented with alternative approaches. Nevertheless, there is a difference in philosophy that is reflected in the percentage of the gross domestic product (GDP) spent on social security, social security legislation, entitlement, disability evaluation, and the levels and amounts of sickness and disability benefits. Over the past 50 years, however, there have been profound economic, social, and political changes, to which social security systems must adapt.

Demographics and Employment

The proportion of the population aged 15 to 64 years (i.e., potentially of working age) in Europe rose slightly from 65% to 67% between 1960 and 1995 (33). The existing small differences among the EU countries are tending to become smaller. During the same period, there was an increase in this age group from 60% to 65% in the United States and from 64% to almost 70% in Japan.

The proportion of the population aged 15 to 64 years who are working fell from 67% to about 60% in Europe between 1960 and 1985 and since then has remained fairly constant (33). In contrast, in the United States, it rose steadily from 63% to 73% between 1960 and 1995, whereas in Japan it fell from 74% to about 70% between 1960 and 1985 and since then has risen again to about 74%. However, different EU countries show different patterns. Between 1960 and 1985, the proportion rose by 12% in Norway and about 6% in Sweden and Denmark, and it fell in every other country, by about 3% to 7% in Finland, the Netherlands, Belgium, Germany, and the United Kingdom and by 13% in France. From 1985 to 1995, the proportion fell by 14% in Finland and by nearly 9% in Sweden, it stayed much the same in most countries, and it rose by 13% in the Netherlands. These changes were much greater and faster than any demographic changes in the age structure of the population, and they depended more on other factors that influenced whether or not people worked.

A key concern about the age structure of the population is that both health care and social security spending is particularly focused on older people and rises rapidly after age 60 years. Data from the United Kingdom for 1991 showed that spending increased about fivefold between persons 50 to 55 years old and those 85 to 90 years old (22). The population is aging, but Hills (22) pointed out that fears of a "demographic time-bomb" are often overstated. Population forecasts (Table 21.1) suggest that the proportion of the population older than 65 years is likely to increase by 3% to 7% by 2020, a change that could increase health and pension expenditure by about 15% to 20%. It is often suggested that this increase in the elderly is also likely to be associated with a fall in the ratio of those of working age to those retired from an average of 4.2 to 3.2. However, the increased number of elderly persons is balanced by a falling number of children, and the proportion of those of working and tax-paying age is likely to change little from an average of 66% to 64% by 2020. Because health and pension expenditure on the elderly makes up something less than 10% to 20% of total public expenditure, such changes in themselves would only produce an increase in individual taxation of a few percentage points. Any demographic effect on retirement is likely to have much less effect than actual working and retirement patterns, political

TABLE 21.1. *National population forecasts*

	Percentage age 65+ yr (%)		Ratio age 15–64/ age 65+ yr	
	2000	2020	2000	2020
Sweden	17.3	22.1	3.7	2.8
Norway	15.3	18.6	4.2	3.4
Finland	14.8	21.8	4.5	2.8
Denmark	14.7	17.6	4.5	3.7
Netherlands	13.6	18.8	5.0	3.5
Belgium	16.7	19.8	3.9	3.2
France	15.9	20.6	4.1	3.0
Germany	16.1	21.7	4.2	3.0
United Kingdom	15.6	22.1	4.2	3.4

Data from *EU demographic statistics 1997: population and social conditions,* series 3A. Luxembourg: Office for Official Publications of the European Communities, 1997 (13).

decisions about taxation in general, and policy and administrative changes in the social security system. There have already been major changes in all these demographics and politics over the past 35 years, and any impact of an aging population over at least the next 20 years is likely to be much less. However, there is a particular concern about the increasing number of the extremely old, aged 85 years or more, 50% of whom need institutional care at some point; this possibility could mean large increases in these costs at municipal levels.

If the number of older people is increasing, one obvious way to try to control the cost of state pensions is to raise the state pension age (29). This suggestion raises problems about the social and political contract of those who have been contributing to the scheme for many years in expectation of existing pension rights. Conversely, changing the terms of the scheme only for new entrants would defer any savings for perhaps 40 years. The solution in the United Kingdom has been to raise the retirement age for women from the present age of 60 years to match the age in men of 65 years, but to do this by progressive stages, with no alteration in pension rights for women born before 1950. A more complicated but perhaps more politically acceptable solution would be to introduce greater flexibility into the pension age. The January 1997 reforms of the Swedish pension scheme introduced a flexible pension age. The earliest age for men and women is 61 years, but with no upper limit. Additional years of contribution generate additional pension rights. Italy is also replacing its unusually early pension age (55 years for women and 60 years for men in 1995) with a flexible age for both sexes between 57 and 65 years. Once again, both Sweden and Italy are phasing in these reforms over many years. The basis of all these flexible schemes is to give financial incentives for people to defer retirement and, conversely, to give financial disincentives to early retirement.

However, the official state pension age is different from the actual retirement age. Table 21.2 shows employment rates with age in various European countries as of 1996 (although it is not possible to estimate or compare possible "black-market" employment). Overall, only 30% of men in Europe worked after age 60 years, and less than 40% of women worked beyond the age of 55 years. There was again marked variation among different European countries. Sweden had by far the highest activity rates with increasing age and the latest retirement in practice, with 59% of men and 50% of women aged 60 to 64 years still working. In the United Kingdom and Denmark, more than 40% of men and 20% to 25% of women aged 60 to 64 years were still

TABLE 21.2. *Employment rates by age*

Age group (yr)	Males				Females			
	45–49	50–54	55–59	60–64	45–49	50–54	55–59	60–64
Sweden	86.2	85.8	76.8	58.5	85.6	83.3	73.7	49.5
Finland	74.5	72.7	46.4	22.1	75.5	74.1	47.6	18.0
Denmark	88.8	83.6	74.1	41.3	79.6	68.5	51.8	19.2
Netherlands	88.7	81.2	58.8	19.6	57.5	46.3	28.8	9.1
Belgium	86.5	77.4	47.0	17.2	53.0	37.7	19.2	5.0
France	87.8	83.6	55.7	11.0	70.6	63.3	40.5	11.2
Germany	87.9	83.8	63.8	26.1	68.2	60.2	41.9	10.3
United Kingdom	86.0	80.3	67.9	43.0	76.2	67.6	52.0	24.8
Total European Union 15	87.3	80.8	61.8	30.0	62.1	53.1	36.6	14.1

Data from *Eurostat labour force survey 1996*. Brussels: Eurostat, 1996.

working. In most other European countries, only 10% to 25% of men and about 5% to 15% of women continued working after age 60 years.

Since the early 1980s, increasing numbers of people have retired earlier, before they are entitled to state pension. This has been partly financed by company pension plans, special arrangements associated with industrial reorganization, personal pension plans, and private savings. For those who do not have access to such financial support, the main alternatives have been sickness and invalidity. Raising the state pension age or changing the financial inducements may not have much effect when so many people chose to retire without them. Rather, such a change may simply transfer more of the cost of retirement provision to these other sources (29).

The last two generations have also seen marked gender changes in employment patterns. The main increase in female employment followed World War II. In Europe, the female proportion of the workforce rose from 32% to 42% between 1960 and 1995. During the same period, it rose from 33% to 46% in the United States, but it remained constant at just over 40% in Japan. However, there are marked differences among different European countries, although these differences are becoming much smaller. In 1960, the rate ranged from 21.5% in the Netherlands to 43.7% in Finland, whereas by 1995 it only ranged from 41.4% in the Netherlands to 47.9% in Sweden. Finland has had one of the highest levels of female employment, with a relatively stable rate throughout. Sweden, Norway, and Denmark increased most rapidly between 1960 and 1985. The other European countries increased more gradually. However, 31% of women work part-time compared with only 5% of men, and this number ranges from 16% in Finland to 68% in the Netherlands (16).

The last two decades have also seen marked changes in unemployment levels. Standardized (by age and sex) unemployment rates in Europe remained below 3% from 1960 until the early 1980s, then rapidly increased to about 10% and have remained high throughout the last 10 years (Table 21.3). In contrast, United States unemployment rates have remained fairly constant at 5% to 6%. Japanese rates have remained at less

TABLE 21.3. *Standardized unemployment rates calculated from unemployment benefits paid[a]*

	1985	1990	1995
Sweden	3.0	1.8	9.2
Norway	2.6	5.3	5.0
Finland	6.1	3.2	16.2
Denmark	7.3[b]	7.7	7.2
Netherlands	8.3	6.2	6.9
Belgium	10.4	6.7	9.9
France	10.1	8.9	11.7
Germany	8.0[b]	6.2[b]	8.2
United Kingdom	11.5	7.1	8.8
Total European Union 15	10.5[b]	8.1[b]	10.8
United States	7.2	5.6	5.6
Japan	2.6	2.1	3.2

[a] Standardized unemployment as defined in the ILO as a percentage of civilian labor force, based on data from the Organisation for Economic Cooperation and Development (OECD) publication *Quarterly Labour Force Statistics.*

[b] Only nonstandardized data available for these countries for these years.

Data from *OECD Historical Statistics 1960–95.* Paris: Organisation for Economic Coperation and Development, 1997.

than 3% since 1960, increasing slightly to 4.1% in 1998. However, this rise occurred at different times in different European countries. The rise occurred first in the Netherlands, Belgium, France, and the United Kingdom, and then to a lesser extent in Denmark and Germany, in the early 1980s. It occurred much later, in the early 1990s, and was of lesser degree in Sweden and Norway. In Finland, the rate increased slightly to about 5% in the early 1980s, remained fairly constant until the early 1990s, and then rocketed to about 18% in 1993. However, these are official figures of recipients of unemployment benefit and are not the same as the numbers of persons who are actually available for and seeking work but are unable to obtain employment. An analysis in the United Kingdom suggested that the true unemployment rate may be about double these unemployment benefit figures (3).

Peak unemployment benefit rates are found in the 20- to 24-year-old age group and then progressively fall with increasing age in most European countries (14). There is a lesser peak in unemployment benefit rates between age 55 and 59 years, most marked in Germany and Finland, where it affects men and women, and to a lesser extent in Sweden, France, and the United Kingdom, where it affects men only (Table 21.4). The slightly higher proportion of unemployment benefits in persons older than 60 years in Sweden and the United Kingdom probably simply reflects the higher proportion still working in that age group (Table 21.2). However, in older workers it is particularly important to stress that these data are only for unemployment benefits paid. Most people in their 50s or early 60s who are faced with loss of their job take other options and do not appear in these official unemployment (benefit) figures. Such people may not be technically "unemployed," but they are still of working age, and given the choice many would prefer still to be in remunerative employment, although they are without a job.

Socioeconomic Comparisons

The GDP gives a rough indicator of the total economic performance of each country. However, purchasing power parity, in which GDP is corrected for purchasing power, is a better indicator of living standards and shows little difference among these countries, with Denmark only slightly higher than the average, and the United Kingdom and Sweden slightly lower than the average (Table 21.5).

Although there are some differences in the age structure of the different national

TABLE 21.4. *Unemployment benefit rates by age groups*

Age group (yr)	Male				Female			
	45–49	50–54	55–59	60–64	45–49	50–54	55–59	60–64
Sweden	6.2	6.2	8.7	9.9	5.1	4.5	6.6	8.8
Finland	12.1	11.4	20.1	—	11.8	9.1	15.6	—
Denmark	5.3	4.7	6.1	5.6	5.5	6.4	6.8	—
Netherlands	3.9	4.3	3.6	—	8.4	6.5	5.6	—
Belgium	5.6	5.0	4.9	—	9.0	6.7	—	—
France	7.5	8.0	9.3	2.8	9.1	8.8	9.1	4.1
Germany	6.8	7.5	13.4	8.2	8.8	10.3	16.4	5.4
United Kingdom	5.8	7.2	9.9	9.0	3.9	4.4	4.2	1.2
Total European Union 15	6.4	7.2	9.9	6.6	8.1	8.0	10.3	4.2

Data from *Eurostat labour force survey 1996.* Brussels: Eurostat, 1996.

TABLE 21.5. *Socioeconomic indicators for six European Union countries in 1995*

Country	Belgium	Denmark	Germany	United Kingdom	Netherlands	Sweden
GDP/capita in US dollars[a]	26,556	33,144	29,542	18,799	25,579	26,096
GDP/capita corrected for PPP	20,714	21,212	20,383	18,235	19,710	17,484
Total employment rate of the population (%)	42.3	53.6	48.0	48.6	48.5	48.4
Unemployment rate as % total labor force[b]	14.1	10.1	10.4	8.3	7.2	7.8
Average age of retirement[c]						
Men	57.6	62.7	0.5	62.7	58.8	63.3
Women	54.1	59.4	58.4	59.7	55.3	62.1

GDP, gross domestic product; PPP, purchasing power parities.

[a] Data from *OECD national accounts: OECD main economic indicators.* Paris: Organization for Economic Cooperation and Development, 1998 (35).

[b] Data from *UN monthly bulletin of statistics.* New York: United Nations, November, 1996 (54).

[c] Data from *OECD labour force statistics.* Paris: Organisation for Economic Cooperation and Development, 1997 (34).

populations, the differences in the employment rates among countries are more marked. Denmark, with the highest GDP per capita in purchasing power parity, has the highest employment rate at 53%, whereas the Belgian rate is 11% lower. The other countries all have similar rates. The unemployment rate is highest in Belgium at 14%, despite the low Belgian employment rate, whereas the Netherlands, Sweden, and the United Kingdom have just over half the Belgian unemployment rate. However, that only includes those receiving unemployment benefits and does not include "hidden" unemployment.

The average age of stopping work and retirement for men is about 63 years in Sweden, Denmark, and the United Kingdom, about $2\frac{1}{2}$ years earlier in Germany, and about 5 years earlier in Belgium and the Netherlands. Sweden has not only one of the highest female work participation rates, but also by far the highest average age of retirement for women at age 62 year, a statistic that reflects the lowest GDP per capita corrected for purchasing power parity and hence the need for more Swedes to work. Women in all the other countries retire on average before age 60 years, and in Belgium and the Netherlands, women retire at about age 54 to 55 years. These average ages of retirement reflect not only the economic necessity for work, but also the social security provisions for retirement pensions and increasingly the availability of alternative exits from the labor market. (This key issue is discussed in more detail later.)

Public Expenditure

Public expenditure and health care indicators are shown in Table 21.6. Average European public expenditure rose from 27.5% of GDP in 1960 to 46% in 1985, and since then it has risen more slowly to 49% in 1995. In contrast, expenditure in the United States was comparable at 24.6% in 1960, but it rose only to 34.4% in 1985 and since that time has not changed. Japan was 13.0% in 1960, only rose to 26.6% in 1985, and since then has only risen slightly further to 28.5% in 1995. However, there is marked variation in different European countries, now ranging from about 42% in

TABLE 21.6. *Public expenditure and health care indicators*

1995	Public expenditure in % of GDP	Health expenditure in % of GDP	Physicians per 100,000 population 1993–1996	Male life expectancy at birth
Sweden	64.0	7.7[b]	285	76.1
Norway	45.8	7.2	300	74.9
Finland	56.3	7.9	339	72.8
Denmark	59.7	6.4	291	72.7
Netherlands	52.1	8.8	252	74.5
Belgium	53.3	8.0	378	73.3
France	50.9	9.9	282	73.8
Germany	46.6	7.7	341	73.3
United Kingdom	42.3[a]	8.2	322	74.2
Total European Union 15	49.2		322	
United States	34.3	14.2		72.6
Japan	28.5			76.6

GDP, gross domestic product.
[a] 1994.
[b] From 1992; the Swedish statistics excluded nursing homes, and if that is included, the figure remains about 8.5% of GDP.

the United Kingdom to 64% in Sweden. Total welfare spending includes social security, health, education, pensions, housing, and personal social services, but since the early 1970s, the share of health and social security has gradually increased.

Health Care

In principle, all citizens of these European countries have access to medical care according to need rather than ability to pay, and there are no or minimal financial barriers, of 4 to 22 ECU per day, to treatment (29,30). All these countries provide arrangements for those who are unable to pay, a group that usually includes those who are unemployed or disabled.

Table 21.6 shows total health expenditure as a proportion of the GDP. Health expenditure in Europe is only about 50% to 60% that in the United States, but it is slightly higher than Japan. At various times over the last decade, Germany, Sweden, and France have had the highest health expenditure as a proportion of GDP, but in terms of purchasing power, Germany has consistently been the highest. There is probably relatively little real difference among most of the other EU countries.

There is some variation in the ratio of physicians to population in different European countries (Table 21.6). However, the number of patient visits per physician is much higher in the United Kingdom than in Sweden. The Netherlands and Finland have much higher numbers of hospital beds, and Germany also has more, whereas the other countries are more or less equal.

There is no evidence that any of these health care arrangements, expenditures, or resources bear any significant relationship with or have much impact on the health of the various nations, at least as measured by general indices of health, as for example male life expectancy at birth (Table 21.6). This applies equally to other health indices such as perinatal and infant mortality, life expectancy at age 65 years, or mortality from ischemic heart disease or cancer. Female statistics show an entirely comparable pattern. So does allowance for health expenditure in purchasing power parity (PPP) (15).

TABLE 21.7. *Relationship between health care expenditure and social security expenditure percentage of gross domestic product based on 1995 data*

	Health expenditure (in rank order)	Social security expenditure
Germany	10.4	18.6
France	9.9	23.2
Netherlands	8.8	25.1
Sweden	8.5	23.4
Norway	8.0	15.8
Denmark	8.0	21.5
Belgium	7.9	24.3
Finland	7.6	23.7
United Kingdom	6.9	15.6
United States	14.1	13.1
Japan	7.2	13.4

Data from *Eurostat yearbook 1997: a statistical eye on Europe 1986–1996.* Brussels: Eurostat, 1997; and *OECD Historical statistics 1960–95.* Paris: Organisation for Economic Co-operation and Development, 1997.

More directly relevant to the current review, Table 21.7 shows that increased expenditure on health care does not reduce social security expenditure. On the contrary, the two are positively related with a correlation coefficient of 0.31 that suggests that they have about 10% of variance in common. This is not surprising. Health care expenditure as a proportion of the GDP is highly and positively correlated with the level of GDP per capita. Thus, the level of health care consumption and of costs is largely a question of the economic welfare situation, rather than of the health of the nation. In general, social security expenditure seems to reflect the same issues.

No comparable data are available at present on health care for back pain in different EU countries, although this information should become available within the next 1 to 2 years when the current ISSA study in Sweden, Denmark, the Netherlands, Belgium, France, Germany, the United States, and Israel is completed.

Social Security Arrangements

European expenditure on social security about doubled between 1960 and 1985 (33), from 9.7% to 17.7% of the GDP, and since that time, it has risen slightly to about 20%. Levels in the United States have shown the same trend but at about half the average European level, doubling between 1960 and 1985 from 5.1% to 10.8 and gradually rising to 13.1% by 1995. The lower level for the United States reflects the greater reliance on individual provision for security. Japanese levels are similar to those in the United States throughout. However, there is marked variation among different European countries. In 1960, social security spending ranged from 5.1% in Finland to 13.5% in France, whereas in 1995, it ranged from about 15% to 16% in the United Kingdom and Norway, 18.6% in Germany, and 23% to 25% in all the other European countries. There is also a difference in trends among different European countries, although to some extent this simply reflects *when* the increase occurred.

TABLE 21.8. *Sickness benefit arrangements in different European countries on 1 July 1996*

Part A	Eligible persons	Qualifying conditions	Sickness certification	Waiting period
Sweden	Employees and self-employed persons >16 yr. Unemployed also eligible	No work period, but minimum income level (ECU 614/yr)	Self-certificate first 7 d, then (family) doctor certificate	1 d
Norway	Employees and self-employed persons >16 yr. Unemployed also eligible	14 d employment or self-employment	?	None
Finland	All residents age 15–64 yr. Unemployed also eligible	Residence in country	Doctor's certificate from day 1	9 d
Denmark	Employees and self-employed persons. Unemployed also eligible	Worked 120 hr in 13 wk	No medical certification	None
Netherlands	All persons age <65 yr in paid employment. Unemployed not eligible?	Membership in approved sickness fund	No medical certification	None (≤2 d)
Belgium	All workers with contract. Voluntary affiliation for unemployed	6 mo employment and contributions	Doctor's certificate from day 1	1 d (none if unemployed)
France	All employees. Voluntary affiliation for unemployed	Sufficient contributions (≈6 mo work)		3 d
Germany	All persons in paid employment. Unemployed also eligible	Membership in sickness fund	Doctor's certificate from third day	None[a]
United Kingdom	Employees: statutory sick pay. Various other groups: incapacity benefit. Others: lower disability	Sufficient contributions (≈2 yr)	Self-certificate first 7 d, then family doctor certificate	3 d

Part B	Amount of benefits (July 1, 1996)[a]	Duration	Benefits taxed
Sweden	75% of earnings. Ceiling ECU 24,360/yr	No formal limit (but converted to disability pension)	Fully liable
Norway	100% of covered earnings. Self-employed and temporarily employed, 65% of assessed earnings after 14 d waiting period. Maximum 6× base amount of 38,000 NEK	52 wk, then disability pension or rehabilitation allowance	Fully liable
Finland	No earnings: ECU 11/d. Complex formula on earnings: ≈80% of earnings	50 wk in 2 yr	Fully liable
Denmark	100% (?) of earnings maximum ECU 352/wk. Unemployed = previous benefits	52 wk in 18 mo	Fully liable
Netherlands	70% of daily wage maximum ECU 97/d	1 yr	Generally fully liable to tax
Belgium	60% of earnings maximum ECU 55/d	1 yr	Fully liable
France	50% of earnings maximum ECU 35/d	1 yr but 3 yr for protracted sickness	80–90% of benefits taxable
Germany	80% of normal earnings, but not exceeding net earnings	76 wk over 3 yr; after 1 yr adjusted as pension	Tax free
United Kingdom	Statutory sick pay: basic ECU 63/wk. Incapacity benefit: basic ECU 52/wk; higher if adult or child dependents	Statutory sick pay 4 d–28 wk. Short-term incapacity benefit: 28 wk	Fully liable

[a] No waiting period in Germany if due to work injury or disease or if hospital treatment required.

Data from MISSOC. *Social protection in the member states of the union: situation on July 1st 1994 and evolution.* Brussels: European Commission Directorate—General Employment, Industrial Relations and Social Affairs, 1995; and MISSOC. *Social protection in the member states of the union: situation on July 1st 1995 and evolution.* Brussels: European Commission Directorate—General Employment, Industrial Relations and Social Affairs, 1996.

Sickness Benefits

Differences in the social security systems of these European countries concern not only obvious linguistic and cultural differences, but also differences in attitudes and behavior and in constitutional and administrative thinking and practice, as reflected in sickness benefits (Table 21.8). In some countries, the focus is on general security (e.g., Sweden, Denmark, the United Kingdom), whereas in others it is on income security (e.g., Germany, the Netherlands) (36). All citizens are eligible for sickness benefits in some countries (e.g., Sweden, Finland, Denmark), whereas in others only those who work are eligible (e.g., France, Germany), or there may be different benefits for employees and others (the United Kingdom). There are also marked differences in the ease of obtaining benefits. There are no qualifications required for eligibility in Finland and the Netherlands, whereas most other countries require a minimum period of work and/or contributions. There is extreme variation in the requirements for medical certification of sickness. In Belgium, strict rules for medical certification are applied from the first day, whereas in Denmark certification is not compulsory, and in the Netherlands it is completely absent. Sweden and the United Kingdom take an intermediate position, with self-certification for up to 7 days and medical certification only necessary thereafter. There are no waiting days to commence benefits in Denmark, the Netherlands, and Germany; most countries have 1 to 3 days, and Finland has 9 days. However, these days are sometimes then paid retrospectively, and in the Netherlands, employers do have the option of applying up to a 2-day waiting period. Finally, the financial consequences of work incapacity from sickness also differ, although these are complex and are considered in more detail later (Table 21.8 part B). These various differences reflect not only different cultural traditions, but also different welfare goals.

Invalidity Benefits

Table 21.9 shows the arrangements for longer-term invalidity benefits in various European countries. Invalidity benefit arrangements show great variations among the countries. For instance, the initiative to apply for an invalidity pension may come from the employer, from the employee, or from the social security agency. There are also differences regarding the minimum degree of loss of earning capacity required; the Swedish and the Dutch systems accept low rates of partial disability (25% and 15%) compared with the average 50% to 67% required loss of working capacity. The type of pension also differs: It is a flat rate in the United Kingdom; earnings related in Germany, Belgium, and the Netherlands; and mixed in Sweden and Denmark. As a whole, the arrangements in Germany, Belgium, and the Netherlands are the most favorable.

In Finland, Belgium, the Netherlands, and the United Kingdom, sickness benefits and invalidity benefits are linked, and after exhaustion of sickness benefits, the claimant more or less automatically receives invalidity benefit. In the other countries, invalidity pensions are separate, at least in principle. In Sweden, sickness benefits may continue indefinitely, and in France they may continue for several years. However, claimants in Sweden, Denmark, France, and Germany may change to an invalidity pension at any time, as soon as their incapacity is considered to be permanent. This means that invalidity benefits may be viewed as either protracted sick pay or as early retirement. In theory, this approach may have considerable consequences on the emphasis on work resumption or rehabilitation, although in practice under any system, once someone is receiving invalidity benefits, the chances of return to work are low.

TABLE 21.9. *Invalidity benefit arrangements in different European countries on 1 July 1996*

	Minimum level of incapacity	Start	Initiate claim	Degrees of invalidity	Duration	Benefits level percentage of earnings
Sweden	25%	When fulfill conditions	Claimant	4	To age 65 yr	65%
Norway	15%	When fulfill conditions	Claimant	2	To age 65 yr	Up to 100% of base amount 38,000 NEK
Finland	Disability pension 60% Partial disability pension 40% Early retirement age 58+ yr No level specified[a]	After 1 yr sickness benefits		3	To age 65 yr	Flat rate
Denmark	50%	When accept permanent incapacity	Claimant	3	To age 67 yr	Flat rate
Netherlands	25%	After 52 wk incapacity	Claimant	7	To age 65 yr	9–73%
Belgium	66.7%	End of primary period of incapacity	Employer	2	To retirement age	40–65%
France	66.7%	When fulfill conditions		3	To age 60 yr	30–70%
Germany	Occupational 50% General 100%	When fulfill conditions	Employer	1	To age 65 yr	Up to 100%
United Kingdom	"Incapable of all work"	After 28 wk incapacity	Dept. of social security	1	Male age 65 yr, female 60 yr	Flat rate[b]

[a] Early retirement age 58+ yr in Finland if: "incapable of continuing their present job because of work-related stress or fatigue or other factors."

[b] Actual total benefits and income received is much higher (Department of Social Security, personal communication).

Data from MISSOC. *Social protection in the member states of the union: situation on July 1st 1994 and evolution.* Brussels: European Commission Directories—General Employment, Industrial Relations and Social Affairs, 1995; MISSOC. *Social protection in the member states of the union: situation on July 1st 1995 and evolution.* Brussels: European Commission Directorate—General Employment, Industrial Relations and Social Affairs, 1996; and Prins R, Veerman TJ, Koster MK. *Work incapacity in six countries: facts and figures 1980–1995.* Leiden: AS/tri, 1998.

Employment Injury Benefits

Almost all European countries, with the exception of the Netherlands, still make special arrangements for state benefits for work-related injuries and occupational diseases. These are generally more generous than the corresponding sickness and invalidity benefits, with no qualifying conditions apart from being employed, no waiting periods, higher benefit levels, no time limit, and various supplementary benefits and allowances. Table 21.10 summarizes these arrangements.

Actual Benefits Received

Tables of sickness, invalidity, and employment injury benefits generally only show the basic levels of benefits and are oversimplified, so they often give a false impression of what people who are incapacitated with back pain actually receive. In all countries, the social security arrangements are extremely complex because they have developed over time to meet many differing needs and political compromises. Many of the apparently generous wage replacement rates have a ceiling that may mean that higher-

TABLE 21.10. *Benefits for work-related injuries and occupational diseases in different European countries on 1 July 1996*

	Temporary incapacity		Permanent incapacity	
	Full wages continued	Benefit level (% of gross earnings)	Minimum loss of earning capacity	Pension (% of gross earnings)
Sweden	No	≤100%	1/15	≤100%
Norway	100% of covered earnings	Sickness benefits up to 52 wk	15%	100% of base amount 38,000 NEK
Finland	No	Sickness benefits for 4 wk, then 100%	Working capacity 10% + loss of earnings 5%	≤85% 70% after age 50 yr
Denmark	No	≤100%	15%	≤80%
Netherlands	No special arrangements: standard sickness and invalidity benefits			
Belgium	30 d	Up to 90%	No minimum	1–100%
France	No	60% for 28 d, then 80%	No minimum	≤100%
Germany	6 wk	80%	20%	≤67%
United Kingdom	No	Flat rate[a]	No minimum	Flat rate[a]

[a] In the United Kingdom, employment injury benefit is paid *in addition to* rather than as an alternative to sickness and invalidity benefits.

Data from, MISSOC. *Social protection in the member states of the union: situation on July 1st 1995 and evolution.* Brussels: European Commission Directorate—General Employment, Industrial Relations and Social Affairs, 1996; and Prins R, Veerman TJ, Koster MK. *Work incapacity in six countries: facts and figures 1980– 1995.* Leiden: AS/tri, 1998.

paid workers do not receive anything like that level of income replacement. There is anecdotal evidence that in at least some countries such as France (Nachemson, personal communication), under certain assessment systems, back pain may in practice be rated as (much) less than 100% incapacity. Claimants may be eligible for more than one type of benefit, with differing criteria for entitlement. Certain benefits lead to additional entitlement to various supplemental housing, child, and other benefits, and other benefits in kind and municipal spending. Different taxation provisions also have a major impact. Purchasing power and what must be bought out of disposable income vary widely. These factors make it unreliable to compare raw wage replacement rates. Whiteford (56) provided a critical review of the limitations of wage replacement rates and the need to allow for much more than the basic social security benefit rates.

In addition, these are only the basic state benefit arrangements. Many groups of workers and unions have negotiated more generous terms, both for short-term sickness and for disability pension arrangements. In most European countries, most salaried public sector employees such as health care workers, civil servants, educators, and police workers receive relatively generous sickness benefits, usually with no waiting period and with full salary for up to 6 months or more. Permanent invalidity is considered compulsory early retirement, and the benefits form part of the employment pension scheme. In Sweden, Denmark, and the Netherlands, employees in the public sector have much the same arrangements as in the private sector. However, in Germany and the United Kingdom, about 50% of public employees do not have any special coverage and simply fall under the basic state benefit system.

Taking all these factors into account, Olsson et al. (36) suggested that for many employees, being sick for 1 week has little effect on disposable income, and there is actually relatively little difference among EU countries. In particular, these investigators pointed out that the common assumption that sickness benefits in Sweden are the most generous is no longer true, if it ever was. Moreover, for employment injury, they found that Sweden was about average, whereas the German and Danish systems overcompensated for lost working capacity, and the Netherlands and the United Kingdom considerably undercompensated. In comparison, one review of the income of disabled people in the United Kingdom found that the actual benefits received were about double the basic, flat-rate benefit and allowing for other income, many disabled workers may have a net income of 50% to 75% of average national earnings (DSS, personal communication).

Sickness Certification, Adjudication, and Appeals Procedures

The relations among sickness, incapacity for work, sickness certification, and social benefits are complex. The Clinical Standards Advisory Group (10) considered three possible situations. First, back pain may be the direct cause of time lost from work, job loss, and unemployment, leading to sickness certification and sickness benefits. Second, the physical, psychologic and social ill effects of unemployment may interact with and may aggravate back pain and disability. Third, people with back pain who lose their job (for whatever reason) may be more likely to receive sickness certification and benefits. These correspond broadly to three routes of entry to invalidity benefits identified in a DSS study in the United Kingdom (46):

Condition-led entry: The nature and severity of the illness and disability lead to long-term or permanent incapacity. Discontinuing benefits depends on the nature of the incapacity and treatment received and the availability of employment.

Employment-led entry: Restricted employment opportunities combined with illness or disability (and often also age) cause loss of employment or inability to gain work and hence the start of benefits. The main barriers to discontinuing benefits are employment opportunities, availability of rehabilitation or retraining, and age.

Self-directed entry: Some interaction among the person's condition, employment opportunities, and motivation to continue or to gain employment results in the perception of sickness benefits as a possible option. This could be either with the support of the family doctor or negotiated with the family doctor. The main barriers to discontinuing benefits are age, low motivation, and restricted employment opportunities, often related to the person's condition. Discontinuing benefits largely depends on external triggers. This usually takes the form of an independent medical review by the DSS or the family doctor's decision to stop sickness certification.

A parallel DSS study in the United Kingdom (46) found that many complex factors influenced a family doctor's judgments of the patient's capacity for work when the physician was issuing a sickness certificate. The patient's medical condition and its impact on employment potential were always high on the list. However, it was almost immediately linked to a whole range of nonmedical factors. These included the patient's prospects of finding work, age, motivation to find work, financial and psychologic consequences of returning to unemployment or job search, and potential for rehabilitation or training.

Capacity and incapacity for work depend on complex interactions among the worker's medical condition and physical capabilities, ergonomic demands of the job, and psychosocial factors (17). The factors that influence stopping work may be different from those that influence staying off and going back to work. The social process of becoming disabled and starting sickness benefits may occur insidiously and unconsciously, rather than as a conscious decision. Once a person is assigned invalidity status, however, that may be almost irreversible in the current economic climate. This is especially so if the person is approaching retirement age anyway.

Emmanuel (12) considered methods of controlling admissions and continued receipt of benefits in social security benefit programs. One obvious solution is to lower the level of benefits, to reduce expenditure directly and also indirectly by lowering demand, and the duration of benefits. However, that approach also affects those who are truly disabled and unable to work and thus limits its political acceptability. Another solution is to offer incentives to employers to keep or take on disabled workers or disincentives to dismissing them. However, there are often loopholes to such systems, and there is little proof of their effectiveness. Emmanuel (12) focused more on ways to improve direct controls:

- The definition and operationalization of criteria for admission to and continued receipt of benefits.
- Efforts to return people to the workforce.
- Separating the administrators of the benefits system from conflicting interests.
- Improving administrative efficiency.
- Focusing on criteria for receiving benefits. This is the most fundamental and critical issue in directing benefits to those who need them and in justifying social support from the taxpayer. Unfortunately, concepts and definitions of incapacity to work because of sickness and disability are difficult to define and are certainly not well designed in social security legislation.

Bloch (6,7) compared the disability pension claim processing and appeals procedures in Sweden, the United Kingdom, the Netherlands, Germany, the United States, and Canada, in 1992 and 1993. He considered that all countries use similar procedures to make initial disability assessments, although they differ in how they structure the process. Thereafter, there is variation in whether assessments are carried out by agency or by outside physicians. All countries have at least one level of appeal on factual and legal issues, although the procedure varies and there is continuing debate on the value of an internal administrative review of eligibility decisions. However, there are no hard data on how these various systems influence the number of claims, the process of claims, the numbers accepted, the number of appeals, or the final outcomes.

Rehabilitation

Nocon and Baldwin (32) gave a brief review of the rehabilitation literature. The origins of rehabilitation lie in a number of separate developments since the First World War and whose roots are evident in the continuing debate about the aims and nature of rehabilitation. Modern rehabilitation represents not only a medical perspective but also social, psychologic, and work-related aspects. There is an emerging consensus on the following:

- The primary objective of rehabilitation involves restoration (to the maximum degree possible) either of function (physical or mental) or role (within the family, social network, or workforce).
- Rehabilitation usually requires a mixture of clinical, therapeutic, and social interventions that also address issues relevant to a person's physical and social environment.
- Effective rehabilitation needs to be responsive to users' needs and wishes, purposeful, involve a number of agencies and disciplines, and be available when required.

However, rehabilitation is often a function of services, not necessarily a service in its own right. MISSOC (30) compared the statutory provisions for rehabilitation in various EU countries (Table 21.11). Statutory provisions do not necessarily reflect what happens in practice, however. Berkowitz et al. (4,5) made a detailed study of rehabilitation arrangements in Sweden, Belgium, the Netherlands, France, Germany, and Israel in the late 1980s for the United States Social Security Administration. The focus was not on the disability benefits system itself, but rather on the relationship between it and the rehabilitation program. In some countries, of which Belgium is the premier example but similar to United States, the benefits system and rehabilitation program are administered quite separately. In contrast, in countries such as the Netherlands and Israel, rehabilitation specialists are part of the disability assessment team. There, claimants for disability benefit do not apply for rehabilitation, but the benefit system automatically assesses their rehabilitation potential and needs, and refusal to accept rehabilitation may lead to reduction in benefits. The ISSA's *Report XII* (23) also compared the quality, effectiveness, and efficiency of rehabilitation measures in Germany, the United States, Australia, and Israel.

Berkowitz considered that Sweden provided lessons on the need for efficient rehabilitation. Rehabilitation resources are finite and must be used rationally to provide the maximum benefit and cost-benefit ratio. This requires early identification of those in need of rehabilitation and accurate assessment of rehabilitation potential, for which Sweden had the major advantage of one of the first completely integrated benefits systems with readily accessible information. Sweden has made a particular effort to

TABLE 21.11. *Statutory arrangements for rehabilitation in various European Union countries as at 1 July 1996*

Sweden	Rehabilitation programs for age 16–64 yr provided by local sickness benefit insurance office; rehabilitation benefits as sickness benefits; appliances and aids provided for age <65 yr by local health authorities and for >65 yr by local municipal authorities
Finland	Pension institutions provide rehabilitation services, which has to make sure the applicant's prospects of rehabilitation have been investigated before making a disability pension determination; a rehabilitation allowance is payable for the period of rehabilitation
Denmark	Measures to lessen effect of invalidity: Assistance for special medical care Maintenance allowance for vocational rehabilitation Appliances and aids supplied by local authority
Netherlands	Law of 11 December 1975: Possibility for the person concerned of measures to maintain, restore, or improve capacity for work, such as rehabilitation, training, or retraining; measures may also be taken to improve living conditions
Belgium	Functional and occupational retraining, in accordance with decision of panel of doctors, in specialized establishments
France	Vocational retraining in specialized vocational retraining centers or establishments, subject to psychotechnical examination, with the social security funds contributing to the costs; pensions or part of pensions continued
Germany	Medical benefits and occupational training as well as other measures including transitional benefits
United Kingdom	Medical therapy and rehabilitation supplied by the National Health Service; vocational assessment and rehabilitation and supported employment provided through the social security services; allowances payable during rehabilitation and retraining

Data from MISSOC. *Social protection in the member states of the union: situation on July 1st 1995 and evolution.* Brussels: European Commission Directorate—General Employment, Industrial Relations and Social Affairs, 1996.

TABLE 21.12. *Swedish rehabilitation projects in the 1990s*

Project name	Aim of rehabilitation	Report(s)	Problems of evaluation
Arbetslivsfonden	Better rehabilitation for return to work	Yes group	No adequate control workplaces Before-and-after measurements of official statistics of sickness days not reliable when unemployment has increased from <2% to >10% plus big changes in sickness benefits and the control system
Dagmar	Special funding to the health care sector in speed rehabilitation by cutting waiting time for treatment (mainly for persons 16–64 yr)	Yes	No control groups (most reports) or inadequate control groups; no conclusions can be drawn
FINSAM	Better and faster rehabilitation from coordination even financially between the health care and the local sickness benefit offices	Yes	Control groups questionable in many cases, e.g., the city of Stockholm compared with rural villages dominated by farmers in southern Sweden in one of the projects
SOCSAM (total financial coordination)	Better and faster rehabilitation from coordination even financially among health care, municipality, and sickness benefit offices	Not published yet	

coordinate the medical, social, psychologic, and work-related aspects to provide more holistic rehabilitation. In the 1990s, there was further drive for financial coordination among the different rehabilitation elements in the public sector.

Many of these Swedish rehabilitation projects are completed and have been evaluated, although often in an unstructured manner (Table 21.12). Unfortunately, so far, almost all the reports of the results have the common weakness of lack of adequate control groups. As an example, Arbetslivsfonden spent more than 3,000 Million SEK on rehabilitation projects for 25,000 enterprises and public organizations. Of more than 3,000 different projects, only two attempted to compare the results with a control group. One of these used as its control group an outdated version of the traditional rehabilitation support given by each local office of the National Social Security Board. The only project with an adequate control group has not yet published its result. The summary report on these 3,000 projects—which was critical and questioned the actual effects of rehabilitation—was completed but was not published by the organization that sponsored the report.

The different rehabilitation projects in Sweden in the 1990s had lofty and laudable ambitions, but although some reports claimed major benefits for individuals and for society, these claims were not properly tested scientifically and were not substantiated by proper controlled studies (26,51).

Social Security Changes in European Countries from 1980 to 1995

During the 1980s and early 1990s, the general public and political perception in Europe was that welfare costs were rising, or could rise in future, and there was a danger that they could get out of control. As long as economic times were good, society could afford welfare, but whenever the national economy stagnated, with fears of falling revenue and increased social costs of unemployment, the perception grew more acute. By the early 1990s, there was a growing debate throughout Europe about a welfare crisis and an apocalyptic fear that welfare would not survive, at least in its present form (29,36,40,41,47). Average public expenditure in Europe did rise by about 10% of the GDP between the mid-1970s and the mid-1980s, although it then remained more or less constant until 1991, when it rose another 2% to 3% between 1991 and 1993 (33). However, average social security expenditure only rose by about 4% to 5% of the GDP between the early 1970s and the mid-1980s, it remained static up to 1991, and then it increased another 3% by 1995 (33). In considering these trends, however, allowance must be made for falling GDP as a result of economic recession in Sweden in the early 1990s. Figures 21.5 and 21.6 show that sickness benefit costs, at least to the state, were actually falling, and in most countries invalidity benefits remained about the same. The two exceptions were the United Kingdom, which had a progressive rise in invalidity costs from the early 1980s, and Sweden, which had rising costs of both sickness and invalidity benefits from about 1987. So to some extent this welfare crisis was more a perception than a reality, although it may be argued that the social pressures and potential for much greater increases were always present and were only forestalled by legislative or administrative checks.

MISSOC (29) summarized several approaches to meeting these problems:

- Cutting benefit costs, either through direct cuts or by restricting access to benefits, or to a lesser extent by making the schemes more efficient.
- Privatization, or partnership with the private sector, to shift some of the costs from government to the employer or to private insurance schemes.
- Targeting social security benefits to the most needy or deserving and thereby it might be possible to improve benefits to those selected groups, which the private sector often has difficulty covering.
- Restructuring the contributions to widen the financial basis of statutory schemes and restructuring both contributions and benefits to remove some of their more negative effects.

By 1994–95, MISSOC (29) reported that the situation was beginning to improve, with rising output and falling unemployment in most European countries. More people were contributing to the mandatory social security schemes, and although the funding of many schemes was still not in balance, they considered the worst was over. "State sponsored pay-as-you-go social security has survived its most severe test since the 1930s" (29).

By 1996, recovery was slow and uneven, unemployment remained high, and the rising cost of social security remained a concern for Europe (30). Nevertheless, there was now little argument that social security was a fundamental and essential part of a modern society and that it would survive in some form or other for the foreseeable future. The debate now focuses more on the goals and effects of social security (9). Some argue that social protection is a disincentive that holds back society economically. Others argue that social protection is important for social cohesion, political stability, and an efficient labor market. A high level of social protection is only possible in a relatively wealthy society, but strong social protection may be a necessary investment that aids labor flexibility and upgrading, to launch and sustain economic growth. The debate now is about exactly what social security can and should aim to achieve and how to structure the social security system to achieve these goals.

MISSOC (30) also looked more specifically at trends and policy changes in invalidity pensions. They suggested a general tendency for the number of invalidity pensions to increase, and in a worsening economic and employment situation, employers become more selective. Unemployed people with any form of sickness or disability appear to give up hope of reemployment and prefer to claim invalidity benefits, which are generally financially better and are also less restrictive than unemployment benefits. This approach is closely linked with the tendency to earlier retirement. MISSOC (30) considered that this trend had been encouraged by social security authorities, either tacitly or overtly, to improve job vacancies for young people. By 1996, there were deliberate attempts to reverse that policy throughout Europe.

All member states are trying to disentangle the medical and employment criteria that have become intertwined in the assessment of disability. The aim is to return to the original concept in which incapacity for work is measured purely on medical grounds without reference to actual employment possibilities. Invalidity pensions should also no longer be seen as a permanent exit from the labor force. Instead, the new emphasis is on review of invalidity status, rehabilitation, and return to work.

Sickness and Invalidity Benefit Statistics and Trends

Eurostat Yearbook 1996 (15) gave data on the relative changes in basic state benefit levels from 1985 to 1994 (Table 21.13). Sickness benefits levels rose in real terms in most countries by about 20% to 30%, although they only rose about 10% in Denmark compared with more than 40% in Belgium. Invalidity benefits rose about 15% to 20% in most countries, but they hardly rose at all in Belgium compared with more than 40% in Denmark and more than 75% in the United Kingdom, although the entire situation in the United Kingdom has changed since 1993 with the introduction of the completely new incapacity benefit to replace the invalidity benefit. These changes appear to reflect a harmonization of social security systems across Europe. Changes in the level of employment injury benefits are much more dramatic. Most countries made little change in real terms, but at one extreme Germany increased the level by 36%, whereas at the other extreme, the United Kingdom was stated to reduce the level by 44%. However, in the United Kingdom, employment injury benefit is only a supplement to the basic sickness benefit, and this change does not reflect total benefit

TABLE 21.13. *Relative level of sickness and invalidity benefits in 1994 at 1985 prices, taking 1985 as 100*

	Sickness benefits (%)	Invalidity benefits (%)	Work-related accident (%)
Denmark	109	145	114
Netherlands	120	114	120
Belgium	143	103	94
France	128	121	92
Germany	118	—	136
United Kingdom[a]	133	176	56

[a] Data only available for 1993.

Data from *Eurostat yearbook 1996: a statistical eye on Europe 1985–1995.* Brussels: Eurostat, 1996.

levels. Unfortunately, this analysis did not include Sweden or other Scandinavian countries. The sequential changes in sickness and invalidity benefit levels in Sweden are described in *Eurostat Yearbook 1996,* but without detailed sources and methodology, it is not possible to produce comparable data to include in Table 21.13.

AS/tri (43) provided the most up-to-date comparative statistics on losses of work capacity resulting from short-term sickness and employment injury in six European countries (Table 21.14). Most of the data are for 1995, although data for the United Kingdom for that year were distorted by major changes in the benefits scheme, so 1996 data were used instead (11). In most countries, women show slightly higher sickness benefit rates, although in Germany women have marginally lower rates. In most countries, sickness benefit rates rise with increasing age, most markedly in Denmark and Germany and least in Belgium. This increase begins from about age 45 to 55 years in men and 40 to 50 years in women. The apparent fall in the sickness benefit rate in some countries after age 55 to 60 years probably reflects varying rates of changing from sickness benefits to invalidity pensions.

AS/tri (11,43) also provided the best comparative statistics on total incapacity benefits in six European countries in 1990 and 1995 (Table 21.15). This is the sum of sickness, invalidity, and employment injury benefits with a number of corrections and standardization to each country's data in an attempt to make the figures more comparable. Einerhard et al. (11) give detailed methodology. Most of the countries

TABLE 21.14. *Loss of work capacity from short-term sickness and employment injury, by age and gender in 1995 (%)*

				Male		
Age (yr)	Belgium	Denmark	Germany	United Kingdom	Netherlands	Sweden
16–19	2.8	1.0	3.1	3.6	2.9	1.3
20–24	2.7	2.8	3.7	2.6	4.2	2.0
25–29	2.6	4.6	3.4	3.3	3.9	2.5
30–34	3.1	4.5	3.9	2.6	4.1	3.0
35–39	3.0	5.0	4.4	3.1	5.0	3.5
40–44	3.5	6.1	4.8	2.8	4.7	3.7
45–49	3.6	7.0	5.7	3.1	5.8	4.1
50–54	4.0	8.2	7.2	4.2	5.2	5.1
55–59	3.0	9.6	8.1	5.1	8.2	6.7
60–64	1.3	7.2	11.1	5.1	5.2	8.0
				Female		
Age (yr)	Belgium	Denmark	Germany	United Kingdom	Netherlands	Sweden
16–19	2.5	0.7	3.1	1.0	4.2	1.5
20–24	3.2	3.3	3.6	3.8	6.3	2.9
25–29	3.1	5.0	3.3	2.6	6.7	3.8
30–34	3.4	6.8	3.6	3.8	6.5	4.6
35–39	5.5	8.8	4.1	4.3	6.9	4.9
40–44	6.3	10.5	4.8	5.1	6.1	5.2
45–49	5.3	12.3	5.6	4.4	7.2	5.7
50–54	5.1	13.6	7.0	5.9	6.7	6.6
55–59	2.8	15.6	7.5	6.8	11.2	(7.9)
60–64	2.5	—	9.5	—	—	9.5

Data from Prins R, Veerman TJ, Koster MK. *Work incapacity in six countries: facts and figures 1980–1995.* Leiden: AS/tri, 1998, with permission (43).

TABLE 21.15. *Total incapacity benefits by gender, standardized to the Netherlands for age (%)*

	1990					
	Male			Female		
Incapacity benefits	Temporary	Long-term permanent	Total	Temporary	Long-term permanent	Total
Belgium	3.1	4.0	7.0	4.8	4.3	9.0
Denmark	3.7	3.7	7.4	5.4	3.5	8.9
Germany	5.2	3.3	8.5	4.5	2.4	6.9
United Kingdom	2.3	3.3	5.6	2.8	3.0	5.9
Netherlands	6.4	8.8	15.2	7.9	7.5	15.5
Sweden	5.3	3.4	8.7	7.0	3.1	10.1
	1995					
	Male			Female		
Incapacity benefits	Temporary	Long-term permanent	Total	Temporary	Long-term permanent	Total
Belgium	3.0	4.1	7.1	3.9	4.4	8.3
Denmark	5.0	4.1	9.1	7.5	3.8	11.2
Germany	4.6	3.1	7.6	4.2	2.4	6.6
United Kingdom	3.1	4.8	7.9	4.0	4.2	8.2
Netherlands	4.4	7.6	12.0	6.1	7.0	13.1
Sweden	3.3	3.7	7.0	4.3	3.5	7.8

Data from Einerhand HGK, Kool G, Prins R, et al. *Sickness and invalidity arrangements: facts and figures from 6 European countries.* The Hague: Ministrie van Sociale Zaken en Wergelengeheid, 1994, with permission.

show similar rates, which have hardly changed between 1990 and 1995. The exception is the Netherlands, which consistently has nearly double the average rate of incapacity benefits. Sweden was slightly above average and the United Kingdom was slightly below average in 1990, but both had come closer to the average by 1995. Denmark was about average in 1990, but it had risen slightly above average in 1995.

These are official statistics of incapacity *benefits paid,* rather than actual work loss or sickness absence. Despite all the efforts at standardization, that depends on entitlement, and the arrangements vary in each country (Tables 21.8 and 21.9). In countries where the first weeks of benefit are paid by the employer and are not reimbursed, such as the United Kingdom and Sweden, official statistics may omit these people. Conversely, in countries where people who are not working are entitled to some sickness and invalidity benefits, such as the United Kingdom, Denmark, and Finland, those receiving sickness and invalidity benefits may be counted even though they are not working in any event. Further, the duration of sickness benefits and the point of transfer to invalidity benefit or retirement pension vary in each country. As the Clinical Standards Advisory Group (10) showed in their analysis of the United Kingdom statistics, these social security statistics of incapacity benefits paid may bear little relationship with actual absence from work resulting from sickness.

Bearing these limitations in mind, it is still possible to draw some tentative conclusions. The different incapacity benefit rates do not appear to be due to any identifiable difference in the labor force or health indicators, but they are more likely to be at least partly due to differences in the social security systems or the culture in each country (2). The way in which the sickness and invalidity benefit systems are structured and operated, and the possible mechanisms of early retirement, are likely to play a role in determining the numbers who use the system, how long they continue to receive benefits, and whether they effectively leave the labor force. At the same time, each population may have different attitudes to work, sickness, and benefits. AS/tri (43) provides further data on trends in incapacity benefits in six European countries from 1980 to 1995, in each case taking the 1980 level as 100.

Figure 21.1 shows trends in the number of spells of sickness benefits paid. The sickness benefit spells dropped in all countries except Sweden during the first half of the 1980s. In Belgium and Germany, there was little or no change in the sickness benefit system from 1980 to 1990, and the number of spells of sickness benefit fell by about 40% and 20%, respectively, over the entire period. The United Kingdom, Sweden, and the Netherlands showed sudden and considerable changes in the number of spells resulting from substantial changes in the sickness benefit system, the most important of which was to make employers provide sick pay for the first period of sickness. In the United Kingdom, progressively longer initial periods of sickness were excluded from the official statistics in the early 1980s. In Sweden, the numbers increased about 50% during the second part of the 1980s. At that time, the unemployment rate was extremely low in Sweden (less than 2%), and sickness benefits became generous (from 1987: 90% of salary and payment from the first day of sickness). However, from 1992, sickness benefit levels were reduced several times, and employers took responsibility for the first 2 weeks of sickness absence, which were omitted from official statistics. At the same time, the unemployment rates rose markedly in Sweden. In the early 1990s, there was a sharp decline in sickness benefit spells, and by 1992, Sweden had one of the greatest relative improvements of reduction of sickness absence over the entire 15-year period.

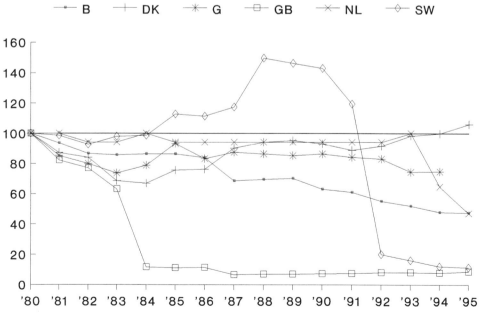

FIGURE 21.1. Sickness benefit spells per 100 insured, 1980 to 1995 (1980 = 100). (From AS/tri, Leiden, with permission [43].)

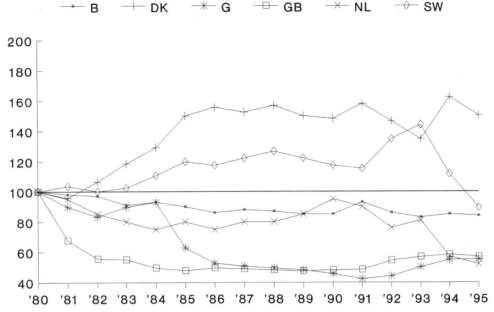

FIGURE 21.2. New disability benefit recipients per 1,000 insured, 1980 to 1995 (1980 = 100). (From AS/tri, Leiden, with permission [43].)

Figure 21.2 shows the incidence of new recipients of disability benefits. In Sweden and Denmark, the incidence has grown steadily since 1980, although in Sweden it has fallen rapidly since 1993 to just below the starting level. However, in absolute numbers, Denmark is still just below the European average (Table 21.14). The incidence in Belgium has gradually fallen slightly without any dramatic change. The United Kingdom, Germany, and the Netherlands showed a sharp drop at different times. The incidence in the United Kingdom incidence fell in the early 1980s when there was a substantial change in the complete benefits system. The German incidence fell in the mid-1980s when some categories of insured were excluded from benefits. The incidence in the Netherlands fell in the early 1990s when stricter eligibility criteria and assessment methods were introduced. Even so, the Netherlands still has by far the highest rate in absolute terms (Table 21.14). The Swedish incidence also fell in the early 1990s, when stricter assessment criteria were introduced, and by 1995, it was more or less back to the starting level in 1980.

Figure 21.3 shows a different pattern in the total numbers receiving disability benefits, however. For most countries, the number remained more or less constant from 1980 to 1995. Swedish numbers increased by about 25% over the 15-year period. In the United Kingdom, the number more than doubled, not because of any increase in the annual numbers of persons who started receiving invalidity benefits, but rather because of an increasing duration of invalidity that was initially considered to be linked to the high level of unemployment in the 1980s. In Germany, in contrast, there was a gradual fall from 1984 to 1992, which has been attributed to the change in eligibility and the possibility of early old-age pensions. This decrease leveled since 1992, after German reunification.

Figures 21.4 and 21.5 show the relative expenditures on sickness and disability

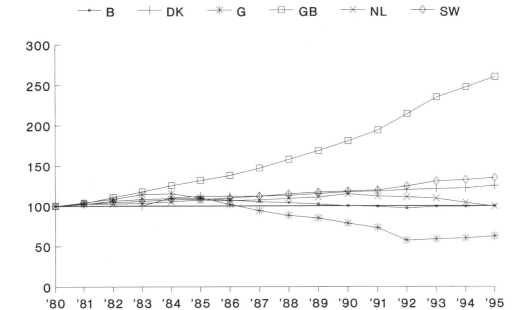

FIGURE 21.3. Number of disability benefit recipients per 1,000 insured, 1980 to 1995 (1980 = 100). (From AS/tri, Leiden, with permission [43].)

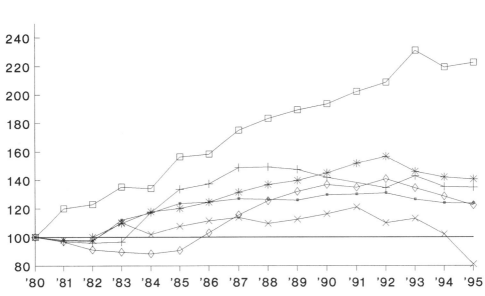

FIGURE 21.4. Sickness benefits paid as a percentage of the gross domestic product from 1980 to 1993 (1980 = 100). (From AS/tri, Leiden, with permission [43].)

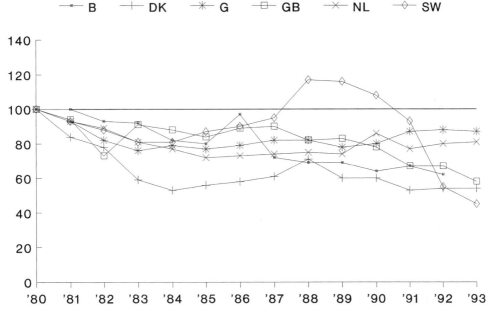

FIGURE 21.5. Disability benefits paid as a percentage of the gross domestic product from 1980 to 1993 (1980 = 100). (From AS/tri, Leiden, with permission [43].)

benefits from 1980 to 1993 as a percentage of the GDP. Figure 21.4 shows that, in most countries, the cost of sickness benefits paid by the state fell by 10% to 45%, although in many countries this simply reflects a shift of costs to employers. The exception is Sweden, where the rapid rise in costs in the late 1980s and sharp fall in the early 1990s reflected the number of spells of sickness benefits. Figure 21.5 shows that there was virtually no change in the cost of disability benefits from 1980 to 1993 in four of the six countries. In the United Kingdom, however, the cost almost doubled, whereas in Sweden it increased about 50%. This all largely reflected the numbers of persons receiving disability benefits (Fig. 21.3). The rise in costs in Sweden was about 50% relative to the GDP, but the Swedish GDP was actually negative for 3 years, whereas benefits were fixed relative to salaries and not to changes in the GDP.

The AS/tri review gave few data on individual causes of sickness or invalidity, but it did point out that in most countries, three main diagnostic groups accounted for the large majority of new recipients of invalidity benefit: musculoskeletal disorders, cardiovascular disorders and mental disorders. Figure 21.6 shows the relative increase in the proportion of new recipients of disability benefits accounted for by musculoskeletal disorders. Most countries showed a gradual rise of 10% to 50% between the early to mid-1980s and the early 1990s and a leveling or slight fall from about 1992 to 1993, although most were still about 20% to 40% higher by 1995. Only the Netherlands managed to return to a lower level than in 1980, although again, its absolute rates of invalidity remain much higher than those of any other country. The marked exception to this overall trend was the United Kingdom, where the proportion of new recipients of disability benefits who had musculoskeletal disorders was already rising from 1980, more than doubled from 1980 to 1995, and showed no fall up to that point. There is no obvious explanation why the pattern of musculoskeletal disorders should be so

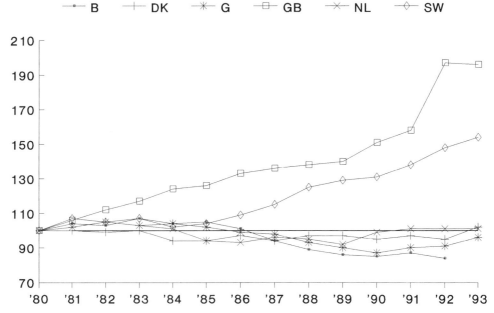

FIGURE 21.6. Proportion of new disability benefit recipients with musculoskeletal disorders, 1980 to 1995 (1980 = 100). (From AS/tri, Leiden, with permission [43].)

different in the United Kingdom. In the United Kingdom, most of this increase is for back pain, but this difference from other EU countries does mean that the exponential increase in DSS benefits paid for back pain in the United Kingdom is probably not representative of other EU countries.

Benefit Levels Versus Incapacity Rates

Attempts are sometimes made to rank sickness absence rates against benefit levels, often using single sets of selected figures. That is a limited perspective of basic state benefit levels and state benefits paid, which is only part of the entire picture of sickness absence. Such crude listings do not allow for the complexity of the benefits systems. As previously noted, in practice there may be much less difference in the net effect on income in the "usual case." As also previously noted, official statistics reflect benefits paid and may not be an accurate reflection of absence from work resulting from sickness. This is not the entire picture, and the relationship of such figures with the whole picture may vary in different countries and over time. For example, in Germany it may be close to the whole picture, whereas in the United Kingdom it is a small part of the picture and gives a misleading impression (10). With these qualifications, Table 21.16 compares the basic statutory benefit level with official statistics of benefits paid and shows little obvious relationship between short-term and long-term benefit levels and the corresponding work incapacities in these six European countries. There is a particularly striking contrast between Germany and the Netherlands, which both have the most generous levels of benefits, yet Germany has the lowest and the Netherlands the highest levels of long-term disability. Perhaps more relevant, through most of this period the Netherlands had one of the most generous and Germany one

TABLE 21.16. *Benefit levels versus incapacity*

	Sickness benefit level in rank order[a]	Amount of short-term incapacity[b]		Invalidity benefits level[a]	Amount of long-term incapacity[b]	
		1990	1995		1990	1995
Germany	Normal earnings	5.0	4.5	≤100%	3.3	3.1
Belgium	100%	3.8	3.3	60–100%	4.2	4.4
Netherlands	Normal earnings	7.1	5.2	9–73%	8.9	8.0
Sweden	100–75%	6.1	3.8	65%	3.5	3.9
Denmark	100%	4.4	6.0	Flat rate	3.8	4.2
United Kingdom	Flat rate	2.6	3.5	Flat rate	3.4	4.9

[a] Data from MISSOC. *Social protection in the member states of the union: situation on July 1st 1995 and evolution.* Brussels: European Commission Directorate—General Employment, Industrial Relations and Social Affairs, 1996.

[b] Data from Prins R, Veerman TJ, Koster MK. *Work incapacity in six countries: facts and figures 1980–1995.* Leiden: AS/tri, 1998.

of the strictest social security systems in terms of eligibility, claims procedures, and decision-making processes. It would also be more relevant to compare the net effect of sickness on the "usual case." Unfortunately, such data are not available at present, although we hope that they will be available in due course from the ISSA study. It would also be of interest to compare sickness and invalidity benefits for persons who are not working with the alternative benefits they would otherwise receive, such as unemployment or basic income support.

Retirement

Rates of early retirement vary greatly in each country, but there is no clear pattern among work activity rates, unemployment rates, and both short-term and long-term work incapacity with increasing age (Table 21.17). Sweden, Denmark, and the United Kingdom have the latest retirement in practice, but despite that they do not have particularly high unemployment, sickness absence rates, or long-term incapacity rates among older workers. In the Netherlands, the high level of long-term or permanent incapacity does appear to be a common mechanism of early retirement in place of relatively low rates of unemployment in older workers (36). Belgium, with one of the earliest retirement patterns, has among the lowest levels of unemployment and short-term sickness absence among older workers, although these workers do have higher than average long-term incapacity. Denmark, with the oldest official retirement age, does not have particularly high levels of unemployment or sickness among older workers. In Germany, there are several ways of early exit from the labor force; men can receive an earlier old-age pension once they have paid pension contributions for 35 years, and women can receive a pension when they have paid contributions for 10 out of 20 years of work. Yet despite that, Germany has higher than average unemployment and long-term incapacity rates among older workers. There are clearly major differences in these patterns in each country, but it is not simply a matter of older workers' moving among these various alternative mechanisms of retirement. Rather, older workers in some countries appear to show different cultural patterns of work, sickness, claiming of benefits, and retirement.

TABLE 21.17. *Relationship among retirement, official retirement age, unemployment, sickness, and incapacity in different European Union countries*

		Males			
	Official retirement age	Employment rate, age 55–59 yr (in rank order)	Unemployment rate, 55–59 yr	Short-term sickness absence, age 55–59 yr	Long-term work incapacity, age 55–59 yr[a]
Sweden	65 (1993)	76.8	8.7	6.7	13.4
Denmark	67	74.1	6.1	9.6	12.0
United Kingdom	65	67.9	9.9	5.1	13.1
Germany	65 flexible	63.8	13.4	8.1	17.7
Netherlands	65	58.8	3.6	8.2	32.9
Belgium	60–65	47.0	4.9	3.0	15.7
		Females			
	Official retirement age	Employment rate, age 55–59 yr (in rank order)	Unemployment rate, 55–59 yr	Short-term sickness absence, age 55–59 yr	Long-term work incapacity, age 55–59 yr[a]
Sweden	65	73.7	6.6	(7.9)	15.5
United Kingdom	60	52.0	4.2	6.8	14.8
Denmark	67	51.8	6.8	15.6	15.4
Germany	65	41.9	16.4	7.5	18.3
Netherlands	65	28.8	5.6	11.2	32.7
Belgium	60–65	19.2	–	2.8	18.7

[a] 1990 to 1991 from Einerhand HGK, Kool G, Prins R, et al. *Sickness and invalidity arrangements: facts and figures from 6 European countries.* The Hague: Ministrie van Sociale Zaken en Wergelengeheid, 1994.
Data from *EU demographic statistics 1997: population and social conditions.* series 3A. Luxembourg: Office for Official Publications of the European Communities, 1997; *OECD Historical statistics 1960–95.* Paris: Organisation for Economic Cooperation and Development, 1997; and Prins R, Veerman TJ, Kosper MK. *Work incapacity in six countries: facts and figures 1980–1995.* Leiden: AS/tri, 1998.

Sweden

Olsson et al. (36), Folkesson et al. (18), MISSOC (29,30), and Svensson and Brorsson (52) reviewed changes in the Swedish social security system during the late 1980s and 1990s and their impact on trends of sickness absence and benefits paid. Traditionally, the "Scandinavian model" of social security or "Nordic welfare society" is based on economic prosperity and high living standards. It is generally accepted that society should and will take good care of its citizens when they are ill, unemployed, old, or are otherwise in economic need (36).

In Sweden before the 1980s, the adjudication of work injury was based on purely medical grounds. However, several judicial decisions made way for a more legal and administrative interpretation (49). The possibility of obtaining work, often a question of age, became as important as medical reasons. The improved economic situation in Sweden in the mid-1980s allowed the government to increase benefits for sickness absence and to remove the first waiting day without benefits. These changes were followed by an increased number of claims for sickness benefits that overwhelmed the local social security offices. As a consequence, more people continued to be listed as sick and received benefits for longer periods, often doing little more than passive waiting. This situation was aggravated by diminishing support for rehabilitation efforts by the local social security offices. There were gradual increases in the number of benefits for work-related injuries (Table 21.18) and in the average duration of sickness

TABLE 21.18. *Benefits for work-related injuries in Sweden from 1980 to 1998*

Year	Total current benefits	New benefits approved	Percentage of new claims approved (%)
1980	189,964	22,271	66.0
1981	182,036	24,044	64.6
1982	178,022	24,226	67.4
1983	186,419	25,545	71.7
1984	203,748	28,974	73.7
1985	218,022	38,632	75.1
1986	233,828	49,551	80.4
1987	244,133	64,382	87.2
1988	260,352	73,488	88.1
1989	248,287	78,313	86.0
1990	222,961	78,447	82.9
1991	191,043	79,285	79.6
1992	155,661	67,636	72.3
1993	232,158	57,457	64.0
1994	132,634	31,917	51.9
1995	118,517	15,668	49.8
1996	113,948	9,179	55.7
1997	108,334	7,800	62.7

Data from Riksförsäkringsverket (RFV). *RFV Informerrar. I-s I 1997:8.* Stockholm: RFV, 1997, with permission (44).

absence, particularly in the number of longer periods of sickness absence (Table 21.19). This situation was particularly harmful to persons who needed active rehabilitation, such as those with back pain. They lost their social links with the workforce and their employment skills, with diminishing prospects of reemployment. This led to gradually increasing numbers of invalidity pensions throughout the 1980s even though invalidity benefit levels had not been increased (39,40). Thus, in the 1980s, sickness absence and longer-term invalidity became more or less accepted and tolerated in a time of economic prosperity and high employment.

TABLE 21.19. *Total number of cases of sickness benefit lasting longer than 1 year and ongoing disability or temporary disability pensions*

Year	Sickness benefit	Disability pension	Total
1980	19,000	292,000	311,000
1985	30,000	323,000	353,000
1990	75,000	361,000	436,000
1991	76,000	367,000	443,000
1992	71,000	383,000	454,000
1993	53,000	414,000[a]	467,000[a]
1994	47,000	422,000	469,000
1995	45,000	420,000	465,000
1996	47,000	419,000	466,000
1997	42,000	423,000	465,000

[a] This includes people with only a supplementary pension.
Data from Riksförsäkringsverket (RFV). *RFV Informerrar. I-s I 1997:8.* Stockholm: RFV, 1997, with permission (45).

By 1990, there were some major problems in the Swedish social security system (29):

- Pension systems out of line with economic growth.
- Wrong incentives.
- No coordinated administrative responsibility for prevention, benefit payments, and rehabilitation.
- Lack of incentives for employers to participate in prevention and rehabilitation.
- Occupational injury insurance out of control.
- Compensation levels different in similar schemes.
- Total costs out of control because of all these problems.

The changed interpretation of work injury and the increasing rate of sickness absence led the Swedish government to convene a special council of rehabilitation (1985) and a commission on work environment (1989). This led to gradual change in the accepted grounds for sickness-related absenteeism and early retirement. The general rule became that sickness-related absenteeism should be based on the working capacity of the individual (*arbetslinjen*). Palme (39) reviewed the political debate in Sweden after the election of a coalition government in 1991, although he emphasized that the reforms had already begun and were also fueled by the economic recession. The first legislative step was to restrict early retirement pension to medical reasons and not on labor-related grounds alone, and in practice there was increasing demand for medical reasons for all sickness and invalidity. The definition of work injury was also changed in 1993. Now an injury or disease is only accepted as the result of harmful influence at work if there are stronger grounds for that presumption than the contrary. Previously, this rule of evidence had been formulated the other way around, in a unique "reverse" burden of proof (29).

From 1991, progressive cuts were made in the level of sickness benefit, and legislation also limited the extent of any collective agreement (Table 21.20). In 1993, a waiting day was introduced for sickness benefits, the level of sickness benefits was cut further, and all types of pensions were reduced. There was a specific further cut in the level of sickness benefit for those who were still absent more than 1 year and were not receiving medical treatment or any form of rehabilitation. Employees also had to start paying sickness benefit contributions of 0.95% of gross earnings. The most radical changes were in short-term industrial injury benefits, which between 1991 and July 1, 1993 were progressively made the same as sickness benefits and were effectively abolished. However, if work injury leads to permanent loss of working capacity of more than one-fifteenth, this loss is still compensated by 100% wage replacement. Palme (39) also pointed to proposed changes that were never implemented. In particular, two attempts to abolish partial pension plans were blocked on both occasions.

TABLE 21.20. *Changes of sickness benefits in Sweden from 1990 to 1996 as a percentage of the wage replacement rate*

Days of sickness	1990	March 1991	January 1992	April 1993	July 1993	January 1996
1	90	65	75	0	0	0
2–3	90	65	75	75	75	75
4–14	90	80	90	90	90	75
15–90	90	80	80	80	80	75
91–365	90	90	90	80	70/80	75
365+	90	90	90	80	70/80	75

To improve the work environment and to reduce the risk of work injury, an important change was made in the law in 1991. The employer now had direct legal responsibility for providing a safe working environment. An employer's responsibility for vocational rehabilitation and for work replacement was also strengthened. From 1992, employers had to take over paying sick benefits for the first 2 weeks of sickness absence. This change imposed a new and more powerful type of financial incentive and control function on employers to minimize injury and sickness.

There were also changes at the local administrative level of the Swedish RFV. From 1992, each local RFV office was made responsible for the coordination of rehabilitation measures, in each individual case of sickness absence, as well as on a general level. The government also allocated special resources to the local RFV offices to purchase vocational rehabilitation resources, which in practice were often used for physical therapy. Some local projects integrated the organization of sickness benefits, social security (at the municipality level), work inspection authorities, and health care.

In the budget for the fiscal year 1997, the Swedish government stated that balancing the finances was the most important prerequisite for a stable welfare policy. All benefits and allowances in the social security system had to be designed to support employment and to reduce unemployment (30). In 1996, a government committee report on disability and invalidity pensions called for a clearer separation of unemployment and disability benefits. The more favorable treatment of people older than 60 years who had labor market difficulties was abolished.

Various government committees have proposed changes to make rehabilitation efforts more successful. It is suggested that the different parties involved in rehabilitation must cooperate in more effective ways to make rehabilitation as efficient as possible, and perhaps this is the best way to reduce social security costs. As previously noted, however, these projects cannot be evaluated properly because of lack of effective control groups.

The characteristics of persons who are on long-term sickness absence are in some ways different from the average member of the Swedish labor market (44). Among those who have long-term sickness absence are higher percentages of women, those aged 50 years or older, and the unemployed. Rehabilitation and reemployment become more difficult during periods of high unemployment, as in Sweden from 1990 to 1996.

These problems through the 1980s and the effects of social security reforms in the 1990s are reflected in the statistics for back pain. Tables 21.21 and 21.22 show the increase in the incidence and duration of work loss resulting from back pain, although

TABLE 21.21. *Increase in the incidence and duration of work loss from back pain in Göteborg, Sweden*

Year	Percentage of workers losing time from work with back pain (%)	Average days lost per annum (d)
1970	1	20
1975	3	22
1980	4	25
1987	8	36
1992	8	39
1997	5	36

TABLE 21.22. *Millions of days per annum of sickness benefit absence from neck and back pain in Sweden, based on a sample from Göteborg, Sweden*

Year	Low back pain	Neck and shoulder pain	Combinations	Total
1987	13.4	9.3	5.3	28.0
1995	10.6	8.2	3.0	21.8
1996	4.5	9.2	4.1	17.8

Data from Nachemson A, personal communication.

this is based on limited statistics for one area that may not be representative of the whole country. Table 21.23 shows the marked increase in the number of early retirements from back pain, particularly between the mid-1980s and 1992 to 1993.

Since the reforms, official RFV statistics show that the time the RFV office took to contact those on long-term sick leave decreased from 100 to 66 days, and the proportion contacted increased from 31% to 60%. For all categories of sickness, there was a cut in the average duration of sickness absence from 242 to 149 days, or almost 3 months. Among those who were employed, the level of early retirement was reduced from 29% to 22%. There were also fewer recurrent cases leading to long-term sickness

TABLE 21.23. *Early retirement and temporary disability pensions in Sweden 1971–1995*

Year	Total early retirements (full + partial) (no. of people)	Total full-time equivalent[a]	Early retirements from back pain (full + partial) (no. of people)
1971	43,984	41,565	3,070
1972	52,370	49,692	4,064
1973	52,148	49,398	4,785
1974	45,931	43,274	4,334
1975	45,457	42,637	4,738
1976	45,306	41,919	5,885
1977	46,350	42,371	6,589
1978	45,144	40,837	6,784
1979	44,278	39,600	7,094
1980	45,289	39,908	6,933
1981	43,615	37,869	6,123
1982	42,286	36,764	5,469
1983	43,338	38,177	5,872
1984	46,792	41,859	6,870
1985	51,009	45,897	7,703
1986	50,106	44,732	8,666
1987	51,691	46,169	7,255
1988	54,135	48,136	8,976
1989	51,991	45,622	11,037
1990	50,493	43,382	11,253
1991	49,554	42,289	10,726
1992	58,382	49,534	12,998
1993	62,465	52,023	13,280
1994	48,531	38,536	9,602
1995	39,204	30,732	8,715
1996	39,245	31,009	6,375
1997	41,198	33,861	6,907

Data from Riksförsäkringsverket (RFV). *RFV Informerrar. I-s I 1997:8.* Stockholm: RFV, 1997, with permission.

absence. However, for musculoskeletal symptoms, in which back pain plays a major part, the results were not so encouraging. For back pain, the median number of days until rehabilitation measures were undertaken actually increased, from 119 to 129 days, and complete recovery in this group fell from 85% to 81%. Although the numbers of persons receiving early retirement for back pain has fallen, they now make up a larger proportion (increased from 11% to 16% of all complete or partial early retirement). Thus, even with official figures, the increased efforts of rehabilitation have been less successful for patients with musculoskeletal disorders than for those with other forms of sickness. An independent study by Jensen (26) showed that only 18% of those in sick leave with back pain for more than 3 months actually received rehabilitation. For those older than 55 years of age, it was only 5%.

DISCUSSION

From a health care perspective, low back pain is not a disease but a common bodily symptom, and low back disability depends more on psychosocial factors than on physical diesease (see Chapters 2, 3, 4, and 8). From an epidemiologic perspective, back pain is not a discrete health problem, but is often associated with other pains, comorbidities, psychologic and stress-related symptoms, and work-related or other social problems (see Chapter 2). From a social perspective, incapacity for work attributed to back pain and social security benefits paid for back pain is a social phenomenon related to the economic and labor market situation (see Chapter 2). These perspectives are not mutually exclusive, but they may represent different views of a complex set of interacting forces.

Incentives and Controls

From economic insurance theory, insurance that gives complete compensation to the individual maximizes the welfare of the individual, whereas perfect control minimizes the cost to society. In reality, it is rarely possible to provide 100% insurance for all events so the individual is always exposed to some loss, and it is often difficult to organize perfect control, with the risk of abuse or even fraud (2). The social security and sickness benefit systems can be analyzed in this framework of financial risk and control. For a working family, the whole complexity of social security and sickness benefits plays a vital part in the family's financial situation, besides the salary.

The rules of the labor market control incentives to employees, and so do the rules of the social security and sickness benefit systems. The rules governing the sickness benefit system can be described as those of financial self-risk for the individual and control of the utilization of benefits. In this context, the average employee acts much like "the economic man," that is, much from the self-interest of the individual, not to be misinterpreted as selfishness or greed. In this context, the types of "signals" transmitted as incentives in the sickness benefit system are vitally important. In a simplified way, this concept can be described in a four-field figure (Fig. 21.7): low and high financial self-risk versus low or high control of utilization of the benefit system.

The sickness benefit system in Sweden in the second half of the 1980s, compared with the second half of the 1990s, provided an illustration of such incentives. In the 1980s, during the period of high economic development, Sweden had high compensation rates of 90% or more, which meant low financial self-risk, and at the same time there was mild control of the utilization of benefits. In the 1990s, however, with a

Financial self-risk

	- Low	- High
Control - Low	Sweden in 1987	
- High		Sweden in 1997

FIGURE 21.7. Incentives from the sickness benefit system: financial self-risk versus control.

general recession of the economy, benefit levels were changed to no compensation for the first day and to 70% (later 75% and from 1998, 80%) for the following days. This change increased the financial self-risk for the individual from 0% to 10% up to 100% for the first day, and from 0% to 10% up to 25% to 30% for the following days. At the same time, employers took over the control function from the local sickness benefit offices for the first 2 weeks of sickness absence and also the payment of benefits. It was in the interest of the employer that the sickness episode during the first 2 weeks became as short as possible, because the employer now paid the sickness benefits, rather than the government, as previously. There was a significant drop in the utilization rate of the Swedish sickness benefit system from the 1980s to the 1990s. However, the labor market also changed during the same period, from less than 2% unemployment to a situation of more than 8% unemployment and another 4% to 5% out of the ordinary labor market (e.g., in educational programs).

The Swedish example is of general interest because it illustrates the importance of sickness benefit systems to provide a reasonable balance of security and incentives for the individual employee to provide for his or her own economic support. In general terms, if the sickness benefit system is too restrictive, that is, if it puts a high financial self-risk on employees combined with a high rate of control of the utilization of the benefits, there is a risk of forcing some sick people to go to work (21). On the contrary, high compensation leading to no or limited self-risk combined with no or mild control of utilization probably leads to a high degree of utilization of benefits even by some persons with only minor degrees of sickness. An unfortunate limitation of such analysis is that most governments reduce benefits and tighten controls (or vice versa) more or less simultaneously, so it is difficult to separate the relative strength of financial self-risk versus control effects.

Osterweis et al. (37) considered the central question to be whether income maintenance payments in any form undermine motivation to work, and they postulated three disincentive effects:

- The availability of disability benefits acts as an incentive for workers with marginal disabilities to drop out of the workforce and to seek disability benefits instead.
- The receipt of disability benefits acts as a disincentive for the recipient to return to work.
- The receipt or potential receipt of disability benefits acts as a disincentive to rehabilitation.

The foregoing could lead to conflict between two competing social goals:

• Providing economic security to disabled people.
• Keeping as many people as possible in the workforce and returning as many people as possible to work through rehabilitation.

Where the balance point between these two extremes should be, or to put it another way, what incentives and controls should characterize the social security and the sickness benefit systems, is a question of political preferences, and not only of economics. However, without a considered strategy, there is a risk of increasing problems of overutilization, or of underutilization, with all the associated implications on individuals and on society as a whole.

There is considerable evidence throughout this review (see Chapters 2 and 20) that financial incentives are important: money matters. The review of workers' compensation data (see Chapter 2) showed that a 10% increase in compensation levels produced a 1% to 11% increase in the number of claims and a 2% to 11% increase in the duration of claims, a clear although actually modest effect. The Swedish trends reviewed here show that the amount of sickness and disability rose in the 1980s when benefit levels were generous and have fallen since the early 1990s when benefit levels were reduced, and there are many such examples. However, it is not possible to attribute this change simply to the level of benefits because major changes occurred simultaneously in the structure and control mechanisms of the social security system. Moreover, the greatest changes in benefit levels during this period were for relatively short-term sickness absence, but the major trends were in employment injury benefits and in long-term invalidity and early retirement. More detailed examination of these changes suggests that the structure and practice of the benefits system had the most immediate and greatest impact on the different benefits paid. The greatest increases and reductions in the number and costs of benefits appear to have resulted from changes in the control mechanisms (eligibility criteria, the definition and assessment of incapacity, and the claims, adjudication, and appeals procedures).

The present comparison of different EU countries also shows marked differences in the levels of sickness absence in the different countries. There are differences in the social security systems in each country, although despite these differences they all appear to face similar problems even if to varying degree. However, there is no clear relationship between the level of social security benefits and the amount of sickness absence. It may be hypothesized that varying cultural and social attitudes toward work, sickness and benefits, and retirement are all likely to be important, although these are difficult to define or measure, and there is little direct evidence. The aims and regulations of the benefit system and the levels of benefits are set in legislation by political process that reflects democratic pressures. Benefits are delivered by a benefits system whose primary ethos is to control the benefits paid and to direct them to those claimants who are entitled to them. That system is counterbalanced by constant pressure from an appeals system, litigation, and the courts to make the scope and extent of benefits more generous. The net effect of these various pressures has been a steady tendency to increasing numbers and costs of social security benefits in most Western countries, although the extent of this increase varies in different countries and is not as great as sometimes claimed. This rise has been countered by periodic revision of the legislation to tighten the scope of benefits or revision of the mechanics of the benefits system to increase controls and to make it more difficult to receive benefits.

This review provides extensive evidence that the structure of the benefits system has a powerful impact and suggests that the availability of benefits, the ease of obtaining them, and the way in which these factors relate to other alternatives are at least as important and possibly more important than the financial value of these benefits.

Early Retirement

The greatest problem identified in this review of social security in Europe is the increasing number of people taking early retirement on medical grounds, of which nonspecific low back pain is one of the most common examples. In Sweden, back pain now accounts for slightly more than 20% of all such early retirements. There is no evidence of any significant change in the pathologic or physical basis of low back pain or in the incidence of work-related back injuries (see Chapter 2). It varies from country to country whether there is any increase in the incidence of work loss and commencing sickness benefits, and in many countries the major increase is the number of people who then go on to chronic disability and long-term benefits. This is a particular problem in persons more than 50 years of age, in whom it is a mechanism of early exit from the labor force and early retirement.

Actual retirement age is different from the official state pension age. Through the 1990s, increasing numbers of people retired earlier, before they were entitled to state pensions. Differences in the structure of the sickness benefit systems, and the presence of alternative exits from the labor market, may give apparent differences in levels of early retirement in different countries. Overall, only 30% of men in Europe now work beyond the age of 60 years, and fewer than 40% of women work beyond age 55, although there is marked variation among different European countries. Sweden has the highest activity rates with increasing age and the latest retirement in practice, with 59% of men and 50% of women aged 60 to 64 years still working. In many other European countries, only 10% to 25% of men and about 5% to 15% of women continue working after age 60 years. Early retirement has been partly financed by employment pension plans, special arrangements associated with industrial reorganization, personal pension plans, and private savings. For those who do not have access to such financial support, the various rules of the social security systems mean that the main alternative has been invalidity benefits and disability pensions.

This increase has to at least some extent coincided with changed economic circumstances and much higher levels of unemployment. Contrary to what may be expected, unemployment benefits do not appear to be a common mechanism of financial support for early retirement, except in Germany. In the late 1980s and early 1990s, there was considerable speculation that invalidity benefits, early retirement on medical grounds, and ordinary pensions were used in different countries to "hide" unemployment. By 1996, there were deliberate attempts to reverse that policy throughout Europe and to disentangle the medical and employment criteria, which had become intertwined in the assessment of disability (30). The aim now is to return to the original concept in which incapacity for work is measured purely on medical grounds without reference to actual employment possibilities. Invalidity pensions should also no longer be seen as a permanent exit from the labor force. Instead, there is increasing emphasis on review of invalidity status, rehabilitation, and return to work.

A fundamental question is whether or to what extent early retirement is a choice or or is forced on people. Changes in the general economic situation, labor market forces, and reduced employment opportunities for older workers have certainly played a part (Table 21.5). At the same time, there have been major changes in attitudes to work and retirement, and many people now want and plan to retire before the official state retirement age. The amount of early retirement is likely to depend on the balance among individual attitudes and expectations, labor market forces, and the social security system. This situation involves social and political issues about how long people should be expected to work, the financial mechanisms society should provide for retirement, and whether nonspecific low back pain should be an acceptable basis for early retirement. These questions are still unresolved, but the solution to this problem depends on answering these social and political issues rather than biomedical questions or health care for back pain.

Social Exclusion and Disadvantage

Much of the evidence on social disadvantage and back pain is reviewed in Chapter 2, but it should be considered here as highly relevant to the social security findings. The evidence on social class and unemployment and the qualitative social security studies all suggest that social disadvantage is important. This finding is hardly surprising because the primary goal of social security is to provide support to those in need. Olsson et al. (36) pointed out that social insurance systems and incentives in different countries can have a profound effect on the level of marginalization and social exclusion.

The review of studies on social class (see Chapter 2) provides conflicting evidence for a relationship between the prevalence of back pain and lower social class, and any effect is probably weak. There is strong evidence that back pain leads to more work loss in people of lower social class. The relationship with social class is more consistent in men but less clear in women. The main problem is what this means. Social class is a crude index to a host of social, educational, occupational, economic, lifestyle, and psychosocial influences, and corresponding social attitudes and behavior, any and all of which may affect work loss associated with back pain. It is probably partly a matter of manual work, particularly in men. It is probably also a matter of social disadvantage in both men and women, although it is not clear exactly which aspects of that disadvantage are important or how they affect back pain.

The current crisis in social security coincides with a changed economic situation and a marked increase in the level of unemployment. There is little difference in the prevalence of back pain in those who are unemployed; the unemployed do seek slightly more health care for back pain, but there is a much higher level of sickness certification for back pain in the unemployed (Table 2.7 in Chapter 2). A large proportion of sickness and invalidity benefits now goes to people who are not employed, although there may be uncertainty or debate about whether or to what extent their lack of employment results from their back pain. There is strong evidence from several studies in times of relatively low unemployment (less than 5%) that sickness absence resulting from back pain was inversely related to the unemployment rate (see Chapter 2). However, many studies show that when unemployment is high, low back disability rates and various sickness and compensation rates are higher. Thus, lack of employment may have different effects in different situations. When unemployment rates are high and job security is low, there may be more pressure on workers to stay at work when they feel unwell, and that may reduce absenteeism from back pain. However, once someone loses a job or is under threat of layoff, there may be social and financial advantages to sickness and invalidity benefit, and this situation may increase sickness certification for back pain among those who are not employed. Sickness and invalidity benefits and disability pensions are higher than unemployment benefits and basic income support for poverty in all European countries. They have the advantage that they are not means-tested, and in one form or another they are generally unlimited in time. Social support benefits for sickness and disability are probably also now regarded as a right and are more socially acceptable than other social security benefits.

Qualitative studies suggest that, during the process of sickness certification, the physician's judgments about the patient's capacity for work are influenced by many complex factors. The patient's medical condition and its impact on employment potential is always high on the list. However, it is almost immediately linked to a whole range of nonmedical factors, including the patient's prospects of finding work, age, motivation to find work, financial and psychologic consequences of returning to unemployment or job search, and the potential for rehabilitation or training. There may be strong pressure on physicians to issue sickness certificates, and there is strong suspicion that some physicians use sickness certification to assist their socially disadvantaged patients to obtain more financial support.

These three aspects of earlier retirement—the structure of the social security system, social exclusion, and social disadvantage—are interrelated. From a social security perspective, neck pain and back pain do not comprise a discrete health problem, but they are only a symptom of a much more fundamental social problem. Progressively lower employment rates and earlier retirement of older workers may be due to labor market forces and lack of employment opportunities or to changed attitudes to work, retirement, and benefits, or the decision may be personal. The interaction and relative importance of these forces may vary in different social classes and circumstances. The more socially and economically advantaged groups often have a greater element of personal decision. These individuals are likely to have more financial resources to support that choice, even if there may still be other psychosocial consequences. In persons who are disadvantaged socially, educationally, in terms of work skills, and financially, it may be more a matter of labor market forces over which they have no control. There may be few alternative job opportunities, and these persons are likely to have no other financial options but to make the best use of the available social security benefits. These people become trapped into a situation from which there is no ready escape, and they face major problems of social exclusion and disadvantage. Health care for neck or back pain will not solve that problem, but it may actually reinforce and perpetuate disability. Benefits should be directed to those in need, but the underlying problem will not be solved simply by tightening the controls on long-term invalidity benefits. Indeed, in isolation, that would only exacerbate social exclusion and disadvantage. Instead, society needs to address the fundamental social problems of finding useful employment for all citizens of varying skill levels, including putting to use the skills and experience of older workers who are by no means finished. If conventional economic market forces fail to offer traditional contracts of employment, then more innovative alternatives must be sought. The enormous sums at present spent inappropriately on disability benefits could be more usefully redirected to providing and supporting activity for those who are able to be active.

CONCLUSIONS

1. The present review provides extensive evidence that social security systems influence sickness certification, benefit claims, and state benefits received. Everyone responds to economic incentives and disincentives, and benefits unquestionably affect behavior.

2. It is not possible to separate the effects of financial self-risk and control mechanisms in the Swedish trends of sickness and invalidity. Nevertheless, the balance of the evidence in this review suggests that the structure of the social security system and the availability and ease or difficulty of obtaining sickness and invalidity benefits (i.e., the control mechanisms: eligibility criteria; the definition and assessment of incapacity; and the claims, adjudication, and appeals procedures) have at least as strong an effect and possibly a stronger one than the actual financial level of the benefits (i.e., the financial self-risk for the individual).

3. The major problem identified in this review is the increasing number of people more than 50 years old, in whom low back pain is associated with long-term work loss, disability pension, and early retirement. This situation is not unique to back pain, but it forms part of a much larger social issue.

4. There is also strongly suggestive evidence that low back pain and disability, sickness certification, sickness and invalidity benefits, and other benefits are linked to social exclusion and disadvantage, although data are insufficient to quantify the magnitude of these relationships. Again, this is not unique to back pain, but it forms part of a much larger social issue.

5. Sickness and invalidity benefits cannot be considered in isolation, but rather, they are only one element of a much broader social framework. Low back pain and disability, and these trends, occur in a social milieu that includes cultural; demographic; social (particularly social disadvantage); and macroeconomic (the general economic situation, average earnings, and purchasing power) factors and labor market (particularly job availability, unemployment, and early retirement); employment-related sick pay and pension arrangements; psychosocial aspects of work; social security (including alternative benefits); and health care issues. For example, differences in social security systems and benefit levels may not be the direct *cause* of variation in sickness absence, but they may *reflect* wider social changes and national values and customs that have a more direct effect on sickness absence and invalidity. From a social security perspective, neck pain and back pain are only symptoms of much more fundamental social problems of how to provide useful employment and financial reward for all its citizens (particularly those with fewer skills and social disadvantage, as well as older workers) and how to deal with the transition from work to retirement.

6. Too often, policy discussions and decisions in this area are based on assumptions and political dogma. This is not the place, and it is not our intent to offer a personal solution to these social and political problems. This review will have served its purpose if it provides as accurate and reliable a picture as possible of what is really happening, to form a sound basis for future policy discussions and decisions on social security.

REFERENCES

1. Allan DB, Waddell G. An historical perspective on low back pain and disability. *Orthop Scand* 1989;234[Suppl 60]:1–23.
2. Arrow KJ. Uncertainty and the welfare economics of medical care. *Am Econ J* 1963;53:941–73.

3. Beatty C, Fothergill S, Gore T, et al. *The real level of unemployment.* Sheffield, UK: Centre for Regional Economic and Social Research, 1997.
4. Berkowitz M, ed. *Forging linkages: modifying disability benefit programs to encourage employment.* New York: Rehabilitation International, 1990:1–15.
5. Berkowitz M, Dean D, Mitchell P. *Social security disability programs: an international perspective.* New York: World Organization for Disability Prevention and Rehabilitation and World Rehabilitation Fund, 1987.
6. Bloch FS. Assessing disability: a six nation study of disability pension claim processing and appeals. *Int Soc Sec Rev* 1994;47:15–35.
7. Bloch FS. *Disability benefit claim processing and appeals in six industrialized countries.* ISSA occasional papers on social security. Geneva: International Social Security Association, 1994.
8. Bolderson H, Mabbett D, Hudson J, et al. *Delivering social security: a cross-national study.* Social security research report no. 59. London: Her Majesty's Stationery Office, 1997.
9. Commission of the European Communities. *The future of social protection: a framework for a European debate.* COM(95) 466 final documents EN 05. Brussels: Commission of the European Communities, 1995.
10. CSAG (Clinical Standards Advisory Group). *CSAG report on back pain.* London: Her Majesty's Stationery Office, 1994:1–72.
11. Einerhand HGK, Kool G, Prins R, et al. *Sickness and invalidity arrangements: facts and figures from 6 European countries.* The Hague: Ministrie van Sociale Zaken en Wergelegenheid, 1994.
12. Emanuel H. Controlling admission to and stay in social security benefit programmes. In: *ISSA research meeting–social security: a time for redefinition?* Geneva: International Social Security Association, 1994.
13. *EU demographic statistics 1997: population and social conditions,* series 3A. Luxembourg: Office for Official Publications of the European Communities, 1997.
14. *Eurostat labour force survey 1996.* Brussels: Eurostat 1996.
15. *Eurostat yearbook 1996: a statistical eye on Europe 1985–1995.* Brussels: Eurostat, 1996.
16. *Eurostat yearbook 1997: a statistical eye on Europe 1986–1996.* Brussels: Eurostat, 1997.
17. Feuerstein M. A multidisciplinary approach to the prevention, evaluation and management of work disability. *J Occup Rehabil* 1991;1:5–12.
18. Folkesson H, Larsson B, Tegle S. *SOS-rapport 1993:6. Health care and social services in seven European countries.* Stockholm: Socialstyrelsen [National Board of Health and Welfare], 1993.
19. Gordon MS. *Social security policies in industrial countries: a comparative analysis.* Cambridge: Cambridge University Press, 1988.
20. Hadler NM. Work incapacity from low back pain: the international quest for redress. *Clin Orthop* 1997;336:79–93.
21. Henrekson M, Lantto K, Persson M. *Bruk och missbruk av sjukforskringen [Use and misuse of the sickness benefit system].* Stockholm: SNS Forlag, 1992.
22. Hills J. *The future of welfare: a guide to the debate,* rev. ed. York: Joseph Rowantree Foundation, 1997.
23. *ISSA 25th General Assembly report XII: quality, effectiveness and efficiency of rehabilitation measures.* Geneva: International Social Security Association, 1995.
24. *ISSA Social protection in Europe 1993.* Geneva: International Social Security Association, 1993.
25. *ISSA Social protection in Europe 1996.* Geneva: International Social Security Association, 1996.
26. Jensen I. *Kartlaggning av rehabiliterinsatser.* Stockholm: Karolinska Institute, 1998.
27. Lonsdale S. *Invalidity benefit: an international comparison.* London: DSS Social Research Branch, 1993.
28. Marshall TH. *Citizenship and social class and other essays.* Cambridge: Cambridge University Press, 1950.
29. MISSOC. *Social protection in the member states of the union: situation on July 1st 1994 and evolution.* Brussels: European Commission Directorate–General Employment, Industrial Relations and Social Affairs, 1995.
30. MISSOC. *Social protection in the member states of the union: situation on July 1st 1995 and evolution.* Brussels: European Commission Directorate–General Employment, Industrial Relations and Social Affairs, 1996.
31. MISSOC. *Social protection in the member states of the union: situation on July 1st 1996 and evolution.* Brussels: European Commission Directorate–General Employment, Industrial Relations and Social Affairs, 1997.
32. Nocon A, Baldwin S. *Trends in rehabilitation policy.* London: Kings Fund, 1998.
33. *OECD historical statistics 1960–95.* Paris: Organisation for Economic Cooperation and Development, 1997.
34. *OECD labour force statistics.* Paris: Organisation for Economic Co-operation and Development, 1997.
35. *OECD national accounts: OECD main economic indicators.* Paris: Organisation for Economic Co-operation and Development, 1998.
36. Olsson ASE, Hansen H, Eriksson I. *Rapport till expertgruppen for studier i offentlig ekonomi [social security in Sweden and other European countries: three essays].* Stockholm: Finans-Departementet, 1993:51.
37. Osterweis M, Kleinman A, Mechanic D, eds. *Institute of Medicine Committee on Pain, Disability and Chronic Illness Behavior. Pain and disability: clinical behavioral and public policy perspectives.* Washington, DC: National Academy Press, 1987.

38. Otero-Sierra C, Varona W, Chau N, et al. Comparison of the occupational disease compensation systems in France and in Spain. *Arch Mal Prof Med Trav* 1997;58/6:539–551.
39. Palme E. Potential gains from early intervention in sickness absenteeism at the workplace: an overview of the current state of knowledge and trends in Sweden. In: Berkowitz M, ed. *Forging linkages: modifying disability benefit programs to encourage employment.* New York: Rehabilitation International, 1990:77–93.
40. Ploug N, Kvist J. *Recent trends in cash benefits in Europe.* Copenhagen: Danish Institute of Social Research, 1994.
41. Ploug N, Kvist J. *Social security in Europe: development or dismantlement?* The Hague: Kluwer Law International, 1996.
42. Prins R, Veerman TJ, Andriessen S. *Work incapacity in a cross-national perspective: a pilot study on arrangements and data in six countries.* Zoetermeer: The Netherlands, 1992.
43. Prins R, Veerman TJ, Koster MK. *Work incapacity in six countries: facts and figures 1980–1995.* Leiden: AS/tri, 1998.
44. Riksförsäkringsverket (RFV). *Risk–och friskfaktorer–sjukskrivning och rehabilitering i Sverige. RFV Redovisar 1997:6.* Stockholm: RFV, 1997. [Indications of bad and good health-sickness absence and rehabilitation]
45. Riksförsäkringsverket (RFV). *RFV Informerar. I-s I 1997:8.* Stockholm: RFV, 1997.
46. Ritchie J, Snape D. *Invalidity benefit: a preliminary qualitative study of the factors affecting its growth.* London: Social and Community Planning Research, 1993.
47. SBU (Swedish Council on Technology Assessment in Health Care). *Ont I Ryggen: orsaker, diagnostik och behandling.* Stockholm: SBU, 1991. [Back pain; causes, Diagnostic and Treatment Methods]
48. Simanis JG. National expenditures on social security and health in selected countries. *Soc Sec Bull* 1990;53:12–16.
49. Sjuk-och arbetsskadeberedningens expertgrupp. *Sjukpenning, arbetsskada och fortidspension: forutsattningar och erfarenheter.* Stockholm: SOU, 1997. [Sickness benefits, working injury and early retirement; conditions and experiences]
50. Soeters J, Prins R. Health care facilities and work incapacity: a comparison of the situation in the Netherlands with that in six other West European countries. *Int Soc Sec Rev* 1985;38:141–156.
51. Statskontoret (Swedish Agency for Administrative Development). *Perspektiv på rehabilitering [Perspectives on rehabilitation].* Stockholm: Statskontoret, 1997:27.
52. Svensson H, Brorsson J-A. Sweden sickness and work injury insurance: a summary of developments. *Int Soc Sec Rev* 1997;50:75–86.
53. Titmuss R. The social division of welfare. In: *Essays on the welfare state.* London: Unwin, 1958.
54. *UN monthly bulletin of statistics.* New York: United Nations, November, 1996.
55. Wentworth ET. Systematic diagnosis in backache. *J Bone Joint Surg* 1916;8:137–170.
56. Whiteford P. The use of replacement rates in international comparisons of benefit systems. *Int Soc Sec Rev* 1995;48:3–30.

Subject Index